AF601490

The Anesthesiologist as Perioperative Leader

George Tewfik
Editor

The Anesthesiologist as Perioperative Leader

Driving Quality, Efficiency, and Financial Success in Modern Healthcare

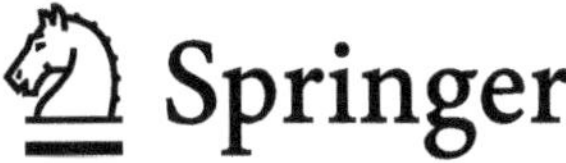

Editor
George Tewfik
Department of Anesthesiology
Rutgers New Jersey Medical School
Newark, NJ, USA

ISBN 978-3-032-18057-5 ISBN 978-3-032-18058-2 (eBook)
https://doi.org/10.1007/978-3-032-18058-2

This Springer imprint is published by the registered company Springer Nature Switzerland AG
The registered company address is: Gewerbestrasse 11, 6330 Cham, Switzerland

Acknowledgments

The success of *The Essential Perioperative Physician* is a direct reflection of the extraordinary expertise, dedication, and generosity of its contributors. I am deeply grateful to the distinguished chapter authors—colleagues and friends from across the American Society of Anesthesiologists—whose scholarship, leadership, and commitment to advancing perioperative medicine have made this volume truly exceptional. Their collective insight spans the breadth of our specialty and exemplifies the highest standards of professional collaboration.

I would also like to extend my sincere appreciation to my colleagues at Rutgers New Jersey Medical School. The support and encouragement from my fellow faculty have been invaluable throughout the development of this project. Their daily dedication to patient care, education, and innovation continually reinforces the importance of anesthesiologists as leaders across the continuum of perioperative care.

I am especially grateful to Dr. Alex Bekker, Professor and Chair of the Department of Anesthesiology at Rutgers New Jersey Medical School. His mentorship, trust, and unwavering support for academic advancement and creative initiative have been essential to bringing this book to life.

Finally, I acknowledge the many healthcare professionals—nurses, surgeons, administrators, trainees, and staff—whose teamwork and partnership elevate anesthesiology and enable the delivery of safe, efficient, and compassionate surgical care. It is our shared commitment to excellence that inspires the continued growth of perioperative medicine.

To all who contributed their time, expertise, and vision—thank you. This book exists because of you.

Contents

Part I The Essential Perioperative Physician: Leadership, Economics, and the Expanding Value of Anesthesiology

1 **Physician Leadership, Anesthesiology's Rise, and Modern Economic Value** 3
George Tewfik

2 **Perioperative Economics: Aligning Efficiency, Quality, and Value in Modern Healthcare** 11
George Tewfik, Bishoy Ezzat, and Rania Aziz

Part II Preoperative Optimization and Perioperative Care Pathways

3 **Anesthesia and Preoperative Testing: A Modern Perspective** 29
Lawrence Chinn, Robert Gubkin, Aditi Master, Jessica Lee, Anoshia Khan, Julia DeLorenzo, and Jonathan Lopez

4 **Optimizing Surgical Readiness: Inpatient vs Outpatient Preoperative Evaluation Models** 43
Justin Calvert and Ivan S. Kim

5 **Preoperative Optimization and Risk Reduction: A Systems-Based Role for Anesthesiologists** 57
Stephen Rivoli, Darryl Brown, Janet Mutschler, John Choi, Alexandra Jankulov, and Rohini Loke

6 **Enhanced Recovery After Surgery: The Anesthesiologist's Role in Accelerating Recovery and Transforming Perioperative Care** 69
Isabelle Nemeh, Daniel Rodriguez-Correa, and Cyrus Ghaderi

Part III The Anesthesiologist as Perioperative Operations Leader

7 **The Science of OR Scheduling: Metrics, Governance, and Staffing Optimization** 85
Fareeda Eraky, Rania Aziz, Faraz Chaudhry, Cynthia Tan, and George Tewfik

8 Perioperative Management of the Surgical Service Line 99
Donna Kucharski

9 Protocol Management for Emergencies by Anesthesiologists 115
Dorothy (Wei Yun) Wang and Anwar Alinani

10 Perioperative Blood Management: The Anesthesiologist's Role in Safer Transfusion Practices 133
Ashley Yager, Sadaf Chaugle, Douglas Nguyen, and Ravi V. Joshi

11 Surgical Site Infection Prophylaxis 159
Eric Reilly and Jazmine Skala-Wade

12 Venous Thromboembolism Prevention: The Role of Anesthesiologists . . . 171
Sharon Sun and Shelby Badani

13 Supply Chain and Fundamentals of Procuring Anesthesia Supplies . . . 183
Jordan Zunder, Matthew Zemel, Cole Crosby, and Rajen Nathwani

14 Medication and Formulary Management: The Hidden Value of Anesthesiologists 195
Gary Haynes

Part IV Postoperative Care and Recovery Management

15 The Post-anesthesia Care Unit: Clinical Stewardship, Systems Leadership, and the Expanding Role of the Anesthesiologist 207
Thomas Doss, Danny Jeong, Apoorva Amudhan, Bishoy Ezzat, and Daisy Munoz

16 Adverse Event Analysis: The Role of the Perioperative Clinician 215
Karolina Brook

17 Acute Pain Services: Clinical Impact, Cost Efficiency, and Hospital Value 229
Julia DeLorenzo, Patrick Discepola, and Jean D. Eloy

Part V Systems of Safety: Technology, Oversight, and Critical Care Leadership in Modern Anesthesiology

18 Crisis Medicine: The Anesthesiologist's Role in Airway, Trauma, and Emergency Preparedness 239
Maeve Muldowney, David A. Leon, and Ireana C. Ng

19 Sedation Governance: The Anesthesiologist's Role in Oversight and Credentialing 253
Charlota Jurcik, Nikhil Kaushal, George Tewfik, and Andres Zuniga

20 Non-operating Room Anesthesia Oversight and Management 273
Aaron N. Primm, Dane Saksa, and Patricia Fogarty Mack

21 Electronic Health Records/Anesthesia Information Management Services 285
Franklin Chiao

22 Quality Management and the Anesthesiologist's Role in Advancing Perioperative Excellence 291
Vilma Joseph and Terry Chambers

23 At the Crossroads of Safety: The Anesthesiologist's Leadership in Preventing Harm 299
Emily Methangkool

24 The Anesthesiologist as Intensivist: Integrating Perioperative and Critical Care Medicine 315
Shivani Patel and Sofia Gilels

25 Peripartum Excellence: The Anesthesiologist's Role in Quality, Safety, and Equity of Maternal Care 323
Sangeeta Kumaraswami, Christine Chen, and Mark Zakowski

Part VI Advancing the Profession of Anesthesiology: Risk, Revenue, Workforce, Policy, and the Future of Perioperative Care

26 Risk Management, Medicolegal Considerations, and the Role of the Anesthesiologist 347
Ashley Eltorai

27 Foundation of Revenue Cycle Management Excellence for Today's Anesthesia Practices 353
Dean Polce and Frank Burns

28 Training the Next Generation: Education, Workforce Development, and the Future of Anesthesiology 363
Yohannes B. Getachew

29 Accountable Care Organizations: Integrating Anesthesiology into Value-Based Care 371
Diana C. Mosquera and Matthew J. Dellaquila

30 Advancing Research in Anesthesiology: A Comprehensive Review . . . 383
Jiang-Hong Ye, Wanhong Zuo, and Zhiyi Zuo

31 Consulting in Perioperative and Anesthesiology Services: Optimizing Operations, Strategy, and Value 413
Jason Klopotowski, Kristen Conway, Leslie Meyer Basham, Supriya Patel, and Joshua S. Miller

32 Advocacy in Action: The Anesthesiologist's Role in Shaping Healthcare Policy and Patient Safety 427
Stacey Watt, Joseph R. Current, John R. Kraus, and Charles J. Assini Jr.

33 Practice Guidelines and Best Practices in Perioperative Care 443
Karen B. Domino

34 Professional Citizenship: How Anesthesiologists Advance Medicine Through Society Engagement 451
Lois A. Connolly, Kraig S. de Lanzac, and Matthew Popovich

Part VII Transforming the Business and Future of Perioperative Care: Innovation, Partnerships, and the Strategic Evolution of Anesthesiology

35 The Hidden Economy of Anesthesiology: Unpaid Work That Sustains Healthcare 467
Thanh-Giang Vu

36 Redesigning Perioperative Care Through Telemedicine and Data Integration 475
Saul Abreu and Dennis Grech

37 After the RFP: Building Sustainable Partnerships Between Anesthesia Practices and Hospitals 487
Shena J. Scott, Jason Greenberg, Joseph W. Szokol, and Jay Mesrobian

38 Anesthesiologists in Hospital Leadership: Bridging the Gap with Regulatory and Accrediting Organizations 497
Michael Simon and Matthew Popovich

39 Anesthesiology and Artificial Intelligence: Leading the Next Transformation in Perioperative Medicine 513
Chris Eixenberger and Vikas O'Reilly-Shah

Index 527

Contributors

Saul Abreu Rutgers New Jersey Medical School, Newark, NJ, USA

Anwar Alinani Department of Anesthesiology and Pain Medicine, University of Washington, Seattle, WA, USA

Apoorva Amudhan Rutgers New Jersey Medical School, Newark, NJ, USA

Charles J. Assini Jr. New York State Society of Anesthesiologists, New York, NY, USA

Rania Aziz Department of Anesthesiology, Rutgers New Jersey Medical School, Newark, NJ, USA

Shelby Badani Department of Anesthesiology, New York-Presbyterian/Weill Cornell Medicine, New York, NY, USA

Leslie Meyer Basham Surgical Directions, Chicago, IL, USA

Karolina Brook Boston University Chobanian & Avedisian School of Medicine, Boston, MA, USA
Boston Medical Center, Department of Anesthesiology, Boston, MA, USA

Darryl Brown Icahn School of Medicine at Mount Sinai, Mount Sinai West and Morningside Hospitals, New York, NY, USA

Frank Burns US Anesthesia Partners, Dallas, TX, USA

Justin Calvert Loma Linda University Medical School, Loma Linda, CA, USA

Riverside University Health System, Moreno Valley, CA, USA

Terry Chambers Department of Anesthesiology, Albert Einstein College of Medicine/Montefiore Medical Center/Moses Campus, New York, USA

Faraz Chaudhry Department of Anesthesiology, Rutgers New Jersey Medical School, Newark, NJ, USA

Sadaf Chaugle Division of Cardiothoracic and Vascular Anesthesiology, University of Texas Southwestern Medical Center (UTSW), Dallas, TX, USA
Department of Anesthesiology & Pain Management, University of Texas Southwestern Medical Center (UTSW), Dallas, TX, USA

Christine Chen Cedars-Sinai Medical Center, Los Angeles, CA, USA

Franklin Chiao Westchester Medical Center Health Network, Valhalla, NY, USA

Lawrence Chinn Rutgers New Jersey Medical School, Newark, NJ, USA

John Choi Icahn School of Medicine at Mount Sinai, Mount Sinai West and Morningside Hospitals, New York, NY, USA

Lois A. Connolly Department of Anesthesiology, Medical College of Wisconsin, Milwaukee, WI, USA

Kristen Conway Surgical Directions, Chicago, IL, USA
Queens University, Knight School of Communication, Charlotte, NC, USA

Cole Crosby Harborview Medical Center, University of Washington Anesthesiology and Pain Medicine, Seattle, WA, USA

Joseph R. Current University at Buffalo, Jacobs School of Medicine and Biomedical Sciences, Buffalo, NY, USA

Kraig S. de Lanzac Department of Anesthesiology, Tulane University School of Medicine, New Orleans, LA, USA
Tulane Lakeside Hospital, Metairie, LA, USA
American Society of Anesthesiologists, Washington, DC, USA

Matthew J. Dellaquila Henry Ford Jackson Hospital, Jackson, MI, USA

Julia DeLorenzo Rutgers New Jersey Medical School, Newark, NJ, USA

Patrick Discepola Department of Anesthesiology, Rutgers New Jersey Medical School, Newark, NJ, USA

Karen B. Domino University of Washington, Seattle, WA, USA

Thomas Doss Rutgers New Jersey Medical School, Newark, NJ, USA

Chris Eixenberger Department of Anesthesiology and Pain Medicine, University of Washington, Seattle, WA, USA

Jean D. Eloy Department of Anesthesiology, Rutgers New Jersey Medical School, Newark, NJ, USA

Ashley Eltorai University of Connecticut School of Medicine, Hartford, CT, USA

Fareeda Eraky Department of Anesthesiology, Rutgers New Jersey Medical School, Newark, NJ, USA

Bishoy Ezzat Rutgers New Jersey Medical School, Newark, NJ, USA

Yohannes B. Getachew, MD MBA Perelman School of Medicine, University of Pennsylvania, Children's Hospital of Philadelphia, Philadelphia, PA, USA
General Anesthesiology, Children's Hospital of Philadelphia, Philadelphia, USA

Cyrus Ghaderi Rutgers New Jersey Medical School, Newark, NJ, USA

Sofia Gilels Montefiore Medical Center, Bronx, NY, USA

Dennis Grech Rutgers New Jersey Medical School, Newark, NJ, USA

Jason Greenberg Department of Anesthesia and Perioperative Care, University of California, San Francisco, San Francisco, CA, USA

Robert Gubkin Rutgers New Jersey Medical School, Newark, NJ, USA

Gary Haynes Tulane University, New Orleans, LA, USA

Alexandra Jankulov Icahn School of Medicine at Mount Sinai, Mount Sinai West and Morningside Hospitals, New York, NY, USA

Danny Jeong Rutgers New Jersey Medical School, Newark, NJ, USA

Vilma Joseph Department of Anesthesiology, Montefiore Medical Center, Weiler Hospital, New York, NY, USA
Department of Anesthesiology, Albert Einstein College of Medicine/Montefiore Medical Center/Moses Campus, New York, USA

Ravi V. Joshi Division of Cardiothoracic and Vascular Anesthesiology, University of Texas Southwestern Medical Center (UTSW), Dallas, TX, USA
Department of Anesthesiology & Pain Management, University of Texas Southwestern Medical Center (UTSW), Dallas, TX, USA

Charlota Jurcik University of Arizona, Banner – University Medical Center, Tucson, AZ, USA

Nikhil Kaushal Rutgers New Jersey Medical School, Newark, NJ, USA

Anoshia Khan Rutgers New Jersey Medical School, Newark, NJ, USA

Ivan S. Kim Loma Linda University Medical Center, Loma Linda, CA, USA

Jason Klopotowski Surgical Directions, Chicago, IL, USA

John R. Kraus University at Buffalo, Jacobs School of Medicine and Biomedical Sciences, Buffalo, NY, USA

Donna Kucharski Southcoast Health, Fall River, MA, USA

Sangeeta Kumaraswami Westchester Medical Center/New York Medical College, Valhalla, NY, USA
ASA Committee on Quality Management and Departmental Administration, ASA Representative to the DNV Healthcare Advisory Board, Schaumburg, IL, USA

Jessica Lee Rutgers New Jersey Medical School, Newark, NJ, USA

David A. Leon Department of Anesthesiology and Pain Medicine and Department of Emergency Medicine, University of California Davis School of Medicine, Sacramento, CA, USA

Rohini Loke Icahn School of Medicine at Mount Sinai, Mount Sinai West and Morningside Hospitals, New York, NY, USA

Jonathan Lopez Rutgers New Jersey Medical School, Newark, NJ, USA

Patricia Fogarty Mack Weill Cornell Medicine, New York Presbyterian Hospital, New York, NY, USA

Aditi Master Rutgers New Jersey Medical School, Newark, NJ, USA

Jay Mesrobian Advocate Aurora Health, Milwaukee, WI, USA

Emily Methangkool Department of Anesthesiology and Perioperative Medicine, University of California, Los Angeles, Los Angeles, CA, USA

Joshua S. Miller Surgical Directions, Chicago, IL, USA

Diana C. Mosquera Northwell, New Hyde Park, NY, USA

Maeve Muldowney Department of Anesthesiology and Pain Medicine, Harborview Medical Center, University of Washington, Seattle, WA, USA

Daisy Munoz Rutgers New Jersey Medical School, Newark, NJ, USA

Janet Mutschler Icahn School of Medicine at Mount Sinai, Mount Sinai West and Morningside Hospitals, New York, NY, USA

Rajen Nathwani Department of Anesthesiology and Pain Medicine, University of Washington, Seattle, WA, USA

Isabelle Nemeh Rutgers New Jersey Medical School, Newark, NJ, USA

Ireana C. Ng Department of Anesthesiology and Pain Medicine, Harborview Medical Center, University of Washington, Seattle, WA, USA

Douglas Nguyen Division of Cardiothoracic and Vascular Anesthesiology, University of Texas Southwestern Medical Center (UTSW), Dallas, TX, USA
Department of Anesthesiology & Pain Management, University of Texas Southwestern Medical Center (UTSW), Dallas, TX, USA

Vikas O'Reilly-Shah Department of Anesthesiology and Pain Medicine, University of Washington, Seattle, WA, USA

Shivani Patel Anesthesia Specialists of Bethlehem, Bethlehem, PA, USA

Supriya Patel Surgical Directions, Chicago, IL, USA

Dean Polce US Anesthesia Partners, Las Vegas, NV, USA

Matthew Popovich American Society of Anesthesiologists, Washington, DC, USA

Aaron N. Primm Department of Anesthesiology, Perioperative Care, and Pain Medicine, NYU Grossman School of Medicine, New York, NY, USA

Eric Reilly Department of Anesthesiology & Pain Medicine, Corewell Health William Beaumont University Hospital, Royal Oak, MI, USA

Stephen Rivoli Icahn School of Medicine at Mount Sinai, Mount Sinai West and Morningside Hospitals, New York, NY, USA

Daniel Rodriguez-Correa Rutgers New Jersey Medical School, Newark, NJ, USA

Dane Saksa UCLA Health, Los Angeles, CA, USA

Shena J. Scott Scott Healthcare Consulting, Inc., Melbourne, FL, USA

Michael Simon HCA Florida Memorial Hospital, Jacksonville, FL, USA

Jazmine Skala-Wade Department of Anesthesiology & Pain Medicine, Corewell Health William Beaumont University Hospital, Royal Oak, MI, USA

Sharon Sun Robert Wood Johnson Hospital, New Brunswick, NJ, USA

Joseph W. Szokol David Geffen School of Medicine at UCLA, Department of Anesthesiology and Perioperative Medicine, UCLA Health, Los Angeles, CA, USA
American Society of Anesthesiologists, Schaumberg, IL, USA
Department of Anesthesiology, Critical Care, and Pain Medicine, NorthShore University HealthSystem, Evanston, IL, USA

Cynthia Tan Department of Anesthesiology, Perioperative Care and Pain Medicine, NYU Langone Health, New York, NY, USA

George Tewfik Department of Anesthesiology, Rutgers New Jersey Medical School, Newark, NJ, USA

Thanh-Giang Vu Washington Permanente Medical Group, Kaiser Permanente, Seattle, WA, USA

Dorothy (Wei Yun) Wang Department of Anesthesiology and Pain Medicine, University of Washington, Seattle, WA, USA

Stacey Watt University at Buffalo, Jacobs School of Medicine and Biomedical Sciences, Buffalo, NY, USA

Ashley Yager Division of Cardiothoracic and Vascular Anesthesiology, University of Texas Southwestern Medical Center (UTSW), Dallas, TX, USA
Department of Anesthesiology & Pain Management, University of Texas Southwestern Medical Center (UTSW), Dallas, TX, USA

Jiang-Hong Ye Department of Anesthesiology, Rutgers University, New Jersey Medical School, Newark, NJ, USA

Mark Zakowski Department of Anesthesiology, Cedars-Sinai Medical Center, Los Angeles, CA, USA
ASA Committee on Obstetric Anesthesia, Past ASA Liaison to ACOG CC-OB, ASA Committee on Quality Management and Departmental Administration, ASA Educational Track Subcommittee on Obstetric Anesthesia, Schaumburg, IL, USA
Society for Obstetric Anesthesia and Perinatology, Lexington, KY, USA
California Society of Anesthesiologists, Sacramento, CA, USA
CSA Foundation for Education, Sacramento, CA, USA

Matthew Zemel Seattle Children's Hospital, Seattle, WA, USA

Jordan Zunder Department of Anesthesiology and Pain Medicine, University of Ottawa, The Ottawa Hospital, Ottawa, ON, Canada

Andres Zuniga Saint Peter's University, Jersey City, NJ, USA

Wanhong Zuo Department of Anesthesiology, Rutgers University, New Jersey Medical School, Newark, NJ, USA

Zhiyi Zuo Department of Anesthesiology, University of Virginia, Charlottesville, VA, USA

Part I

The Essential Perioperative Physician: Leadership, Economics, and the Expanding Value of Anesthesiology

1 Physician Leadership, Anesthesiology's Rise, and Modern Economic Value

George Tewfik

1.1 Introduction

The modern hospital is a complex, dynamic system of interlocking clinical, logistical, and financial processes. In this environment, physicians who combine clinical acumen with systems thinking exert disproportionate influence over outcomes, quality, and institutional sustainability. As surgery grew more sophisticated in the twentieth century, anesthesiologists gradually evolved from technicians into central perioperative architects. Today, the anesthesiologist is increasingly the **essential perioperative physician**—not only responsible for intraoperative safety but also for upstream optimization, downstream recovery, and the economic viability of surgical services. This chapter traces the history of physicians as hospital leaders, the emergence of anesthesiology as a specialty, and the modern economic value proposition of anesthesiologists within health systems.

1.2 Physicians as Hospital Leaders: Historical Trajectory

1.2.1 Early Hospitals and Physician Authority

In the early modern period, hospitals were often charitable or religious institutions. Administration was frequently overseen by clergy, civic boards, or lay trustees; physicians were consulted for care, but rarely held administrative authority. Over time, medicine's scientific advances (e.g. germ theory, antisepsis, and laboratory diagnostics) elevated the epistemic authority of physicians, making them indispensable to hospital operations.

G. Tewfik (✉)
Department of Anesthesiology, Rutgers New Jersey Medical School, Newark, NJ, USA
e-mail: glt31@njms.rutgers.edu

G. Tewfik (ed.), *The Anesthesiologist as Perioperative Leader*,
https://doi.org/10.1007/978-3-032-18058-2_1

By the late nineteenth and early twentieth centuries, leaders such as Sir William Osler at Johns Hopkins and Harvey Cushing in neurosurgery epitomized the physician–scholar–administrator model. In academic centers, departmental chairs and medical school deans gained influence over hospital priorities (e.g., capital allocation, service line development, faculty recruitment). This evolution entrenched the physician as institutional steward, both clinically and operationally.

1.2.2 Mid-twentieth Century: The Rise of the Medical Director and Departmental Leadership

As hospital complexity increased—with critical care units, imaging suites, and multidisciplinary services—physicians assumed roles such as chiefs of service and medical directors. Their purview extended to quality oversight, credentialing, safety initiatives, and interdepartmental coordination. Yet, in many institutions, decision-making remained fragmented: surgeons, internists, cardiologists, and others each held influence over their domains.

Physician leadership academies and training programs (e.g., in healthcare administration, executive MBA) began to emerge in the late twentieth century, signaling formal recognition that clinical leaders needed management skills. Simultaneously, hospitals recognized that physician buy-in on workflow redesign and quality initiatives were critical to success.

Anesthesiologists, by virtue of their cross-disciplinary exposure to every surgical specialty and their global view of perioperative processes, were in an ideal position to bridge siloes—when empowered to lead.

1.3 The Evolution of Anesthesiology as a Specialty

1.3.1 Early Origins and Pre-specialty Era

Efforts to relieve surgical pain date back millennia—alcohol, opium, herbal concoctions, even "stroke to the head" interventions are recorded in ancient texts (e.g., Hippocratic and Ayurvedic). Through the medieval and early modern eras, sedative or analgesic techniques were applied inconsistently, often by nonphysician practitioners or surgeons themselves.

The modern era of anesthesia is often traced to **October 16, 1846**, when William T. G. Morton successfully demonstrated ether anesthesia at Massachusetts General Hospital. This event marked the transition from excruciating surgery to the concept of planned, controlled unconsciousness. In the late nineteenth and early twentieth centuries, anesthetic practices were diffuse: surgeons, dentists, or attendants (often nurses or trainees) would administer ether, chloroform, or early gas mixtures. The field lacked standardized training, formal credentialing, or academic anchoring.

1.3.2 Toward Formal Recognition: Waters, Rovenstine, and the Specialty Movement

In the early decades of the twentieth century, a trio of anesthesiologists—Paul Wood, John Lundy, and Ralph Waters—played pivotal roles in crystallizing anesthesiology's identity and legitimacy. Ralph Waters, in particular, is credited with establishing the first anesthesiology department and residency program at the University of Wisconsin in 1927, thereby institutionalizing training and research in anesthesia. Throughout the 1930s and 1940s, physician anesthetists gradually displaced nonphysician providers. At the same time, anesthesiologists began to assume roles in pain management, postoperative care, critical care, and airway management.

Pioneers such as Harold Griffith (notably introducing curare for muscle relaxation during anesthesia) further advanced anesthetic technique, safety, and mechanistic understanding. In Canada, Griffith also established the first postoperative recovery room, laying groundwork for enhanced post-anesthesia care.

The American Board of Anesthesiology (ABA) attained independent specialty status mid-twentieth century, and anesthesiology certification became a recognized credential distinguishing physician anesthetists from other practitioners. In parallel, residency training structures, academic departments, and subspecialty fellowships matured. By the latter half of the twentieth century, anesthesiology had become a full-fledged medical specialty, contributing not only to surgical care but to perioperative systems, quality, and patient safety.

1.3.3 Perioperative Systems and Organizational Influence

As anesthesia matured, practitioners expanded their remit beyond the operating room. Anesthesiologists developed preoperative evaluation clinics, postoperative recovery units, standardized protocols, and multidisciplinary collaboration in enhanced recovery pathways. They became early adopters of monitoring technologies (e.g., pulse oximetry, capnography), closed-loop ventilation, and simulation training.

Importantly, anesthesiologists' workflow cuts across multiple surgical services, enabling them to assume system-level leadership (e.g., scheduling, resource allocation, quality metrics). In many forward-thinking institutions, they function as perioperative medical directors or surgical service line leaders.

1.4 Economic Value of Anesthesiologists in Contemporary Hospitals

In an era of declining margins, shifting reimbursement models, and value-based care, the economic contribution of anesthesiologists is increasingly measurable—and strategically vital.

1.4.1 Operating Room Efficiency and Throughput

The operating suite is often a hospital's most revenue-intensive unit, generating substantial inpatient, outpatient, and ancillary utilization. Anesthesiologists, through leadership in OR management, can influence:

- On-time starts, by aligning preoperative workflows
- Turnover times, by optimizing staffing and equipment readiness
- Case scheduling and block utilization
- Cancelation and delay mitigation
- Resource allocation (e.g., instruments, staffing)

Even modest improvements in OR block utilization or turnover efficiency can yield significant incremental revenue. Many health systems now prioritize "OR productivity" metrics, and anesthesiology groups are central to those efforts.

1.4.2 Cost Control, Waste Reduction, and Efficiency

Anesthesiologists also help to control perioperative costs. For example:

- Intraoperative drug choice and delivery (e.g., low-flow anesthesia, balanced vs TIVA strategies) significantly affect consumable costs.
- Reduction of anesthetic gas leakage (especially in centralized nitrous oxide pipelines) yields savings, given that inhalational agents may constitute ~5–6% of total drug expenses within anesthesia services.
- Streamlined staffing models, appropriate supervision levels, and team scheduling help reduce labor costs.

In one analysis, anesthesia-related cost reductions of US $13–30 per case (multiplied across ~25 million annual anesthetics) could amount to potential national savings of $350–750 million [1].

Moreover, anesthesia waste is nontrivial: for example, bispectral index monitoring during inhalational anesthesia has been critiqued as adding cost without clear benefit.

1.4.3 Value-Based Care, Quality, and Risk Mitigation

In value-based reimbursement models, outcomes matter. Anesthesiologists contribute to:

- Decreasing perioperative complications (e.g., myocardial infarction, respiratory failure)

- Reducing postoperative nausea and vomiting (PONV), which impacts patient satisfaction and throughput
- Minimizing unplanned readmissions
- Enhancing discharge efficiency

For instance, economic modeling suggests that in ambulatory and inpatient settings, total intravenous anesthesia (TIVA) using propofol may reduce overall cost compared to inhalational anesthesia—largely via reductions in PONV and faster recovery [2].

Similarly, outpatient anesthesia consultation clinics (OPACs) have been shown, in matched-cohort studies, to reduce preoperative admission costs versus traditional inpatient pre-evaluation systems [3].

As anesthesiologists adopt prehabilitation and optimization (e.g., managing comorbidities, reducing delays), they shift the surgical risk profile, resulting in fewer complications and lower downstream resource use [4].

1.4.4 Revenue Preservation, Documentation, and Reimbursement

Accurate documentation of anesthesia time, modifiers, and intraoperative complexity is critical to securing appropriate reimbursement. Anesthesia Information Management Systems (AIMS) and automated charge-capture tools contribute to documentation completeness, compliance, and audit defensibility. Furthermore, as payers scrutinize billing patterns, anesthesiologists must protect against undervaluation or arbitrary reimbursement cuts.

From a cost-effectiveness perspective, earlier reviews note that practice changes that improved outcomes often increased net health expenditures; but acceptable cost-effectiveness thresholds (e.g., $50,000–$100,000 per life-year saved) remain guiding benchmarks. The specialty continues to require rigorous, high-quality economic evaluations in many domains [5]. Nonetheless, anesthesiologists are well-positioned as financial stewards—capable of controlling costs, generating revenue, and improving institutional reputation.

1.4.5 Beyond the OR: Critical Care, Pain, and Perioperative Systems

Many anesthesiology groups oversee intensive care units (ICUs), sedation services, regional anesthesia programs, and chronic pain clinics. These services, when integrated under anesthesiology leadership, contribute both clinical and financial value:

- ICU management improves resource utilization, length of stay, and workflow alignment

- Regional anesthesia and pain services enhance patient satisfaction, reduce opioid use, and often support revenue from procedural volumes
- Anesthesiologists' systems view enables integration of preoperative, intraoperative, and postoperative pathways under a cohesive economic and quality framework

1.5 The Anesthesiologist as the Perioperative Leader

Integrating historical perspective with modern economics, the essential perioperative physician is one who:

1. **Shapes upstream optimization**—participating in preoperative clinics, risk stratification, and resource planning
2. **Commands intraoperative excellence**—applying anesthetic, physiologic, and safety domains
3. **Guides downstream recovery**—through ERAS, PACU, ICU, and early mobilization
4. **Coordinates across surgical services**—linking specialties and aligning priorities
5. **Drives financial sustainability**—balancing cost control, throughput, documentation integrity, and quality outcomes

In effect, the anesthesiologist becomes the bridge between clinical imperatives and institutional viability. As hospitals grapple with regulatory pressures, workforce constraints, and shrinking margins, the ability to deliver safe, efficient, value-based care positions anesthesiology leadership as indispensable.

1.6 Summary and Forward View

In summary:

- The rise of institutional medicine elevated physicians to leadership roles; as disciplines matured, anesthesiology emerged as uniquely positioned to influence perioperative systems.
- The specialty evolved from a technical service into an academic, organizational, and economic force.
- In contemporary health systems, anesthesiologists create value not only through clinical safety, but through throughput, cost control, quality leadership, documentation integrity, and integrated perioperative planning.
- Framing anesthesiology in economic as well as clinical terms strengthens its legitimacy as a leadership domain in hospitals.

In succeeding chapters, we will explore case studies, metrics frameworks, contract models, and implementation strategies that make the vision of the *essential perioperative physician* tangible in real-world settings

References

1. Rinehardt EK, Sivarajan M. Costs and wastes in anesthesia care. Curr Opin Anaesthesiol. 2012;25(2):221–5. https://doi.org/10.1097/ACO.0b013e32834f00ec.
2. Kampmeier T, Rehberg S, Omar Alsaleh AJ, Schraag S, Pham J, Westphal M. Cost-effectiveness of propofol (diprivan) versus inhalational anesthetics to maintain general anesthesia in noncardiac surgery in the United States. Value Health. 2021;24(7):939–47. https://doi.org/10.1016/j.jval.2021.01.008.
3. Lee A, Chui PT, Chiu CH, Gin T, Ho AMH. The cost-effectiveness of an outpatient anesthesia consultation clinic before surgery: a matched Hong Kong cohort study. Perioperat Med. 2012;1(1):3. https://doi.org/10.1186/2047-0525-1-3.
4. Ahmed F, Chithrala B, Barve K, Biladeau S, Clifford SP. Value-based care and anesthesiology in the USA. Cureus. 2023;15(8):e44410. https://doi.org/10.7759/cureus.44410.
5. Teja BJ, Sutherland TN, Barnett SR, Talmor DS. Cost-effectiveness research in anesthesiology. Anesth Analg. 2018;127(5):1196–201. https://doi.org/10.1213/ane.0000000000003334.

Perioperative Economics: Aligning Efficiency, Quality, and Value in Modern Healthcare

2

George Tewfik, Bishoy Ezzat, and Rania Aziz

2.1 Introduction

Perioperative medicine encompasses the spectrum of care delivered before, during, and after surgery, extending beyond the confines of the operating room. As health care systems face mounting pressure to improve quality while controlling costs, the economic implications of perioperative practice have become increasingly significant. Surgical services are among the largest drivers of hospital revenue, but they also represent a major source of expenditure. Within this complex balance, perioperative medicine offers a unique opportunity to influence both sides of the economic equation.

Anesthesiologists, by virtue of their central role in surgical and procedural care, are uniquely positioned to impact hospital efficiency, resource utilization, and patient outcomes [1]. Decisions made in the perioperative setting—from preoperative optimization to postoperative recovery—carry downstream effects on complications, length of stay, readmissions, and overall cost of care. Effective perioperative practices not only improve clinical outcomes but also generate measurable economic value for health systems operating under fee-for-service, bundled payment, or value-based care models.

This chapter explores the multifaceted economic impact of perioperative medicine. We will examine direct and indirect cost drivers, analyze the contribution of perioperative interventions to institutional financial performance, and highlight the strategic value of anesthesiologists as leaders in this domain. By integrating clinical excellence with economic stewardship, perioperative medicine underscores the

G. Tewfik (✉) · R. Aziz
Department of Anesthesiology, Rutgers New Jersey Medical School, Newark, NJ, USA
e-mail: glt31@njms.rutgers.edu

B. Ezzat
Rutgers New Jersey Medical School, Newark, NJ, USA

G. Tewfik (ed.), *The Anesthesiologist as Perioperative Leader*,
https://doi.org/10.1007/978-3-032-18058-2_2

evolving identity of the anesthesiologist as both a clinician and a key contributor to the financial health of modern health care organizations.

2.2 Direct Cost Drivers in Perioperative Care

The perioperative environment is resource-intensive, and even small inefficiencies can translate into substantial financial consequences. Understanding the direct cost drivers within perioperative medicine is essential for hospitals and anesthesiologists seeking to optimize both patient care and institutional economics (Table 2.1).

2.2.1 Operating Room Utilization

Operating room (OR) time is among the most expensive resources in the hospital, with estimates ranging from **$20 to $80 per minute** depending on institutional context [2]. Inefficient scheduling, case delays, and turnover time directly increase costs while limiting throughput. Anesthesiologists play a crucial role in managing OR efficiency through preoperative readiness assessments, case sequencing, and minimizing avoidable delays.

2.2.2 Staffing Models

Labor costs represent a significant portion of perioperative expenditures. The composition of anesthesia teams—whether anesthesiologist-only, anesthesia care team (ACT) models, or hybrid staffing—has economic implications for both cost and quality. Optimal staffing ensures safety while aligning with institutional financial realities. Moreover, variability in staffing across peak and off-peak hours impacts overtime, staffing inefficiencies, and cost-per-case metrics.

Table 2.1 Direct cost drivers in perioperative care

Cost driver	Description	Role of anesthesiologists
Operating room utilization	OR time costs $20–$80/min; inefficiencies reduce throughput	Manage scheduling, readiness, and minimize delays
Staffing models	Labor costs vary by team composition and hours	Optimize team structure and shift coverage
Medications & Supplies	Drug and supply choices affect cost	Promote standardization and cost-effective choices
PACU efficiency	Longer stays increase costs and bottlenecks	Implement protocols for faster recovery/discharge
Cancelations and delays	Lost OR time and disrupted schedules	Lead pre-op clinics and readiness protocols

2.2.3 Medications and Supply Utilization

Pharmaceuticals and disposables contribute directly to perioperative costs. Drug selection (e.g., generic versus branded agents, volatile anesthetics versus total intravenous anesthesia), multimodal analgesia protocols, and judicious use of high-cost agents all influence economic outcomes. Supply chain optimization, including standardization of airway devices, monitoring equipment, and perioperative kits, can generate measurable savings without compromising care.

2.2.4 Post-Anesthesia Care Unit (PACU) Efficiency

The PACU is a major determinant of perioperative resource utilization. Prolonged PACU stays increase staffing costs and reduce bed availability, which can cascade into OR bottlenecks and surgical cancelations. Effective pain and nausea control, early mobilization protocols, and standardized discharge criteria help reduce PACU length of stay and downstream costs.

2.2.5 Cancelations and Delays

Same-day surgical cancelations and intraoperative delays represent substantial economic waste. Lost OR time cannot be recaptured, and cancelations disrupt schedules for patients, surgeons, and staff. Preoperative optimization clinics, efficient communication among surgical teams, and evidence-based protocols for patient readiness significantly mitigate these losses.

2.3 Downstream Cost Implications

While direct perioperative expenses are significant, the downstream consequences of perioperative management often account for the largest share of economic impact (Table 2.2). The quality and efficiency of care delivered during the surgical episode have far-reaching effects on patient recovery, hospital resource use, and overall

Table 2.2 Downstream cost implications of perioperative management

Factor	Economic impact	Mitigation strategy
Postoperative complications	Tens of thousands per complication	Infection control, fluid management, monitoring
Readmissions & ICU escalation	Financial penalties, high resource use	ERAS protocols, early detection, pain control
Length of stay (LOS)	Higher costs, reduced bed availability	Discharge planning, pain programs, coordination
Surgical cancelations	Lost revenue, disrupted staffing	Pre-op optimization, communication protocols

health system expenditures. Data has shown that physician anesthesiologists leading an anesthesia care team leads to an overall improvement in patient outcomes, and that these improvements lead to overall cost savings in our healthcare systems [3].

2.3.1 Preventing Postoperative Complications

Postoperative complications substantially increase costs of care, often dwarfing the expense of the procedure itself. Complications such as surgical site infections, thromboembolic events, or respiratory failure lead to prolonged hospitalizations, increased use of intensive care, and higher rates of readmission. Even a single preventable complication can add **tens of thousands of dollars** to an episode of care. Perioperative interventions—such as optimized fluid management, infection prophylaxis, and vigilant monitoring—represent high-value strategies for cost avoidance.

2.3.2 Readmissions and Escalation of Care

Hospital readmissions are increasingly scrutinized under value-based payment models and are often financially penalized. Patients with poorly managed pain, untreated comorbidities, or unrecognized complications are at heightened risk of readmission. Similarly, escalation of care to an intensive care unit (ICU) significantly amplifies costs. Perioperative optimization, including enhanced recovery after surgery (ERAS) protocols, targeted monitoring, and early identification of deterioration, can reduce these costly outcomes [4].

2.3.3 Impact on Length of Stay

Hospital length of stay (LOS) is a key driver of cost and a critical metric of perioperative efficiency. Prolonged LOS not only increases direct expenses but also limits bed availability for new admissions, constraining hospital revenue potential. Enhanced perioperative pathways, effective discharge planning, and multidisciplinary coordination have been shown to shorten LOS, improving both patient satisfaction and institutional financial performance. The implementation of comprehensive acute pain programs has benefits with countless metrics with economic implications including improved patient experiences and postoperative pain with decreases in opioid consumption, alterations in mental status, surgical wound infection rates, etc. [5].

2.3.4 Surgical Cancelations and Throughput Bottlenecks

The effects of surgical cancelations extend beyond direct OR losses. Cancelations disrupt downstream resources, including PACU and ward staffing, and reduce institutional revenue from scheduled cases. Similarly, throughput bottlenecks—such as delayed PACU discharges or ICU bed shortages—have ripple effects that constrain surgical volume. Anesthesiologists, by facilitating efficient perioperative care and advocating for systems-level improvements, directly influence these downstream dynamics.

2.4 Perioperative Medicine and Value-Based Care

As health systems shift away from fee-for-service models toward value-based payment structures, perioperative medicine has emerged as a focal point for both quality improvement and cost containment (Table 2.3). Because surgical episodes account for a disproportionate share of hospital expenditures and revenue, optimizing perioperative care is central to achieving success in value-based models.

2.4.1 Bundled Payments and Alternative Payment Models

In bundled payment arrangements, a single payment covers the costs of all services related to an episode of care, such as a joint replacement or cardiac surgery. This incentivizes hospitals and providers to reduce unnecessary variation, avoid complications, and minimize readmissions. Perioperative physicians influence nearly every component of the bundle, from preoperative optimization and intraoperative management to postoperative recovery, positioning anesthesiologists as key drivers of cost-effective care.

2.4.2 Pay-for-Performance Incentives

Programs such as Medicare's Hospital Value-Based Purchasing and Quality Payment Program tie reimbursement to performance on safety, efficiency, and patient experience metrics. Perioperative outcomes—including rates of surgical site

Table 2.3 Value-based care levers in perioperative medicine

Payment model	Perioperative influence	Anesthesiologist's role
Bundled payments	Incentivizes reduced variation and complications	Manage entire episode from pre-op to recovery
Pay-for-performance	Ties reimbursement to safety and efficiency metrics	Enhance recovery, pain control, discharge timing
Cost avoidance initiatives	Rewards prevention over treatment	Lead ERAS, opioid-sparing, and prehabilitation

infection, postoperative pain control, and timely discharge—directly affect institutional performance. Anesthesiologists contribute to these measures through enhanced recovery protocols, multimodal analgesia, and standardized monitoring practices.

2.4.3 Cost Avoidance Through Quality Initiatives

Value-based care rewards the prevention of adverse outcomes rather than the treatment of complications. Perioperative initiatives such as ERAS, opioid-sparing analgesia, and prehabilitation programs have demonstrated both clinical benefits and significant cost savings [6, 7]. By reducing LOS, lowering readmissions, and improving patient satisfaction scores, these programs enhance financial performance under risk-sharing models.

2.4.4 Alignment with Health System Priorities

Hospitals engaged in accountable care organizations (ACOs) and integrated delivery networks view perioperative medicine as a strategic priority. Surgical services are often a "front door" for patient entry into health systems; thus, improving perioperative value strengthens both institutional reputation and market competitiveness. Anesthesiologists' leadership in quality and safety initiatives aligns seamlessly with these broader organizational goals.

2.5 Anesthesiologist's Role in Population Health Management

Perioperative medicine extends beyond the surgical episode to influence the broader health of populations. As health systems increasingly embrace population health strategies, anesthesiologists play a vital role in risk reduction, optimization of comorbid conditions, and the prevention of costly complications that drive systemwide expenditures.

2.5.1 Preoperative Optimization of Comorbidities

Chronic conditions such as diabetes, hypertension, and obstructive sleep apnea are strongly associated with increased perioperative risk. Addressing these comorbidities in preoperative clinics improves surgical outcomes and reduces downstream costs. For example, glycemic control in diabetic patients decreases surgical site infections, while optimized cardiac function reduces postoperative morbidity. By identifying and managing risks preoperatively, anesthesiologists prevent costly complications and reduce variability in care. These types of initiatives fit into an overall strategy of pursuing value-based, instead of service volume-based, care in anesthesiology in the USA [8].

2.5.2 Enhanced Recovery After Surgery (ERAS) Protocols

ERAS pathways exemplify the anesthesiologist's contribution to population health by standardizing perioperative care and minimizing complications. Protocols incorporating multimodal analgesia, fluid optimization, early mobilization, and opioid-sparing strategies have been shown to shorten hospital stays, reduce readmissions, and lower overall costs [9]. Importantly, ERAS also enhances functional recovery, benefiting both patients and the health system.

2.5.3 Perioperative Management of High-Risk Populations

Elderly patients, individuals with frailty, and those with multiple comorbidities contribute disproportionately to health care costs. Anesthesiologists are uniquely equipped to assess and stratify perioperative risk, implement individualized care plans, and coordinate multidisciplinary management for these vulnerable groups. Early recognition of risk factors and proactive interventions help reduce ICU admissions, readmissions, and mortality, translating into significant cost savings.

2.5.4 Preventive and Longitudinal Care Impact

Perioperative encounters often represent a critical touchpoint in a patient's broader health trajectory. By identifying undiagnosed conditions—such as untreated hypertension, anemia, or sleep apnea—anesthesiologists contribute to preventive care efforts that improve long-term outcomes and decrease future health expenditures. In this way, perioperative medicine serves as both an immediate economic driver and a contributor to broader population health strategies.

2.6 Health Economics of Innovation and Technology

Technological innovation has transformed perioperative medicine, offering both clinical advantages and economic opportunities (Table 2.4). While the initial investment in new devices or systems can be substantial, their potential to reduce variability, improve outcomes, and enhance efficiency often translates into significant long-term savings. Anesthesiologists are central to evaluating, adopting, and optimizing these technologies within the perioperative environment.

Table 2.4 Technological innovations and economic benefits

Technology/ innovation	Clinical benefit	Economic outcome
Informatics & Dashboards	Early risk detection, standardization	Fewer tests, shorter LOS, fewer complications
AI & Predictive Analytics	Anticipate adverse events	Reduced ICU use, proactive care
Noninvasive monitoring	Improved safety, fewer invasive procedures	Lower complication rates, faster recovery
Telemedicine	Remote assessments and follow-ups	Fewer cancelations, shorter stays

2.6.1 Informatics and Decision-Support Tools

The integration of perioperative informatics—including electronic health record (EHR) dashboards, real-time analytics, and clinical decision support—enables early identification of at-risk patients and standardization of best practices. These systems reduce unnecessary testing, prevent missed diagnoses, and improve communication across surgical teams. From an economic perspective, informatics tools minimize duplication of services, shorten length of stay, and reduce costly complications.

2.6.2 Artificial Intelligence and Predictive Analytics

AI-driven algorithms are increasingly applied to predict adverse events such as hypotension, hypoxemia, or postoperative delirium. Predictive modeling allows for earlier intervention, reducing the incidence of complications that would otherwise extend hospital stays or require intensive care. The economic benefit lies in shifting from reactive to proactive management, decreasing both direct and downstream costs.

2.6.3 Monitoring and Minimally Invasive Technologies

Advances in noninvasive hemodynamic monitoring, cerebral oximetry, and point-of-care ultrasound improve diagnostic accuracy and reduce the need for invasive procedures. These tools not only enhance safety but also lower complication rates, decreasing associated costs. Studies have already shown that initiatives such as using goal-directed fluid therapy lead directly to improved rates of post-surgical morbidity and ICU lengths of stay [10]. Similarly, the adoption of minimally invasive surgical and anesthetic techniques leads to faster recovery, reduced LOS, and higher patient throughput.

2.6.4 Telemedicine and Remote Perioperative Care

Telemedicine platforms allow anesthesiologists to extend perioperative oversight beyond the hospital setting. Virtual preoperative assessments and postoperative follow-ups reduce cancelations, facilitate earlier discharge, and improve patient satisfaction. Economically, telemedicine minimizes resource use while maintaining quality, representing a scalable solution for health systems seeking to manage large patient populations efficiently.

2.6.5 Cost-Benefit Considerations of Innovation

Despite clear advantages, adoption of new technologies requires careful cost-benefit analysis. Institutions must balance upfront capital expenditures with projected savings from reduced complications, shorter LOS, and increased throughput. Anesthesiologists, as both clinicians and systems leaders, are well-positioned to guide these investment decisions, ensuring that innovation aligns with institutional financial goals.

2.7 Strategic and Institutional Value

Beyond direct and downstream costs, perioperative medicine provides hospitals with significant **strategic and institutional value**. By shaping efficiency, quality, and reputation, anesthesiologists and perioperative teams influence a hospital's competitive position in increasingly complex health care markets.

2.7.1 Hospital Throughput and Capacity Management

Operating rooms and perioperative units are major revenue centers, but their value is maximized only when patient flow is efficient. Anesthesiologists' leadership in optimizing OR scheduling, PACU turnover, and ICU utilization enhances hospital throughput. Improved capacity management increases surgical volume without requiring additional infrastructure, thereby strengthening financial performance.

2.7.2 Institutional Reputation and Market Competitiveness

High-quality perioperative care translates into fewer complications, reduced mortality, and improved patient experiences—outcomes that directly affect hospital rankings, public reporting, and referral patterns. Institutions known for superior perioperative outcomes attract both patients and surgical talent, reinforcing market position and long-term financial growth.

2.7.3 Integration with Strategic Priorities

Hospitals increasingly prioritize initiatives such as value-based care, population health, and service line development (e.g., orthopedics, cardiac surgery). Perioperative medicine aligns closely with these priorities by delivering both cost control and quality improvements. Anesthesiologists, positioned across service lines, provide the systems-level perspective necessary to integrate perioperative initiatives with institutional strategy.

2.7.4 Anesthesiologists as Institutional Leaders

In addition to their clinical role, anesthesiologists contribute as administrators, committee leaders, and innovators in perioperative services. Their expertise in safety, quality improvement, and resource management positions them as key stakeholders in institutional decision-making. By bridging clinical care and economic strategy, anesthesiologists enhance not only patient outcomes but also the hospital's long-term sustainability.

2.8 Case Studies

The economic impact of perioperative medicine is best illustrated through real-world examples. Across diverse health systems, perioperative interventions have consistently demonstrated measurable improvements in both clinical outcomes and financial performance.

2.8.1 Enhanced Recovery After Surgery (ERAS) Pathways

Implementation of ERAS protocols in colorectal surgery has reduced length of stay by **2–3 days** on average, decreased complication rates, and generated cost savings estimated at **$3000–$6000 per patient episode** [11]. Similar benefits have been documented in orthopedic, gynecologic, and urologic procedures, underscoring the broad applicability of these pathways.

2.8.2 Preoperative Optimization Clinics

Institutions that establish preoperative assessment and optimization clinics report reductions in same-day cancelations, fewer unplanned ICU admissions, and improved surgical readiness [12]. These interventions translate into cost savings by reducing wasted OR time, preventing postoperative complications, and improving patient throughput.

2.8.3 Perioperative Anemia Management

Programs targeting preoperative anemia—through iron supplementation, erythropoiesis-stimulating agents, or restrictive transfusion practices—have decreased transfusion rates, shortened LOS, and improved outcomes. From an economic perspective, reducing allogeneic transfusions lowers direct costs while avoiding transfusion-related complications.

2.8.4 Multidisciplinary Perioperative Teams

Hospitals that integrate anesthesiologists, surgeons, nurses, and allied health professionals into perioperative teams report higher levels of efficiency and quality. For example, perioperative surgical homes (PSH) have shown reductions in readmissions, improved patient satisfaction, and significant reductions in overall episode costs [13].

2.8.5 Comparative Institutional Outcomes

Comparisons across institutions reveal that hospitals with structured perioperative medicine programs consistently outperform peers on metrics such as LOS, complication rates, and readmissions. These outcomes not only improve financial performance but also enhance institutional reputation and competitiveness in the health care marketplace.

2.9 Challenges and Barriers

Despite compelling evidence that perioperative medicine improves both outcomes and economic performance, significant challenges remain in fully realizing its potential. These barriers are multifactorial, spanning data limitations, organizational complexity, and entrenched cultural practices.

2.9.1 Limitations in Economic Data

While numerous studies demonstrate associations between perioperative interventions and improved outcomes, precise attribution of cost savings remains difficult. Variability in methodologies, institutional differences in accounting, and lack of standardized metrics make it challenging to generalize results across health systems. Without robust and reproducible data, it can be difficult to justify investment in perioperative programs to hospital administrators.

2.9.2 Fragmentation of Care and Misaligned Incentives

Perioperative care involves multiple stakeholders—surgeons, anesthesiologists, nurses, administrators—each operating within distinct incentive structures. Fee-for-service payment models reward procedural volume rather than complication prevention or care coordination, limiting the financial motivation to implement perioperative innovations. Misalignment of incentives across departments often hampers collaborative efforts to reduce costs and improve efficiency.

2.9.3 Resistance to Change

Cultural and organizational inertia can undermine the adoption of perioperative best practices. Surgeons and anesthesiologists accustomed to traditional workflows may be reluctant to adopt standardized pathways such as ERAS or perioperative surgical homes. Similarly, staff may resist new documentation, monitoring, or communication requirements. Overcoming these barriers requires leadership, education, and demonstration of both clinical and economic value.

2.9.4 Resource Constraints

The implementation of perioperative programs often requires upfront investment in personnel, technology, and infrastructure. Smaller hospitals and resource-limited settings may struggle to allocate funds or staff to establish preoperative clinics, adopt advanced monitoring, or implement robust data collection systems. Without external support or long-term financial planning, these barriers can perpetuate disparities in access to high-quality perioperative care.

2.9.5 Policy and Regulatory Hurdles

Health policy and regulatory frameworks may lag behind clinical innovation. For example, reimbursement models may not adequately recognize the economic value of perioperative optimization or telemedicine-based assessments. Similarly, accreditation standards may impose rigid requirements that do not align with emerging models of team-based perioperative care. Advocacy is needed to ensure that policy keeps pace with innovation.

2.10 Future Directions

The economic role of perioperative medicine will continue to expand as health care systems pursue strategies to deliver higher-quality care at lower cost. Emerging technologies, evolving payment models, and growing recognition of anesthesiologists as systems leaders will shape the next phase of development.

2.10.1 Expansion of Perioperative Surgical Homes (PSH)

The PSH model integrates multidisciplinary care across the surgical continuum, aligning incentives for quality and efficiency. Future iterations are likely to incorporate more robust data analytics, patient engagement platforms, and integration with population health initiatives. Broader adoption could position anesthesiologists at the center of institutional efforts to improve both outcomes and financial sustainability. The PSH model has been shown to improve resource utilization, amongst other metrics, when implemented successfully by physician anesthesiologists [14].

2.10.2 Integration of Predictive Analytics and Artificial Intelligence

Predictive modeling tools will play an increasingly important role in stratifying risk, preventing complications, and guiding individualized perioperative pathways. By identifying high-risk patients early, health systems can focus resources where they have the greatest impact, reducing costly adverse outcomes and optimizing resource utilization.

2.10.3 Telemedicine and Remote Optimization

The rapid growth of telemedicine provides an avenue for expanding preoperative optimization and postoperative follow-up beyond hospital walls. Virtual perioperative clinics can improve access, decrease cancelations, and shorten hospital stays, while reducing overall costs. Future models may leverage hybrid in-person and virtual care to maximize both efficiency and patient satisfaction.

2.10.4 Policy and Payment Reform

As bundled payments, accountable care organizations, and other alternative payment models mature, perioperative medicine will play a pivotal role in aligning clinical care with economic incentives. Anesthesiologists must engage with policymakers, payers, and professional societies to ensure that perioperative contributions are recognized and appropriately reimbursed.

2.10.5 Emphasis on Patient-Centered Outcomes

Future models of perioperative economics will extend beyond length of stay and cost-per-case to incorporate functional recovery, quality of life, and long-term outcomes. By prioritizing patient-centered metrics, perioperative medicine will align with broader health system goals of population health management and value-based care.

2.11 Conclusion

Perioperative medicine represents one of the most powerful levers for influencing both the quality and the economics of modern health care. By addressing direct cost drivers such as operating room efficiency, staffing, and PACU utilization, and by reducing downstream burdens including complications, readmissions, and prolonged length of stay, anesthesiologists contribute to substantial financial value for hospitals and health systems. Beyond these measurable savings, perioperative initiatives strengthen institutional reputation, market competitiveness, and strategic alignment with value-based care.

Anesthesiologists are uniquely positioned at the intersection of clinical expertise and systems-level management. Their leadership in preoperative optimization, enhanced recovery pathways, and innovative models such as perioperative surgical homes demonstrates the potential to improve outcomes while simultaneously reducing costs. As health systems evolve toward bundled payments, accountable care organizations, and patient-centered models, the influence of perioperative medicine will only grow.

The future success of perioperative medicine will depend on continued innovation, robust data collection, and active engagement with policymakers and institutional leaders. By embracing these roles, anesthesiologists can ensure that perioperative medicine remains a cornerstone of both clinical excellence and economic sustainability in health care.

References

1. Mahajan A, Esper SA, Cole DJ, Fleisher LA. Anesthesiologists' role in value-based perioperative care and healthcare transformation. Anesthesiology. 2021;134(4):526–40. (In eng). https://doi.org/10.1097/aln.0000000000003717.
2. Childers CP, Maggard-Gibbons M. Operating room efficiency: cost per minute and strategies to improve throughput. JAMA Surg. 2018;153(4). https://doi.org/10.1001/jamasurg.2017.6233.
3. Abenstein JP, Long KH, McGlinch BP, Dietz NM. Is physician anesthesia cost-effective? Anesth Analg. 2004;98(3):750–7. Table of contents. (In eng). https://doi.org/10.1213/01.ane.0000100945.56081.ac.
4. Ljungqvist O, Scott M, Fearon KC. Enhanced recovery after surgery: a review. JAMA Surg. 2017;152(3):292–8. (In eng). https://doi.org/10.1001/jamasurg.2016.4952.

5. Gray CF, Smith C, Zasimovich Y, Tighe PJ. Economic considerations of acute pain medicine programs. Tech Orthop. 2017;32(4):217–25. (In eng). https://doi.org/10.1097/bto.0000000000000241.
6. Ljungqvist O, Thanh NX, Nelson G. ERAS-value based surgery. J Surg Oncol. 2017;116(5):608–12. (In eng). https://doi.org/10.1002/jso.24820.
7. Memtsoudis SG, Poeran J, Mazumdar M. Regional anesthesia and outcomes after total joint arthroplasty: a population-based study of costs and complications. Anesthesiology. 2013;118(5):1046–58. https://doi.org/10.1097/ALN.0b013e318286061d.
8. Ahmed F, Chithrala B, Barve K, Biladeau S, Clifford SP. Value-based care and anesthesiology in the USA. Cureus. 2023;15(8):e44410. (In eng). https://doi.org/10.7759/cureus.44410.
9. Greco M, Capretti G, Beretta L, Gemma M, Pecorelli N, Braga M. Enhanced recovery in colorectal surgery: a meta-analysis of economic and clinical outcomes. World J Surg. 2014;38(6):1531–41. https://doi.org/10.1007/s00268-013-2416-8.
10. Benes J, Giglio MT, Cecconi M. Economic impact of perioperative goal-directed hemodynamic therapy: systematic review. Crit Care. 2014;18(5):584. https://ccforum.biomedcentral.com/counter/pdf/10.1186/s13054-014-0584-z.pdf.
11. Feldheiser A, Aziz O, Baldini G, Cox BP, Fearon KC, Feldman LS, Gan TJ, Kennedy RH, Ljungqvist O, Lobo DN, Miller T, Radtke FF, Ruiz Garces T, Schricker T, Scott MJ, Thacker JK, Ytrebø LM, Carli F. Enhanced Recovery After Surgery (ERAS) for gastrointestinal surgery, part 2: consensus statement for anaesthesia practice. Acta Anaesthesiol Scand. 2016 Mar;60(3):289-334. https://doi.org/10.1111/aas.12651. Epub 2015 Oct 30. PMID: 26514824; PMCID: PMC5061107.
12. Ferschl MB, Tung A, Sweitzer B, Huo D, Glick DB. Preoperative clinic visits reduce operating room cancellations and delays. Anesthesiology. 2005 Oct;103(4):855-9. https://doi.org/10.1097/00000542-200510000-00025. PMID: 16192779.
13. American Society of A. Perioperative surgical home: anesthesiology-led care coordination to improve value. ASA; 2013. https://www.asahq.org.
14. Vetter TR, Goeddel LA, Boudreaux AM, Hunt TR, Jones KA, Pittet JF. The perioperative surgical home: how can it make the case so everyone wins? BMC Anesthesiol. 2013;13:6. (In eng). https://doi.org/10.1186/1471-2253-13-6.

Part II

Preoperative Optimization and Perioperative Care Pathways

3 Anesthesia and Preoperative Testing: A Modern Perspective

Lawrence Chinn, Robert Gubkin, Aditi Master, Jessica Lee, Anoshia Khan, Julia DeLorenzo, and Jonathan Lopez

3.1 Introduction

Anesthesiology and perioperative care have evolved significantly, with pre-admission testing (PAT) emerging as a cornerstone of modern perioperative clinics. The origins of PAT trace back to mid-twentieth-century efforts to improve surgical outcomes by identifying and addressing patient-specific risks before surgery. Early practices heavily relied on routine laboratory and diagnostic tests for all patients, often leading to unnecessary testing and increased healthcare costs [1]. Over time, PAT evolved into a more targeted and evidence-based approach, emphasizing the importance of tailoring evaluations to the patient's medical history, comorbidities, and the complexity of the surgical procedure [2].

The establishment of dedicated perioperative clinics refined PAT by centralizing evaluations and fostering collaboration among anesthesiologists, surgeons, and other healthcare providers [3]. These clinics aimed to optimize patient health, reduce surgical delays, and enhance efficiency. In the context of value-based healthcare, anesthesia and PAT play pivotal roles in improving patient outcomes while optimizing costs. By reducing complications, minimizing delays, and prioritizing evidence-based practices, PAT aligns with the broader goals of healthcare systems striving for efficiency, safety, and patient-centered care [4].

3.2 The Role of Anesthesiologists in Perioperative Care

Anesthesiologists are at the forefront of perioperative medicine, performing key responsibilities beyond the operating room. They screen patients, stratify risks, and determine appropriate surgical settings such as inpatient facilities, ambulatory

L. Chinn (✉) · R. Gubkin · A. Master · J. Lee · A. Khan · J. DeLorenzo · J. Lopez
Rutgers New Jersey Medical School, Newark, NJ, USA
e-mail: chinnlw@njms.rutgers.edu

G. Tewfik (ed.), *The Anesthesiologist as Perioperative Leader*,
https://doi.org/10.1007/978-3-032-18058-2_3

surgical centers, and non-operating room anesthesia (NORA) locations. Evaluating readiness for surgery by considering medical and social factors, anesthesiologists optimize patient safety, surgical scheduling, and provide cost-effective care [5]. Their tailored anesthetic plans reduce complications and improve outcomes.

3.3 Strategic Preoperative Evaluation: Risk Mitigation and Cost-Effectiveness in Perioperative Care

In the era of value-based healthcare, efficient and evidence-guided preoperative evaluation has become central to surgical planning and patient optimization. While early perioperative practices relied heavily on routine laboratory and diagnostic testing, such approaches have been shown to increase healthcare costs without a corresponding improvement in patient outcomes. A strategic, patient-specific approach to preoperative assessment—particularly for low-risk procedures—has demonstrated equal or superior safety outcomes while curbing unnecessary resource utilization.

3.3.1 Risk Mitigation Through Patient-Centered Evaluation

Preoperative assessments serve a crucial role in identifying perioperative risks, optimizing comorbidities, and enhancing communication among surgical teams. However, broad application of standardized testing protocols often leads to redundant investigations, patient inconvenience, and potential harm due to false-positive findings. Clinical guidelines now emphasize history-based, individualized risk stratification models to guide testing and perioperative planning.

The American Society of Anesthesiologists (ASA) updated its practice advisory to encourage directed, rather than routine, evaluations. This guidance supports testing only when it is likely to affect patient management, especially in the setting of low- to intermediate-risk surgery [6]. A Cochrane review focusing on cataract surgery—a prototypical low-risk procedure—found that routine testing did not improve outcomes and should not be standard practice [7].

3.3.2 Cost Implications and Avoidance of Financial Waste

The financial implications of unnecessary preoperative testing are considerable. Numerous studies have demonstrated that indiscriminate testing not only increases direct costs but can also contribute to downstream expenditures due to follow-up testing and surgery delays. In an analysis of Medicare claims, nearly 60% of laboratory and radiologic tests ordered before low-risk ambulatory surgeries were deemed potentially avoidable [8].

Kirkham et al. found that implementing evidence-based preoperative assessment protocols for low-risk procedures significantly reduced costs while preserving safety and workflow efficiency [9]. Furthermore, structured preoperative clinics, particularly those led by anesthesiologists, have been associated with reductions in day-of-surgery cancelations, improved documentation, and enhanced patient satisfaction [10].

3.3.3 Safety Outcomes: Minimal Impact from Reduced Testing

Critically, efforts to streamline preoperative evaluations have not compromised patient safety. In a review by Smetana and Macpherson, the elimination of routine preoperative testing in asymptomatic patients undergoing elective surgery showed no increase in intraoperative or postoperative complications [11]. Similar conclusions were reached in a large observational study by Wijeysundera et al., which found that limiting consultations and testing to indicated cases did not adversely affect outcomes [12].

Such findings reinforce that preoperative interventions should be guided by clinical judgment, risk prediction tools, and the nature of the surgical procedure. These tools enable clinicians to stratify patients appropriately and make informed decisions about additional evaluation or specialist referral.

3.3.4 Guideline-Driven Frameworks for Directed Testing

Modern perioperative pathways emphasize the use of validated tools such as the ASA physical status classification and the American College of Surgeons NSQIP Surgical Risk Calculator. These allow for tailored decision-making that prioritizes high-value interventions and minimizes the risks of over-testing. Shared decision-making between anesthesiologists, surgeons, and patients ensures that care remains both patient-centered and aligned with best practices. The physical and clinical characteristics incorporated into these commonly used risk assessment tools are summarized in Table 3.1.

Thorough preoperative evaluations mitigate risks and prevent unnecessary testing. Directed care aligns with evidence-based guidelines and minimizes financial waste. Focused care not only minimizes costs but also has negligible impact on complication rates, highlighting the value of strategic preoperative management [13, 14].

Table 3.1 Physical and clinical characteristics incorporated in each risk assessment tool

Characteristic	ASA classification	RCRI	Gupta MICA index	ACS NSQIP risk calculator
Age	✗	✗	✓	✓
Gender	✗	✗	✗	✓
Comorbidities (e.g., HTN, DM, CHF, CAD)	✓ (subjective)	✓	✓	✓
ASA Physical Status Score	N/A	✗	✓	✓
Type of Surgery/Procedure	✗	✓ (high-risk surgery)	✓	✓
Functional Status (independent vs. dependent)	✗	✗	✗	✓
Serum Creatinine/Renal Function	✗	✓	✓	✓
Emergency Surgery Indicator	✗	✗	✓	✓
Diabetes requiring insulin	✓ (general health impact)	✓	✗	✓
History of Stroke or TIA	✗	✓	✓	✓
History of MI, Angina, or Cardiac Intervention	✓ (broadly considered)	✓	✓	✓
Smoking Status	✗	✗	✗	✓
Dyspnea/COPD/Pulmonary Disease	✓ (subjective inclusion)	✗	✓	✓
Laboratory Values (e.g., Hct, Na, Albumin)	✗	✗	✗	✓ (if available)
Sepsis/Infection Status	✗	✗	✗	✓
Expected Operative Time	✗	✗	✗	✓

3.4 Enhancing Efficiency and Reducing Costs

Anesthesiologists directly impact operating room efficiency by ensuring patients are optimized before surgery, thus minimizing cancelations and delays. Techniques such as regional anesthesia, which may be planned in preoperative clinics, further enhance efficiency and offers cost-saving advantages by reducing the need for post-anesthesia care unit (PACU) resources, lowering anesthesia-controlled operating room times, and enabling faster recovery and discharge. These benefits, coupled with the reduced likelihood of postoperative complications, underscore how anesthesiology optimizes healthcare resource utilization while prioritizing patient safety and satisfaction [15].

Preoperative evaluations also extend to addressing comorbid conditions such as hypertension, cardiac diseases, diabetes, and pulmonary diseases. These clinics, often led by anesthesiologists, prepare patients for surgery by identifying and managing preoperative risks, leading to fewer ICU admissions, shorter hospital stays, and fewer readmissions. Chronic diseases may be evaluated by the anesthesiologist, or the associated clinician, and further interventions planned. These may include modification of medications or referral to appropriate specialists. Tailored strategies to optimize health not only minimize healthcare costs, they improve outcomes [16, 17].

3.5 Collaboration, Communication, and the Flow of Information: A Critical Component of the Pre-admission Testing Process

Anesthesiologists facilitate coordination between patients, surgeons, and specialists, fostering trust and improving adherence. Their detailed discussions with patients provide clarity on procedural expectations and alleviate anxiety. Anesthesiologists also convey pertinent health updates to surgical teams, addressing potential risks before affecting the surgical schedule. Effective communication enhances procedural efficiency, reduces miscommunications in complex interdisciplinary cases thereby improving safety and outcomes.

A successful pre-admission testing (PAT) process relies not only on clinical expertise but fundamentally on the efficient, timely, and structured flow of information across the perioperative team. Effective communication among anesthesiologists, surgeons, primary care providers, nursing staff, and patients ensures that pertinent clinical data—such as past medical histories, medication lists, laboratory and diagnostic results, and specialist consultations—are gathered, reviewed, and integrated into the perioperative plan well in advance of surgery.

Efficient information flow enables early identification of high-risk conditions, timely medical optimization, and appropriate surgical planning, significantly decreasing the risk of same-day cancelations and unexpected intraoperative complications. In contrast, fragmented or delayed communication often results in redundant testing, overlooked comorbidities, unanticipated perioperative management challenges, and increased healthcare costs. Clear documentation, coordinated data sharing, and systematic case reviews are essential components of a robust PAT process.

Ferschl et al. (2005) demonstrated that patients evaluated in a structured preoperative clinic—where clinical information was centralized and reviewed systematically—experienced significantly fewer day-of-surgery cancelations and delays compared to patients assessed through decentralized processes [18]. Their findings emphasized that when information transfer is reliable and thorough, medical optimization can occur proactively rather than reactively, safeguarding operating room efficiency and enhancing patient outcomes.

Further supporting this, Blitz et al. (2016) found that patients who attended preoperative evaluation clinics had a significantly lower risk of in-hospital postoperative mortality. The benefit was largely attributed to improved information capture, earlier detection of comorbidities, and enhanced preparation enabled by cohesive team communication [19].

Altogether, these findings illustrate that optimizing the flow of information within the PAT process is not a peripheral concern, but a central pillar of patient safety and surgical efficiency. Institutions that invest in standardized communication protocols, integrated health IT systems, and multidisciplinary coordination are better positioned to deliver high-value, complication-free perioperative care. The strength of any pre-admission testing program lies not only in its clinical rigor but also in how effectively information is gathered, communicated, and applied. When data flows seamlessly between all members of the surgical team, the result is not just operational efficiency, but improved medical management, reduced unnecessary testing, and enhanced patient satisfaction. Ultimately, enhancing the flow of information in the PAT process is not merely a logistical task—it is a patient safety imperative. By ensuring that all perioperative team members have access to complete, accurate, and timely information, surgical teams can optimize preparation, reduce variability, and promote more predictable and efficient surgical care. A well-designed, information-driven PAT process transforms preoperative evaluation into a strategic asset for health systems committed to safety, quality, and value.

3.6 Utilizing Modern Technology: Electronic Health Records (EHR)

The effective use of the electronic health record (EHR) is a cornerstone of anesthesiologists' efforts to provide safe and efficient care. These systems consolidate critical patient information such as medical history, surgical clearances, allergies, medications, vital signs, and informed consents into a single accessible platform. EHR systems consolidate patient information, enabling holistic assessment, weigh surgical risks and anticipate potential complications. By streamlining data into one centralized location, EHR systems enhance efficiency of chart review and support optimal preoperative planning, resulting in improved patient outcomes.

Modern EHR platforms incorporate safeguards like red flag alerts to assist anesthesiologists in identifying risks such as drug interactions or allergies acting as a secondary layer of protection against medical errors [20]. Additionally, advanced monitors and automated charting technologies enable continuous tracking of vital signs reducing manual workload and enabling earlier detection of complications allowing anesthesiologists to focus on patient-centered care and safety [21].

AI-driven clinical decision support (CDS) systems may help drive the algorithm by which PAT functions and orders tests and consults. Modern EHR platforms incorporate safeguards like red flag alerts to assist anesthesiologists in identifying risks such as drug interactions or allergies, acting as a secondary layer of protection against medical errors [22]. Additionally, advanced monitors and automated charting technologies enable continuous tracking of vital signs, reducing manual workload and enabling earlier detection of complications, allowing anesthesiologists to focus on patient-centered care and safety.

As these technologies continue to evolve, their integration into the preoperative workflow has the potential to transform PAT into a dynamic, data-driven process.

AI-powered CDS tools can continuously analyze patient demographics, comorbidities, medication profiles, and procedural risks to recommend personalized preoperative evaluations. This approach reduces variability in clinical decision-making and ensures adherence to evidence-based guidelines. EHR-based automation can also streamline documentation, flag incomplete assessments, and prompt real-time follow-up actions, thus minimizing delays [23]. When paired with predictive analytics and machine learning algorithms, PAT systems can not only identify patients at higher risk for postoperative complications but also propose proactive interventions well before surgery [24]. As a result, anesthesiologists are empowered to allocate their attention to complex clinical judgments, enhancing the safety and efficiency of perioperative care in increasingly sophisticated surgical environments.

3.7 Developing Specialized Perioperative Guidelines

Anesthesiologists are integral to perioperative care, encompassing the preoperative, intraoperative, and postoperative theaters. Leveraging their expertise in physiology, pharmacology, and pathology, they assess patients' overall physiological status to determine their fitness of surgery and anesthesia. Anesthesiologists use tools like the ASA Physical Status Classification, the Revised Cardiac Risk Index (RCRI), the Gupta Myocardial Infarction and Cardiac Arrest (MICA) index, as well as the American College of Surgeons (ACS) National Surgical Quality Improvement Program (NSQIP) Surgical Risk Calculator to assess perioperative risk [15–18]. Selecting and interpreting these tools appropriately in individual patients requires an understanding of the clinical characteristics they incorporate (Table 3.1). Managing comorbidities, reducing unnecessary testing, and implementing pathways for conditions like hypertension, anemia, and sleep apnea improves outcomes.

Metabolic conditions and perioperative anemia require particular attention. Strategies such as intravenous iron supplementation has been shown to reduce transfusion needs in gynecological patients [25], and protocols on GLP-1RA medication management mitigate perioperative risks related to ketoacidosis and delayed gastric emptying [26, 27].

3.8 Preparing for the Postoperative Setting

Anesthesiologists continue to play a critical role postoperatively, and the successful planning for postoperative care often starts before surgery. Anesthesiologists ensure patient comfort and safety through effective pain management. They prevent complications through careful pharmacologic management and monitoring. Their oversight extends into post admission health maintenance and monitoring patients' recovery progress ensuring continuity of care.

The American Society of Anesthesiologists (ASA) emphasizes specific strategies for older adults, recommending comprehensive preoperative evaluations for patients aged 65 or older to mitigate risks such as postoperative delirium. Studies have shown that frailty and cognitive impairment are strong predictors of postoperative delirium in older adults, and incorporating these domains into preoperative evaluations improves risk stratification and prevention efforts [28]. Additionally, a systematic review and meta-analysis found that preoperative malnutrition is a significant predictor of POD [29]. These findings underscore the importance of comprehensive preoperative evaluations that include assessments of frailty, cognitive function, and nutritional status to mitigate the risk of POD [30].

3.9 Genetic Profiling for Anesthetic Management

The integration of personalized medicine into anesthesiology through genetic profiling is revolutionizing anesthetic care. Pharmacogenomics—the study of genetic influences on drug responses—optimizes efficacy while minimizing adverse effects by tailoring anesthetic regimens to individual genetic profiles. This approach mitigates risks such as prolonged sedation, respiratory depression, and inadequate pain relief [31]. Understanding genetic markers, particularly cytochrome P450 (CYP450) enzyme variations, is central to this strategy, as they significantly impact the pharmacokinetics of many anesthetic agents.

Propofol, metabolized by CYP2B6, exemplifies how genetic variability can alter drug metabolism. CYP2B6 polymorphisms affect propofol clearance rates, influencing sedation depth and duration. Similarly, ketamine, processed via CYP2B6 and CYP3A4, demonstrates reduced clearance in patients with the CYP2B6 allele, particularly those with chronic pain, increasing the likelihood of side effects like dizziness and hallucinations [32]. Midazolam, predominantly metabolized by CYP3A4 and CYP3A5, is also influenced by genetic variants like CYP3A422 and POR*28, which reduce enzymatic function, prolonging sedation and recovery times [33]. For opioids such as tramadol and codeine, genetic polymorphisms in CYP2D6 alter analgesic efficacy, with poor metabolizers experiencing inadequate pain relief and ultra-rapid metabolizers at risk for exaggerated effects [34].

Pharmacogenomics also extends to antiemetics like ondansetron, commonly used to manage postoperative nausea. CYP2D6 ultra-rapid metabolizers may require dosage adjustments or alternative antiemetics to maintain efficacy [35]. By reducing interpatient variability, pharmacogenomics-based anesthesia enables more precise and safer care.

Genetic profiling transforms anesthetic practice by enabling highly individualized care. Routine pharmacogenetic testing, particularly for high-risk patients, aids anesthesiologists in identifying genetic variations that influence drug metabolism, thereby optimizing drug selection, dosage, and timing. This approach minimizes adverse effects, reduces intraoperative complications, and enhances overall safety and efficacy [36].

Advancements in artificial intelligence (AI) further enhance pharmacogenomics by integrating real-time pharmacokinetic modeling with genetic data. AI-based tools may offer predictive insights into individual drug responses, assisting anesthesiologists in delivering precise, data-driven care. Together, pharmacogenomics and

AI are poised to establish personalized anesthesia as a standard of care, reducing variability in patient outcomes and promoting safety. As research progresses, integrating genetic profiling into routine preoperative assessments could further improve surgical success rates and set new benchmarks for precision healthcare.

The fusion of genetic profiling with anesthetic management marks a new era in personalized medicine. This innovative approach, enhanced by advancements in artificial intelligence, not only has the potential to optimize drug efficacy but also significantly reduces the risk of adverse effects and intraoperative complications. By tailoring anesthetic care to individual genetic profiles, we are setting new standards in precision healthcare, ultimately leading to safer and more effective surgical outcomes. As this field continues to evolve, the potential to transform anesthetic practice and improve patient care becomes increasingly evident, heralding a future where personalized anesthesia is the norm.

3.10 Expanding Preoperative Evaluations

Preoperative optimization plays a vital role in improving surgical outcomes, reducing perioperative risks, and controlling healthcare costs. Programs like the Presurgical Optimization Clinic demonstrate success in targeted interventions, such as smoking cessation, nutritional rehabilitation, and weight management, which enhance recovery and reduce complications [37]. Expanding these programs across healthcare institutions can lead to reduced morbidity, shorter hospital stays, and enhanced patient satisfaction [38]. Notably, the Perioperative Enhancement Team (POET) at Duke University uses a multidisciplinary approach to address modifiable risk factors like diabetes and anemia, improving surgical outcomes. Preoperative glycemic control reduces surgical site infections [39], while anemia management lowers transfusion requirements and perioperative morbidity [40, 41].

3.10.1 Operational and Economic Impact of Preoperative Optimization Programs

Structured preoperative optimization programs have consistently demonstrated significant improvements in workflow efficiency, surgical preparedness, and institutional cost savings. The impact of such optimization on total episode-of-care spending is illustrated in Fig. 3.1, which compares healthcare costs for surgical patients who underwent structured preoperative optimization versus usual care. A case study by the American College of Surgeons showed that the implementation of a hospital-based preoperative clinic integrating Enhanced Recovery After Surgery (ERAS) protocols and structured optimization pathways reduced day-of-surgery cancelations from 4.9% to 0.95% [42]. This multidisciplinary approach centralized risk assessment and chronic disease management, facilitating coordinated care among anesthesiologists, surgeons, and internists while improving operating room (OR) scheduling predictability and resource utilization.

	Without Preoperative Optimization	With Preoperative Optimization
Average Cost per Patient	$15,6382	$12,3952
Complication Rate	20%	10%
Length of Hospital Stay	7 days	5 days
Readmission Rate	15%	5%

Fig. 3.1 Comparison of Healthcare Spending on Surgical Patients With and Without Preoperative Optimization (HFMA. Integrating care to improve surgical outcomes and reduce costs. Available from: https://www.hfma.org/operations-management/61399/; Leeds I, et al. Assessing the societal cost-effectiveness of preoperative optimization. Available from: https://meetings.ssat.com/abstracts/2019/140.cgi; VanDenBerg T, et al. On all accounts: cost-effectiveness analysis of limited preoperative optimization efforts before colon cancer surgery. Available from: https://schaeffer.usc.edu/research/on-all-accounts-cost-effectiveness-analysis-of-limited-preoperative-optimization-efforts-before-colon-cancer-surgery/)

Similarly, a prospective study conducted at a tertiary care facility in an underserved area evaluated the impact of introducing a structured preoperative checklist on surgery cancelations due to patient-related factors. The study found that the use of the checklist significantly reduced cancelations attributed to incomplete workups or unoptimized medical conditions—from 15.4% in the control group to 4.7% post-implementation ($p = 0.000$) [43]. This outcome demonstrates how structured screening tools can facilitate early identification of barriers to surgery, enhance patient readiness, and improve coordination among preoperative care teams, ultimately reducing last-minute cancelations and supporting more efficient surgical throughput.

Further evidence of the cost-effectiveness of these strategies is demonstrated in a recent study from the *Journal of Anesthesia, Analgesia and Critical Care*, which evaluated a value-based preoperative assessment program in a tertiary care center. The transition from routine to indication-based testing, alongside targeted interventions for anemia, diabetes, and anticoagulant management, resulted in annual cost savings of approximately €90,000 or over $100,000 in USD [44]. Additionally, the program reduced patient throughput time in preoperative clinics and alleviated administrative burden, underscoring the dual benefit of optimized clinical care and resource efficiency. Collectively, these findings support the integration of structured preoperative optimization pathways as a best practice model for improving surgical workflow, reducing avoidable cancelations, and generating measurable institutional savings.

Internists play an important role in preoperative evaluations by identifying and mitigating surgical risks. However, gaps in their knowledge of anesthesia-related assessments highlight the need for enhanced education and structured protocols. Strengthening collaboration among internists, anesthesiologists, and surgeons could bridge these gaps, leading to improved outcomes and fewer complications [45].

3.11 Economic Contributions of Anesthesiologists to Healthcare Savings

As illustrated in Fig. 3.1, proactive, anesthesiologist-led optimization can shift spending away from preventable downstream complications toward efficient preoperative care. Anesthesiologist-led preoperative clinics and perioperative management strategies have demonstrated significant cost-saving benefits across healthcare systems. These savings stem from reductions in unnecessary testing, improved surgical efficiency, and optimized patient outcomes.

3.11.1 Preoperative Clinics and Testing

Preoperative clinics directed by anesthesiologists have been shown to reduce redundant laboratory tests and consultations, leading to substantial financial savings. For example, a study found that implementing preoperative evaluation clinics reduced preoperative testing costs by 30%, saving approximately $200,000 annually in a single institution [46]. Similarly, another study highlighted that preoperative clinics decreased same-day surgical cancelations by 50%, which can save hospitals an estimated $100,000 to $300,000 annually depending on surgical volume [1]. These clinics also streamline patient preparation, ensuring that only clinically necessary tests are performed, thereby reducing wasteful expenditures.

3.11.2 Additional Examples of Cost Savings

Standardized pathways, such as the Perioperative Surgical Home (PSH) model, have demonstrated significant cost savings in surgical care. For instance, a community-based health system implementing the PSH model for hip and knee replacements reported an average savings of $4205 per surgical episode, along with a 35% decrease in 30-day readmissions [47].

Ambulatory Surgery Centers (ASCs), particularly those led by anesthesiologists, offer a cost-effective alternative to inpatient settings. Studies have shown that procedures performed in ASCs can be approximately 35% less expensive in total cost compared to those in hospital outpatient departments. This cost reduction is primarily attributed to shorter procedure times and more efficient resource utilization [42, 48].

Eliminating low-value preoperative testing has also been identified as a significant opportunity for cost savings. By adhering to evidence-based guidelines and avoiding unnecessary tests, healthcare systems can reduce expenditures without compromising patient safety. For example, implementing protocols to minimize unwarranted preoperative tests has led to substantial financial savings across various institutions [49].

3.12 Conclusion

Anesthesiologists play a central role in optimizing perioperative care by leading targeted pre-admission testing, developing individualized anesthetic plans, and fostering multidisciplinary collaboration. Their involvement is instrumental in reducing surgical delays, minimizing perioperative complications, and achieving significant healthcare cost savings. Moreover, the integration of electronic health records, regional anesthesia techniques, and pharmacogenomic profiling has advanced the delivery of personalized, patient-centered care.

As surgical procedures grow more complex and patient comorbidities become increasingly prevalent, the anesthesiologist's expertise in perioperative risk stratification, preoperative optimization, and postoperative recovery will become even more vital. Expanding the use of structured optimization programs and embracing emerging technologies will not only improve patient outcomes but also enhance healthcare system efficiency. Looking ahead, innovations in precision medicine will further elevate the role of anesthesiologists, positioning them at the forefront of advancing patient safety and value-based surgical care.

References

1. Blitz JD, Mabry C. Designing and running a preoperative clinic. Anesthesiol Clin. 2018;36(4):479–91.
2. Davenport DL, Henderson WG, Khuri SF, Mentzer RM. Preoperative risk factors and surgical complexity are more predictive of costs than postoperative complications. Ann Surg. 2005;242(2):463–71.
3. Fleisher LA, Beckman JA, Brown KA, et al. 2014 ACC/AHA guideline on perioperative cardiovascular evaluation and management of patients undergoing noncardiac surgery. Circulation. 2014;130(24):e278–333.
4. Aronson S, Westover J, Guinn N, et al. A perioperative medicine model for population health: an integrated approach for an evolving clinical science. Anesth Analg. 2018;126(2):682–90.
5. Friedlander DF, Krimphove MJ, Cole AP, et al. Where is the value in ambulatory versus inpatient surgery? Ann Surg. 2019;273(5):909–16.
6. Apfelbaum JL, Connis RT, Nickinovich DG, Pasternak LR, Arens JF, Caplan RA, et al. Practice advisory for preanesthesia evaluation: an updated report by the American Society of Anesthesiologists. Anesthesiology. 2012;116(3):522–38.
7. Keay L, Lindsley K, Tielsch J, Katz J, Schein OD. Routine preoperative medical testing for cataract surgery. Cochrane Database Syst Rev. 2009;(2):CD007293.
8. Benarroch-Gampel J, Sheffield KM, Duncan CB, et al. Preoperative laboratory testing in patients undergoing elective, low-risk ambulatory surgery. Ann Surg. 2012;256(3):518–28.
9. Kirkham KR, Wijeysundera DN, Pendrith C, et al. Preoperative testing before low-risk surgical procedures. Anesth Analg. 2011;112(6):1390–8.
10. Ferschl MB, Tung A, Sweitzer BJ, Huo D, Glick DB. Preoperative clinic visits reduce operating room cancellations and delays. Anesth Analg. 2005;100(6):1425–30.
11. Smetana GW, Macpherson DS. The case against routine preoperative laboratory testing. Med Clin N Am. 2003;87(1):7–40.
12. Wijeysundera DN, Austin PC, Beattie WS, Hux JE, Laupacis A. Outcomes and processes of care related to preoperative medical consultation. BMJ. 2010;340:b252.
13. Issa MRN, Isoni NFC, Soares AM, Fernandes ML. Preanesthesia evaluation and reduction of preoperative care costs. Braz J Anesthesiol. 2011;61(1):60–71.

14. Taylor GA, Oresanya LB, Kling SM, Saxena V, Mutter O, Raman S, et al. Rethinking the routine: preoperative laboratory testing among American Society of Anesthesiologists class 1 and 2 patients before low-risk ambulatory surgery in the 2017 National Surgical Quality Improvement Program cohort. Surgery [Internet]. 2021;171(2):267–74.
15. Graff V, Kumar A, Patel H. Cost-effectiveness of regional anesthesia techniques. Reg Anesth Pain Med. 2023;48(1):55–63.
16. Haq ZA, Murthy P, Malik I, et al. Detection of comorbid illnesses during pre-anesthesia evaluation. J Anesth. 2015;27(5):256–8.
17. Van Klei WA, Hoff RG, Van Aarnhem EE, et al. Effects of the introduction of the WHO "Surgical Safety Checklist" on in-hospital mortality: a cohort study. Ann Surg. 2012;255(1):44–9. https://doi.org/10.1097/SLA.0b013e31823779ae.
18. Ferschl MB, Tung A, Sweitzer B, et al. Preoperative clinic visits reduce operating room cancellations and delays. Anesthesiology. 2005;103(4):855–9.
19. Blitz JD, Kendale SM, Jain SK, Cuff GE, Kim JT, Rosenberg AD. Preoperative evaluation clinic visit is associated with decreased risk of in-hospital postoperative mortality. Anesthesiology. 2016;125(2):280–94.
20. Ayaad O, Alloubani A, ALhajaa EA, et al. The role of electronic medical records in improving the quality of health care services. Int J Med Inform. 2019;127:63–8.
21. Rowland BA, Motamedi V, Michard F, Saha AK, Khanna AK. Impact of continuous and wireless monitoring of vital signs on clinical outcomes: a propensity-matched observational study of surgical ward patients. Br J Anaesth [Internet]. 2024; [cited 2025 Jan 25]; Available from: https://pubmed.ncbi.nlm.nih.gov/38135523
22. Silow-Carroll S, Edwards JN, Rodin D. Using electronic health records to improve quality and efficiency: the experiences of leading hospitals. Issue Brief (Commonw Fund). 2012;17(1):40.
23. Xue B, Li D, Lu C, King CR, Wildes T, Avidan MS, Kannampallil T, Abraham J. Use of machine learning to develop and evaluate models using preoperative and intraoperative data to identify risks of postoperative complications. JAMA Network Open. 2021;4(3):e212240.
24. You SB, Hirschman KB, Stawnychy MA, Song J, Sang E, Pitcher K, Oh S, O'Connor M, Garren P, Bowles KH. Qualitative study of the context of health information technology in sepsis care transitions: facilitators, barriers, and strategies for improvement. J Am Med Dir Assoc. 2025;26(7):105606. https://doi.org/10.1016/j.jamda.2025.105606.
25. Ellermann I, Bueckmann A, Eveslage M, et al. Treating anemia in the preanesthesia assessment clinic: results of a retrospective evaluation. Anesth Analg. 2018;127(5):1202–10.
26. Joshi GP, LaMasters T, Kindel TL. Preprocedure care of patients on GLP-1 receptor agonists: a multisociety clinical practice guidance. Anesthesiology. 2024;140(2):212–8.
27. Thompson A, Fleischmann KE, Smilowitz NR, et al. Guideline for perioperative cardiovascular management for noncardiac surgery: a report of the American College of Cardiology/American Heart Association Joint Committee on Clinical Practice Guidelines. Circulation. 2024;150(19)
28. Dammavalam V, Murphy J, Johnkutty M, Elias M, Corn R, Bergese S. Perioperative cognition in association with malnutrition and frailty: a narrative review. Front Neurosci. 2023;17:1275201.
29. Dong B, Wang J, Li P, Li J, Liu M, Zhang H. The impact of preoperative malnutrition on postoperative delirium: a systematic review and meta-analysis. Perioperat Med. 2023;12(1):55.
30. Gong S, Qian D, Riazi S, et al. Association between the FRAIL scale and postoperative complications. Anesth Analg. 2022;136(2):251–61.
31. Chou WY, Wang CH, Liu PH, Liu CC, Tseng CC, Jawan B. Human opioid receptor A118G polymorphism affects intravenous patient-controlled analgesia morphine consumption after total abdominal hysterectomy. Anesthesiology. 2006;105(2):334–7.
32. Li Y, Jackson KA, Slon B, Hardy JR, Franco M, William L, Poon P, Coller JK, Hutchinson MR, Currow DC, Somogyi AA. CYP2B6* 6 allele and age substantially reduce steady-state ketamine clearance in chronic pain patients: impact on adverse effects. Br J Clin Pharmacol. 2015;80(2):276–84.
33. Elens L, Nieuweboer AJ, Clarke SJ, Charles KA, de Graan AJ, Haufroid V, van Gelder T, Mathijssen RH, van Schaik RH. Impact of POR* 28 on the clinical pharmacokinetics of CYP3A phenotyping probes midazolam and erythromycin. Pharmacogenet Genomics. 2013;23(3):148–55.

34. Zeng S, Qing Q, Xu W, Yu S, Zheng M, Tan H, Peng J, Huang J. Personalized anesthesia and precision medicine: a comprehensive review of genetic factors, artificial intelligence, and patient-specific factors. Front Med. 2024;11:1365524.
35. Bell GC, Caudle KE, Whirl-Carrillo M, Gordon RJ, Hikino K, Prows CA, Gaedigk A, Agundez JA, Sadhasivam S, Klein TE, Schwab M. Clinical Pharmacogenetics Implementation Consortium (CPIC) guideline for CYP2D6 genotype and use of ondansetron and tropisetron. Clin Pharmacol Ther. 2017;102(2):213.
36. Manolio TA, Chisholm RL, Ozenberger B, Roden DM, Williams MS, Wilson R, Bick D, Bottinger EP, Brilliant MH, Eng C, Frazer KA. Implementing genomic medicine in the clinic: the future is here. Genet Med. 2013;15(4):258–67.
37. Delaney LD, Howard R, Palazzolo K, Ehlers AP, Smith S, Englesbe M, Dimick JB, Telem DA. Outcomes of a presurgical optimization program for elective hernia repairs among high-risk patients. JAMA Netw Open. 2021;4(11):e2130016.
38. Aronson S, Westover J, Guinn N, Setji T, Wischmeyer P, Gulur P, Hopkins T, Seyler TM, Lagoo-Deendayalan S, Heflin MT, Thompson A. A perioperative medicine model for population health: an integrated approach for an evolving clinical science. Anesth Analg. 2018;126(2):682–90.
39. Jacober SJ, Sowers JR. An update on perioperative management of diabetes. Arch Intern Med. 1999;159(20):2405–11.
40. Williams ML, He X, Rankin JS, Slaughter MS, Gammie JS. Preoperative hematocrit is a powerful predictor of adverse outcomes in coronary artery bypass graft surgery: a report from the Society of Thoracic Surgeons Adult Cardiac Surgery Database. Ann Thorac Surg. 2013;96(5):1628–34.
41. Wu WC, Schifftner TL, Henderson WG, Eaton CB, Poses RM, Uttley G, Sharma SC, Vezeridis M, Khuri SF, Friedmann PD. Preoperative hematocrit levels and postoperative outcomes in older patients undergoing noncardiac surgery. JAMA. 2007;297(22):2481–8.
42. American College of Surgeons. A hospital-based preoperative clinic: Patient optimization with ERAS and Strong for Surgery [Internet]. Available from: https://www.facs.org/quality-programs/qi-resources/case-studies/a-hospital-based-preoperative-clinic-patient-optimization-with-enhanced-recovery-after-surgery-and-strong-for-surgery/
43. Mremi A, Mwashambwa MY, Chalya PL, et al. Effectiveness of a preoperative checklist in reducing surgery cancellations due to patient factors at Muhimbili National Hospital, Tanzania. Tanzan J Health Res. 2024;25(4):1550.
44. Cecconi M, Goretti G, Pradella A, Meroni P, Pisarra M, Torzilli G, Montorsi M, Spinelli A, Zerbi A, Castoro C, Casale P. Value-based preoperative assessment in a large academic hospital. J Anesth Analg Crit Care. 2024;4(1):42.
45. Lepage MA, Lecavalier A, Baldini G, Sun NZ, Bessissow A. Preoperative risk assessment and optimization integrating surgical and anesthetic principles and practices: a national survey for internists. Perioperat Med. 2025;14(1):6.
46. Pollard JB. Economic aspects of an anesthesia preoperative evaluation clinic. Curr Opin Anesthesiol. 2002;15(2):257–61.
47. American Society of Anesthesiologists. First-of-its-kind perioperative surgical home initiative demonstrates significant improvements in patient outcomes and cost savings [Internet]. 2016. Available from: https://www.asahq.org/about-asa/newsroom/news-releases/2016/02/first-of-its-kind-perioperative-surgical-home-initiative
48. American Academy of Orthopaedic Surgeons. Ambulatory surgery centers are more cost-effective than hospitals for certain orthopaedic procedures. AAOS Now Daily Edition [Internet]. 2024; Available from: https://www.aaos.org/aaosnow/2024/aaos-now-daily-edition%2D%2Dwednesday/research/research06/
49. LifeWire. Perioperative Surgical Home, the “Google Home” of Healthcare [Internet]. 2018. Available from: https://lifewiregroup.com/Blog/ArticleID/49/Perioperative-Surgical-Home-the-%E2%80%9CGoogle-Home%E2%80%9D-of-Healthcare

4 Optimizing Surgical Readiness: Inpatient vs Outpatient Preoperative Evaluation Models

Justin Calvert and Ivan S. Kim

4.1 Introduction

The preoperative evaluation plays a vital role in modern healthcare, serving as the foundation for determining a patient's readiness for surgery and recovery. While the primary purpose is to identify potential barriers to safe anesthesia administration, these evaluations also provide an opportunity for patient education, counseling, obtaining informed consent, and optimizing modifiable conditions to improve perioperative and long-term health outcomes [1]. Rather than functioning as a simple medical clearance, the preoperative evaluation is a tailored process designed to develop the most appropriate anesthetic plan with the goals of enhancing safety, improving outcomes, preventing complications, and maximizing patient comfort. These critical evaluations can be performed in a variety of ways, and in two main settings: inpatient vs outpatient. This chapter will explore various models, contrasting the advantages and disadvantages with each of these settings.

4.2 History

The evolution of the preoperative evaluation process reflects broader transformation of healthcare delivery over the past 20 years. Before that, preoperative assessments were largely ad hoc, often contributing to day-of-surgery cancelations and increased perioperative risks [2, 3]. The traditional model involved routine hospitalization one or more days before surgery to allow time for evaluation and testing [4, 5]. In this

J. Calvert (✉)
Loma Linda University Medical School, Loma Linda, CA, USA

Riverside University Health System, Moreno Valley, CA, USA
e-mail: jtcalvert@llu.edu

I. S. Kim
Loma Linda University Medical School, Loma Linda, CA, USA

G. Tewfik (ed.), *The Anesthesiologist as Perioperative Leader*,
https://doi.org/10.1007/978-3-032-18058-2_4

system, anesthesiologists frequently met patients for the first time on the night before surgery.

However, growing cost pressures and the pursuit of greater efficiency drove the shift toward outpatient preoperative assessments, leading to the development of dedicated Preanesthesia Clinics (PACs). Typically led by anesthesiologists, these clinics implement a variety of evaluation programs and practice models, now incorporating telemedicine, mid-level care extenders, and digital assessment tools [2]. Although economic pressures have largely shifted preoperative evaluations to the outpatient setting, inpatient assessments still play a role in urgent or emergent surgeries and for select high-risk patients [4].

As the healthcare landscape has evolved, with shrinking reimbursements, an aging population burdened by chronic disease, advances in surgical procedures and technology, and more high-risk patients undergoing surgery, the role of the anesthesiologist has had to adapt as well [6, 7]. Today, anesthesiologists are stepping beyond traditional operating room boundaries, with an expanding role as perioperative medicine consultants and leaders, integrating their unique blend of both medical and surgical expertise into system-wide quality improvement initiatives [8–11].

4.3 Core Functions of Preoperative Evaluation

Preoperative evaluations serve multiple critical functions within the surgical care pathway. While details regarding the setting and model may vary, the core components remain consistent across all approaches. These include risk stratification, anesthetic planning, patient education, and an informed consent process. In recent years, there has also been a growing emphasis on care coordination and medical optimization as integral parts of the preoperative process.

Preoperative risk stratification involves identifying factors associated with perioperative complications. A comprehensive history, physical exam, and appropriate testing form the foundation of this evaluation, but standardized patient questionnaires and validated scoring systems are increasingly applied to enhance risk assessment [8, 12–14]. These systems vary widely, ranging from general risk indices to specialized organ- and disease-based assessment. Risk tools come in two main forms: risk scores and risk prediction models. Risk scores assign weighted values to predictive factors to allow broad comparison among patients often differentiating them into high vs low risk categories, whereas risk prediction models use individualized patient data to estimate the probability of specific outcomes [15, 16].

General Risk Assessment Tools:

- American Society of Anesthesiologists Physical Status (ASA PS) classification
- American College of Surgeons National Surgical Quality Improvement Program (ACS NSQIP) surgical risk calculator
- Physiological and Operative Severity Score for the Study of Mortality and Morbidity (POSSUM)

Cardiac Risk Assessment Tools:

- Revised Cardiac Risk Index (RCRI)
- Gupta perioperative Myocardial Infarction or Cardiac Arrest (MICA) calculator

Additional Assessment Tools:

- Duke Activity Status Index (DASI)
- Assess Respiratory Risk in Surgical patients in Catalonia (ARISCAT) risk index
- Clinical Frailty Scale
- Mini-Cog cognitive assessment

No single risk prediction tool can capture all aspects of perioperative risk for all patients. Understanding the strengths, limitations, and when/how to apply each tool is essential. Used in conjunction with a thorough history and exam, these instruments can help identify high-risk patients, support shared decision-making, improve patient education, and guide targeted preoperative optimization strategies.

Anesthetic planning typically follows risk prediction. A thorough assessment addresses anesthesia-specific concerns that could impact intraoperative management or postoperative recovery, allowing for appropriate preparation and mitigation of identified risks [1, 4]. This planning process focuses on the selection of anesthetic technique, airway and hemodynamic management strategy, and anticipated intraoperative procedures or therapies [9, 17, 18]. Ongoing refinement of these processes has made anesthesia care remarkably safe in recent years, with anesthesia-related mortality improving from 1:10,000 in 1985 to less than 1:200,000 today [19, 20].

Patient education is another essential component of the preoperative visit. It serves to reduce anxiety and improve patient engagement by familiarizing patients with the anesthetic plan, reviewing potential risks and expected outcomes, and providing an opportunity to address anesthesia-related questions [3, 8, 19]. In addition to anesthesia-specific information, PACs also provide detailed logistical guidance for the day of surgery, including medication management, arrival times, fasting protocols, and more [9, 12]. Written materials or multimedia resources are often provided at PAC visits to enhance patient understanding. This process has been shown to reduce anxiety and decrease cancelations due to logistical factors and patient preparation [8, 21].

A comprehensive discussion of the risks, benefits, and alternatives of surgery and anesthesia is central to the informed consent process [22, 23]. Transparent communication ensures that patients fully understand potential complications and likely perioperative outcomes, empowering them to participate meaningfully in shared decision-making. Eliciting and understanding patient values and health outcome priorities, which are often misunderstood if not explicitly discussed, are essential to aligning care plans with individual goals [21, 24].

Care coordination represents another fundamental function of preoperative evaluation. Anesthesiologists use information gathered during assessment to communicate relevant risks and management plans to the broader care team, ensuring seamless transitions and continuity across the perioperative continuum [10, 19]. Effective coordination relies on a multidisciplinary approach, involving anesthesiologists, surgeons, consultants, nursing staff, pharmacists, physical therapists, case managers, social workers, as well as patients and their families [25]. Alternative care models such as the Perioperative Surgical Home (PSH) have built on this collaborative framework, emphasizing team-based, comprehensive care from surgical decision through post-discharge recovery [26, 27].

Anesthesiologists are commonly faced with the decision of determining whether patients are "cleared for surgery," meaning "Can the patient go to surgery now?" This question is deceptively simple, however a more meaningful and nuanced question would be: "Is the patient in the best possible condition for surgery, and if not, what can be done to move them in that direction in the timeframe allowed based on the surgical urgency?" This perspective shift has led to greater emphasis on preoperative optimization, with anesthesiologists and PACs taking a leading role in addressing modifiable perioperative risk factors. These efforts include optimizing chronic comorbidities such as anemia, cardiac disease, diabetes, pain syndromes, malnutrition, obesity, and sleep apnea. Lifestyle interventions including prehabilitation efforts focused on dietary modification, exercise, and smoking cessation are also being implemented by anesthesiologists following preoperative evaluation [1, 4, 11, 28].

4.4 Preoperative Evaluation Models

4.4.1 Inpatient Evaluations

Historically, perioperative care was primarily surgeon-directed. Anesthesiologists performed only inpatient assessments, while much of the preoperative preparation and optimization was managed by the surgeon, primary care physician, and other specialists [5]. Patients were typically admitted to the surgical service shortly before surgery, at which point the anesthesiologist would conduct an inpatient preoperative evaluation (IPE) and order any necessary labs, studies, or consults. In some cases, patients would spend several days in the hospital before surgery undergoing workup [9].

More recently, new models for managing inpatient surgical patients have emerged include co-management and anesthesia consult services. Under these systems, surgical teams partner with hospitalist services, often comprised of internists, geriatricians, or anesthesiologists to collaboratively manage both the patient's underlying medical comorbidities as well as the surgical conditions throughout their hospital stay. These services provide recommendations for preoperative optimization, assist with management of existing medical conditions or postoperative complications, and aid in discharge planning [10, 29].

4.4.2 Advantages

While the classic preadmission model is no longer as common, there are some advantages to this process, particularly for high-risk patients. The IPE allows for comprehensive assessment and management by a multidisciplinary team, which is especially valuable for patients with significant risk factors that could affect their outcome and recovery [4]. The inpatient environment also provides immediate access to diagnostic testing and consultation by subspecialists that may not be readily accessible in an outpatient setting. Furthermore, IPE is often the only option for urgent procedures, trauma-related surgeries, and situations where critical stabilization or monitoring are necessary.

4.4.3 Disadvantages

The obvious disadvantage of IPE is the high cost and associated burden on healthcare systems. According to the American Hospital Association, hospitalization is one of the most expensive types of health care utilization, with an average adjusted cost of $14,101 per inpatient stay at community hospitals in 2019, averaging $3,025/day [30]. Worse, preadmission stays are often poorly reimbursed [31]. Additionally, overuse of IPEs and extended inpatient preoperative times can exacerbate the already severe problem of emergency department (ED) boarding. Boarding describes the situation where admitted patients remain in the ED for prolonged periods, awaiting inpatient bed placement. These delays can last from several hours to even weeks, further straining hospital capacity and patient flow [32].

4.4.4 Outpatient Evaluations

The concept of anesthesiologists performing outpatient preoperative evaluations (OPEs) to enhance preoperative care is not new. Alfred Lee, a surgeon turned anesthesiologist, wrote in 1949, "I think that an anesthetic outpatient department could contribute considerably to preventive medicine... To see the patient the evening before operation or even two or three days before that, is not enough. He should be seen as soon as possible after his name is added to the waiting list" [33]. Modern OPEs can be structured in several ways and offer numerous advantages in the current healthcare environment [8].

4.5 Outpatient Models

4.5.1 Preanesthesia Clinics (PACs)

Anesthesiologist-led outpatient PACs have become an increasingly more common setting for preoperative evaluation [8, 34]. These clinics can be hospital-based or free-standing and criteria for evaluation vary by institution. Some organizations evaluate all surgical patients in-person, while others selectively assess higher-risk patients, using preoperative screening algorithms or triage tools [12, 31, 35, 36].

The clinical teams involved in the OPE process can include a variety of healthcare workers, each with unique roles and scopes of practice:

- Medical assistants (MAs) are unlicensed individuals who work under the supervision of a licensed physician or nurse practitioner and perform administrative and basic clinical tasks like scheduling or obtaining vital signs.
- Nurses, both Licensed Vocational Nurses (LVNs) and Registered Nurses (RNs) can perform patient assessments, document histories and symptoms, perform diagnostic tests, and provide patient education.
- Nurse Practitioners (NPs) are advanced practice nurses with master's or doctoral training who can perform comprehensive exams, order tests and consults, and prescribe treatments, either in conjunction with physicians or independently, depending on location.
- Physician Assistants, similarly to NPs can perform patient evaluations, diagnose conditions, and manage treatment plans, with physician collaboration [37].

While these clinics are often led by anesthesiologists, other systems exist run by primary care providers or even nurse-only models [8, 36].

More advanced OPE systems such as Duke University's Perioperative Enhancement Team (POET) or Riverside University's Perioperative Optimization Clinic (POC) have been established to also address specific modifiable risk factors such as anemia, obstructive sleep apnea, and malnutrition before surgery [28]. These specialized visits are distinct from the standard preanesthesia assessments in that they are separately reportable Evaluation and Management (E/M) services which require referral and are billed independently [1, 22]. These systems can benefit from multidisciplinary partnerships with departments including hematology, cardiology, nutrition, and physical therapy to assist with care coordination and preoperative optimization. Unlike typical preanesthesia visits this process is performed weeks to months before surgery to allow for meaningful disease modification [3, 22, 28].

4.6 Technology in Preoperative Evaluation

Advancements in technology have also impacted the preoperative evaluation process. In the wake of the COVID-19 pandemic, the use of telemedicine accelerated for many specialties, including anesthesiology. While pandemic isolation enhanced telehealth adoption, advantages were found for both patients and clinicians. A 2021 study out of UCLA evaluated appointment completion rates for in-person vs telemedicine preoperative visits. They found that 81% of patients completed telemedicine visits compared to 76% of those with in-person appointments. There was also a significant decrease in appointment cancelation rates in the telemedicine group compared to in-person, of 12.5% vs 19.4% [38]. Studies also showed a high degree of patient satisfaction with telemedicine visits [39]. Furthermore, surgical plans developed during telemedicine encounters remained unchanged even after in-person examinations [40]. Even virtual airway examinations have been found to have strong agreement with in-person airway evaluations [41].

Technological innovation extends beyond just telehealth. Artificial intelligence (AI) holds substantial promise for the future of perioperative evaluation, offering several different use cases. Large Language Models (LLMs) are already being used to streamline clinical documentation using ambient scribes to generate notes from provider-patient interactions [42]. Automated chart review and AI guided patient education are other likely uses for LLMs [43]. Moving forward, personalized risk prediction models using machine learning and deep neural networks may fundamentally shift how we quantify preoperative risk by analyzing and integrating vast clinical datasets [44–47]. While the potential benefits are significant, widespread adoption will require addressing important ethical, legal, and logistical challenges regarding data privacy, transparency, and clinical accountability.

4.7 Advantages

4.7.1 Reduction in Day-of-Surgery Delays and Cancelations

OPEs have consistently demonstrated reductions in day-of-surgery (DOS) delays and cancelations [3, 4, 8]. While surgical cancelation rates can vary significantly between institutions, they represent a significant cost to organizations, with lost revenue averaging between $900 and $1700 per operating room hour [12, 48].

A 2005 study from the University of Chicago compared case cancelation rates of first-start cases and found notable differences between patients evaluated in OPE clinics vs those assessed on the DOS. For same-day surgeries, the cancelation rate was 8.4% for OPE patients compared to 16.2% for those without prior evaluation. For all operating room cases, cancelation rates were 5.3% vs 13% respectively. These improvements occurred despite OPE patients on average being older and having higher ASA PS scores [49]. Similar results have been reported across different institutions and practice models. Stanford University Hospital experienced significant reduction in annual DOS cancelations from 1.96% to 0.21% after implementation of OPEs, while a Veterans Affairs Hospital saw reduced cancelation rate from 26.6% to 6.6% for outpatient surgeries, within 6 months after implementing OPEs [34, 50].

4.8 Reduction of Preoperative Testing

Anesthesiologist-directed OPEs have proven effective in reducing unnecessary preoperative testing and associated healthcare costs [3, 4, 8]. Increased focus on healthcare waste has prompted a reduction in preoperative testing in recent years, yet a

2016 study in Anesthesiology found that routine testing still often occurs for even low risk procedures [51].

Issa et al. evaluated 200 patients scheduled for elective surgery or diagnostic procedures whose preoperative care was surgeon-directed. These same patients also underwent OPE where anesthesiologists evaluated the necessity of ordered labs and referrals. This study revealed that 55.8% of orders were not indicated, representing 50.8% of the total examination costs. The cost of surgeon-directed preoperative care was found to be significantly higher than anesthesiologist-directed care [52]. Similarly, Power and Thackray reported that with the introduction of anesthesia-led OPEs, there were significant reductions in preoperative testing, including electrocardiograms, chest radiographs, and blood tests, ultimately decreasing preoperative investigation costs by 38% [53]. Stanford found that OPE directed testing for outpatients and to-be-admitted patients resulted in potential cost-reduction of ~1 million dollars in one year ($112.09 per patient) [50].

Beyond cost considerations, over testing can directly harm patients through unnecessary follow-up procedures. A 1987 study investigated the effects of preoperative chest radiographs on 606 patients and found that 64% of radiographs lacked appropriate indications. Moreover, only 1 of the 386 unindicated exams revealed clinically significant findings, however 3 led to further invasive testing, including one thoracotomy, with no subsequent discovery of disease [50]. This phenomenon of low-value care cascades persists today. A 2022 study evaluated veterans undergoing low to intermediate-risk surgery and found that unnecessary preoperative testing not only remained common but led to additional unnecessary services, generating costs of over $150 per patient [54].

4.9 Reduction in Length of Hospital Stay & Admission to Higher Level of Care

Length of stay (LOS) is a key efficiency metric for hospitals and researchers. As mentioned earlier, even one additional day of admission can ultimately cost thousands of dollars [30]. Kamal et al. studied orthopedic joint surgery, evaluating postoperative admission to the intensive care unit (ICU) and intermediate care unit (HDU), as well as average LOS. They found a significant reduction in LOS in the HDU from 2.1 to 1.6 days ($p = 0.01$) and in the ICU from 2.3 days to 1.9 days ($p = 0.01$) after implementing an OPE [55]. Furthermore, a 2005 study by Mendes reviewed performance indicators of a hospital for 5 years after the introduction of OPEs and found a significant decrease in mean hospital stay from 6.2 to 5.0 days ($p \leq 0.001$) [56]. Decreased LOS not only helps to reduce costs, but also creates opportunity for further revenue generation as well as addresses the growing problem of patient boarding.

4.10 Reduction in Anxiety

The perioperative period is one of the most stressful experiences for patients, with anxiety often peaking in the preoperative phase. Mild anxiety is a normal physiological response, but as anxiety levels increase, negative perioperative effects occur including increased anesthetic medication use, immunosuppression, and delayed wound healing [57]. Furthermore, high anxiety before surgery is an independent predictor of high postoperative pain [58]. Decreased preoperative anxiety levels are a frequently reported benefit of OPEs [8, 9, 19]. A Swiss study by Klopfenstein et al. compared anxiety levels using two validated measures and found anxiety levels were significantly reduced in patients undergoing OPE compared to those undergoing evaluation on the night before surgery [59].

4.11 Disadvantages of Outpatient Evaluations

Despite their many advantages, OPEs have certain limitations compared to IPEs. One major drawback is limited access to immediate diagnostic tests and treatments. Outpatient workup can be prolonged due to multiple factors including scheduling, need for prior authorizations, and other logistical issues. There is also increased risk of incomplete or scattered medical records if a patient is receiving care from multiple organizations, which could result in missing critical information during the OPE process. Outpatient workups are also significantly more reliant on patient compliance, stressing the need for patient and family education. Patient actions and behavior such as fasting times, transportation, and preoperative medication use are tightly controlled in the inpatient setting, whereas these controls do not exist for outpatient. Another challenge is the financial investment needed to initiate and subsequently staff an OPE, which often requires partnership with hospitals [12, 31]. Despite these drawbacks, the benefits of a well-run OPE for patients, organizations, and the larger healthcare system far outweigh their associated costs.

4.12 Why Anesthesiologists Should Lead

Anesthesiologists are uniquely positioned to lead the preoperative evaluation process due to their expertise and understanding of surgery, physiology, and medicine [4, 8, 13]. Anesthesiology residents have been shown to have significantly higher perioperative care education and knowledge compared to primary care residents due to dedicated preoperative rotations and focus [60]. Anesthesiologists are trained to complete each of the core preoperative functions, and their mastery is demonstrated by numerous studies revealing that anesthesiologist-directed preoperative clinics have significant benefits, including reduced surgical cancelations, fewer complications, improved resource utilization, and decreased healthcare costs [9, 35, 52, 61]. Anesthesiologist-led preoperative evaluations enhance patient comfort and safety, optimize surgical outcomes, and improve healthcare efficiency, addressing the strategic priorities for healthcare improvement [23, 62].

Anesthesiologists serve as the essential bridge between primary care physicians, who focus on chronic disease management, and the surgical teams, who concentrate on procedural techniques and acute surgical issues. This unique positioning makes anesthesiologists the ideal perioperative physicians.

References

1. Blitz J. Preoperative evaluation in the 21st century. Anesthesiology. 2023;139(1):91–103. https://doi.org/10.1097/aln.0000000000004582.
2. Jonker P, Hoeks VS, Heijkoop È, Stolker R-J, Korstanje J-W. Alternatives to the in-person anaesthetist-led preoperative assessment in adults undergoing low-risk or intermediate-risk surgery. Eur J Anaesthesiol. 2023;40(5):343–55. https://doi.org/10.1097/eja.0000000000001815.
3. van Klei WA, Moons KGM, Rutten CLG, et al. The effect of outpatient preoperative evaluation of hospital inpatients on cancellation of surgery and length of hospital stay. Anesth Analg. 2002;94(3):644. https://doi.org/10.1097/00000539-200203000-00030.
4. Halaszynski TM, Juda R, Silverman DG. Optimizing postoperative outcomes with efficient preoperative assessment and management. Crit Care Med. 2004;32(Supplement):S76–86. https://doi.org/10.1097/01.ccm.0000122046.30687.5c.
5. Gropper MA, Eriksson LI, Fleisher LA, Cohen NH, Leslie K, Johnson-Akeju O. Miller's Anesthesia, 2-Volume Set. 10th ed. Elsevier Health Sciences; 2024. p. 51–7.
6. Fowler AJ, Wahedally MAH, Abbott TEF, Prowle JR, Cromwell DA, Pearse RM. Long-term disease interactions amongst surgical patients: a population cohort study. Br J Anaesth. 2023;131(2):407–17. https://doi.org/10.1016/j.bja.2023.04.041.
7. Koike M, Yoshimura M, Mio Y, Uezono S. The effects of a preoperative multidisciplinary conference on outcomes for high-risk patients with challenging surgical treatment options: a retrospective study. BMC Anesthesiol. 2021;21(1) https://doi.org/10.1186/s12871-021-01257-1.
8. Tariq H, Ahmed R, Kulkarni S, et al. Development, functioning, and effectiveness of a preoperative risk assessment clinic. Health Serv Insights. 2016;9(Suppl 1):1–7. https://doi.org/10.4137/HSI.S40540.
9. Silvay G, Zafirova Z. Ten years experiences with preoperative evaluation clinic for day admission cardiac and major vascular surgical patients. Semin Cardiothorac Vasc Anesth. 2015;20(2):120–32. https://doi.org/10.1177/1089253215619236.
10. Stier G, Ramsingh D, Raval R, et al. Anesthesiologists as perioperative hospitalists and outcomes in patients undergoing major urologic surgery: a historical prospective, comparative effectiveness study. Perioperat Med. 2018;7(1) https://doi.org/10.1186/s13741-018-0090-y.
11. Aronson S, Murray S, Martin G, et al. Roadmap for transforming preoperative assessment to preoperative optimization. Anesth Analg. 2020;130(4):811–9. https://doi.org/10.1213/ane.0000000000004571.
12. Bader AM, Sweitzer BJ, Kumar A. Nuts and bolts of preoperative clinics: the view from three institutions. Cleve Clin J Med. 2009;76(10 suppl 4):S104–11. https://doi.org/10.3949/ccjm.76.s4.17.
13. Kitts JB. The preoperative assessment: who is responsible? Can J Anaesth. 1997;44(12):1232–6. https://doi.org/10.1007/bf03012768.
14. Riggs KR, Segal JB. What is the rationale for preoperative medical evaluations? A closer look at surgical risk and common terminology. Br J Anaesth. 2016;117(6):681–4. https://doi.org/10.1093/bja/aew302.
15. Moonesinghe SR, Mythen MG, Das P, Rowan KM, Grocott MPW. Risk stratification tools for predicting morbidity and mortality in adult patients undergoing major surgery:

qualitative systematic review. Anesthesiology. 2013;119(4):959–81. https://doi.org/10.1097/ALN.0b013e3182a4e94d.

16. Stones J, Yates D. Clinical risk assessment tools in anaesthesia. BJA Educ. 2019;19(2):47–53. https://doi.org/10.1016/j.bjae.2018.09.009.
17. Basic Standards for Preanesthesia Care. www.asahq.org. https://www.asahq.org/standards-and-practice-parameters/basic-standards-for-preanesthesia-care
18. Sroka R, Gabriel E, Al-Hadidi D, Nurkin S, Urman RD, Quinn TD. A novel anesthesiologist-led multidisciplinary model for evaluating high-risk surgical patients at a comprehensive cancer center. J Healthc Risk Manag. 2018;38(3):12–23. https://doi.org/10.1002/jhrm.21326.
19. Kristoffersen EW, Opsal A, Tveit TO, Berg RC, Fossum M. Effectiveness of pre-anaesthetic assessment clinic: a systematic review of randomised and non-randomised prospective controlled studies. BMJ Open. 2022;12(5):e054206. https://doi.org/10.1136/bmjopen-2021-054206.
20. The Anesthesia Patient Safety Foundation (APSF): A 35 year commitment to patient safety. Anesthesia Patient Safety Foundation. https://www.apsf.org/article/the-anesthesia-patient-safety-foundation-apsf-a-35-year-commitment-to-patient-safety/
21. Kristoffersen EW, Opsal A, Tveit TO, Fossum M. Knowledge, safety, and teamwork: a qualitative study on the experiences of anaesthesiologists and nurse anaesthetists working in the preanaesthesia assessment clinic. BMC Anesthesiol. 2022;22(1) https://doi.org/10.1186/s12871-022-01852-w.
22. ASA Committee on Economics. Distinguishing Between a Pre-Anesthesia Evaluation and a Separately Reportable Evaluation and Management Service. www.asahq.org. Published November 2020. https://www.asahq.org/quality-and-practice-management/managing-your-practice/timely-topics-in-payment-and-practice-management/distinguishing-between-a-pre-anesthesia-evaluation-and-a-separately-reportable-evaluation-and-management-service
23. Grocott MPW, Plumb JOM, Edwards M, Fecher-Jones I, Levett DZH. Re-designing the pathway to surgery: better care and added value. Perioperat Med. 2017;6(1) https://doi.org/10.1186/s13741-017-0065-4.
24. Festen S, van Twisk YZ, van Munster BC, de Graeff P. “What matters to you?” Health outcome prioritisation in treatment decision-making for older patients. Age Ageing. 2021;50(6) https://doi.org/10.1093/ageing/afab160.
25. Kuiper BI, Janssen LMJ, Versteeg KS, et al. Does preoperative multidisciplinary team assessment of high-risk patients improve the safety and outcomes of patients undergoing surgery? BMC Anesthesiol. 2024;24(1) https://doi.org/10.1186/s12871-023-02394-5.
26. Kain ZN, Vakharia S, Garson L, et al. The perioperative surgical home as a future perioperative practice model. Anesth Analg. 2014;118(5):1126–30. https://doi.org/10.1213/ane.0000000000000190.
27. Harrison TG, Ronksley PE, James MT, et al. The Perioperative Surgical Home, Enhanced Recovery After Surgery and how integration of these models may improve care for medically complex patients. Can J Surg. 2021;64(4):E381–90. https://doi.org/10.1503/cjs.002020.
28. Aronson S, Westover J, Guinn N, et al. A perioperative medicine model for population health. Anesth Analg. 2018;126(2):682–90. https://doi.org/10.1213/ane.0000000000002606.
29. Shaw M, Pelecanos AM, Mudge AM. Evaluation of Internal Medicine Physician or Multidisciplinary Team Comanagement of Surgical Patients and Clinical Outcomes. JAMA Netw Open. 2020;3(5):e204088. https://doi.org/10.1001/jamanetworkopen.2020.4088.
30. AHA Annual Survey Database™ | AHA Data. www.ahadata.com. https://www.ahadata.com/aha-annual-survey-database
31. Lew E, Pavlin DJ, Amundsen L. Outpatient preanaesthesia evaluation clinics. Singapore Med J. 2004;45(11):509–16.
32. Canellas MM, Jewell M, Edwards JL, Olivier D, Jun-O’Connell AH, Reznek MA. Measurement of cost of boarding in the emergency department using time-driven activity-based costing. Ann Emerg Med. 2024;84(4) https://doi.org/10.1016/j.annemergmed.2024.04.012.
33. Alfred Lee J. The anaesthetic out-patient clinic. Anaesthesia. 1949;4(4):169–74. https://doi.org/10.1111/j.1365-2044.1949.tb05837.x.

34. Pollard JD, Zboray AL, Mazze RI. Economic benefits attributed to opening a preoperative evaluation clinic for outpatients. Anesth Analg. 1996;83(2):407–10. https://doi.org/10.1097/00000539-199608000-00035.
35. Blitz JD, Kendale SM, Jain SK, Cuff GE, Kim JT, Rosenberg AD. Preoperative evaluation clinic visit is associated with decreased risk of in-hospital postoperative mortality. Anesthesiology. 2016;125(2):280–94. https://doi.org/10.1097/aln.0000000000001193.
36. Zafar JE, Chan KT, Ryder LJ, et al. Information technology-enhanced telehealth consultations reduce preoperative evaluation center visits in a bariatric surgery population. Healthcare. 2023;11(3):309. https://doi.org/10.3390/healthcare11030309.
37. U.S. Bureau of Labor Statistics. U.S. Bureau of Labor Statistics. Bls.gov. Published August 29, 2024. https://www.bls.gov/
38. Le DQ, Burton BN, Tejeda CJ, Jalilian L, Kamdar N. Improvement in adherance to anesthesia preoperative appointment with telemedicine: a retrospective analysis. Cureus. 2024;16(5):e60805. https://doi.org/10.7759/cureus.60805.
39. Orrange S, Patel A, Mack WJ, Cassetta J. Patient satisfaction and trust in telemedicine during the COVID-19 pandemic (Preprint). JMIR Hum Factors. 2021;8(2) https://doi.org/10.2196/28589.
40. Eyrich NW, Andino JJ, Ukavwe RE, et al. The lack of a physical exam during new patient telehealth visits does not impact plans for office and operating room procedures. Urology. 2022;167:109–14. https://doi.org/10.1016/j.urology.2022.06.017.
41. Sigal I, Dayal P, Hoch JS, Mouzoon JL, Morrow E, Marcin JP. Travel, time, and cost savings associated with a university medical center's video medical interpreting program. Telemed E-Health. 2020;26(10):1234–9. https://doi.org/10.1089/tmj.2019.0220.
42. Lonsdale H, Burns ML, Epstein RH, et al. Strengthening discovery and application of artificial intelligence in anesthesiology: a report from the Anesthesia Research Council. Anesthesiology. 2025;142(4):599–610. https://doi.org/10.1097/aln.0000000000005326.
43. Han L, Char DS, Aghaeepour N, et al. Artificial intelligence in perioperative care: opportunities and challenges. Anesthesiology. 2024;141(2):379–87. https://doi.org/10.1097/aln.0000000000005013.
44. Bonde A, Varadarajan KM, Bonde N, et al. Assessing the utility of deep neural networks in predicting postoperative surgical complications: a retrospective study. Lancet Digit Health. 2021;3(8):e471–85. https://doi.org/10.1016/s2589-7500(21)00084-4.
45. Graeßner M, Jungwirth B, Frank E, et al. Enabling personalized perioperative risk prediction by using a machine-learning model based on preoperative data. Sci Rep. 2023;13(1) https://doi.org/10.1038/s41598-023-33981-8.
46. Harris C, Pimpalkar A, Aggarwal A, et al. Preoperative risk prediction of major cardiovascular events in noncardiac surgery using the 12-lead electrocardiogram: an explainable deep learning approach. Br J Anaesth. 2025; https://doi.org/10.1016/j.bja.2025.07.085.
47. Xu H, Fu C, Zhao W, et al. Anesthesia transformed: AI pioneering a new era in perioperative medicine. Anesthesiol Perioperat Sci. 2025;3(1) https://doi.org/10.1007/s44254-025-00091-9.
48. Dexter F, Marcon E, Epstein RH, Ledolter J. Validation of statistical methods to compare cancellation rates on the day of surgery. Anesth Analg. 2005;101(2):465–73. https://doi.org/10.1213/01.ane.0000154536.34258.a8.
49. Ferschl MB, Tung A, Sweitzer B, Huo D, Glick DB. Preoperative clinic visits reduce operating room cancellations and delays. Anesthesiology. 2005;103(4):855–9. https://doi.org/10.1097/00000542-200510000-00025.
50. Fischer SP. Development and effectiveness of an anesthesia preoperative evaluation clinic in a teaching hospital. Anesthesiology. 1996;85(1):196–206. https://doi.org/10.1097/00000542-199607000-00025.
51. Kirkham KR, Wijeysundera DN, Pendrith C, et al. Preoperative laboratory investigations. Anesthesiology. 2016;124(4):804–14. https://doi.org/10.1097/aln.0000000000001013.
52. Issa MRN, Isoni NFC, Soares AM, Fernandes ML. Preanesthesia evaluation and reduction of preoperative care costs. Braz J Anesthesiol. 2011;61(1):60–71. https://doi.org/10.1016/s0034-7094(11)70007-1.

53. Power LM, Thackray NM. Reduction of preoperative investigations with the introduction of an anaesthetist-led preoperative assessment clinic. Anaesth Intensive Care. 1999;27(5):481–8. https://doi.org/10.1177/0310057x9902700508.
54. Pickering AN, Zhao X, Sileanu FE, et al. Prevalence and cost of care cascades following low-value preoperative electrocardiogram and chest radiograph within the veterans health administration. J Gen Intern Med. 2022; https://doi.org/10.1007/s11606-022-07561-x.
55. Kamal T, Conway R, Littlejohn I, Ricketts D. The role of a multidisciplinary pre-assessment clinic in reducing mortality after complex orthopaedic surgery. Ann R Coll Surg Engl. 2011;93(2):149–51. https://doi.org/10.1308/003588411x561026.
56. Mendes FF, da Mathias LAST, Duval Neto GF, Birck AR. Impact of preoperative outpatient evaluation clinic on performance indicators. Rev Bras Anestesiol. 2005;55(2) https://doi.org/10.1590/s0034-70942005000200004.
57. Baagil H, Baagil H, Gerbershagen MU. Preoperative anxiety impact on anesthetic and analgesic use. Medicina. 2023;59(12):2069. https://doi.org/10.3390/medicina59122069.
58. Liu Q, Li L, Wei J, Xie Y. Correlation and influencing factors of preoperative anxiety, postoperative pain, and delirium in elderly patients undergoing gastrointestinal cancer surgery. BMC Anesthesiol. 2023;23(1) https://doi.org/10.1186/s12871-023-02036-w.
59. Klopfenstein CE, Forster A, Van Gessel E. Anesthetic assessment in an outpatient consultation clinic reduces preoperative anxiety. Can J Anesth. 2000;47(6):511–5. https://doi.org/10.1007/bf03018941.
60. Adesanya AO, Joshi GP. Comparison of knowledge of perioperative care in primary care residents versus anesthesiology residents. Baylor Univ Med Cent Proc. 2006;19(3):216–20. https://doi.org/10.1080/08998280.2006.11928165.
61. Tsen LC, Segal S, Pothier M, Hartley LH, Bader AM. The effect of alterations in a preoperative assessment clinic on reducing the number and improving the yield of cardiology consultations. Anesth Analg. 2002;95(6):1563–8. https://doi.org/10.1097/00000539-200212000-00016.
62. Vetter TR, Boudreaux AM, Jones KA, Hunter JM, Pittet JF. The perioperative surgical home. Anesth Analg. 2014;118(5):1131–6. https://doi.org/10.1213/ane.0000000000000228.

5 Preoperative Optimization and Risk Reduction: A Systems-Based Role for Anesthesiologists

Stephen Rivoli, Darryl Brown, Janet Mutschler, John Choi, Alexandra Jankulov, and Rohini Loke

5.1 Introduction: The Imperative for Optimization and the Anesthesiologist's Leadership Role

Physician anesthesiologists stand at the intersection of profound healthcare challenges and opportunities. The demographic landscape of the USA features an increasing and rapidly aging population, with projections indicating a doubling of the elderly subset by 2050 [1, 2]. This shift inevitably drives a greater demand for surgical services, often for patients presenting with a higher burden of complex, chronic comorbidities such as cardiovascular disease, pulmonary disease, diabetes, and obesity. A significant percentage of inpatient surgeries are already performed on individuals whose underlying health issues predispose them to higher complication rates, prolonged hospitalizations, and a diminished capacity for regaining independence post-surgery [3]. Adding to this clinical complexity is the ongoing strain of rising healthcare costs, which consume a substantial and growing portion of the national gross domestic product (GDP) [4]. This economic reality forces healthcare systems and administrators to constantly find innovative strategies that enhance efficiency, control costs, and simultaneously improve the quality and safety of patient care.

In this demanding environment, the traditional model where anesthesiologists focus primarily on the intraoperative phase of care proves inadequate. A paradigm shift toward proactive, comprehensive **perioperative optimization** is not merely beneficial but essential. This transformation requires leadership, systems-based thinking, and a deep understanding of both clinical medicine and healthcare delivery—qualities inherent to the specialty of anesthesiology. This unique training provides a robust foundation for **Anesthesiologist Leadership** in this domain. Beyond technical expertise in anesthesia and critical care, the discipline of perioperative

S. Rivoli (✉) · D. Brown · J. Mutschler · J. Choi · A. Jankulov · R. Loke
Icahn School of Medicine at Mount Sinai, Mount Sinai West and Morningside Hospitals, New York, NY, USA

G. Tewfik (ed.), *The Anesthesiologist as Perioperative Leader*,
https://doi.org/10.1007/978-3-032-18058-2_5

medicine emphasizes rigorous attention to patient safety, data interpretation, rapid decision-making under pressure, and effective communication within complex, interdisciplinary teams [5]. Anesthesiologists function as integrators, coordinating with surgeons, nurses, specialists, pharmacists, and technicians across diverse clinical settings—from the operating room and ICU, to labor and delivery and outpatient clinics. This constant practice in team-based care and process management cultivates skills directly applicable to leading system-level improvements. This vital role may come to the forefront in public health crises, such as the COVID-19 pandemic, further demonstrating the capacity of physician anesthesiologists for leadership in resource allocation, protocol development, critical care management, and cross-specialty collaboration [6]. This background uniquely positions anesthesiologists not just as perioperative physicians, but as perioperative *leaders*, driven to enhance outcomes for individual patients while simultaneously improving the efficiency and value of the healthcare system.

5.2 Preoperative Assessment: The Comprehensive Foundation

The cornerstone of effective **Perioperative Optimization** is a meticulous and comprehensive **Preoperative Assessment**. This process extends far beyond a simple "clearance for surgery"; it is an opportunity to develop a deep understanding of the patient's physiological status, identify potential risks, and initiate strategies for mitigation. Specifically, the specialty has moved away from the word "clearance" or obtaining for "clearance," because the meaningful anesthesia clearance for surgery happens just prior to surgery during in-person assessment. The patient may present markedly different on the day of their procedure than how they appeared in prior assessments. The preoperative assessment typically includes a detailed medical and surgical history, focusing on the severity and stability of comorbidities; a thorough physical examination directed at relevant organ systems; a review of pertinent laboratory data; and the interpretation of ancillary diagnostic tests (e.g., ECG, echocardiography, PFTs), judiciously selected based on the patient's condition and the anticipated surgical stress [7]. Effective assessment requires not only clinical acumen but also strong coordination skills, as input from other medical specialists is often necessary to fully evaluate complex conditions.

Crucially, a truly comprehensive assessment acknowledges the profound impact of non-medical factors as well. Social determinants of health (SDOH)—encompassing socioeconomic status, educational attainment, neighborhood environment, access to nutritious food and transportation, health literacy, and social support networks—are increasingly recognized as powerful predictors of surgical outcomes [8]. Patients facing social vulnerability experience higher rates of postoperative complications, prolonged hospital stays, increased readmission rates, and even higher mortality following various surgical procedures [8]. Therefore, **Anesthesiologist Leadership** in the preoperative sphere includes advocating for and implementing systematic screening for SDOH within the assessment process.

This might involve integrating validated screening tools into pre-anesthesia clinic (PAC) workflows or collaborating with hospital administration to establish clear referral pathways to social work, case management, or community-based resources. While more research is needed to fully delineate the impact of specific SDOH interventions [9, 10], acknowledging and addressing these factors is an ethical imperative and a critical component of holistic patient preparation.

Many institutions utilize a pre-anesthesia clinic (PAC) model for conducting these assessments. While efficient for gathering information close to the surgical date, traditional PAC structures may primarily focus on immediate risk identification rather than long-term optimization [11]. Transforming the PAC from a clearance center into an "optimization hub" requires **Anesthesiologist Leadership**. This involves establishing protocols for earlier patient referral, creating dedicated pathways for specific optimization needs, and fostering robust multidisciplinary collaboration [11]. The program at Duke University serves as an example, demonstrating how referring patients early allows for targeted interventions in specialized clinics (e.g., anemia, diabetes, smoking cessation, frailty) to be managed collaboratively. Such integrated models, though resource-intensive, demonstrably improve outcomes, such as reducing transfusion requirements and shortening hospital stays for patients undergoing preoperative anemia treatment [12], clearly illustrating the value proposition of this proactive, coordinated approach.

5.3 Prehabilitation: Building Resilience Before Surgery

A key strategy within proactive optimization is **Prehabilitation**. This involves implementing targeted interventions *before* surgery to enhance the patient's physiological and psychological reserve, thereby improving their ability to withstand surgical stress and accelerating recovery [13, 14]. The rationale is compelling: patients with low functional capacity entering surgery face significantly higher risks of mortality, complications, and prolonged hospital stays [13]. **Prehabilitation** typically employs a multimodal strategy involving:

1. **Physical Exercise**: Tailored programs focusing on aerobic capacity, strength training, and balance or flexibility exercises, designed to improve overall fitness and functional reserve [13, 15]. Home-based programs have also shown promise. [16].
2. **Nutritional Optimization**: Assessing nutritional status and providing interventions, such as dietary counseling or supplementation (e.g., high-protein supplements, immunonutrition), to counteract catabolism, support wound healing, and bolster immune function [14, 15].
3. **Psychological Support**: Addressing preoperative anxiety and stress through education, counseling, mindfulness techniques, or cognitive behavioral therapy to enhance coping mechanisms and mental resilience [13, 15].
4. **Behavior Modification**: Incorporating programs for smoking cessation or alcohol reduction, where applicable [17].

As perioperative leaders, anesthesiologists are ideally positioned to champion and integrate **Prehabilitation** programs. This involves leading the development of screening protocols within the PAC to identify suitable candidates, coordinating the multidisciplinary team (physiotherapists, dietitians, psychologists, and surgeons), advocating for institutional resources, and ensuring prehabilitation goals align with the overall perioperative plan [13]. While the certainty of evidence continues to evolve for specific outcomes and populations [15], systematic reviews and meta-analyses increasingly suggest potential benefits, including reduced postoperative complications, improved functional capacity, shorter lengths of stay, and enhanced quality of life [14–16]. **Prehabilitation** represents a paradigm shift toward actively preparing patients, rather than simply assessing them, embodying the principles of proactive **Perioperative Optimization**.

5.4 Perioperative Risk Stratification: Informing Personalized Care

Individualized **Risk Stratification** serves as the critical link between assessment and tailored management [18]. It involves synthesizing patient-specific factors and procedural risks to predict the likelihood of adverse outcomes, thereby guiding clinical decisions and facilitating informed patient consent [19]. Numerous tools exist, ranging from general assessments to highly specific calculators [19, 20]. The ASA Physical Status classification, despite its age and subjectivity [21, 22], remains a cornerstone [23]. Its strength lies in its simplicity and its proven correlation with overall morbidity and mortality [18]. A higher ASA score reliably flags patients needing more intensive evaluation and resource allocation, influencing decisions about monitoring, staffing, and postoperative disposition (e.g., ICU vs. ward) [18]. However, its limitations—subjectivity, lack of procedural specificity, and inability to reflect optimization efforts—necessitate its use in conjunction with other tools [18, 22].

The Revised Cardiac Risk Index (RCRI) provides more specific cardiac risk prediction for noncardiac surgery [24, 25]. By evaluating factors like ischemic heart disease, heart failure, diabetes, kidney disease, cerebrovascular history, and surgical risk level, it helps categorize patients' risk for major adverse cardiac events (MACE) [24]. This stratification directly informs decisions regarding further cardiac testing, the initiation or continuation of cardioprotective medications such as beta-blockers [24], and the intensity of intra- and postoperative monitoring. While valuable, the RCRI also has limitations, excluding certain conditions and exhibiting variable predictive power in specific cohorts [24, 25]. More comprehensive, procedure-specific calculators like the ACS NSQIP Surgical Risk Calculator provide detailed, individualized risk estimates across a spectrum of potential complications [4]. Other scores like P-POSSUM, SORT, and NELA are often used in specific contexts, such as emergency surgery [20]. **Anesthesiologist Leadership** involves not only applying these tools appropriately but also critically interpreting their results within the context of the individual patient and the planned procedure, moving beyond a simple score to a nuanced risk assessment. Furthermore, the integration of artificial intelligence (AI) and machine learning holds significant potential [26]. AI algorithms could potentially analyze vast datasets to provide more accurate, dynamic risk predictions, possibly even adapting intraoperatively based on real-time physiological data, although challenges in data contextualization and validation remain [26].

5.5 Avoiding Preventable Perioperative Harm: A Multifaceted Approach

Leveraging the insights gained from comprehensive assessment and **Risk Stratification** [3, 27], anesthesiologists implement multifaceted strategies to actively *prevent* specific perioperative harms throughout the pre-, intra-, and postoperative phases of care. This preventative focus is central to **Anesthesiologist Leadership** in patient safety and **Quality Improvement (QI)**.

Addressing cardiovascular risk involves not only identifying high-risk patients [1] but also acting on that information. Optimization may include adjusting medications such as beta-blockers [28] or statins, ensuring appropriate management of hypertension, or coordinating further cardiac evaluation [27]—interventions aimed at preventing MACE like myocardial infarction [28, 29] and stroke [30, 31]. The significant mortality and cost associated with these events [32, 33] underscore the value of prevention. Similarly, for respiratory complications, identifying patients with chronic obstructive pulmonary disease (COPD), asthma, or obstructive sleep apnea (OSA) [34] leads to interventions including smoking cessation support [35, 36], optimization of inhaler therapy [37], CPAP initiation for OSA [38], and planning for lung-protective ventilation strategies intraoperatively [36] to prevent costly and potentially preventable, complications (PPCs) [32]. Venout thromboembolism (VTE) prevention involves translating risk scores (e.g., Caprini) into action through appropriate pharmacological and mechanical prophylaxis [39] and promoting early mobilization within enhanced recovery after surgery (**ERAS**) pathways [40], mitigating the substantial costs and morbidity of deep vein thrombosis (DVT) and pulmonary embolism (PE) [41, 42]. Preventing surgical site infections (SSIs) requires a bundled approach informed by risk factors: ensuring tight glycemic control in diabetics [43], administering timely and correct antibiotic prophylaxis [44], addressing malnutrition, and collaborating on skin preparation; these interventions contribute to reductions of infection rates and associated costs [45–47]. Identifying patients at risk for acute kidney injury (AKI) allows for preventative strategies like maintaining euvolemia and avoiding nephrotoxic agents [48], while recognizing delirium risk factors prompts multimodal prevention protocols [49].

Intraoperatively, vigilance is paramount. Meticulous preoperative airway assessment directly informs anesthetic strategy, ensuring preparedness with advanced equipment and techniques to prevent catastrophic loss of airway [50]. Continuous hemodynamic monitoring allows for early detection and treatment of instability, preventing downstream organ ischemia. Anesthesiologists carefully titrate anesthetic depth, using tools processed EEG monitoring when appropriate, to balance the risks of awareness and excessive anesthetic exposure [51]. Goal-directed fluid therapy (GDFT) strategies help optimize intravascular volume, reducing complications associated with both hypovolemia and hypervolemia [52]. Active temperature management is employed to maintain normothermia, preventing its detrimental effects on coagulation, wound healing, and infection risk [53]. Quantitative neuromuscular monitoring ensures complete reversal of blockade, preventing residual weakness and respiratory compromise post-extubation [54]. Lastly, meticulous patient positioning throughout the procedure prevents nerve damage and pressure injuries.

Postoperatively, the focus shifts to facilitating recovery and managing immediate risks. Implementing multimodal pain regimens provides effective analgesia while minimizing opioid side effects, enabling earlier mobilization and reducing complications [55]. Prophylactic antiemetic strategies, guided by risk assessment, mitigate postoperative nausea and vomiting (PONV) [56]. Anesthesiologists continue to collaborate with nursing and surgical teams to promote early ambulation [40] and ensure clear, structured communication during patient handovers to maintain continuity of care and prevent errors [57, 58]

5.6 Patient Pathways, ERAS, and Value-Based Care: Leading System Change

The principles of **Perioperative Optimization** are most effectively realized through structured, integrated **Patient Pathways** that standardize care while allowing for personalization [59]. **Anesthesiologist Leadership** is crucial in the design, implementation, and continuous refinement of these pathways, particularly within the frameworks of **ERAS** and **Value-Based Care**. **ERAS** protocols bundle multiple evidence-based interventions (e.g., preoperative counseling, carbohydrate loading, optimized fluid management, opioid-sparing multimodal analgesia, early feeding and mobilization, etc.) to attenuate the surgical stress response, reduce complications, and accelerate functional recovery [40]. As anesthesiologists, we are deeply involved in implementing and adapting many core ERAS components related to anesthesia and pain management [52, 60]. We work collaboratively to customize these pathways based on individual patient needs identified during **Preoperative Assessment** and **Risk Stratification**, ensuring that standardization does not preclude necessary individualization [40].

This system-based approach aligns directly with **Value-Based Care**, which aims to deliver the highest quality outcomes at the lowest possible cost [61]. By reducing complications (like SSIs, VTE, PPCs) and shortening length of stay, optimization strategies, **Prehabilitation**, and **ERAS** pathways directly contribute to **Cost Reduction (Healthcare)** [32, 41, 62, 63]. Anesthesiologists contribute to **Value-Based Care** not only through clinical implementation but also by leading **Quality Improvement (QI)** initiatives. This involves establishing key performance indicators (KPIs) related to perioperative outcomes (e.g., complication rates, length of stay (LOS), readmissions, and patient satisfaction), tracking performance using dashboards, analyzing data to identify areas for improvement, and leading multidisciplinary teams to implement changes [64, 65]. This expertise in data analysis and systems-based thinking allows perioperative physician anesthesiologists to effectively champion these QI assessments. Furthermore, anesthesiologists participate in designing value-based payment bundles, ensuring that care pathways are efficient, evidence-based, and financially sustainable [66, 67]. Integrating these approaches requires robust systems, leveraging electronic health records and potentially predictive analytics [65], optimizing operating room scheduling [68], and ensuring seamless care transitions through proactive discharge planning [65]. Our leadership ensures these complex systems function cohesively, fostering collaboration among all stakeholders [64, 69].

5.7 Conclusion: The Anesthesiologist as Perioperative Leader and Value Generator

The modern physician anesthesiologist's influence extends far beyond the traditional confines of the operating room. As this chapter has detailed, **Anesthesiologist Leadership** is integral to the successful implementation and continuous improvement of **Perioperative Optimization**. Through meticulous **Preoperative Assessment**, insightful **Risk Stratification**, proactive **Prehabilitation**, vigilant intraoperative care, and the strategic design of **Patient Pathways** within **ERAS** and **Value-Based Care** models, we actively prevent harm and enhance recovery. Our unique skill set, combining clinical expertise with a systems-oriented perspective, allows us to effectively lead multidisciplinary teams, champion **Quality Improvement (QI)** initiatives, and demonstrate significant **Cost Reduction** achieved through optimized perioperative care. By embracing this comprehensive role, we not only improve safety and outcomes for individual patients but also generate substantial value for the healthcare system, solidifying our position as essential leaders in shaping the future of high-quality, efficient surgical care [64, 69].

References

1. U.S. Census Bureau. U.S. population grows at fastest pace in more than two decades. 2024 Dec 20 [cited 2025 Mar 01]. Available from: https://www.census.gov/library/stories/2024/12/population-estimates.html
2. Pallin DJ, Espinola JA, Camargo CA Jr. US population aging and demand for inpatient services. J Hosp Med. 2014;9(3):193–6. https://doi.org/10.1002/jhm.2145.
3. Aronson S, Martin G, Gulur P, Lipkin ME, Lagoo-Deenadayalan SA, Mantyh CR, et al. Preoperative optimization: a continued call to action. Anesth Analg. 2020;130(4):808–10. https://doi.org/10.1213/ANE.0000000000004492.
4. Centers for Medicare & Medicaid Services. National health expenditure data: historical. 2024 [cited 2025 Mar 23]. Available from: https://www.cms.gov/data-research/statistics-trends-and-reports/national-health-expenditure-data/historical

5. Accreditation Council for Graduate Medical Education. Program Requirements for Graduate Medical Education in Anesthesiology. [07/01/2025]. Available from: https://www.acgme.org/globalassets/pfassets/programrequirements/2025-reformatted-requirements/040_anesthesiology_2025_reformatted.pdf
6. Weingarten TN, Gajic O. The next next wave: how critical care might learn from the past to improve the future. Anesth Analg. 2022;135(5):807–9. https://doi.org/10.1213/ANE.0000000000006159.
7. American Society of Anesthesiologists Task Force on Preanesthesia Evaluation. Practice advisory for preanesthesia evaluation: a report by the American Society of Anesthesiologists Task Force on Preanesthesia Evaluation. Anesthesiology. 2002;96(2):485–96. https://doi.org/10.1097/00000542-200202000-00037.
8. Diallo MS, Hasnain-Wynia R, Vetter TR. Social determinants of health and preoperative care. Anesthesiol Clin. 2024;42(1):87–101. https://doi.org/10.1016/j.anclin.2023.07.002.
9. Diallo M, Tan J, Heitmiller E, Vetter T. Achieving greater health equity: an opportunity for anesthesiology. Anesth Analg. 2022;134(6):1175–84. https://doi.org/10.1213/ANE.0000000000005937.
10. Palmer RC, Ismond D, Rodriquez EJ, Kaufman JS. Social determinants of health: future directions for health disparities research. Am J Public Health. 2019;109(S1):S70–1. https://doi.org/10.2105/AJPH.2019.304964.
11. Aronson S, Murray S, Martin G, Blitz J, Crittenden T, Lipkin ME, et al. Roadmap for transforming preoperative assessment to preoperative optimization. Anesth Analg. 2020;130(4):811–9. https://doi.org/10.1213/ANE.0000000000004571.
12. Guinn NR, Fuller M, Murray S, Aronson S, Duke Perioperative Enhancement Team (POET). Treatment through a preoperative anemia clinic is associated with a reduction in perioperative red blood cell transfusion in patients undergoing orthopedic and gynecologic surgery. Transfusion. 2022;62(3):569–78. https://doi.org/10.1111/trf.16847.
13. Carli F. Prehabilitation for the anesthesiologist. Anesthesiology. 2020;133(3):645–52. https://doi.org/10.1097/ALN.0000000000003331.
14. Molenaar CJL, Papen-Botterhuis NE, Herrle F, Slooter GD. Prehabilitation, making patients fit for surgery – a new frontier in perioperative care. Innov Surg Sci. 2019;4(4):132–8. https://doi.org/10.1515/iss-2019-0017. PMID: 33977122; PMCID: PMC8059351
15. McIsaac DI, Kidd G, Gillis C, et al. Relative efficacy of prehabilitation interventions and their components: systematic review with network and component network meta-analyses of randomised controlled trials. BMJ. 2025;388:e081164. Published 2025 Jan 22. https://doi.org/10.1136/bmj-2024-081164.
16. D'Amico F, Dormio S, Veronesi G, et al. Home-based prehabilitation: a systematic review and meta-analysis of randomised trials. Br J Anaesth. 2025;134(4):1018–28. https://doi.org/10.1016/j.bja.2025.01.010.
17. Coffman CR, Howard SK, Mariano ER, Kou A, Pollard J, Boselli R, et al. A short, sustainable intervention to help reduce day of surgery smoking rates among patients undergoing elective surgery. J Clin Anesth. 2019;58:35–6. https://doi.org/10.1016/j.jclinane.2019.04.034.
18. Matthews L, Levett DZH, Grocott MPW. Perioperative risk stratification and modification. Anesthesiol Clin. 2022;40(1S):e1–e23. https://doi.org/10.1016/j.anclin.2022.03.001.
19. Adeleke I, Chae C, Okocha O, Sweitzer B. Risk assessment and risk stratification for perioperative complications and mitigation: where should the focus be? How are we doing? Best Pract Res Clin Anaesthesiol. 2021;35(4):517–29. https://doi.org/10.1016/j.bpa.2020.11.010.
20. Bedford JP, Redfern OC, O'Brien B, Watkinson PJ. Perioperative risk scores: prediction, pitfalls, and progress. Curr Opin Anaesthesiol. 2025;38(1):30–6. https://doi.org/10.1097/ACO.0000000000001445. (Verify Publication Details)
21. Hurwitz EE, Simon M, Vinta SR, et al. Adding examples to the ASA-Physical Status classification improves correct assignments to patients. Anesthesiology. 2017;126(4):614–22. https://doi.org/10.1097/ALN.0000000000001581.

22. Sankar A, Johnson SR, Beattie WS, Tait G, Wijeysundera DN. Reliability of the American Society of Anesthesiologists physical status scale in clinical practice. Br J Anaesth. 2014;113(3):424–32. https://doi.org/10.1093/bja/aeu100.
23. Mayhew D, Mendonca V, Murthy BVS. A review of ASA physical status – historical perspectives and modern developments. Anaesthesia. 2019;74(3):373–9. https://doi.org/10.1111/anae.14510.
24. Smilowitz NR, Berger JS. Perioperative cardiovascular risk assessment and management for noncardiac surgery: a review. JAMA. 2020;324(3):279–90. https://doi.org/10.1001/jama.2020.784.
25. Neuman MD, Liu J. Reassessing the Revised Cardiac Risk Index in the modern perioperative setting. Br J Anaesth. 2020;125(6):880–8. https://doi.org/10.1093/bja/aez384.
26. Bignami E, Panizzi M, Bellini V. Artificial intelligence for personalized perioperative medicine. Cureus. 2024;16(1):e53270. https://doi.org/10.7759/cureus.53270.
27. Thompson A, Fleischmann KE, Smilowitz NR, de Las Fuentes L, Mukherjee D, Aggarwal NR, et al. AHA/ACC/ACS/ASNC/HRS/SCA/SCCT/SCMR/SVM Guideline for perioperative cardiovascular management for noncardiac surgery: a report of the american college of cardiology/american heart association joint committee on clinical practice guidelines. Circulation. 2024;150(19):e351–e442. https://doi.org/10.1161/CIR.0000000000001285.
28. Auerbach AD, Goldman L. Beta-blockers and reduction of cardiac events in noncardiac surgery: scientific review. JAMA. 2002;287(11):1435–44. https://doi.org/10.1001/jama.287.11.1435.
29. Devereaux PJ, Sessler DI. Cardiac complications in patients undergoing major noncardiac surgery. N Engl J Med. 2015;373(23):2258–69. https://doi.org/10.1056/NEJMra1502824.
30. Smilowitz NR, Gupta N, Ramakrishna H, Guo Y, Berger JS, Bangalore S. Perioperative major adverse cardiovascular and cerebrovascular events associated with noncardiac surgery. JAMA Cardiol. 2017;2(2):181–7. https://doi.org/10.1001/jamacardio.2016.4792. PMID: 28030663; PMCID: PMC5563847
31. Boehme AK, Esenwa C, Elkind MS. Stroke risk factors, genetics, and prevention. Circ Res. 2017;120(3):472–95. https://doi.org/10.1161/CIRCRESAHA.116.308398.
32. Stokes SM, Scaife CL, Brooke BS, Glasgow RE, Mulvihill SJ, Finlayson SRG, Varghese TK. Hospital costs following surgical complications: a value-driven outcomes analysis of cost savings due to complication prevention. Ann Surg. 2022;275(2):e375–81. https://doi.org/10.1097/SLA.0000000000004243.
33. Strilciuc S, Grad DA, Radu C, Chira D, Stan A, Ungureanu M, et al. The economic burden of stroke: a systematic review of cost of illness studies. J Med Life. 2021;14(5):606–19. https://doi.org/10.25122/jml-2021-0361.
34. Miskovic A, Lumb AB. Postoperative pulmonary complications. Br J Anaesth. 2017;118(3):317–34. https://doi.org/10.1093/bja/aex002.
35. Mills E, Eyawo O, Lockhart I, Kelly S, Wu P, Ebbert JO. Smoking cessation reduces postoperative complications: a systematic review and meta-analysis. Am J Med. 2011;124(2):144–154.e8. https://doi.org/10.1016/j.amjmed.2010.09.013.
36. Neto AS, Simonis FD, Barbas CSV, et al. Lung-protective ventilation with low tidal volumes and the occurrence of pulmonary complications in patients without acute respiratory distress syndrome: a systematic review and individual patient data analysis. Crit Care Med. 2015;43(10):2155–63. https://doi.org/10.1097/CCM.0000000000001189.
37. Duggan EW, Carlson K, Umpierrez GE. Perioperative hyperglycemia management: an update. Anesthesiology. 2017;126(3):547–60. https://doi.org/10.1097/ALN.0000000000001515.
38. Kaw R, Chung F, Pasupuleti V, Mehta J, Gay PC, Hernandez AV. Meta-analysis of the association between obstructive sleep apnea and postoperative outcome. Br J Anaesth. 2012;109(6):897–906. https://doi.org/10.1093/bja/aes302.
39. Gould MK, Garcia DA, Wren SM, et al. Prevention of VTE in nonorthopedic surgical patients: antithrombotic therapy and prevention of thrombosis, 9th ed: American College

of Chest Physicians Evidence-Based Clinical Practice Guidelines. Chest. 2012;141(2 Suppl):e227S–77S. https://doi.org/10.1378/chest.11-2297.
40. Ljungqvist O, Scott M, Fearon KC. Enhanced recovery after surgery: a review. JAMA Surg. 2017;152(3):292–8. https://doi.org/10.1001/jamasurg.2016.4952.
41. Steinle T, Lees M. Economic burden of venous thromboembolism: a systematic review. J Med Econ. 2011;14(1):65–74. https://doi.org/10.3111/13696998.2010.546465.
42. Heit JA. Epidemiology of venous thromboembolism. Nat Rev Cardiol. 2015;12(8):464–74. https://doi.org/10.1038/nrcardio.2015.83. Epub 2015 Jun 16. PMID: 26076949; PMCID: PMC4624298. https://pmc.ncbi.nlm.nih.gov/articles/PMC4624298/
43. van den Berghe G, Wouters P, Weekers F, et al. Intensive insulin therapy in critically ill patients. N Engl J Med. 2001;345(19):1359–67. https://doi.org/10.1056/NEJMoa011300.
44. Bratzler DW, Dellinger EP, Olsen KM, et al. Clinical practice guidelines for antimicrobial prophylaxis in surgery. Am J Health Syst Pharm. 2013;70(3):195–283. https://doi.org/10.1093/ajhp/70.3.195.
45. Zimlichman E, Henderson D, Tamir O, et al. Health care-associated infections: a meta-analysis of costs and financial impact on the US health care system. JAMA Intern Med. 2013;173(22):2039–46. https://doi.org/10.1001/jamainternmed.2013.9763.
46. Rosemurgy A, Whitaker J, Luberice K, Rodriguez C, Downs D, Ross S. A cost-benefit analysis of reducing surgical site infections. Am Surg. 2018;84(2):254–61.
47. Anderson DJ, Podgorny K, Berríos-Torres SI, et al. Strategies to prevent surgical site infections in acute care hospitals: 2014 update. Infect Control Hosp Epidemiol. 2014;35(Suppl 2):S66–88. https://doi.org/10.1086/676022.
48. Kheterpal S, Tremper KK, Englesbe MJ, et al. Predictors of postoperative acute renal failure after noncardiac surgery in patients with previously normal renal function. Anesthesiology. 2007;107:892–902. https://doi.org/10.1097/01.anes.0000290938.99444.fd.
49. Inouye SK, Westendorp RG, Saczynski JS. Delirium in elderly people. Lancet. 2014;383(9920):911–22. https://doi.org/10.1016/S0140-6736(13)60688-1.
50. Apfelbaum JL, Hagberg CA, Caplan RA, et al. American Society of Anesthesiologists. Practice guidelines for management of the difficult airway: an updated report by the American Society of Anesthesiologists Task Force on Management of the Difficult Airway. Anesthesiology. 2013;118:251–70. https://doi.org/10.1097/ALN.0b013e31827773b2.
51. Punjasawadwong Y, Phongchiewboon A, Bunchungmongkol N. Bispectral index for improving anaesthetic delivery and postoperative recovery. Cochrane Database Syst Rev. 2014;(6):CD003843. https://doi.org/10.1002/14651858.CD003843.pub2.
52. Feldheiser A, Aziz O, Baldini G, et al. Enhanced Recovery After Surgery (ERAS) for gastrointestinal surgery. Part 2: Consensus statement for anaesthesia practice. Acta Anaesthesiol Scand. 2016;60(3):289–334. https://doi.org/10.1111/aas.12651.
53. Sessler DI. Perioperative thermoregulation and heat balance. Lancet. 2016;387(10038):2655–64. https://doi.org/10.1016/S0140-6736(15)00981-2.
54. Naguib M, Brull SJ, Kopman AF, et al. Consensus statement on perioperative use of neuromuscular monitoring. Anesth Analg. 2018;127(1):71–80. https://doi.org/10.1213/ANE.0000000000002670.
55. Chou R, Gordon DB, de Leon-Casasola OA, et al. Management of Postoperative Pain: A Clinical Practice Guideline From the American Pain Society, the American Society of Regional Anesthesia and Pain Medicine, and the American Society of Anesthesiologists' Committee on Regional Anesthesia, Executive Committee, and Administrative Council. J Pain. 2016;17(2):131–57. https://doi.org/10.1016/j.jpain.2015.12.008.
56. Gan TJ, Diemunsch P, Habib AS, et al. Consensus guidelines for the management of postoperative nausea and vomiting. Anesth Analg. 2014;118(1):85–113. https://doi.org/10.1213/ANE.0000000000000001.
57. Segall N, Bonifacio AS, Schroeder RA, et al. Can we make postoperative patient handovers safer? A systematic review of the literature. Anesth Analg. 2012;115(1):102–15. https://doi.org/10.1213/ANE.0b013e318253af4b.

58. Martins FZ, de Lima LB, Trevilato DD, Hemesath MP, de Magalhães AMM. Protocols for postanesthesia care unit handoff and patient safety: a scoping review. J Adv Nurs. 2025;81(7):3528–44. https://doi.org/10.1111/jan.16673.
59. Grocott MPW, Mythen MG, Pearse RM. Perioperative medicine: the future of anaesthesia? Br J Anaesth. 2012;108(5):723–6. https://doi.org/10.1093/bja/aes124.
60. Scott MJ, Baldini G, Fearon KC, et al. Enhanced Recovery After Surgery (ERAS) for gastrointestinal surgery. Part 1: Pathophysiological considerations. Acta Anaesthesiol Scand. 2015;59(10):1212–31. https://doi.org/10.1111/aas.12601.
61. Porter ME. What is value in health care? N Engl J Med. 2010;363(26):2477–81. https://doi.org/10.1056/NEJMp1011024.
62. Goldfield N, Kelly WP, Patel K. Potentially preventable events: an actionable set of measures for linking quality improvement and cost savings. Qual Manag Health Care. 2012;21(4):213–9. https://doi.org/10.1097/QMH.0b013e31826d1d3a.
63. Macario A, Vitez TS, Dunn B, McDonald T. Where are the costs in perioperative care? Analysis of hospital costs and charges for inpatient surgical care. Anesthesiology. 1995;83(6):1138–44. https://doi.org/10.1097/00000542-199512000-00002.
64. Vetter TR, Goeddel LA, Boudreaux AM, Hunt TR, Jones KA, Pittet JF. The Perioperative Surgical Home: how anesthesiology can collaboratively achieve and leverage the triple aim in health care. Anesth Analg. 2014;118(5):1131–6. https://doi.org/10.1213/ANE.0000000000000230.
65. Grocott MP, Mythen MG. Perioperative medicine: the value proposition for anesthesia?: A UK perspective on delivering value from anesthesiology. Anesthesiol Clin. 2015;33(4):617–28. https://doi.org/10.1016/j.anclin.2015.07.003.
66. Vetter TR, Boudreaux AM, Jones KA, Hunter JM Jr, Pittet JF. The perioperative surgical home: how anesthesiology can collaboratively achieve and leverage the triple aim in health care. Anesth Analg. 2014;118(5):1131–6. https://doi.org/10.1213/ANE.0000000000000228.
67. Ahmed F, Chithrala B, Barve K, Biladeau S, Clifford SP. Value-based care and anesthesiology in the USA. Cureus. 2023;15(8):e44410. Published 2023 Aug 30. https://doi.org/10.7759/cureus.44410.
68. Wachtel RE, Dexter F. Influence of the operating room schedule on tardiness from scheduled start times. Anesth Analg. 2009;108(6):1889–901. https://doi.org/10.1213/ane.0b013e31819f9f0c.
69. Cannesson M, Kain Z. The perioperative surgical home: an innovative clinical care delivery model. J Clin Anesth. 2015;27(3):185–7. https://doi.org/10.1016/j.jclinane.2015.01.006.

6 Enhanced Recovery After Surgery: The Anesthesiologist's Role in Accelerating Recovery and Transforming Perioperative Care

Isabelle Nemeh, Daniel Rodriguez-Correa, and Cyrus Ghaderi

6.1 Introduction

6.1.1 Definition and Origins of ERAS

Enhanced Recovery After Surgery (ERAS) refers to a patient-centered, multimodal, evidence-based approach to perioperative care designed to enhance recovery outcomes, minimize complications, and shorten hospital stays. Initially conceptualized by Danish surgeon Henrik Kehlet, ERAS was first applied in colorectal surgery procedures [1]. Kehlet aimed to improve surgical recovery by reducing unnecessary interventions and focusing on physiological and psychological recovery. Over time, the principles of ERAS have proven to be highly effective, expanding into other surgical fields such as orthopedics, gynecology, urology, cardiac surgery, and bariatrics [2].

The ERAS protocol embodies a paradigm shift in surgical care, transitioning away from traditional practices that emphasized prolonged hospital stays, long periods of fasting, and heavy reliance on opioid analgesics. The focus of ERAS is on achieving faster recovery through a combination of medical, nutritional, and physical interventions, while avoiding unnecessary medical interventions [1]. This protocol aims to optimize patient outcomes across the entire perioperative spectrum, from preoperative preparation through postoperative recovery.

6.1.2 Evolution of Perioperative Care Paradigms

The traditional model of perioperative care was often guided by rigid, one-size-fits-all practices, involving long periods of fasting before surgery, excessive intravenous

I. Nemeh (✉) · D. Rodriguez-Correa · C. Ghaderi
Rutgers New Jersey Medical School, Newark, NJ, USA
e-mail: ikn3@njms.rutgers.edu

G. Tewfik (ed.), *The Anesthesiologist as Perioperative Leader*,
https://doi.org/10.1007/978-3-032-18058-2_6

fluid administration, and opioid-based pain management. These practices were intended to reduce complications but often resulted in longer hospital stays and increased perioperative risks. For example, prolonged fasting led to insulin resistance and dehydration, while excessive fluid administration contributed to pulmonary edema and delayed wound healing. Furthermore, opioid-based pain management, while effective for pain control, often resulted in increased risk of ileus, delayed mobilization, and prolonged recovery. ERAS departs from conventional practices, advocating for individualized care that emphasizes early mobilization, nutritional optimization, reduced opioid use, and goal-directed fluid management. ERAS principles have been shown to significantly reduce postoperative complications, shorten hospital stays, and improve overall recovery.

6.1.3 Importance of a Multidisciplinary Approach

A core component of ERAS is the involvement of a multidisciplinary team, including anesthesiologists, surgeons, nurses, physiotherapists, dietitians, and other healthcare professionals [1]. This collaboration is essential to ensure the full spectrum of ERAS protocols is followed, achieving the goal of optimizing patient recovery outcomes. Each specialist contributes to various aspects of the patient's care, from preoperative education and nutritional optimization, to postoperative mobilization and pain management. Anesthesiologists play a pivotal role in ERAS through preoperative optimization, intraoperative management, and implementation of opioid-sparing analgesic strategies. The integration of multiple healthcare specialists ensures a holistic approach and that every facet of the patient's recovery is addressed in a coordinated manner.

ERAS protocols require institutional commitment to continuous quality improvement. Hospitals and surgical centers must invest in training, monitoring, and auditing practices to ensure that all aspects of the ERAS pathway are adhered to, and improved, over time. The collaboration between various healthcare professionals, along with institutional support, is fundamental to the successful implementation and sustainability of ERAS protocols in clinical practice.

6.2 Physiologic Basis of ERAS

ERAS protocols are built on the understanding that surgery triggers significant physiological stress, including hormonal shifts, inflammation, and metabolic disruptions. Traditional perioperative practices often worsen these responses, leading to complications like delayed healing and muscle breakdown. ERAS aims to optimize the body's natural recovery mechanisms by reducing these stressors. Through strategies such as carbohydrate loading, goal-directed fluid therapy, and multimodal pain management, ERAS protocols support a more balanced physiological response, helping to promote faster recovery and improve patient outcomes.

6.2.1 Surgical Stress Response

If left unchecked, the initial physiologic responses of the body to surgical trauma can lead to complications such as delayed healing, organ dysfunction, and impaired immune function. The key components of the stress response include, but are not limited to:

- **Increased Cortisol Levels**: Cortisol is released by the adrenal glands in response to surgical trauma. Elevated cortisol levels mobilize energy stores by increasing glucose production, enhancing the breakdown of fats and proteins, and promoting gluconeogenesis in the liver. While this helps provide energy for recovery, the catabolic effect of cortisol can result in muscle breakdown and delayed wound healing, both of which are counterproductive to a rapid recovery [3, 4]. Excessive cortisol can impair metabolic recovery, particularly in patients with pre-existing metabolic abnormalities like diabetes [4].
- **Cytokine Release**: After surgery, the body releases pro-inflammatory cytokines such as interleukin-6 (IL-6) and tumor necrosis factor-alpha (TNF-α). These cytokines promote inflammation, and excessive release can lead to systemic inflammation, impaired tissue healing, and increased risk of complications like infection or organ dysfunction [3].
- **Insulin Resistance**: Cells become less responsive to insulin due to the release of stress hormones such as cortisol, catecholamines, and glucagon. As a result, glucose uptake is impaired, leading to hyperglycemia. This metabolic shift makes it more difficult for the body to regulate blood sugar, which can hinder recovery, particularly in patients with diabetes or those who are prone to infection or delayed wound healing [3].
- **Muscle Breakdown**: One of the most detrimental effects of surgery is catabolism, or muscle breakdown. Increased cortisol levels, coupled with reduced insulin sensitivity, result in the breakdown of muscle protein. This leads to postoperative weakness, difficulty with mobility, and increased risk of postoperative falls and pressure ulcers. ERAS protocols aim to reduce these catabolic effects by focusing on early mobilization, nutritional support, and optimized fluid management [4].

6.2.2 Metabolic and Inflammatory Implications of Traditional Approaches vs ERAS

Traditional perioperative practices exacerbate the body's inflammatory response and metabolic alterations. In contrast, ERAS relies on a combination of multimodal interventions designed to optimize the body's physiological state. These include practices such as:

- **Prolonged Fasting**: In the traditional model of perioperative care, patients were required to fast for 8 to 12 h before surgery. Prolonged fasting leads to muscle catabolism, insulin resistance, and delayed recovery. ERAS protocols promote shorter fasting periods avoiding these complications.

- **Immobilization**: Traditionally, patients were advised to stay in bed following surgery, but this practice can result in muscle atrophy, impaired circulation, and delayed recovery. ERAS protocols encourage early mobilization preventing pneumonia, DVT, and ileus, all of which can extend the hospital stay and delay recovery [4].
- **Excessive Intravenous Fluids**: Overhydration leads to tissue edema, which impairs wound healing and contributes to complications like pulmonary edema, ileus, and increased intra-abdominal pressure. Dilution of serum electrolyte concentrations can lead to imbalances that disrupt organ function. It is the role of the anesthesiologist to follow ERAS protocols and use *Goal-Directed Fluid Therapy (GDFT)*, a more individualized approach that adjusts fluid administration based on patient-specific parameters like stroke volume variation (SVV) and pulse pressure variation (PPV). This approach prevents fluid overload, enhances tissue perfusion, promote faster recovery and reduces postoperative complications [4].
- **Opioid-Sparing Strategies**: Traditional opioid-based pain management, while effective for pain control, often resulted in increased risk of ileus, delayed mobilization, and prolonged recovery. ERAS protocols prioritize the use of multimodal analgesia to minimize opioid use, which has been shown to have numerous benefits, including improved postoperative recovery and reduced risk of opioid-related complications such as nausea, vomiting, or prolonged sedation.

6.3 Key Components of ERAS Protocols

A structured, patient-centered approach, ERAS addresses all three phases of perioperative care. In this section, we will explore each key component of the ERAS protocol in more detail and discuss its implementation.

6.3.1 Preoperative Phase

6.3.1.1 Education and Counseling

One of the core components of ERAS is preoperative education and counseling. Patient education helps set realistic expectations, reduces anxiety, and improves overall compliance with the recovery process. Evidence suggests that patients who are well-informed about their upcoming procedure tend to experience reduced levels of postoperative pain and anxiety, and report shorter hospital stays and faster recoveries [5].

Effective education includes providing information about the surgery itself, the expected recovery process, pain management strategies, the benefits of early mobilization, starting an exercise program, and smoking cessation [6, 7]. Many ERAS programs incorporate preoperative education sessions, either in person or through digital platforms. Nurses, physiotherapists, and dietitians often play a crucial role in delivering this information in a way that is tailored to individual patient needs.

Additionally, some ERAS protocols include the use of preoperative counseling tools such as videos, leaflets, or interactive apps to deliver education about the protocol in a more patient-friendly and engaging manner. Research shows that digital tools for patient education can help improve understanding and adherence to the ERAS pathway, reducing stress and improving postoperative outcomes [5].

6.3.1.2 Nutritional Optimization

Preoperative nutritional support is critical for improving patient outcomes, particularly for those at risk of malnutrition or those who are obese. Malnutrition can increase the risk of infections, delay wound healing, and lead to complications like anastomotic leakage, while obesity is linked to increased surgical risks and longer recovery times. Protein supplementation in patients with negative nitrogen balance improves wound healing [8].

To address these issues, ERAS emphasizes preoperative nutritional screening, followed by intervention when necessary. Patients with identified nutritional deficits may be prescribed oral nutritional supplements or be provided with an individualized diet plan aimed at improving their nutritional status prior to surgery. In addition, preoperative *carbohydrate loading* where patients consume a carbohydrate-rich drink 2–3 h before surgery has been shown to improve postoperative glucose control, providing energy for recovery and minimizing the stress response. Carbohydrate loading also improves insulin sensitivity, reduces stress response, improves postoperative muscle function, provides glycogen stores for recovery, and improves patient satisfaction, avoiding prolonged fasting times [4]. This approach supports faster gastrointestinal recovery, maintains muscle protein synthesis, and stabilizes blood glucose levels, leading to reduced postoperative complications and shorter hospital stays [9].

6.3.1.3 Minimizing Fasting Times

ERAS protocols advocate for reducing fasting times of 2 h following ingestion of clear liquids, 4 h after breast milk, 6 h following a light meal, and >8 h post ingestion of a fatty meal prior to undergoing general, regional anesthesia, or sedation [10]. This minimizes the metabolic stress caused by fasting, improves insulin sensitivity, and preserves muscle mass during the perioperative period [10].

It is essential that patients are informed about the modified fasting protocol well in advance to avoid confusion and anxiety. Evidence shows that this approach improves postoperative glucose control, reduces the risk of insulin resistance, and enhances recovery, particularly for patients with metabolic disorders such as diabetes [9, 10].

6.3.1.4 Assessment of Obstructive Sleep Apnea (OSA) Enhances Perioperative Management Strategies

The rising prevalence and the large heterogeneity of OSA in its severity underscores the importance of evidence-based screening methods and monitoring algorithms

[11, 12]. For instance, a simple STOP-BANG preoperative screening method can impact an anesthesiologist's choice of using neuromuscular blocking agents, analgesics, and local or regional vs systemic anesthesia [13]. OSA has different phenotypes that impact postoperative management strategies [14].

6.3.2 Intraoperative Phase

6.3.2.1 Goal-Directed Fluid Therapy

Goal-Directed Fluid Therapy (GDFT) to individualize patient's fluid needs based on specific parameters such as SVV and PPV is an essential part of the ERAS protocol. Therefore, improving tissue perfusion while preventing fluid overload, and minimizing complications like acute kidney injury (AKI) [15].

GDFT may require sophisticated monitoring equipment and necessitates a proactive approach from anesthesiologists. This may involve the use of invasive monitoring techniques such as central venous pressure (CVP) measurements or non-invasive methods like ultrasound-guided estimation of fluid responsiveness. It is also essential to educate other involved healthcare providers on the importance of goal-directed fluid management, as it requires ongoing adjustments based on real-time patient data.

Clinical evidence demonstrates that GDFT leads to better postoperative outcomes, including improved recovery of organ function and reduced incidence of complications like respiratory failure and acute kidney injury [15].

6.3.2.2 Anesthesia Techniques

One of the hallmarks of ERAS is the use of regional anesthesia techniques, including epidural anesthesia, peripheral nerve blocks (e.g., TAP blocks), and spinal anesthesia. These techniques provide superior pain relief compared to traditional opioid-based analgesia and minimize the body's stress response while avoiding the opioid-related side effects, such as nausea, vomiting, ileus, and respiratory depression. Use of regional anesthesia also enhances recovery by allowing patients to mobilize more quickly and resume normal gastrointestinal function [16].

It is essential to select the appropriate anesthetic technique based on the type of surgery and patient characteristics. For example, epidural anesthesia or transabdominal plane (TAP) blocks may be favored in abdominal surgeries, while peripheral nerve blocks are increasingly utilized in joint replacement procedures.

Furthermore, total intravenous anesthesia (TIVA) is commonly used to minimize postoperative nausea and vomiting (PONV), a frequent and unpleasant complication of surgery, when using specific medications such as inhaled anesthetics. By using intravenous anesthetic agents like propofol and avoiding volatile anesthetics, TIVA reduces the incidence of PONV due to its more stable effect on the central nervous system and lower emetogenic potential. Prophylactic use of antiemetic medications such as ondansetron, a 5-HT3 receptor antagonist, and dexamethasone, a corticosteroid, along with TIVA are significantly effective in reducing PONV [17].

In addition, TIVA reduces bleeding during endoscopic sinus surgery and has less hemodynamic fluctuations with better blood pressure control. Similar observations have been made in other surgical interventions such as C-section and orthognathic surgeries [18, 19].

6.3.3 Postoperative Phase

6.3.3.1 Early Mobilization

Early mobilization is a critical component of ERAS that aims to prevent complications such as deep vein thrombosis (DVT), pulmonary embolism (PE), pneumonia, and ileus. ERAS emphasizes mobilizing within hours of surgery, to enhance circulation, improve lung function and accelerate return of gastrointestinal motility [9, 10].

Nurses, physiotherapists, and participation in structured rehabilitation program play an essential role in encouraging and assisting patients with these early activities.

6.3.3.2 Multimodal Pain Management

Pain management is an essential component of ERAS to optimize recovery, minimize opioid-related complications, and facilitate early mobilization. ERAS protocols prioritize multimodal analgesia including non-opioid medications such as acetaminophen, NSAIDs, gabapentinoids, and ketamine, along with regional anesthesia. This approach minimizes the need for opioids while still providing effective pain control [5].

6.3.3.3 Early Enteral Nutrition

ERAS protocol emphasizes the importance of early enteral nutrition to promote faster recovery, short hospital stays and reduce complications. Traditionally, abdominal surgery patients were often kept on prolonged fasting and required nasogastric (NG) tubes for decompression after surgery causing potential ileus and malnutrition. Instead, early enteral nutrition, typically within hours of surgery, provides essential nutrients and supports gut function. This early feeding helps maintain the integrity of the gastrointestinal tract, reduces the risk of infection, and enhances immune function.

6.4 ERAS in Different Surgical Specialties

ERAS protocols have revolutionized the approach to perioperative care across various surgical specialties. These evidence-based protocols incorporate core principles of ERAS and significantly improve recovery outcomes, reduce complications, and shorten hospital stays and may be applied to various surgical disciplines.

6.4.1 Colorectal Surgery

Colorectal surgery is the specialty with the most extensive evidence base, making it the foundation of ERAS practices. Systematic reviews demonstrate significant improvements in patient outcomes, including reduced rates of surgical site infections, anastomotic leaks, and postoperative ileus, while also leading to a marked reduction in hospital stay from an average of 7–10 days to around 3–5 days [2]. Key ERAS components in colorectal surgery include preoperative carbohydrate loading, intraoperative goal-directed fluid therapy, and the use of epidural analgesia or multimodal pain management strategies to reduce opioid consumption and improve postoperative mobilization. By minimizing the body's stress response and optimizing physiological recovery, ERAS has proven to be a valuable tool in enhancing patient outcomes in colectomies and rectal resections.

6.4.2 Orthopedic Surgery

In orthopedic surgery, particularly in total hip and knee arthroplasty (THA and TKA), ERAS protocols have become a standard part of perioperative care. The main focus of ERAS in orthopedic surgery is multimodal pain management, and early mobilization. Studies have demonstrated that ERAS protocols in TKA and THA patients result in a significant reduction in the need for opioid analgesics, reducing the risk of opioid-related side effects such as nausea, constipation, and sedation [5]. Additionally, early mobilization, typically within 24 h of surgery, has been shown to significantly improve functional outcomes, decrease the risk of DVT, and speed up rehabilitation. Moreover, the integration of regional anesthesia techniques, such as femoral nerve blocks or spinal anesthesia, allows achieving these outcomes by minimizing the need for systemic opioids and facilitating quicker recovery of motor function [20].

6.4.3 Gynecologic and Urologic Surgery

ERAS protocols have also been successfully implemented in gynecologic and urologic surgeries, including hysterectomy and prostatectomy. In these fields, ERAS focuses on reducing opioid use, minimizing hospital stays, and improving postoperative recovery times. In hysterectomy patients, ERAS protocols emphasize the use of regional anesthesia, multimodal analgesia (including non-opioid analgesics), early oral feeding and mobilization to promote faster recovery [21]. Studies have shown that ERAS significantly reduces opioid consumption and hospital length of stay, contributing to better overall recovery and a reduction in postoperative complications, such as urinary retention and wound infections [22]. Similarly, for prostatectomy patients, ERAS protocols help minimize opioid-related side effects, improve functional recovery, and reduce the risk of complications such as ileus and deep vein thrombosis [22].

6.4.4 Cardiac and Thoracic Surgery

One of the key strategies in cardiothoracic surgery is early extubation, which helps reduce the risk of respiratory complications. Lung-protective ventilation strategies, such as using lower tidal volumes and reducing the duration of mechanical ventilation, are integral components of ERAS protocols in this cohort [25]. Early extubation, often within 6 h post-surgery, has been shown to significantly reduce the incidence of ventilator-associated pneumonia and other pulmonary complications, thus speeding up recovery and reducing the length of hospital stay [23]. In addition, multimodal pain management helps minimize the stress response and aids in early mobilization, further improving recovery and reducing complications like atelectasis, DVT, and pneumonia [24].

6.4.5 Bariatric and Hepatobiliary Surgery

ERAS protocols have also been successfully adapted for bariatric and hepatobiliary surgeries, such as gastric bypass and liver resections. These types of surgeries often have long recovery times and a higher risk of complications due to the invasiveness of the procedures and the underlying comorbidities of the patients. ERAS in bariatric surgery typically includes preoperative carbohydrate loading, early oral feeding, and multimodal pain management to promote recovery and minimize complications like nausea, vomiting, and wound infections [25]. Studies have shown that ERAS in bariatric surgery results in a significant reduction in hospital length of stay, improved postoperative mobility, and a reduction in complications like pneumonia and thrombosis [25]. Similarly, in hepatobiliary surgery, including liver resections, ERAS protocols help optimize postoperative recovery by reducing the use of opioids, promoting early ambulation, and encouraging early enteral nutrition. This approach accelerates recovery, reduces the risk of complications like infections and bile leaks, and improves overall patient outcomes [26].

6.4.6 Sinus Surgery

Nose and paranasal sinuses are lined with vascular mucosa that bleeds easily with surgical trauma. The endoscopic approach has made significant advancements in this discipline; however, visualization with endoscopes requires a relatively dry surgical field. Utilization of TIVA over inhalant anesthetics, as part of ERAS, demonstrated a superior effect in controlling bleeding compared to head elevation, lowering BP or use of vasoactive topicals alone [27]. The reduction in bleeding often leads to shorter surgical time; the shorter time of exposure to anesthetics enhances patient's recovery post operatively.

6.4.7 Facing Challenges and Relying on Outcomes to Move Forward

ERAS reduces hospital stay by 30–50% and lowers complication rates. Dissemination of these ongoing evidence-based data sets supporting ERAS can help alleviate institutional and cultural resistance. Education and quality improvement can ease the concerns of reluctant surgeons who are accustomed to traditional approaches and it will also demonstrate the cost-saving potentials of ERAS to those who are concerned with the costs of implementing a new approach. ERAS reduces turnover time and increases caseloads for a given operating room with shorter hospital stay offsetting the costs of training nurses and purchasing new equipment if necessary.

There is ongoing research and innovations including personalized ERAS pathways based on machine learning and perioperative remote patient monitoring using wearables. These will further enhance anesthesia delivery and potentially eliminate extra costs currently associated with perioperative care. Anesthesiologists need to continue championing ERAS by working with surgeons and hospital administrators to standardize ERAS pathways and establish institution-wide guidelines [28].

The overall approach to promote ERAS may include training residents, nurses, and other perioperative staff on ERAS principles as well as conducting audits and data analysis to refine protocols over time. Task forces made up of physicians and nurses can insure adherence and continuous improvement in protocols. Using electronic medical records, ERAS compliance tracking can be automated. The task force can also contribute to material and methods in educating patients and raising the community awareness about quality approaches. These outreach activities may include patients as team members to promote the new paradigm shift in health care facilities. Lastly there is a need to standardize the ERAS protocols across hospitals [29, 30]. This will allow measurable metrics in progress as well as transparency across different institutions.

6.5 Conclusion

The physiologic basis of ERAS highlights how the protocol works to counteract the body's natural stress response to surgery, optimize metabolic function, and reduce inflammatory complications. By incorporating multimodal interventions that address both the surgical stress response and postoperative recovery, ERAS has optimized perioperative care across all stages of surgery employing a comprehensive evidence-based approach. The key components—preoperative education, nutritional optimization, goal-directed fluid therapy, regional & TIVA anesthesia techniques, multimodal pain management, and early mobilization—work together to accelerate recovery, reduce complications, and shorten hospital stays. ERAS protocols have been successfully implemented across a variety of surgical specialties, as evidence continues to accumulate, the application of ERAS protocols will be refined and adopted to other surgical fields transforming the way perioperative care is delivered globally. The implementation of ERAS requires collaboration across multidisciplinary teams and a commitment to continuous quality improvement with anesthesiologists playing a central role. Future advances in digital health, precision medicine, and AI-guided perioperative care will further refine ERAS protocols.

References

1. Kehlet H, Wilmore DW. Multimodal strategies to improve surgical outcome. Am J Surg. 2002;183(6):630–41. https://doi.org/10.1016/s0002-9610(02)00866-8. PMID: 12095591
2. Ljungqvist O, Scott M, Fearon KC. Enhanced recovery after surgery: a review. JAMA Surg. 2017;152(3):292–8. https://doi.org/10.1001/jamasurg.2016.4952. PMID: 28097305
3. Desborough JP. The stress response to trauma and surgery. Br J Anaesth. 2000;85(1):109–17. https://doi.org/10.1093/bja/85.1.109. PMID: 10927999
4. Minto G, Mythen MG. Perioperative fluid management: science, art or random chaos? Br J Anaesth. 2015;114(5):717–21. https://doi.org/10.1093/bja/aev067. Epub 2015 Mar 19. PMID: 25794505
5. Gustafsson UO, Scott MJ, Hubner M, Nygren J, Demartines N, Francis N, Rockall TA, Young-Fadok TM, Hill AG, Soop M, de Boer HD, Urman RD, Chang GJ, Fichera A, Kessler H, Grass F, Whang EE, Fawcett WJ, Carli F, Lobo DN, Rollins KE, Balfour A, Baldini G, Riedel B, Ljungqvist O. Guidelines for perioperative care in elective colorectal surgery: enhanced recovery after surgery (ERAS®) society recommendations: 2018. World J Surg. 2019;43(3):659–95. https://doi.org/10.1007/s00268-018-4844-y. PMID: 30426190
6. Liu D, Zhu L, Yang C. The effect of preoperative smoking and smoke cessation on wound healing and infection in post-surgery subjects: a meta-analysis. Int Wound J. 2022;19(8):2101–6. https://doi.org/10.1111/iwj.13815. Epub 2022 Apr 22. Retraction in: Int Wound J. 2025;22(4):e70421. doi:10.1111/iwj.70421. PMID: 35451193; PMCID: PMC9705191
7. Wong J, Lam DP, Abrishami A, Chan MT, Chung F. Short-term preoperative smoking cessation and postoperative complications: a systematic review and meta-analysis. Can J Anaesth. 2012;59(3):268–79. https://doi.org/10.1007/s12630-011-9652-x. Epub 2011 Dec 21. PMID: 22187226
8. Demling RH. Nutrition, anabolism, and the wound healing process: an overview. Eplasty. 2009;9:e9. Epub 2009 Feb 3. PMID: 19274069; PMCID: PMC2642618
9. Carli F, Zavorsky GS. Optimizing functional exercise capacity in the elderly surgical population. Curr Opin Clin Nutr Metab Care. 2005;8(1):23–32. https://doi.org/10.1097/00075197-200501000-00005. PMID: 15585997
10. Martindale RG, McClave SA, Taylor B, Lawson CM. Perioperative nutrition. J Parenter Enteral Nutr. 2013;37:5S–20S. https://doi.org/10.1177/0148607113496821.
11. Bae E. Preoperative risk evaluation and perioperative management of patients with obstructive sleep apnea: a narrative review. J Dent Anesth Pain Med. 2023;23(4):179–92. https://doi.org/10.17245/jdapm.2023.23.4.179. Epub 2023 Jul 29. PMID: 37559666; PMCID: PMC10407451
12. Auckley D, Singh M. Protocolizing perioperative OSA screening and management: moving in the right direction. J Clin Sleep Med. 2022;18(8):1895–6. https://doi.org/10.5664/jcsm.10154. PMID: 35702018; PMCID: PMC9340586
13. Chung F, Abdullah HR, Liao P. STOP-bang questionnaire: a practical approach to screen for obstructive sleep apnea. Chest. 2016;149(3):631–8. https://doi.org/10.1378/chest.15-0903. Epub 2016 Jan 12. PMID: 26378880
14. Altree TJ, Chung F, Chan MTV, Eckert DJ. Vulnerability to postoperative complications in obstructive sleep apnea: importance of phenotypes. Anesth Analg. 2021;132(5):1328–37. https://doi.org/10.1213/ANE.0000000000005390. PMID: 33857975

15. Miller TE, Roche AM, Mythen M. Fluid management and goal-directed therapy as an adjunct to Enhanced Recovery After Surgery (ERAS). Can J Anaesth. 2015;62(2):158–68. https://doi.org/10.1007/s12630-014-0266-y. Epub 2014 Nov 13. PMID: 25391735
16. Mancel L, Van Loon K, Lopez AM. Role of regional anesthesia in Enhanced Recovery After Surgery (ERAS) protocols. Curr Opin Anaesthesiol. 2021;34(5):616–25. https://doi.org/10.1097/ACO.0000000000001048.
17. Ahmadzadeh Amiri A, Karvandian K, Ashouri M, Rahimi M, Ahmadzadeh AA. Comparação entre anestesia intravenosa e inalatória na náusea e vômito pós-operatórios em laparotomia: estudo clínico randomizado [Comparison of post-operative nausea and vomiting with intravenous versus inhalational anesthesia in laparotomic abdominal surgery: a randomized clinical trial]. Braz J Anesthesiol. 2020;70(5):471–6. https://doi.org/10.1016/j.bjan.2020.04.019. Epub 2020 Sep 6. PMID: 33032806; PMCID: PMC9373333
18. Little M, Tran V, Chiarella A, Wright ED. Total intravenous anesthesia vs inhaled anesthetic for intraoperative visualization during endoscopic sinus surgery: a double blind randomized controlled trial. Int Forum Allergy Rhinol. 2018;8(10):1123–6. https://doi.org/10.1002/alr.22129. Epub 2018 Sep 10. PMID: 30198644
19. Shimada K, Iwagami M, Makito K, Shigemi D, Uda K, Ishimaru M, Komiyama J, Morita K, Matsui H, Fushimi K, Yasunaga H, Tanaka M, Tamiya N. The comparison of caesarean section bleeding between volatile and total intravenous anaesthesia in a Japanese nationwide database. Eur J Anaesthesiol Intensive Care. 2023;2(2):e0021. https://doi.org/10.1097/EA9.0000000000000021. PMID: 39917593; PMCID: PMC11783640
20. Goode VM, Morgan B, Muckler VC, Cary MP Jr, Zdeb CE, Zychowicz M. Multimodal pain management for major joint replacement surgery. Orthop Nurs. 2019;38(2):150–6. https://doi.org/10.1097/NOR.0000000000000525. PMID: 30768538; PMCID: PMC6727971
21. O'Neill AM, Calpin GG, Norris L, Beirne JP. The impact of enhanced recovery after gynaecological surgery: a systematic review and meta-analysis. Gynecol Oncol. 2023;168:8–16. https://doi.org/10.1016/j.ygyno.2022.10.019.
22. Zhao Y, Zhang S, Liu B, et al. Clinical efficacy of enhanced recovery after surgery (ERAS) program in patients undergoing radical prostatectomy: a systematic review and meta-analysis. World J Surg Onc. 2020;18:131. https://doi.org/10.1186/s12957-020-01897-6.
23. McCarthy C, Fletcher N. Early extubation in enhanced recovery from cardiac surgery. Crit Care Clin. 2020;36(4):663–74. https://doi.org/10.1016/j.ccc.2020.06.005. Epub 2020 Aug 13. PMID: 32892820
24. Kelava M, Alfirevic A, Bustamante S, Hargrave J, Marciniak D. Regional anesthesia in cardiac surgery: an overview of fascial plane chest wall blocks. Anesth Analg. 2020;131(1):127–35. https://doi.org/10.1213/ANE.0000000000004682.
25. Huh YJ, Kim DJ. Enhanced recovery after surgery in bariatric surgery. J Metab Bariatr Surg. 2021;10(2):47–54. https://doi.org/10.17476/jmbs.2021.10.2.47. Epub 2021 Oct 21. PMID: 36683671; PMCID: PMC9847637
26. Lillemoe HA, Aloia TA. Enhanced recovery after surgery: hepatobiliary. Surg Clin North Am. 2018;98(6):1251–64. https://doi.org/10.1016/j.suc.2018.07.011. Epub 2018 Aug 24. PMID: 30390857; PMCID: PMC6345553
27. De Sousa MA. Effect of anesthesia on endoscopic sinus surgery hemostasis: a state-of-the-art review. Cureus. 2023;15(7):e42467. https://doi.org/10.7759/cureus.42467. PMID: 37637628; PMCID: PMC10450361
28. Feldheiser A, Aziz O, Baldini G, et al. Enhanced Recovery After Surgery (ERAS) for gastrointestinal surgery. Part 2: Consensus statement for anesthesia practice. Acta Anaesthesiol Scand. 2016;60(3):289–334.
29. Thiele RH, Rea KM, Turrentine FE, et al. Standardization of care: impact of an enhanced recovery protocol on length of stay, complications, and direct costs after colorectal surgery. J Am Coll Surg. 2015;220(4):430–43.

30. Scott MJ, McEvoy MD, Gordon DB, et al. American Society for Enhanced Recovery and Perioperative Quality Initiative joint consensus statement on perioperative opioid minimization in opioid-naive patients. Anesth Analg. 2017;125(5):1406–13.

Part III

The Anesthesiologist as Perioperative Operations Leader

7 The Science of OR Scheduling: Metrics, Governance, and Staffing Optimization

Fareeda Eraky, Rania Aziz, Faraz Chaudhry, Cynthia Tan, and George Tewfik

7.1 Introduction

Anesthesiologists sit at the center of perioperative operations, bridging clinical judgment with day-to-day organization of people, rooms, and information. This chapter frames the operating room (OR) as both a major revenue engine and a major cost center, grounds decisions in economic reality (fixed vs. variable costs and contribution margin), and uses key performance indicators (KPIs) (utilization, first-case readiness, turnover time, cancellations, and off-hours use) to guide action. We compare historical scheduling modalities with modern principles such as hybrid/block models, data-informed block assignment and release, and day-of case placement rules. We also review anesthesiologist-led operational leadership and the smart use of dashboards and electronic health record (EHR) workflows. Finally, we address add-on/emergency cases and after-hours policies, tying every operational change back to safety, surgeon and patient experience, optimizing favorable financial performance.

7.2 The Economics and Metrics of OR Utilization

The operating room is a complex environment requiring continuous interaction between anesthesiologists, surgeons, nurses, turnover teams, and, most importantly, patients. It is also a source of both high revenue and cost expenditure, often accounting for 35–40% of a hospital's costs and 60–70% of its revenue [1]. Cost of health

F. Eraky (✉) · R. Aziz · F. Chaudhry · G. Tewfik
Department of Anesthesiology, Rutgers New Jersey Medical School, Newark, NJ, USA
e-mail: fwe5@njms.rutgers.edu

C. Tan
Department of Anesthesiology, Perioperative Care and Pain Medicine, NYU Langone Health, New York, NY, USA

G. Tewfik (ed.), *The Anesthesiologist as Perioperative Leader*,
https://doi.org/10.1007/978-3-032-18058-2_7

care delivery is a major area of investigation, especially in the operating room. Although variability exists, historical cross-sectional longitudinal analysis estimated the mean cost of OR time as $36–37 per minute. Note that 40–45% of this cost was attributed to “indirect” components—described as costs from non-revenue centers outside the OR, such as security or parking allocated to the department [2]. This component is often not modifiable through changes in OR utilization and efficiency, which is relevant to the discussion in this chapter. Direct costs accounted for $20–21 per minute and include wages, benefits, supplies, and other miscellaneous categories. This study did not include costs from anesthesia administration, implants and tissue factors, blood bank operations, or radiographic and pathologic tests into the cost per minute of OR use [2].

A similar concept is highlighted by contrasting fixed and variable costs. Fixed costs attributed to buildings, salaried staff, and equipment are independent of case volume, whereas variable costs (disposable items, medications, etc.) are not [3]. Cost-effective use of operating rooms requires minimizing hours of under-utilized OR time to widely distribute fixed costs, while avoiding hours of over-utilized OR time. Under-utilized OR time refers to unused allocated hours. Over-utilized OR time is defined as time used outside of the number of allocated hours and is recorded in multiple studies to be a significant contributor to increased expenditure [4]. Furthermore, its contribution increases in significance as a day of scheduled cases approaches. This phenomenon is significant because under-utilization has a negligible increase in cost during a working day as compared to significant over-utilized time. As such, it is crucial to explore ways to more efficiently utilize allocated OR time daily.

Contribution margin, as discussed by Dr. Macario in the Journal of Clinical Anesthesia, is also important to consider in the context of OR economics. It is calculated by subtracting variable costs from the revenue generated from a case. A financial point of view deems a safe case with a positive contribution margin as worth doing. This reasoning comes into play when making decisions regarding add-on cases and block release schedules, discussed later in this chapter.

- Key performance indicators: utilization, turnover time, case start times, cancellations

To assess OR utilization and generate plans to increase efficiency, key performance indicators (KPI) must be identified. Allocated OR time, under-utilized time, and over-utilized time have been discussed above and serve as performance indicators in the context of inefficiency calculations (hours of under-utilized OR time multiplied by the cost per hour of under-utilized OR time, plus hours of over-utilized OR time multiplied by the cost per hour of over-utilized OR time) [4]. However, additional measures exist to assess OR performance.

First-case start accuracy is a commonly discussed and targeted performance indicator. It describes delays in start time of the first case and is used to assess the efficiency of preoperative processes. Many hospitals allow a 5-min grace period for case start times [5]. Dexter et al. suggest that first-case start times are often incorrectly used to assess outcomes and ineffectively targeted to improve OR efficiency [6]. This conclusion is based on the mixed evidence correlating delayed first-case starts to OR efficiency and increased hours of over-utilized OR time. Dexter et al. reported a lack of definitive correlation between first case start time and OR over-utilization when controlling for workload, and Pandit et al. found no correlation between late starts and late case completions [6, 7]. However, it remains a reflection of the effectiveness of preoperative preparation and readiness and can impact patient satisfaction or cancellations [8]. As such, the etiologies of delayed starts, as well as methods to improve first-case on-time starts will be discussed in this chapter.

Cancellations are another KPI assessed in the operational management of ORs. Cancellations are costly to healthcare institutions due to the possible creation of under-utilized time [9]. They also impact patient care and impose financial, emotional, and logistical burdens on patients [9]. Multiple studies have been conducted to assess causes of cancellations and ways to reduce their occurrence. The most commonly identified cause of surgical cancellation is change in medical condition prior to induction of anesthesia [10]. Other possible causes identified include airway problems, patient opinion or schedule, resource availability, or a lack of need for the procedure [10, 11]. This chapter discusses strategies to reduce surgical case cancellations including enhanced preoperative testing, accurate prediction of case length, and changes in cancellation policies.

Turnover time (TOT) is an important KPI to discuss in the context of OR metrics and improvement as it has significant impacts on utilization. TOT is defined as the time between which one patient is wheeled out of the OR until the next patient is wheeled in, however some studies describe it as the time between one closure and the following case incision [6, 12]. TOT varies significantly between hospitals and depends on factors like staffing, case complexity, surgeon involvement in the preparation process, equipment availability, and type of surgery. A reduction in TOT has been estimated to have a financial impact of over $2.5 million per OR per year by increasing the average throughput from 2.8 to 4 cases per day [12]. There are multiple strategies that have been identified to reduce TOT, including separating rooms by service or specialty, streamlining handover, and standardization of the process. Further discussion of these strategies will take place later in this chapter.

It is important to consider these metrics alongside each other rather than using just one to assess efficiency or utilization. Saving time is valuable when it prevents over-utilization **or** allows for an additional safe case with a positive contribution margin. Beyond the significant financial benefits, increased efficiency means increased patient/surgeon satisfaction, safety, morale, and staff retention. Although we explored the direct relationship between cost and OR management, these positive outcomes result in additional indirect financial benefit through factors like increasing hospital marketability and staff retention.

7.3 Governance and Structure of OR Management

Overview

The governance of operating rooms (ORs) defines how perioperative services are organized, how decisions are made, and how competing priorities are reconciled. Strong governance aligns the interests of surgeons, anesthesiologists, nursing, and administrators toward shared institutional goals: safety, efficiency, patient satisfaction, and financial sustainability. The structure of OR governance varies by institution, but nearly all successful models share three essential features:

1. A **Perioperative Services Committee (PSC)** with multidisciplinary oversight.
2. A clearly empowered **Medical Director of Perioperative Services (MDPS)**—most often an anesthesiologist.
3. **Collaborative operational dyads** linking surgical, nursing, and administrative leadership.

1. **The Perioperative Services Committee (PSC)**

The PSC (also called the OR Committee or Surgical Services Committee) is the **primary decision-making and policy-setting body** for perioperative operations. It is responsible for establishing operational policies, optimizing surgical scheduling, approving block allocations, and adjudicating disputes among surgical services.

Composition:
- Chair: Medical Director of Perioperative Services (typically anesthesiologist)
- Voting Members: Chief of Surgery, OR Nursing Director, Business/Finance Administrator
- Nonvoting Members: OR Manager, Scheduler, Infection Prevention, Quality, Materials Management

Core Responsibilities:
- Develop and enforce **OR scheduling policies** (block release, add-on criteria, cancellation rules).
- Review **performance metrics**—first-case on-time starts, turnover times, utilization rates, and delay causes.
- Oversee **equipment standardization** and capital requests.
- Review **staffing plans** and perioperative budgets.
- Evaluate quality and patient safety initiatives.

The PSC typically reports to the **Chief Medical Officer (CMO)** or **Hospital Operations Council**, integrating perioperative issues into broader institutional strategy.

2. **The Role of the Medical Director of Perioperative Services (MDPS)**

The MDPS acts as the **chief integrator** of perioperative operations, bridging the clinical, administrative, and financial domains of surgical services. This position is increasingly recognized as a **physician executive role**, with a scope akin to a service-line COO.

Key Functions:

- **Operational leadership**: Oversee OR scheduling, staffing, and daily flow management.
- **Strategic planning**: Align perioperative performance with hospital capacity management and service-line growth.
- **Quality and safety oversight**: Implement performance dashboards, root cause analysis, and peer review.
- **Financial stewardship**: Monitor utilization, budget adherence, and anesthesia subsidy economics.
- **Data governance**: Ensure the integrity and use of perioperative metrics from AIMS/EHR systems.
- **Conflict resolution**: Serve as a neutral intermediary between surgeons, anesthesiology, and nursing.

Skill Set:

Effective MDPS leaders combine **clinical credibility** with training in **healthcare management, quality improvement, or business administration**. The ASA and AORN jointly recommend leadership training in lean process improvement, data analytics, and interdepartmental negotiation.

3. **Collaboration Among Surgery, Nursing, and Administration**

Successful perioperative governance depends on **shared governance**—a model emphasizing mutual accountability and data transparency among surgical, anesthesia, and nursing leadership (Fig. 7.1).

Joint metrics—like **OR utilization, first-case on-time starts**, and **PACU hold times**—should be **shared, reviewed, and acted upon** at monthly PSC meetings (sample metrics in Table 7.1). Institutions that embed **real-time dashboards** (Epic OpTime or custom analytics) demonstrate measurable improvements in throughput and cost control.

Discipline	Primary Focus	Governance Contribution
Surgery	Case access, block ownership, service-line growth	Defines case prioritization and elective volume strategy
Anesthesiology	Safety, throughput, resource utilization	Oversees scheduling fairness, efficiency metrics, and staffing plans
Nursing	Workflow, staffing, infection control	Ensures operational feasibility and team readiness
Administration	Financial performance, capacity management	Aligns perioperative metrics with institutional goals

Fig. 7.1 Sample of organizational shared governance that outlines the focus and contributions of various specialties to perioperative function

Table 7.1 Sample perioperative dashboard layout *(Performance Metrics Dashboard for PSC Oversight)*

Metric	Definition	Target/ Benchmark	Responsible stakeholders	Reporting frequency
First-Case On-Time Start Rate	% of scheduled first cases that start within 5 min of scheduled time	>85%	MDPS, Surgery, Nursing	Weekly
Turnover Time	Time between patient exit and next patient entry	<25 min	Nursing, Anesthesia	Weekly
Block Utilization	Percentage of allocated block time used productively	>80%	Surgical Services, Administration	Monthly
Case Cancellation Rate	% of cases cancelled within 24 h	<3%	PSC (multidisciplinary)	Monthly
PACU Boarding Time	Average time PACU patients wait for inpatient beds	<60 min	Nursing, Bed Management	Weekly
Staffing Match Index	Ratio of available anesthesia staff to scheduled cases	>95%	Anesthesia Department	Daily
Equipment Downtime	% of cases delayed due to equipment issues	<1%	Biomedical/OR Manager	Monthly

7.4 Scheduling Models and Principles

Suggested optimal levels of utilization for ORs are between 75% and 80% [13]. Scheduling of elective cases is complex and involves short, medium, and long-term decision making ranging from real-time changes based on add-on caseload to dedicating OR time to services months in advance [14]. The management of block schedules typically follows one of three systems: block, open, and modified/hybrid scheduling strategies. Block systems allocate OR time and resources to certain services/providers who can schedule their cases within those timeframes. Open schedules allow flexibility for surgeons to schedule any cases in any OR at any time. Modified/hybrid schedules combine the simplicity and organization of block schedules with the flexibility of open schedules, with many organizations in the country using a hybrid schedule [13, 14]. Block schedules are usually modified after a review periods of a couple months based on historical average use by the block occupant [13]. However, this does not take into consideration the extent of over or under-utilization by surgeons/services. Hosseini et al. proposed the use of a linear-programming-based block allocation model that addresses variability in demand over 12 months rather than average use over a shorter period [13].

Aside from the medium-term allocations, block release can frequently occur on the day of surgery. Block release may be voluntary, but predetermined release times have been commonly used to give away unused block time based on how far in advance a service schedules cases [15]. A service that schedules cases weeks in advance would have a predetermined release time that is more distant from the operating day. With regards to case placement on the day of surgery, Dexter et al. recommend the following strategies to prevent under or over utilization: prioritizing scheduling within allocated block time before creating overtime elsewhere, not using overtime if another service has open block time, and shuffling cases between a service's own blocked ORs to prevent overtime. Based on these measures, the authors recommend against the use of predetermined release time without assessing a day's demands [16].

7.5 Anesthesiologist's Operational Leadership

The preoperative period is a heavily investigated topic due to its impact on OR efficiency and utilization. Case readiness has significant effects on individual patients as well as the overall OR schedule. Key performance indicators including first-case-on-time starts and cancellations are strongly influenced by optimized preoperative testing, patient education, provider availability and the use of well-defined preoperative protocols. Anesthesiologists are often considered leaders of the preoperative process on the day of surgery as they evaluate patients, prepare the OR, and make decisions on cancellations and delays. In fact, multiple studies have linked anesthesiologist availability and supervision ratios to case delays and patient safety. Having a ratio of one anesthesiologist per three rooms makes it unlikely for first cases to begin on time while ensuring adequate supervision during critical periods [17]. The financial benefits of having a supervision ratio of 1:3 are also offset by the need of an additional provider to help provide breaks [17]. Epstein et al. recommend a supervision ratio of 1:2 with an extra floating anesthesiologist at the beginning of the day, or implementation of staggered starts [17]. Beyond the day of surgery, increased involvement of anesthesiologists in preoperative testing and optimization has positive impacts on efficiencies and KPIs.

After surgeon/anesthesiologist unavailability, incomplete preoperative patient testing or evaluation and need for sedation or anxiety medications are the most common causes of case cancellations [18]. Fischer et al. explore the idea of heavily involving anesthesiologists in the preoperative testing process. The study describes the process of developing an anesthesiologist-run preoperative testing clinic and its effects on patient care and KPIs in the OR. At this clinic, clinicians reviewed the patients' medical record, prescribed and completed required tests on site, and provided recommendations to surgeons on how to best optimize patients for their procedures. After implementation of this strategy, the investigators found an 87.9% decrease in same day cancellations and a 55.1% decrease in tests ordered, reducing costs for patients and hospitals. Starting to review medical records during clinic instead of on the day of admission reduced delays and costs to the hospital. This process is also more convenient for patients as it allows them to complete their preoperative evaluation at one location under the oversight of one physician [19]. Furthermore, patient education at anesthesiology-run preoperative clinics ensures patient readiness and decreases the likelihood of cancellations due to unexpected violations of anesthesia-related instructions regarding fasting, reporting time, and medication use [5].

Aside from efficient preoperative testing, changes implemented in the immediate perioperative period on the day of surgery can reduce cancellation rates and increase on-time starts. Cases are often delayed or cancelled due to factors including staff unavailability, inadequate preoperative testing, poor patient preparation, transport delay, missing paperwork, and equipment readiness [5]. Alter et al. explored the implementation of preoperative "team huddle" 15 min prior to the start of a case with the goal of reducing delays caused by staff tardiness. The intervention involved documenting reasons for delay in the EHR to be reviewed weekly by a committee responsible for sending emails to staff with late arrivals. The huddle aimed to mitigate issues caused by the lack of standardized reporting time for many OR staff and improve communication between interdisciplinary teams [8]. It is recommended that a thorough discussion of the case and equipment selection be done during the huddle since a statistically significant relationship exists between room readiness and on-time starts [5, 20]. Although this setup is not ideal for attending anesthesiologists responsible for more than one OR, the authors propose that the buffer between the huddle start time and case start allows physicians to attend more than one huddle. The study reported an improvement of on-time starts from 58% to 80% [8].

Attempting to implement a staggered start to prevent delays caused by anesthesiologists juggling multiple rooms failed, possibly due to underestimating the time needed for a safe induction and creating confusion in the schedule [8]. Some studies suggest that specifically targeting surgeon punctuality has a significant relationship to on-time starts and equipment readiness [5, 8, 20]. Even with the introductions of protocols to promote efficiency, delayed and overtime surgeries will occur. It is suggested that cancelling overtime cases is less profitable than completing them, and changes in cancellation policy to reflect this concept could be financially beneficial. However, effects on morale and staff retention should be taken into consideration in these situations [9]. Lastly, dedicating an OR for emergency cases has been shown to decrease cancellation rates, which will be discussed later in this chapter.

7.6 Turnover Time and Throughput Improvement

Throughput, an industrial metric used to assess the flow of material through a system, has been applied to assess and improve OR efficiency. As such, other business models like Six Sigma and Lean Methodology have been used in OR management and coordination [20]. Six Sigma methodologies are used to define, measure, analyze, improve, and control issues and interventions [20]. Lean strategies identify the patient as the "customer" and explore ways to eliminate waste in OR throughput, while providing satisfactory service [21]. Value Stream Mapping (VSM), a specific lean management method, was used to decrease patient waiting time and turnover time in one study by Schwarz et al. Based on this model, non-value adding parts of OR flow, like waiting time, were minimized. One example from this investigation was the use of an anesthesia induction room outside the room for inducing and intubating the patient while staff finalized the room setup. The investigation showed a statistically significant 21% decrease in throughput time and turnover time in the group utilizing VSM-based workflow, compared to the non-optimized group. This has a potentially significant impact on revenue as the authors estimated the possibility of conducting an additional 1257 cases annually without additional cost [22].

Six Sigma methodologies are also promising in the operational management of OR efficiency and utilization, and were shown to decrease turnover time in a study that targeted reducing waste related to transportation, motion, waiting, and overproduction [20, 21]. Fairbanks et al. experimented with using the PACU as a staging center prior to cases instead of a "holding" ward or area on a different floor. This resulted in a decrease in holding time and turnover time, as well as well as an increase in on-time starts. The authors attributed this to eliminating transport time and phone calls to determine patient readiness and increased availability of anesthesiologists and surgeons to answer OR staff questions or administer medications or nerve blocks [20].

Turnover time was also shown to significantly decrease in rooms with the same specialty cases, anesthesiologist, surgeon, and nursing staff for consecutive procedures, although it tends to be influenced by case complexity as well [23]. This improved workflow and preparedness is likely due to the staff's familiarity with case types, surgeon preferences on positioning and equipment, and an established collaborative team. The standardization of handoffs has also been explored as a means of improving turnover time and throughput. The use of checklists and a standardized protocol separating physical patient and equipment handoff from information transfer resulted in a statistically insignificant decrease in handoff time [24]. However, it was shown to positively influence quality of care and decrease omission of information. This was primarily achieved by aligning prioritized information of the PACU and OR staff. Most importantly, standardized handoffs increased safety and quality of care without negatively impacting turnover time of overall throughput.

7.7 Leveraging Data and Technology

The Data-Driven Operating Room

Modern operating rooms are information ecosystems. Every patient encounter, case delay, turnover event, and staffing decision generates data that can be captured, analyzed, and used to improve performance. The perioperative environment—rich in structured timestamps, physiological data, and workflow events—has become one of the most digitally instrumented areas in healthcare. Leveraging this data effectively requires an integration of **real-time monitoring tools, predictive analytics, and interoperable electronic health records (EHRs)** to transform raw information into operational intelligence.

Real-Time OR Management Software and Dashboards

Real-time OR management platforms have evolved from simple case tracking boards into sophisticated, analytics-enabled command centers. These systems—such as Epic OpTime Analytics, Cerner Dynamic Documentation, and specialized platforms like LiveData, iQueue for Operating Rooms (LeanTaaS), or Surgical Directions' OR Control Tower—aggregate live data from scheduling, anesthesia records, and nursing documentation to provide a unified operational view.

Key functionalities include:

- **Live Case Tracking**: Visualization of case progress, turnover times, and room status across all operating suites.
- **Alerting and Escalation**: Automated notifications for delayed starts, missing consents, or equipment readiness issues.
- **Throughput Analytics**: Real-time dashboards showing OR utilization, room idle time, and staffing efficiency.
- **Decision Support**: AI-enabled forecasting modules that identify underutilized blocks, suggest reallocation, or predict overcapacity.

These systems enable a "mission control" model for perioperative leadership, allowing anesthesiologists, nurse managers, and administrators to coordinate dynamically. For example, when a procedure runs long, the dashboard can automatically suggest moving a subsequent case to a parallel room or extending anesthesia coverage, avoiding idle staff and patient cancellations. Hospitals that adopt such technology consistently report reductions in **first-case delays by 15–30% and turnover time improvements of 10–20%**.

Predictive Analytics to Optimize Scheduling

Traditional OR scheduling relies heavily on historical averages and subjective input from surgeons. Predictive analytics introduces a data science framework that uses machine learning algorithms to anticipate case duration, staff availability, and patient flow bottlenecks. Inputs include procedure codes, surgeon-specific time distributions, anesthesia type, and historical turnover data.

Applications include:

- **Case Duration Prediction**: Statistical modeling (e.g., random forests or gradient boosting) to forecast case length more accurately than static time estimates.
- **Dynamic Block Allocation**: Algorithms analyze utilization trends and recommend reassignments to maximize OR capacity.
- **Cancellations and No-Show Forecasting**: Predictive models identify cases at risk for same-day cancellations, enabling proactive intervention (e.g., confirming consent, verifying labs, or ensuring anesthesia clearance).
- **Staffing Forecasts**: Anticipating peak periods to align anesthesia provider and nursing schedules with expected demand.

The Role of Electronic Health Records in Workflow Coordination

Electronic Health Records (EHRs) are the digital backbone of perioperative communication. When properly integrated, the EHRlinks preoperative assessment, intraoperative documentation, and postoperative care into a seamless continuum. Yet EHRs can also create bottlenecks if data is siloed or inaccessible to operational systems.

Modern perioperative EHR modules now provide:

- **Preoperative Readiness Indicators**: Flags for incomplete evaluations, labs, or consents, visible to scheduling staff and anesthesiologists in real time.
- **Automated Handoffs**: Structured, standardized handoff templates (SBAR or IPASS) embedded in anesthesia documentation improves continuity and safety.
- **Cross-System Interoperability**: Integration with patient flow and bed management software ensures that PACU discharge readiness automatically triggers inpatient bed requests.
- **Metadata Utilization**: EHR metadata—such as time stamps, keystrokes, and documentation intervals—can be analyzed to identify workflow inefficiencies and cognitive load.

When combined with OR dashboards, EHR-integrated analytics create a **closed-loop feedback system**: data flows from the point of care to management dashboards and back to frontline providers, allowing rapid cycle improvement. For anesthesiologists, this integration elevates their role from proceduralists to **information stewards and systems leaders**, capable of shaping the operational and financial performance of the entire surgical enterprise.

Data and technology have transformed perioperative medicine from a reactive to a predictive discipline. By adopting real-time dashboards, predictive analytics, and EHR-integrated workflows, anesthesiologists can drive measurable improvements in **efficiency, safety, and economic value**. The perioperative physician's future role will hinge not only on clinical skill but on fluency in interpreting and leveraging data to design smarter, more resilient surgical systems.

7.8 Managing Emergency and After-Hours Cases

Aside from existing challenges for OR scheduling due to patient, staff, and resource management, unpredictable emergent cases add a layer of complexity to the process [14]. Policies regarding scheduling emergent cases and balancing them with elective caseload have been a major area of research [25]. Logistical management of the OR must be rooted in the delivery of safe, effective, efficient, and equitable care. Debates often occur between major strategies used to manage add-on cases. Some hospitals schedule add-on cases after completion of elective cases or by rearranging elective case schedules [25]. Others dedicate an OR for emergent/urgent add-on cases [25, 26]. Heng et al. suggest that this dedicated OR should be available for add-on cases of multiple services due to some hospitals having inadequate volume to dedicate the room to one service. This is in contrast to having a dedicated surgical team for the OR from one specific service, which could mitigate issues surrounding surgeon availability [25].

While prompt completion of urgent and emergent operations promotes patient safety, it should aim to be done in a way that positively impacts OR utilization and minimizes harm to those scheduled for elective procedures. Many investigations compared scheduling policies using simulation models; however, recent experimental studies suggest that dedicating an operating room for add-on cases is the superior strategy [26]. Veen-Berkx et al. compared 2 centers with a dedicated room for emergencies to one where the emergency OR was converted to a "virtual team" with allocated capacity in all elective ORs. The investigation found that closing the dedicated emergency OR increased utilization *and* overtime, as compared to the control centers with a dedicated OR that saw increased utilization with *decreased* overtime. Additionally, the ratio of cancellations attributed to the addition of an emergency case decreased in centers with a dedicated room [26]. Given the cost of over-utilization and over time, these findings favor the utilization of a separate OR room for emergencies to increase OR efficiency. A similar study found that implementation of a dedicated OR significantly improved waiting time for priority three emergency cases (those whose waiting time is recommended to be <12 h). The average waiting time dropped from 11 h and 8 min under the management of a "virtual emergency team" to 10 h and 5 min using a dedicated emergency OR resulting in a 6% increase in the number of patients who got surgery within their recommended timeframe [25]. With regard to OR utilization and elective cases, this intervention resulted in a statistically significant decrease in cancellations caused by emergency cases from 1.5% to 0.7% and a decrease in emergent cases performed in the evening or nighttime [25].

7.9 Anesthesiologists as Change Agents

As one of the key players in OR management, anesthesiologists are in a unique position to lead cultural changes toward accountability and efficiency. Their mastery of balancing structure and flexibility is necessary in managing complex OR schedules. As physicians, anesthesiologists have a unique understanding of both the surgical process and operational management. As shown by Fischer et al., initiatives led by anesthesiologists, like the creation of a preoperative clinic, have significant positive impacts on OR utilization, institutional finances, patient outcomes, and patient satisfaction [19]. Additionally, the creation of an anesthesiologist-led preoperative huddle has been shown to decrease delays and promote on-time starts [8]. Furthermore, both interventions promoted a sense of team work and promoted a sense of collaboration with surgical colleagues [8, 19]. The role of anesthesiologists in leading OR schedule management varies across institutions with involvement often being greater at academic centers [27].

7.10 Summary and Key Takeaways

Effective perioperative leadership by anesthesiologists promotes OR efficiency and positive patient outcomes through fewer preventable cancellations, more reliable starts, faster but safer turnovers, and fewer hours of over-utilized time. The throughline of this chapter is an integration of disciplined economics with practical governance. Some discussed concepts include allocating and releasing blocks with variability in mind, defining clear problems with interventions, and prioritizing moves that either avoid overtime or enable an additional safe case with a positive contribution margin. Standardized handoffs and Lean/VSM keep flow predictable, real-time dashboards and accountable huddles sustain change, and a thoughtfully staffed daytime add-on pathway protects both elective and urgent care. Taken together, these strategies build trust with surgical colleagues, improve staff morale and retention, and strengthen institutional finances, showcasing the strategic value of anesthesiologists as the essential perioperative physicians.

References

1. Ramme AJ, Hutzler LH, Cerfolio RJ, Bosco JA. Applying systems engineering to increase operating room efficiency. Bull Hosp Jt Dis (2013). 2020;78(1):26–32. https://www.ncbi.nlm.nih.gov/pubmed/32144960.
2. Childers CP, Maggard-Gibbons M. Understanding costs of care in the operating room. JAMA Surg. 2018;153(4):e176233. https://doi.org/10.1001/jamasurg.2017.6233.
3. Macario A. What does one minute of operating room time cost? J Clin Anesth. 2010;22(4):233–6. https://doi.org/10.1016/j.jclinane.2010.02.003.
4. Dexter F, Epstein RH. Operating room efficiency and scheduling. Curr Opin Anaesthesiol. 2005. https://journals.lww.com/co-anesthesiology/pages/articleviewer.aspx?year=2005&issue=04000&article=00015&type=Fulltext.
5. Rothstein DH, Raval MV. Operating room efficiency. Semin Pediatr Surg. 2018;27(2):79–85. https://doi.org/10.1053/j.sempedsurg.2018.02.004.
6. Dexter F, Epstein RH. Fundamentals of operating room allocation and case scheduling to minimize the inefficiency of use of the time. Perioper Care Oper Room Manag. 2024. https://www.sciencedirect.com/science/article/abs/pii/S240560302400013X.
7. Pandit JJ, Abbott T, Pandit M, Kapila A, Abraham R. Is 'starting on time' useful (or useless) as a surrogate measure for 'surgical theatre efficiency?'. Anaesthesia. 2012;67(8):823–32. https://doi.org/10.1111/j.1365-2044.2012.07160.x.

8. Alter J, Estright A, Platten M, et al. Improving on-time surgical starts through a perioperative stop and huddle. Perioper Care Oper Room Manag. 2025;38. https://www.sciencedirect.com/science/article/pii/S2405603024000918.
9. van Veen-Berkx E, Elkhuizen SG, van Logten S, et al. Enhancement opportunities in operating room utilization; with a statistical appendix. J Surg Res. 2015;194(1):43–51.e1–2. https://doi.org/10.1016/j.jss.2014.10.044.
10. Lau HK, Chen TH, Liou CM, Chou MC, Hung WT. Retrospective analysis of surgery postponed or cancelled in the operating room. J Clin Anesth. 2010;22(4):237–40. https://doi.org/10.1016/j.jclinane.2009.10.005.
11. Turunen E, Miettinen M, Setala L, Vehvilainen-Julkunen K. Elective surgery cancellations during the time between scheduling and operation. J Perianesth Nurs. 2019;34(1):97–107. https://doi.org/10.1016/j.jopan.2017.09.014.
12. MacMillan L, Madura GM, Elliot M, et al. What affects operating room turnover time? A systematic review and mapping of the evidence. Surgery. 2025;181:109263. https://doi.org/10.1016/j.surg.2025.109263.
13. Hosseini N, Taaffe KM. Allocating operating room block time using historical caseload variability. Health Care Manag Sci. 2015;18(4):419–30. https://doi.org/10.1007/s10729-014-9269-z.
14. Al Amin M, Baldacci R, Kayvanfar V. A comprehensive review on operating room scheduling and optimization. Oper Res. 2024;25(1). https://doi.org/10.1007/s12351-024-00884-z.
15. Patterson P. A few simple rules for managing block time in the operating room. OR Manager. 2004;20(11):1, 9–10, 12. https://www.ncbi.nlm.nih.gov/pubmed/15581240.
16. Dexter F, Traub RD. How to schedule elective surgical cases into specific operating rooms to maximize the efficiency of use of operating room time. Anesth Analg. 2002;94(4):933–42, table of contents. https://doi.org/10.1097/00000539-200204000-00030.
17. Epstein RH, Dexter F. Influence of supervision ratios by anesthesiologists on first-case starts and critical portions of anesthetics. Anesthesiology. 2012;116(3):683–91. https://doi.org/10.1097/ALN.0b013e318246ec24.
18. Wright JG, Roche A, Khoury AE. Improving on-time surgical starts in an operating room. Can J Surg. 2010;53(3):167–70. https://www.ncbi.nlm.nih.gov/pubmed/20507788.
19. Fischer SP. Development and effectiveness of an anesthesia preoperative evaluation clinic in a teaching hospital. Anesthesiology. 1996;85(1):196–206. https://doi.org/10.1097/00000542-199607000-00025.
20. Fairbanks CB. Using Six Sigma and Lean methodologies to improve OR throughput. AORN J. 2007;86(1):73–82. https://doi.org/10.1016/j.aorn.2007.06.011.
21. Robinson ST, Kirsch JR. Lean strategies in the operating room. Anesthesiol Clin. 2015;33(4):713–30. https://doi.org/10.1016/j.anclin.2015.07.010.
22. Schwarz P, Pannes KD, Nathan M, et al. Lean processes for optimizing OR capacity utilization: prospective analysis before and after implementation of value stream mapping (VSM). Langenbecks Arch Surg. 2011;396(7):1047–53. https://doi.org/10.1007/s00423-011-0833-4.
23. Sarpong K, Kamande S, Murray J, et al. Consecutive surgeon and anesthesia team improve turnover time in the operating room. J Med Syst. 2022;46(3):16. https://doi.org/10.1007/s10916-022-01802-6.
24. McFarlane A. The impact of standardised perioperative handover protocols. J Perioper Pract. 2018;28(10):258–62. https://doi.org/10.1177/1750458918775555.
25. Heng M, Wright JG. Dedicated operating room for emergency surgery improves access and efficiency. Can J Surg. 2013;56(3):167–74. https://doi.org/10.1503/cjs.019711.
26. van Veen-Berkx E, Elkhuizen SG, Kuijper B, Kazemier G, Dutch Operating Room Benchmarking C. Dedicated operating room for emergency surgery generates more utilization, less overtime, and less cancellations. Am J Surg. 2016;211(1):122–8. https://doi.org/10.1016/j.amjsurg.2015.06.021.
27. Marjamaa RA, Kirvelä OA. Who is responsible for operating room management and how do we measure how well we do it? Acta Anaesthesiol Scand. 2007;51(7):809–14. (In eng). https://doi.org/10.1111/j.1399-6576.2007.01368.x.

Perioperative Management of the Surgical Service Line

8

Donna Kucharski

8.1 Introduction

A surgical service line is the organization and coordination of patient care around a set of similar or related surgical procedures typically using ICD-10 procedure codes. The range and expanse of a service line varies by the entity creating or considering the service line. Entities may be interested in only those elements where there is financial control and responsibility including the transference of risk or organizations taking financial risk. Others, such as professional organizations, may use a definition that includes all aspects which influence patient long-term outcomes. The surgical service line spans the perioperative events from preoperative through the intraoperative, immediate postoperative and short- and long-term recovery. This service line will include operational, financial, and strategic management of the patient pathway elements that serve the organizational strategy.

The surgical service line exists within the management system of a hospital or health care system possessing clinical, operational, financial, and strategic elements of the organization. Administration of the operational, financial, and strategic aspects of the service line are often opaque to the clinical providers involved. The opacity often renders surgeons and anesthesiologists unable to consider and potentially execute changes likely to be advantageous to patient outcomes. By extension physicians are unable to make suggestions concerning the operational and financial well-being of the enterprise. Michael Nurok, MBChB, Thoralf Sundt, MD, Robert S. Kaplan, PhD, and Bruce Gewertz, MD wrote in a 2021 Annals of Surgery *Surgical Perspectives* article of the progress toward value-based care which "create(s) incentives for hospitals to reduce their costs without affecting the quality of the services [1]. These authors also emphasize the need for "more strategic and deliberate partnerships between administrators and clinicians, particularly surgeons, interventionalists and perioperative physicians whose work relies on a large portion of hospital

D. Kucharski (✉)
Southcoast Health, Fall River, MA, USA

G. Tewfik (ed.), *The Anesthesiologist as Perioperative Leader*,
https://doi.org/10.1007/978-3-032-18058-2_8

material and human resources." Physicians hold the clinical expertise and expert knowledge for best evidence-based clinical care although they may not have the financial and accounting knowledge to understand the relation of the clinical work to the financial reports. Physicians have moved toward value creation through studies "by defining and achieving relevant quality and utilization metrics that help to reduce cost while maintaining excellent clinical outcomes" [2].

The objective of this chapter is to present some of the current concepts from both of the clinical and administrative viewpoints—first steps in gaining perspective to understand the totality of the health care environment. "Hospital leaders need to appreciate all perioperative processes and phases as parts of an interconnected, integrated whole" [3]. Leaders and managers from all stages of the service line must work together to ensure adequate input, create accountability, and reduce conflict "in a more strategic and deliberate partnership" [1].

8.2 The Perioperative Physicians' Perspective

Physicians' sphere of expertise and immediate influence begins with the knowledge developed surrounding risk and risk mitigation for a variety of conditions and morbidities. The preoperative patient analysis, testing, and potential optimizing interventions can be critically important in those patients found to have high-risk morbidities. Analysis of patient risk in the immediate preoperative time frame should include considerations of the accomplished preoperative diagnostic workup and preconditioning. The operative anesthetic plan intends to minimize morbidities and optimize the post-operative course. Practice guidelines and advisories are developed through coordination of multiple clinical experts of varied experience and training to inform clinicians of evidence-based care. This evidence-based knowledge provides best practice process pathways such as surgical site infection prevention, avoidance of renal dysfunction, optimization of early extubation, and pain control. The surgical service line typically has incorporated many of these routinely applied activities and facilitated their timely and efficient execution. High level execution of these best practices serves to minimize intraoperative variability, similar to that of a high reliability organization (HRO). Sutcliffe [4] notes contextual similarities between High Reliability Organization settings and that of anesthesia and perioperative care: high interdependence of various aspects of the organizational system, a continuously changing environment, non-routine work, interactive complexity, hidden, unanticipated or unintended consequences of small problems.

The advantages of HRO created by optimized protocols include decreased variability and increased constancy and efficiency for improved performance of the organization. However, market changes and patient variability present continuous fluctuation to circumstances that require a constant adaptive strategy on both the intraoperative, perioperative and management levels. Huynh et al. note that "Perioperative care is a two-tiered system composed of factory-like processes and complex adaptive processes" [5]. In addition to the external factors such as regulatory changes and contractional requirements, those patients who carry a high-risk profile due to multiple comorbidities, advanced disease states, or emergency status, require real-time complex care decision making for unique individual patient pathology. The level of care implied in the complex adaptive system is an adaptive skill learned by anesthesiologists and presents the unique care decisions dictated by both the daily variance of the practice environment and each patient's unique physiology. Furthermore, because the function within a Complex Adaptive System differs from a process model, "the relevant measure of this performance is the agility defined as the speed and ease with which providers adapt and learn as context changes" [6].

Incorporation of these principles across the surgical service line requires coordination among a variety of providers. The span of the surgical episode of care begins with the consideration of surgical readiness with internists and specialists to maximize the patient's optimization in any time frame. These time frames may range from hours from an emergency room door to the operating suite when intravascular fluid resuscitation, and pain control are among the few options, to weeks for patient preparation. This longer time horizon includes the possibility of modification of comorbidities such as improved diabetic control, iron deficiency correction, nutritional evaluation and medication optimization.

Each surgical service line should optimize the episode to current evidence to ensure de-implementation of low-value care such as excessive labs and imaging [7]. Common elements of the preoperative efforts include patient history and risk assessment, shared decision-making and planning for anesthesia and surgery, optimization of modifiable conditions, longitudinal care planning of surgical venue, care transitions and discharge planning [8]. The metrics used for evaluation of surgical service line episodes often extend beyond morbidity and cancelation rates. More recent regulatory efforts have focused on readmission rates and cost. Choice of metrics for each surgical service line should present a focus on those interventions most likely to improve patient long and short-term outcomes and prevent postoperative adverse events [8].

Some institutions have the patient volume and resources required to develop and sustain free standing preoperative assessment and optimization processes. Aronson et al. [9] report the evolution of the preanesthesia clinic into the perioperative anesthesia and surgical screeding clinic (PASS) where the readiness of each patient is evaluated considering the planned procedure and morbidities, then referred to the perioperative enhancement team (POET) if advised. The implementation of the PASS clinic occurred in parallel to the preanesthesia clinic, allowing the day-to-day operations of the PAC preoperative anesthesia clinic to allow stable function of the preoperative process as new methodology was developed and tested [9].

The model of implementation in parallel with existing processes illustrates work described by Kotter in Accelerate (XLR8) when a new process is tested in parallel to the existing process to maintain stability of the organization, during which time an agile process is used to develop the new model [10]. There are two important points to make concerning implementation in parallel to existing structure. First, the maintenance of a stable functioning process is facilitated by regular communications and maintenance of current processes that work well [11]. The second consideration is the recognition of the agile process as a Clinical Practice Improvement (CPI) effort. The bridge between new scientific knowledge and evidence-based medicine is the design of a CPI using new knowledge to improve patient outcomes [12]. It is noteworthy that the CPI process is not confined to the clinical working of the surgical service line but is also found at the management levels when dealing with new operations functions, onboarding of new technology and in some financial planning. The agile functions discussed by Kotter for continuous improvement allows the implementation of changes that are dictated by ongoing data and conditions. Amy Edmonson [13] introduced the Learning Organization as "execution as learning" where changes in the work process are tentatively implemented, feedback obtained, and changes tailored for success. The traditional process of "execution as efficiency" implements change designed by persons remote to the work and without the input of those close to the process. The author presents four steps for "execution as learning": first provide the process guidelines, second provide tools for that enable employees to collaborate in real time, third, collect process data, and fourth, institutionalize discipled reflection [13].

8.3 The C-Suite

The C-Suite bears the responsibility of guiding the corporation or enterprise to successfully carry out their strategic plan. That success requires meeting the financial requirements of profitability, regulatory demands and payor demands, while addressing the patients' needs. Within the management system of a hospital or health care system the surgical service line is structured to profitably provide the operational, financial and strategic elements for the patient clinical pathway. As healthcare continues transformation to value, the CEO, COO, and CFO functions have become more integrated as the value transformation demands more consideration of the interdependence of business and clinical aspects created by episodes of care.

The impact of clinical operations on hospital profitability is evaluated to format a surgical service pathway with elements predicted to be profitable. Past underperformance of value-based contracting is thought to be secondary to complexity of health care, misalignment of measures, and inadequate financial incentives [14]. Current work in this space has focused on cost reductions through implementation of best practice methodologies. Earlier research presented evidence that "the occurrence of postsurgical complications was associated with a higher per-encounter hospital contribution margin for patients covered by Medicare and private insurance" [15]. A direct comparison between patients with and without a defined set of complications demonstrated that "patients developing complications stay longer in the hospital and incur increased costs that outpace the increase in received payments" thereby negatively impacting hospital profitability and patient outcomes [16].

The most efficient means of decreasing the cost associated with surgical complications is through prevention. Stokes et al. [17] used ACS NSQIP definitions of outcomes and complications to further define the increased cost of surgical complications through cost evaluation in three models. Groups were compared by ASA status, functional status, and comorbidities. They conclude that "any strategy (preoperative, perioperative, or postoperative) which decreases complication rates will be able to significantly reduce associated costs." Glotzbach et al. illustrated that attainment of "perfect cardiac care" through the use of a 10-point list of goals did improve patient outcomes although the cost savings was not significant. Avoidance of excessive spending on complications is an important advancement [2]. Mahajan and Mythen [18] note the importance of defining and standardizing outcomes after surgery. They present the Core Outcomes Measures in Perioperative and Anesthetic Care noting the five domains of outcomes, derived by consensus: (1)—mortality/survival, (2)—perioperative complications, (3)—resource use, (4)—short-term recovery, and (5)—long-term recovery [19].

Implementation of EBPOM in all stages of the surgical service line both allows for alignment of performance measures and increases their relevance in VBHC. On the clinical level, efforts exist to standardize outcomes and performance measures allowing more fruitful comparisons and potential benchmarking. On the administrative level, monitoring of operational and financial data and continuous improvement activities both informs, and can create, an optimized cost analysis and potentially determine cost effectiveness.

The service line includes clinical, operational, and financial considerations across all departmental considerations involved in the delivery of the given surgical service. A bundled payment is a payment model that groups together all of the services associated with that episode of care. An initial service line evaluation sets the strategic planning and governance footprint. The strategic concerns of the enterprise must be served by the functions of the clinical, operational, and financial arms, yet the strategic goals must be aligned with the functional realities of these arms. Together, they determine a path forward to serve the continuum of care of the population with whom they have established a relationship. As the move from fee-for-service continues, surgical service lines can provide specialty focus for an episode of care. "By focusing on specific procedures or medical conditions and defining an episode of care, bundled payments provide a way for specialty provider organizations to engage in value-based payment in a manner that is aligned with their influence over healthcare expenditures" [20]. These authors also note that more widely defined bundles (episodes) have greater opportunity to improve efficiency and quality but are likely to carry higher financial risks.

Effective decision-making requires good data and analytics. Clinicians need an understanding of both financial performance metrics as well as operational performance metrics to evaluate data and determine responses to strategic questions of direction and adoption.

8.4 Operations

Operational considerations encompass the management of resources needed for the service line processes of patient care including personnel, facilities, space and time, as well as materials while matching demand with resources. Every surgical service line is influenced not only by the participating surgeon and anesthesiologist but also referring physicians, primary care, internists, and specialists. Focusing these numerous variables for the care of unique patients across a service line episode of care requires consideration of the local entity and the patient population. Operations management includes efforts to reduce costs, reduce variability and improve logistical flow, ensure productivity, provide higher quality services, and facilitate business processes. Understanding resource availability will help to identify limitations and determine what changes would be predicted to produce increased value.

Measures of operational performance are used to "characterize the efficiency by which the organization provides services with the resources at hand" [21]. Studies to better characterize elements of operational performance have brought new methodologies with progress and improvement in VBC. Operational excellence of OR management gained traction with studies like the application of the Toyota model in 2011 to cardiac surgery in the healthcare setting [22]. Current work has often been aimed at quantification of operational process and manpower with Time-Driven Activity-Based Costing (TDABC) to enable proper accounting for various workforce levels and optimization of model throughput. A study by Riahl et al. found potential usefulness of machine learning (ML) methods for reaching a more accurate estimation of operation duration compared to current models [23]. A systematic literature review of healthcare supply chain research in 2018 noted that "supply chain operations, performance measurement, inventory management, lean and agile operation, and the use of information technology were well studied, indicating recent areas of highest interest and likely directions of development [24].

Management decision-making begins with the organizational evaluation of existing processes, often using Ishikawa diagrams or process flow mapping, to identify problems or efficiency, bottlenecks, or possible safety gaps in service line processes to be addressed. Criteria and key variables are determined, and the weight of each is considered. Best strategic alignment, highest impact, and highest demand are some of the considerations used to determine first steps. Considerations of competition and market impact of any enterprise investments may include scenario analysis and game theory to evaluate the possible range of outcomes [21]. These initial interventions are considered and "piloted" as a guide to find the optimal decision for high impact.

In the service line model, process mapping evaluates the complete service line from initial patient contact and pre-op evaluation, through the completion of surgery, postoperative, and recovery phases. Optimization will require an understanding of the core and support processes, the workflows, supply chain, capacity planning and quality control. The service line model may have activities outside of the hospital such as patient referral and pre-evaluation from private community primary physicians as well as rehabilitation and post-operative care facilities. The transfer into and out of the hospital system are critical points for management as they can serve to create capacity or create safety hazards. Within the hospital system, process mapping for optimization of capacity planning including first case on time starts, case times, and PACU times, or any limiting step where change is thought to increase productivity can serve to create resource capacity.

Surgical supply chain efficiency is critical to effective hospital management. Cumulative inefficiencies in OR processes can lead to a significant loss of revenue for the hospital, staff dissatisfaction, and patient care disruption [21]. These considerations are often challenged by workforce limitations, scheduling constraints, drug shortages, pharmaceutical costs, regulatory and contractual obligations. These factors further require recurring assessment for the appearance of new threats.

Current work has often been aimed at quantification of manpower with TDABC to enable proper accounting for various workforce levels and for modeling throughput. Najjar et al. [25] present TDABC Costing for Surgical Episodes as an innovation for delivering higher value by maintaining or improving outcomes while reducing costs. They note the traditional top-down hospital accounting systems, using allocation of departmental expense through cost to charge ratio assumes that resource cost is proportional to the charges. The second top-down method used is the relative-value units-based costing based only on the reimbursed costs; this method therefore does not reflect the true resources used. Both of these traditional methodologies are often inaccurate and offer little insight to surgeons and clinical staff on how and where to optimally reduce costs. TDABC applied to surgical episodes measures cost across episodes of care by time and the cost per unit of each resource used in the service line. Najjar offers a three-step model. (1)—Map each process across the episode of care, (2)—Calculate the capacity cost rate for each resource in the process, and (3)—Use capacity cost rate and process times to compute total cost. The calculation process using TDABC can provide insight into inefficiencies across the supply chain and may reveal capacity [26]. If the TDABC accounting process is tailored to focus on the unit of measure that holds the most value, TDABC can serve as a road map to decide where strategic assets should be deployed.

Application of these methods is demonstrated by Martin et al. [27] using TDABC as a key component in the value platform for colonoscopy, TAVR and carpal tunnel release. They determined that both appropriate procedural setting and appropriate application of staff can each provide value to the service line. The authors also note that Activity-Based Costing used in product industry can identify:

1. Unprofitable customer relationships by asking if negotiated contracts are serving the organization.
2. Unprofitable processes, such as limiting low value preop visits for low-risk patients.
3. Poor process design, thereby determining if modifications are needed for special groups such as the frail.

Increasing interest, reports and research surrounding TDABC resulted in numerous associated study designs. To facilitate comparative analysis, a standardized framework was developed through the evaluation of existing literature. A total of 32 useful elements were identified with 23 elements considered essential for system TDABC application in any enterprise effort [28]. These authors further convened a group to launch the international cost standard-set program in a 2022 publication with the intention of developing a standard for best-evidence and potential benchmarking [29].

Balancing the many aspects of service line management requires communication with multiple stakeholders. In order to communicate priorities and promote managerial progress, the use of Key Performance Indicators (KPI) may be used. KPIs help to quantify progress of elements and provide a measurable indicator for understanding the advancement or successful realization of objectives to the group of project members. Evaluation of the current status of the service line and strategic planning to prioritize the next steps should be paired with a choice of KPI's "to facilitate decisions and to improve OR efficiency, safety, and satisfaction" [30]. Usual KPI's for operational OR management are contribution margins, case cancelation rates, start-time delays, or turnover time. The choice of any indicator that appears to negatively patient safety, patient satisfaction or financial margins may identify first line problems to address. In turn, as evidence based clinical practices are implemented, effects on OR operational KPI's could potentially be observed and tracked.

8.5 Finance

Financial performance accounting "measures how a firm uses assets from operations to generate revenue" [31]. The financial performance tells investors or other stakeholders about the general well-being of a firm as a snapshot of its economic health and the job management is doing. The standard financial statements are analyzed to evaluate performance including the balance sheet, the income statement and the statement of cash flow as required by General Accepted Accounting Principles (GAAP). The financial statement analysis is meant to provide information about the overall financial health or financial condition of the organization to inform management for both short- and longer-term planning processes [32].

Financial analysis through use of ratio analysis is routinely used in planning and forecasting. Three broad categories of ratio analysis exist: profitability, operating efficiency and leverage (the use of debt financing). The most important measure of a business's profitability is Return on Equity (ROE). The Return on Equity ratio is often examined in the framework of the Du Pont analysis, a financial analysis tool that deconstructs ROE into three components: profit margin, total asset turnover, and equity multiplier.

$$
\begin{array}{lclclcl}
\text{ROE} & = & \text{Total Margin} & \times & \text{Total asset turnover} & \times & \text{Equity Multiplier} \\
\text{Profitability} & = & \text{Margin} & \times & \text{Efficiency} & \times & \text{Leverage} \\
\dfrac{\text{Net income}}{\text{Total equity}} & = & \dfrac{\text{Net income}}{\text{Total revenues}} & \times & \dfrac{\text{Total revenue}}{\text{Total Assets}} & \times & \dfrac{\text{Total Assets}}{\text{Total equity}}
\end{array}
$$

A study in 1993 by Gapenski sought to define the determinants of hospital profitability [33]. As third-party payers began to incentivize activity in an attempt to control spending, increasing pressure on profitability forced introspection by hospitals when making service decisions. The analysis was intended to define areas of focus for managerial evaluation and action of a hospital's profitability and provide insights for improvement as well as to provide insight to policy makers when considering alternative actions. Gapenski presents a study [33] using data from 1989 that points to cost-reduction strategies derived from length of stay reductions, labor productivity enhancements, overhead cost controls, and substituting capital for labor when possible as the most important factors. In this 1993 study, the authors did not find that for profit (investor owned) hospitals or system status (a member of a health system) had correlation to profitability. Managerial variables including lower age of plant, better debt utilization, offering more services and less labor-intensive activities were all good for profit. Patient variables that were shown to improve profitability included a subacute care mix, the use of swing beds to conclude a hospital admission and a Medicare mix were each found to increase profitability.

In contrast, Turner et al. in 2015, used the DuPont analysis to examine hospital profitability in the US Market using CMS cost report information from 2007 to 2012 [34]. The evaluation found that when stratified by hospital characteristics, the results indicate investor-owned hospitals have higher profit margins, higher efficiency and were substantially more leveraged. Hospitals in systems have higher ROE, margins and efficiency but less leverage. The higher profit margins of investor owned (IO) hospitals may be the result of more effective cost containment or higher contracted payment rates. In conjunction with other studies, lower patient satisfaction at IO facilities would seem to indicate that holding down costs may lead to declines in particular quality HCAHP metrics [34].

Since the passage of the Affordable Care Act (ACA) there is increased focus on access and quality. The Value-Based Purchasing Program for hospitals, quality-based clinician compensation, bundled payment models, readmission reduction program and hospital acquired conditions reduction program are incentivized programs; each developed to improve the efficiency with which medical care is delivered. Akinleye et al. in 2018 [35], looked at the correlation between hospital finances and quality and safety of patient care. Using hospital data from CMMS they found that the composite quality/safety performance score and hospital financial performance were correlated at $p < 0.001$. The composite financial performance score was also correlated with the CMS Value-Based Purchasing Total Performance Score $p = 0.002$. In addition, the Hospital Financial Performance was negatively correlated with composite readmissions as well as various readmission subgroups. The composite financial performance score components include factors interpreted as measuring profitability, asset efficiency, absolute size of assets, debt coverage, capital structure, and uncompensated care or unutilized income and growth. The composite quality/patient safety performance components included the patient experience of care (ten subscales from HCAHPS), timeliness in surgical care improvement, timeliness of stroke care, two emergency indicators, patient safety indicators, and inpatient mortality.

In 2023, Beauvais [36] reported an exploratory analysis of the relation between quality measures and financial performance. Using independent variables including HCAHPS star rating, Hospital Compare Overall rating, and 2021 Total Performance Score against a variety of operational and geographic indicators they revealed that positive Score performance was directly associated with hospital profitability while readmission rate was negatively correlated.. In addition, the group examined the Hospital Value-Based Purchasing sub-domains of clinic outcomes, safety, engagement, and efficiency as independent variable against a variety of dependent variables including total assets per bed, for profit status, surgical case mix index, medical case mix index, and average length of stay. The positive association with profitability gives weight to the continued efforts surrounding patient safety, improved clinical outcomes, engagement and efficiency.

Although clinicians are not likely to be familiar with financial analytic tools, discussions surrounding methodologies and organizational financial priorities can provide insight to clinicians for determining key areas for coordinated efforts. Financial analysis of a surgical service line for strategic planning may consider clinical costs, outcomes, and regulatory and contractual obligations to meet the organizational demands. The use of TDABC (discussed in the previous section) focuses on the quantification of clinical activities, calculated as the capacity cost rate [37], for calculation of resource use. This process is critical for determination of utilization to identify excess capacity or misaligned personnel assignment. "TDABC enables surgeons, other front-line clinicians, administrators, and finance professionals to develop a shared understand of the costs incurred by their clinical care of patients and by their administrative processes" [25].

The use of financial statement analysis provides more granular information required for managerial analysis and decision-making. Operating indicators such as occupancy, patient mix, length of stay, and productivity measures can be attributed to specific surgical service lines and used to identify factors that contribute to the financial conditions and variance analysis. Hospital performance measures including capacity, utilization, patient/payer mix, capital structure, liquidity, revenues, expenses, profitability, productivity, efficiency, and pricing strategies inform hospital operations about current conditions. In a surgical service line, indices specific to acute care beds in service, acute care discharges, average length of stay for acute care, patient and payer mix, gross patient revenue per adjusted discharge, laboratory cost, pharmacy cost, administrative cost, total asset turnover ratio as net patient revenue/total assets for any given surgical service line provide data for analysis and application to improve profitability. The financial approach to the comprehensive analysis of a service line includes the financial performance, expenses, growth potential, and overall contribution of each service line to the hospital's financial health.

8.5.1 The Surgical Service Line

The coordination of the various dimensions of a surgical service line, including the clinical, operational, and financial components is ultimately what is needed to analyze and implement changes for progress and modification. In a report by the research and consulting group Mathematica [38], the group described their work operating distinct learning systems for Medicare ACOs which led to the production of the CMS Care Transformation Kit published January 2021 [39]. The steps for implementation of care transformation begin with a review of the policy guidelines to define the initiative objectives. This work is followed by identification and engagement of the stakeholders, definition of workflows and processes, with selection and engagement of the targeted beneficiary groups. Piloting workflows and processes will be followed by refinement and expansion of the initiative based on measures of implementation, progression, and outcomes [39]. Within a healthcare system, this framework is the work of implementation of the surgical service line where the refinement and expansion is the detail of the patient pathway across the perioperative space. Cannesson and Mahajan [40] write of the vertical and horizontal pathways within a healthcare system as the intersection and integration of the perioperative home and enhanced recovery after surgery programs. Etges et al. [41] and the TDABC Healthcare Consortium present a standardized framework for evaluating surgical enhanced recovery pathways. The framework is meant to standardize the process and allow the framework to support decision making. The vertical integration in the healthcare system of each surgical service line should be layered with the clinically relevant evidence-based care, operational concerns, and the financial data within a strategically advantageous framework for the enterprise. Service line governance is often described as the operational accountability and management of the facilities within the enterprise. Building a surgical service line with integrated activity-based costing and appropriate data collection and accounting data allows full evaluation of the fixed and variable costs. It also adds to the evaluation of workflows by measuring the allocation of personnel, determining most appropriate use and the availability of idle time. These frontline activities, in turn, are evaluated at the executive level for review of market share, the system case mix index, the overall revenue from the service line, profitability and benchmarks for internal financial operational performance. As the surgical service line is evaluated, all aspects are considered for modifications and improvements in clinical care. Operational and strategic realignment should occur to maintain a competitive edge.

The strategic analysis of the surgical service line should be done in the framework of the Balanced Scorecard. The concept of the Balanced Scorecard was introduced by Kaplan and Norton in 2005 [42] and presents a management strategy comprised of four processes:

1. Translating the vision.
2. Communicating and linking.
3. Business planning.
4. Feedback and learning.

Alongside the Value Chain presented by Kaplan and Porter [43], the integration of the surgical service line can be evaluated at both the clinical level and the enterprise level. This is done to allow full vertical integration for both strategic planning and at the clinical level, where evidence-based practice of medicine can be evaluated for effects on enterprise profitability and resource capacity planning can be optimized. A recent evaluation by Kaplan [44] considered using the Balanced Scorecard for health care merger and acquisition integration. The merger of both horizontal and vertical elements of the surgical service line could be integrated within the enterprise an4and Senior executives can use the scorecard to (1) better communicate the new strategy to all employees, (2) align employees' daily work to strategic priorities, and (3) monitor, evaluate, and reward employee performance (4) the information provides a basis for regular strategy review management meetings. These actions are designed to keep the organization focused on effective strategy implementation during the critical post-merger years [44].

As senior executives seek to integrate surgical service lines within the enterprise, the realization of the need for the continuous change of new clinical information should be considered when choices are made. Allowance for plasticity of the processes will serve to keep competitive change easily accessible. There remains the need to improve healthcare value-based decision-making through methodologic transparency of various assessments and continued efforts of consensus-based measures that reflect IOM's quality framework [45]. This work by Craig et al., focused on the quality aspects of the value-based universe of healthcare, identifies measure and maps them to the Donabedian conceptualization of measures as structure, process or outcomes, as well as the STEEEP (safety, timeliness, effectiveness, efficiency, equity, and patient centeredness) framework for quality measures. These authors notably consider adjusted operating profit margin, hospital-specific designations, and percent of Medicare beneficiaries of all ages with diabetes or heart disease. They specifically recognize the need for fiscal insights for true value-based decisions and care and encourage further development of a focus on a hospitals' ability to support the expansion of programs.

The organization of surgical service lines into entities that allow internal transparency as well as methodologies for change, serve to strengthen an organization's ability to adapt for internal improvement initiatives as well as the ability to adapt to external forces of regulation and payor demands. External transparency provides access as policy analysis continues to develop. Towse and Fenwick published a work "Setting out the conditions in which performance-based risk-sharing arrangements work for both parties" [46]. The authors encourage product development with steps to make risk-sharing more practical, so that payers consider it as an option. A strong service line structure allows the analysis to develop insight for change and gives confidence in the hospitals' ability to implement and monitor the changes mandated by any risk-sharing agreement. The reality of continued analysis of health systems speaks to the range of conditions in which health systems exist and function.

Risk-sharing agreements, governmental mandates and payor conditions of participation all place demands on any hospital system involved. Health system efficiency is a priority concern regardless of organizational size or type. Mbau et al. [47] examined evidence concerning health system efficiency over a range of settings and a variety of applications. Healthcare managers and leadership must consider the external factors affecting their organization that are largely outside their control-external policy makers, payor organizations, socioeconomic factors. Promoting reforms that are most suitable for the given health care system efficiency must be equalized with promoting health care interventions to promote best care of chronic conditions as well as those promoting best treatments and wellness. The authors go on to encourage engaging health system decision makers and implementors to understand their organization and identify content-appropriate inputs and outputs for efficiency.

Understanding the nuances of both the financial status and operational functions is essential to position any organization for best market performance. The surgical service lines, using best evidence-based medical care, serves the function of providing methodology for excellent patient outcomes in the current Value-Based healthcare environment. Each anesthesiologist is the provider in the clinic or OR where the care delivered is the care that protects the patient's being and physiology and returns them to normal life. That delivery of care needs to be optimized in whatever delivery system you practice. This optimization of delivery is a part of operational efficiency, managed and financed within the hospital administration. Advocating for and participating in a surgical service line or other patient care pathway and offering input into methodology as well as management discussions is critical. Understanding the needs of your organization is terms of operational efficiency, budgetary constraints, and strategic direction may not be openly available. Seeking this information within a patient-centered framework proves interest but also might be delivering information to the management that will make your value evident.

References

1. Nurok M, et al. Surgeon and administrators co-create value. Ann Surg. 2021:e630–1. https://doi.org/10.1097/SLA.0000000000005183.
2. Glotzbach JP, et al. Value- driven cardiac surgery: achieving "perfect care" after coronary artery bypass grafting. J Thorac Cardiovasc Surg. 2018;156:1436–48. https://doi.org/10.1016/j.jtcvs.2018.2818.03.177.
3. Mazurek M. Improving operations, from preop to postop. J Healthc Manag. 2024;69(1). https://doi.org/10.1097/JHM-D-23-00238.
4. Sutcliffe K. Building cultures of high reliability. Lessons from the high reliability paradigm. Anesthesiol Clin. 2023;41:707–17. https://doi.org/10.1026/j.anclin.2023.03.012.
5. Huynh T, et al. The perioperative surgical home: high-reliability or ultra-safe organization? Int Anesthesiol Clin. 57(1):32–44. https://doi.org/10.1097/AIA.0000000000000214.

6. Mahajan A, et al. A hospital is not just a factory, but a complex adaptive system- implications for perioperative care. Anesth Analg. 2017;125:333–41. https://doi.org/10.1213/ANE.0000000000002144.
7. Pitt S, Dossett L. Deimplementation of low-value care in surgery. JAMA Surg. 2022;157(11):977–8. https://doi.org/10.1001/jama.2021.3308.
8. Koepke EJ. Systems of care delivery and optimization in the preoperative arena. Anesthesiol Clin. 2023;41:833–45. https://doi.org/10.1016/j.anclin.2023.03.014.
9. Solomon A, et al. Roadmap for transforming preoperative assessment to preoperative optimization. Anesth Analg. 2020;130(4):811–9. https://doi.org/10.1213/ANE.0000000000004571.
10. Kotter JP. Accelerate: building strategic agility for a faster-moving world. Harvard Business Review Press; 2014. ISBN 978-1-62527-174-7.
11. Goodall A. Creating stability is just as important as managing change. HBR.org. 9 July 2024. Reprint HO8A5H.
12. Schwann NM, et al. Clinical practice improvement: mind the gap or fall into the chasm. Anesth Analg. 2019;128(1). https://doi.org/10.1213/ANE.0000000000003877.
13. Edmondson A. The competitive imperative of learning. Harv Bus Rev. 2008:2–10.
14. Boone C, et al. Value-based contracting in clinical care. JAMA Health Forum. 2024;5(8):e242020. https://doi.org/10.1001/jamahealthforum.2024.2020.
15. Eappen S, et al. Relationship between occurrence of surgical complications and hospital finances. JAMA. 2013;309(15):1599–606.
16. Haidar S, et al. Impact of surgical complications on hospital costs and revenues: retrospective database study of Medicare claims. J Comp Eff Res. 2023:e230080. https://doi.org/10.57264/cer-2023/0080.
17. Stokes S, et al. Hospital costs following surgical complications. A value-driven outcomes analysis of cost savings due to complication prevention. Ann Surg. 2022;275:e375–81. https://doi.org/10.1097/SLA.0000000000004243.
18. Aman M, Mythen M. Innovations in practices and technologies that will shape perioperative medicine. Anesth Analg. 2023;136(4):623–6. https://doi.org/10.1213/ANE0000000000006439.
19. Harvie DA, et al. Understanding outcomes after major surgery. Anesth Analg. 2023;136:665–4. https://doi.org/10.1213/ANE.0000000000006438.
20. Carol B, et al. What are bundled payments and how can they be used by healthcare organizations? 2023. Retrieved 29 Feb 2025 from https://www.milliman.com/en/insight/what-are-bundled-payments-and-how-can-they-be-used-by-healthcare-organizations.
21. Langabeer JR II, Helton J. Health care operations management, a system perspective. 3rd ed. Jones & Bartlett Learning, LLC; 2021.
22. Culig MH, et al. Improving patient care in cardiac surgery using Toyota production system based methodology. Ann Thorac Surg. 2011;91:394–400. https://doi.org/10.1016/j.athorasur.2010.09.032.
23. Riahl, et al. Improving preoperative prediction of surgery duration. BMC Health Serv Res. 2023;23(1):1343. https://doi.org/10.1186/s12913-023-10264-6.
24. Dixit A, et al. A systematic literature review of healthcare supply chain and implication of future research. Int J Pharm Healthc Market. 2019;13(4):405–35. https://doi.org/10.1108/IJPHM-05-2018-0028.
25. Najjar P, et al. Time-driven activity based costing for surgical episodes. JAMA Surg. 2017;152(1):96–7. https://doi.org/10.1001/jamasurg.2016.3356.
26. Jalalabadi F, et al. Activity-based costing. Semin Plast Surg. 2018;32:182–6. https://doi.org/10.1055/s-0038-1672208.
27. Martin J, et al. Using time-driven activity based costing as a key component on the value platform: a pilot analysis of colonoscopy, aortic valve replacement and carpal tunnel release procedures. J Clin Med Res. 10(4):314–20. https://doi.org/10.14740/jocmr3350w.
28. Etges AP, et al. A standardized framework to evaluate the quality of studies using TDABC in healthcare: the TDABC in Healthcare Consortium Consensus Statement. BMC Health Serv Res. 2020;20:1107. https://doi.org/10.1186/s12913-020-05869-0.

29. Etges AP, et al. Cost standard set program: moving forward to standardization of cost assessment based on clinical condition. J Comp Eff Res. 2022;11(17):1219–23. https://doi.org/10.2217/cer-2022-0169.
30. Kaye AD, Ulman R, Fox CJ III. Operating room leadership and perioperative practice management. Cambridge; 2019. p. 78.
31. https://www.investopedia.com/terms/f/financialperformance.asp#toc-the-bottom-line.
32. Reiter K, Song P. Gapenski's healthcare finance. An introduction to accounting and financial management. 7th ed. Chicago: Health Administration Press; 2021.
33. Gapenski LC. The determinants of hospital profitability. Hosp Health Serv Adm. 1993;38(1):63–80.
34. Turner J, et al. A decomposition of hospital profitability; an application of DuPont analysis to the US market. Health Serv Res Manag Epidemiol. 2015;2:1–10.
35. Akinleye DD, et al. Correlation between hospital finance and quality and safety of patient care. PLoS One. 2018. https://doi.org/10.1371/journal.pone/2.
36. Beauvais B, et al. An exploratory analysis of the association between hospital quality measures and financial performance. Healthcare. 2023;11:2785. https://doi.org/10.3390/healthcare11202758.
37. Definition of capacity cost. https://www.accountingtools.com/articles/what-are-capacity-costs.html. Accessed 18 May 2025.
38. Mathematica. Project: 2013–2020. Learning systems for accountable care organizations. Prepared for the US Department of Health and Human Services, CMMS.
39. CMS ACO learning system for ACO's. Care Transformation Tool Kit. 2021.
40. Cannesson M, Mahajan A. Vertical and horizontal pathways: intersection and integration of enhanced recovery after surgery and the perioperative surgical home. Anesth Analg. 2018;127(5):1275–7. https://doi.org/10.1213/ANE.0000000000003506.
41. Etges AP, et al. A standardized framework for evaluating enhanced recovery pathways: a recommendations statement from the TCABD in Health-care Consortium. J Health Econ Outcomes Res. 2021;8(1):116–24. https://doi.org/10.36469/jheor.2021.24590.
42. Kaplan RS, Norton D. Using the balanced scorecard as a strategic management system. Harv Bus Rev. 2005.
43. Kaplan RS, Porter M. How to solve the cost crisis in health care. Harv Bus Rev. 2011.
44. Kaplan RS. Using the balanced scorecard for successful health care M&A integration. NEJM Catal Innov Care Deliv. 2020. https://doi.org/10.1056/CAT.20.0286.
45. Craig T, et al. US hospital performance methodologies: a scoping review to identify opportunities for crossing the quality chasm. BMC Health Serv Res. 2020;20:640. https://doi.org/10.1186/s12913-020-05502-z.
46. Towse A, Fenwick E. It takes 2 to Tango. Setting out the conditions in which performance-based risk-sharing arrangements work for both parties. Value Health. 2024;27(8):1057–965. https://doi.org/10.1016/j.jval.2024.03.2196.
47. Mbau R, et al. Analyzing the efficiency of health systems: a systematic review of the literature. Appl Health Econ Health Policy. 2023;21:205–24. https://doi.org/10.1007/s40258-022-00785-2.

9 Protocol Management for Emergencies by Anesthesiologists

Dorothy (Wei Yun) Wang and Anwar Alinani

9.1 Malignant Hyperthermia (MH)

9.1.1 Clinical Overview

Malignant hyperthermia (MH) is a rare genetic condition which can result in a life-threatening, hypermetabolic syndrome comprised of severe muscle rigidity and metabolic derangements when a susceptible individual is exposed to inhaled anesthetics or depolarizing muscle relaxants such as succinylcholine [1]. The most common cause is a mutation in the ryanodine receptor type 1 (RYR1) gene, which is transmitted in an autosomal dominant fashion, and leads to an excessive release of calcium from the sarcoplasmic reticulum of skeletal muscles upon exposure to triggering agents [1]. Malignant hyperthermia is considered a medical emergency as it can become fatal if not treated appropriately and in a timely manner.

The most important first steps after the recognition of the possibility of MH are to stop the offending agent and administer treatment. The primary treatment of choice for MH that is FDA-approved for both adults and children is dantrolene, a post-synaptic muscle relaxant [2]. The initial dose of dantrolene is 2.5 mg/kg via intravenous administration, potentially followed by additional boluses of 1–2.5 mg/kg if symptoms persist. Following initial treatment, additional intravenous dantrolene at 1 mg/kg can be administered every 6 hours for 24 hours [2].

D. (Wei Yun) Wang (✉) · A. Alinani
Department of Anesthesiology and Pain Medicine, University of Washington, Seattle, WA, USA
e-mail: weiyun@uw.edu; aalinani@uw.edu

G. Tewfik (ed.), *The Anesthesiologist as Perioperative Leader*,
https://doi.org/10.1007/978-3-032-18058-2_9

9.1.2 Protocol Development

Protocol development should start with thorough research on up-to-date scientific evidence, professional society guidelines, Centers for Medicare and Medicaid Services (CMS) requirements, institutional policies and practices, financial analyses of treatment and reimbursement costs, and feasibility of implementation. Some practical elements to consider include involvement of multidisciplinary stakeholders, availability of funding, ease of use for end-point providers, long-term sustainability, and evaluation processes.

Multidisciplinary stakeholders, such as representatives from the operating room (OR), nursing staff and pharmacy staff, should be involved in decisions concerning the location of the MH cart and the appropriate personnel to maintain the cart by restocking used items and checking expiration dates for supplies and medications. In addition to the recommended items, the MH cart can also carry cards that can be distributed with specific instructions for each type of provider, including OR circulating nurse, scrub technician, anesthesia technician, and the surgical team. A new protocol is ideally tested via mock multidisciplinary exercise to assess for ease of use and sustainability. A quality improvement process should be built into the protocol for review of guideline updates and any reported issues.

9.1.3 CMS Requirements

The Social Security Act (the Act) mandates the establishment of minimum health and safety and standards that must be met by providers and suppliers participating in the Medicare and Medicaid programs. These standards are found in the 42 Code of Federal Regulations. The Secretary of the Department of Health and Human Services has designated CMS to administer the standards compliance aspects of these programs [3].

To receive Medicare and/or Medicaid reimbursement for services, hospitals are required to be compliant with federal requirements outlined in the Medicare Conditions of Participation (CoP) established by CMS in accordance with the Social Security Act. The CMS designates State Agencies to perform surveys to ensure that these standards for minimum health and safety are met by providers and suppliers participating in the Medicare and Medicaid programs through a process known as certification [4].

CMS stipulates that governing policies for surgical care for Critical Access Hospitals (CAH) should include those on the topic of malignant hyperthermia, and they must be in accordance with acceptable standards of medical practice [5]. CMS also expects an Ambulatory Surgical Center (ASC) to have medication supplies and equipment required to treat emergency conditions (such as MH) if the risk exists thereof, in accordance with nationally recognized guidelines [6].

9.1.4 Clinical Guidelines

Broad clinical guidelines include temperature monitoring during anesthesia care, usage of non-triggering anesthetic agents, diligent preparation of the anesthesia machine and workstation in patients susceptible to MH, and of course, the timely administration of dantrolene in patients suspected of having an MH episode. The Malignant Hyperthermia Association of the United States (MHAUS) recommends a stock of 700 mg of dantrolene on hand, which is 36 vials of Dantrium® or Revonto® with 20 mg per vial, or 3 vials of Ryanodex® with 250 mg per vial [7, 8]. Facilities that meet criteria to stock dantrolene should also prepare an MH cart [7, 8]. Items for stock in an MH cart as recommend by the MHAUS are listed in Fig. 9.1.

For preparation of the anesthetic workstation for MH patients, or patients at risk of MH, the MHASU recommends flushing the anesthetic machine circuit according to manufacturer's recommendations, disconnecting the vaporizers from the machine, using a new breathing circuit, and replacing the carbon dioxide absorber [7]. An acceptable alternative is using a commercially available activated charcoal filter following a 90 s flush with high fresh gas flows. Lastly, although likely not cost-effective, it is also acceptable to use a dedicated anesthesia machine or critical care unit ventilator that has never been exposed to volatile anesthetic agents [7].

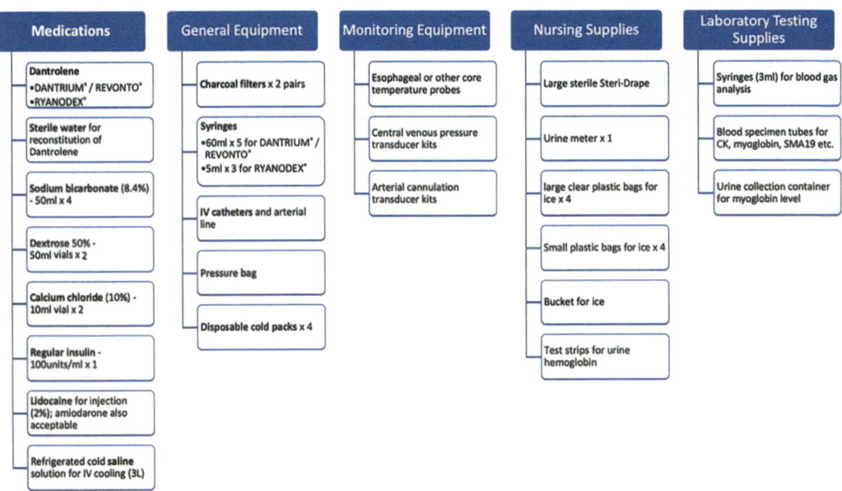

Fig. 9.1 Items for the MH cart as recommended by the MHAUS [8]. (Created with ChatGPT)

9.1.5 Financial Considerations

Cost calculations should generally take into consideration an estimated number of MH cases at the facility based on the number of surgeries and/or procedures requiring general anesthesia, the incidence of MH pertaining to the patient population, and the fatality of the condition [9]. Regarding the cost of an MH cart, parameters that should be considered include the cost of dantrolene and other supportive care medications, the cost of the supplies within the MH cart, and the personnel cost of cart maintenance.

According to a 2018 cost analysis study, the annual cost of one MH cart is estimated to be $2016, accounting for the cost of 20 mg vials of dantrolene ($84 per vial × 36 vials for a 3-year shelf life), an MH cart ($1400–$3200 based on supplier for 10–16 years of use), other various monitoring and testing equipment and supplies, and maintenance cost based on 15 min of nursing time per week (at $42.68 hourly wage) and 15 min of pharmacist time per month (at $71.68 hourly wage) [9]. The 250 mg vials of dantrolene is simpler to mix for administration but more expensive than the 20 mg vials. They range from $2000 to $3000 per vial, making the required amount (three vials) approximately $2000–$3000 per year (assuming a 3-year shelf life).

Another cost-effectiveness study from 2014 reported that stocking 36 vials of 20 mg dantrolene at every ASC in the USA would save 33 lives per year at an incremental cost-effectiveness of approximately $200,000 per life saved, which is considered cost-effective when compared with the estimated value of statistical life used by US regulatory agencies [10].

9.2 Local Anesthetic Systemic Toxicity (LAST)

9.2.1 Clinical Overview

Local anesthetic systemic toxicity (LAST) is another potentially fatal condition that can be encountered in the practice of anesthesia. It most commonly results from the administration of an exceedingly large dose of local anesthetic medication(s) or inadvertent intravenous administration of local anesthetics other than lidocaine [1]. Time to symptom onset can be variable, ranging from minutes to hours [11]. Symptoms include mental status changes such as confusion, agitation, lethargy, tinnitus, and perioral numbness. If not treated promptly, seizure, coma, arrhythmias, and respiratory arrest can also occur. The prevailing theories of pathophysiology involve inhibition of essential ion channels and conduction pathways in both the cardiovascular and central nervous systems [1, 11].

Initial treatment consists of administration of intravenous lipid emulsions (ILE), such as Intralipid® 20%, as well as supportive treatment such as airway management and circulatory support. ILE should be given at a bolus of 1.5 mL/kg followed by an infusion of 0.25 mL/kg/min until 15 min after hemodynamic stability is achieved [11]. Additional boluses can be given, and the infusion rate can be increased to

0.5 mL/kg/min if life-threatening symptoms do not subside. The maximum cumulative dose is 12 mL/kg [11]. Benzodiazepines can be used to treat seizures associated with LAST, such as midazolam 0.05–0.1 mg/kg [1]. In the case of cardiac arrest, the standard ACLS algorithm should be followed, with the exception that the bolus dose of epinephrine should be 1 mcg/kg or less [11]. Cardiopulmonary bypass can also be considered in extreme or treatment-resistant presentations [11].

9.2.2 Protocol Development

When designing a protocol for LAST, in addition to the usual considerations given to clinical guidelines, regulatory requirements, and cost, education should also be a key component, since LAST is a relatively newly coined term as an anesthetic emergency. As such, it presents as a foreign concept and protocol to non-anesthesia clinical staff. Before a protocol can be designed and implemented, buy-in from hospital, OR, and pharmacy administrative leadership is paramount for funding, planning, and personnel support. The protocol needs to clearly delineate the department and personnel that is responsible for kit assembly and maintenance. The most common practice is having anesthesia staff, such as an anesthesia technician, certified nurse anesthetist (CRNA), or a regional anesthesia team nurse, take responsibility for designing the LAST kit and checking it regularly for drug and supply restock needs. Common protocol pitfalls include OR staff not knowing where the ILE is stored, ILE being expired when needed, and lack of visual protocol nearby to guide timely clinical treatment decisions in emergencies.

An anesthesia-led multidisciplinary approach with educational programs for other OR staff needs to be implemented to familiarize staff with the concept of LAST, the immediate treatment, and their role in assisting with the resuscitation of patients suspected of having LAST. The utilization of mock exercises can greatly enhance knowledge retention and overall protocol compliance. Such LAST education programs for non-anesthesia clinical staff are especially crucial for smaller centers where there may not be another anesthesia team member who can be of immediate assistance when a patient is suspected of LAST. Even when there is a protocol in place and all relevant staff have received the necessary education, continuous assessment and review is crucial for quality improvement, maintaining cost-effectiveness and prevention of lapse in protocol adherence with staff turnover.

9.2.3 CMS Requirements

While there is no specific mention of LAST in CMS requirements, the general expectation is that Critical Access Hospitals (CAH) have policies and procedures for administering local anesthetics as well as immediate availability of medications for treating emergency conditions (such as LAST) [5]. Additionally, CAH policies must include policies for reporting adverse drug reactions and errors in the administration of drugs (such as local anesthetics) [5]. Similar guidelines on the administration of drugs by qualified personnel and the reporting of drug adverse reactions and errors exist for Ambulatory Surgical Centers (ASC) [6]. Although LAST and ILE for its treatment are not specifically mentioned, the CMS expect an ASC to have medication supplies and equipment required to treat emergency conditions if the risk exists thereof [6]. It is reasonable to expect an ASC that uses more than minimal amounts of local anesthetics either for surgical or peripheral nerve block purposes to carry ILE for treatment in the event of LAST.

9.2.4 Clinical Guidelines

The American Society of Regional Anesthesia and Pain Medicine (ASRA) recommends early administration of ILE for the treatment of LAST [12]. A LAST rescue kit should include 1000 ml of ILE, several large syringes and needles for administration, standard IV tubing, and the ASRA LAST checklist [12]. This checklist is a treatment visual aid with a detailed medication type and dosage decision tree. It can be found on the ASRA website and is freely available for practical and educational purposes. In addition, it is recommended that local anesthetic dosing be part of the "surgical pause/time-out" discussion, such that the surgical, anesthesia and nursing team are aware of the total amount of local anesthetic the patient has received and/or will receive to prevent LAST from local anesthetic overdose [12]. Ongoing awareness and communication as such are especially important when multiple teams participating in patient care have the potential to administer local anesthetic, examples of which include subcutaneous lidocaine for IV start by nursing staff in the preoperative area, performance of peripheral nerve blockade by the regional anesthesia team, use of lidocaine on induction by the OR anesthesia team, surgical site infiltration with bupivacaine by the surgical team at the end of the surgery, and potential use of lidocaine patches or a postoperative lidocaine infusion by the acute pain team.

9.2.5 Financial Considerations

Intralipid® 20% is the most commonly used ILE for the treatment LAST. It costs approximately $50 for a 250 mL bag per hospital pricing, with a shelf life of approximately 1 year. Smaller centers can be cost-effective by using nearly expired ILE as total parenteral nutrition (TPN) or cycling it to tertiary centers for such purposes [13]. Aside from the direct cost of treatment, there is unfortunately a paucity of data on the cost and economic ramifications of LAST, such as lost OR time, increased hospital length of stay, intensive care unit stay, the cost of other medications and supplies used for treatment, as well as patient disability and missed labor [14]. Although there has not been any official analysis comparing the theoretical cost per life saved to the accepted value of statistical life, any examination of such undertaking which considers the clinical severity of LAST, the cost and effectiveness of intralipid, and the simplicity of recommended kit supplies would most certainly yield results in favor of the cost-effectiveness of regularly stocking a LAST treatment kit.

9.3 Code Blue

9.3.1 Introduction

In-hospital cardiac arrest or hemodynamic compromise represents a significant challenge in any healthcare setup, and is associated with substantial morbidity and mortality. A "Code Blue" is a commonly used term to signal a medical emergency which usually involves a cardiac or respiratory arrest, and the need for immediate resuscitation [15]. It is a hospital-wide alert and incorporates rapid response teams (RRT) from diverse disciplines that can provide immediate and high acuity care [16]. The timely and effective response to a Code Blue event is crucial in improving patient outcomes [17]. RRTs can also be in place to identify and intervene in cases of patient deterioration before a full cardiac arrest occurs, potentially preventing the need for a Code Blue activation. Sometimes these early rapid response triggers are indistinguishable from a true Code blue event. For the scope of this chapter, a wide definition of hemodynamic instability is considered for triggering "Code blue", incorporating any medical emergency that points toward an acute threat to life. This chapter will explore the multifaceted relationship between anesthesiology and Code Blue events, encompassing the anesthesiologist's role, cost implications, strategies for improvement, design considerations for new healthcare setups, and directions for the future.

9.3.2 The Role of the Anesthesiologist in Code Blue

Anesthesiologists possess many unique skillsets that make them invaluable members of the Code Blue team, be it in the operating room (OR) or any areas outside of the OR. In the perioperative setting, anesthesiologists continuously monitor vital signs and recognize early physiological deterioration, often intervening before the situation becomes irreversible. Their deep understanding of patient physiology and the intricacies of hemodynamic shifts during a procedure positions them well to generate timely and robust responses to this early derangement. Their prowess with cardiovascular physiology, pharmacology, airway management, rapid peripheral and central intravenous access and, when indicated, coordination during extracorporeal membrane oxygenation (ECMO) /ECPR initiation, is widely appreciated.

In the intraoperative code blue, also referred to as "Anesthesia STAT" events, the anesthesiologist assumes the code leadership by default, coordinating surgeons, nurses, and ancillary responders. Not infrequently even emergencies outside of the OR end with anesthesia as the lead. In these high-pressured settings, rapid decision-making and seamless adaptation to evolving circumstances are critical skills in which anesthesiologists excel. Finally, anesthesiologists can facilitate a seamless transition to intensive care units (ICU) after emergency events and ensure continuity of appropriate care and treatment plans.

9.3.3 Common Code Blue Protocols

Different institutions may define their rapid response protocols differently based on available services, resources and institutional limitations. For example, a level 1 trauma center may have extensive medical intervention capabilities such as ECPR or ECMO, whereas an ambulatory day surgery center would have far less resources. What is common to most facilities would be an incorporation of the Basic life support (BLS) and Advance life support (ALS) protocols as their blueprints for any proposed service area-based emergency algorithms [18]. Secondly, "Code Blue" protocols in the perioperative setting may be specialized according to the intricacies of the involved service areas. An example of such a model can be seen in the practices of obstetric or regional anesthesia, where local anesthesia toxicity (LAST) would be high on the list of differential diagnoses and the response may center around having appropriatel therapies such as lipid emulsion readily available. In contrast, a code blue protocol in the cardiac intensive care unite (ICU) or cardiac catheterization lab may focus more on have an ECPR/ECMO consult service readily available and on standby. Providing such combinations of different code blue service area priorities is beyond the scope of this chapter, but a list of common etiologies responsible for hemodynamic collapse in the perioperative settings is shown in Fig. 9.2 followed by a simple code blue protocol (Fig. 9.3) common in ambulatory day care units [19].

9.3.4 Costs of Rapid Response System and How to Make Them Efficient

RRT and Code Blue events impose substantial direct and indirect costs on healthcare systems [23]. Although there are no formal studies to identify this burden quantitatively, from an organizational point of view, there is no doubt that the financial burden of these services is significant for the following reasons:

- Assembling and deploying a multidisciplinary team of physicians (anesthesiologists, intensivists, emergency doctors, hospitalists), nurses, respiratory therapists, pharmacists, and support staff require immediate mobilization as well as prolonged engagement of all these departments, which drives up personnel expenses.
- The consumables and devices which are essential to resuscitation, defibrillators, ventilators, intubation kits, emergency medications, and, in advanced cases, extracorporeal support equipment all need availability (inventory), maintenance, hands-on troubleshooting, replacements, storage, and other supply chain related intricacies.
- There are opportunity costs accrued whenever clinicians are diverted from routine duties or scheduled procedures to these emergent and catastrophic events.

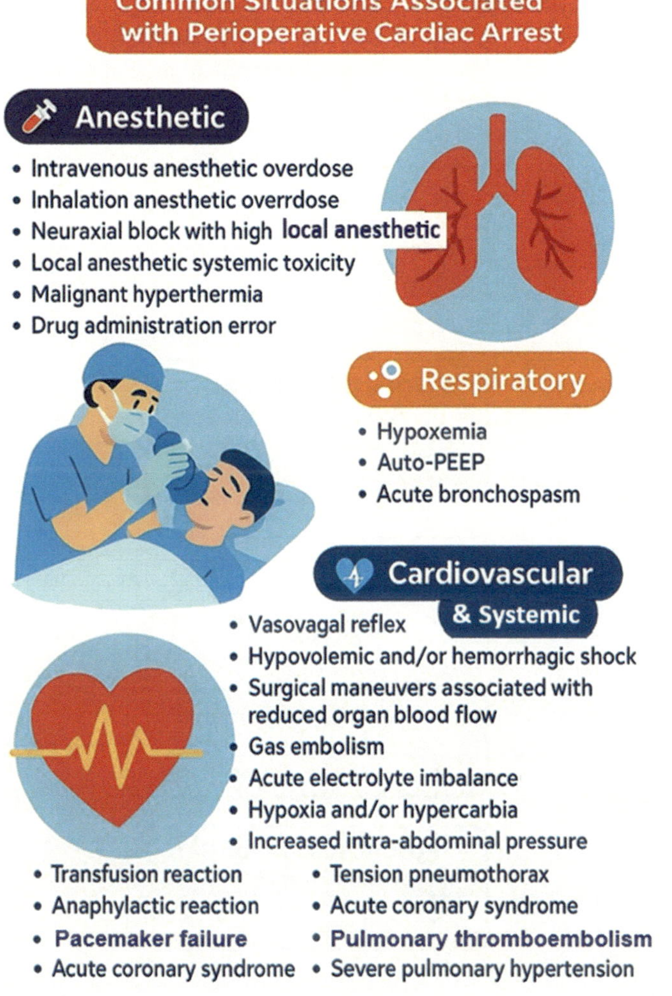

Fig. 9.2 Common causes of perioperative cardiac arrest. (Compiled by Anwar Alinani)

- Post RRT resource allocation: patients who survive cardiac arrest often need extended ICU stays, mechanical ventilation, and other resource-intensive therapies.
- Lastly, these events can also bring in legal claims or liability costs by virtue of being a consequence of or associated with negative outcomes.

Improving the efficiency of Code Blue responses and reducing their associated costs requires a comprehensive, multi-pronged, multidisciplinary strategy that can be organized around the following values:

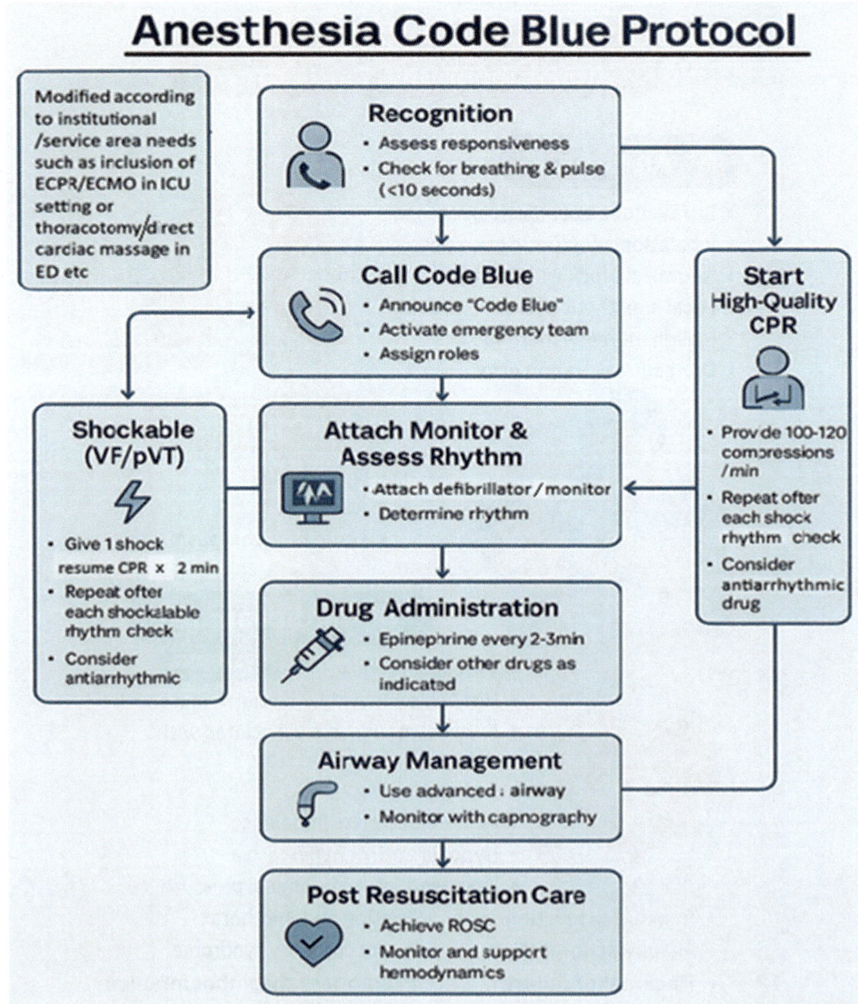

Fig. 9.3 Illustration of a sample Code Blue protocol for anesthesiology. (Illustrated by Anwar Alinani Based on common BLS/ALC algorithms) [18–22]

1. Prevention through robust Rapid Response Systems: tracking andtriggering early warning signs help identify and stabilize at-risk patients before a full arrest occurs [24].
2. Rigorous adherence to standardized, evidence-based protocols (e.g., ACLS guidelines), as well as frequent protocol reviews ensures consistency and effectiveness [25].
3. High-quality CPR training reinforced through simulation-based modalities and walk-through exercises builds team confidence and minimizes prolonged,

resource-intensive interventions. These training exercise should have clear structured communication, be simple and include pre-assigned roles to keep every team member informed and focused [26].

4. Once return of spontaneous circulation (ROSC) is achieved, immediate post resuscitation care needs special attention. Teams should focus on keys elements of this phase, such as acute metabolic derangements, targeted temperature management, and early neurologic assessments, as they may improve outcomes more effectively, compared with de-escalation of care post-ROSC [14].
5. Equally important is the organizational focus on resource allocation by maintaining well-stocked, readily accessible code carts, and supplementing them with mobile "Code Blue bags" in remote or high-need areas [24].
6. Finally, regular audits of response times, protocol adherence, and patient outcomes—paired with timely feedback and quality-improvement initiatives—create a culture of continuous learning as well as improved processes [25].

9.3.5 The Future of Rapid Response Teams (RRT)

As healthcare evolves, rapid response systems and Code Blue protocols are bound to become more proactive, personalized, and data driven. Advances in machine learning and predictive analytics will continue to help shift emphasis from reaction to anticipation and prevention through early warning alerts. At the same time, deeper insights into arrest pathophysiology can foster a more personalized approach to resuscitation, which means tailoring pharmacologic therapy, compression depth, and ventilation strategies to each patient's characteristics and arrest etiology [27]. Telemedicine and remote monitoring managed through artificial intelligence (AI) driven advances can extend expert oversight to even the most resource-limited settings. Early integration of advance care planning and end-of-life discussions will continue to play a prominent role and ensure resuscitative efforts align with patient wishes and reduce unnecessary interventions. Post-arrest care will likewise evolve, with a growing focus on cerebral resuscitation techniques such as optimized hemodynamic targets and neuroprotective strategies to prioritize not just survival, but meaningful neurological recovery [24]. Finally, a system-wide standardization of data collection and reporting would enable robust benchmarking, further research endeavors, and the contribute to the sharing of best practices across institutions [25].

9.4 Operating Room Fires

9.4.1 Introduction

Fires in the operating room are rare but devastating events with significant consequences for patients, the surgical team, and the hospital system [28]. These occurrences can lead to severe burns, inhalation injuries, disfigurement, and even death [28]. While the exact incidence is difficult to quantify due to the lack of mandatory national reporting in some regions, estimates in the USA suggest approximately 600–650 on-patient fires occur annually, resulting in at least two to three patient deaths per year [29]. Furthermore, surgical fires are an increasing source of surgical liability claims, rising from less than 1% in the late 1980s to almost 5% between 2000 and 2009 [29]. The potential for catastrophic outcomes in otherwise healthy individuals undergoing routine procedures underscores the critical importance of understanding the causes and implementing effective prevention strategies [30]. Airway fires represent the most commonly reported incidents and occur most frequently during head and neck, procedures. Examples of common high-risk procedures include tracheostomy, adenotonsillectomy, cutaneous surgery, ophthalmic procedures (e.g., cataract surgery), and Burr hole surgery [31–35].

9.4.2 The Fire Triad and Fire Prevention Algorithm

The occurrence of a fire necessitates the simultaneous presence of three key components, collectively known as the "fire triad" (Fig. 9.4): an oxidizer, an ignition source, and a fuel [31]. In the OR, common oxidizers include oxygen and nitrous oxide, both of which enhance combustion [36, 37]. Ignition sources are diverse, with electrocautery being the most frequent culprit, responsible for up to 90% of surgical fires [19]. Other ignition sources include lasers, heated probes, drills, fiber-optic light cables, and defibrillator paddles [36]. Fuels in the OR can be varied, encompassing alcohol-based skin preparation solutions (a significant contributor), surgical drapes, gowns, gauze, endotracheal tubes, the patient's hair, and even gastrointestinal gases [34, 36, 37].

Recognizing the interplay of these elements, several professional organizations, including the Joint Commission (JCI), the American Society of Anesthesiologists (ASA), and the Anesthesia Patient Safety Foundation (APSF), have developed guidelines and "fire prevention algorithms" to mitigate the risk [28, 38, 40]. A graphic compilation of common points from these protocols is given in Fig. 9.5.

9.4.3 Closed Claims Database Outcomes and Areas for Improvement

A review of the American Society of Anesthesiologists Closed Claims Database revealed that electrocautery was the ignition source in 90% of fire claims; most of these fires occurred during head, neck, or upper chest procedures (high fire risk procedures). Oxygen served as the oxidizer in 95% of electrocautery-induced fires, with open delivery systems being used in 84% of these cases. Notably, 81% of electrocautery-induced fires occurred during monitored anesthesia care (MAC), and

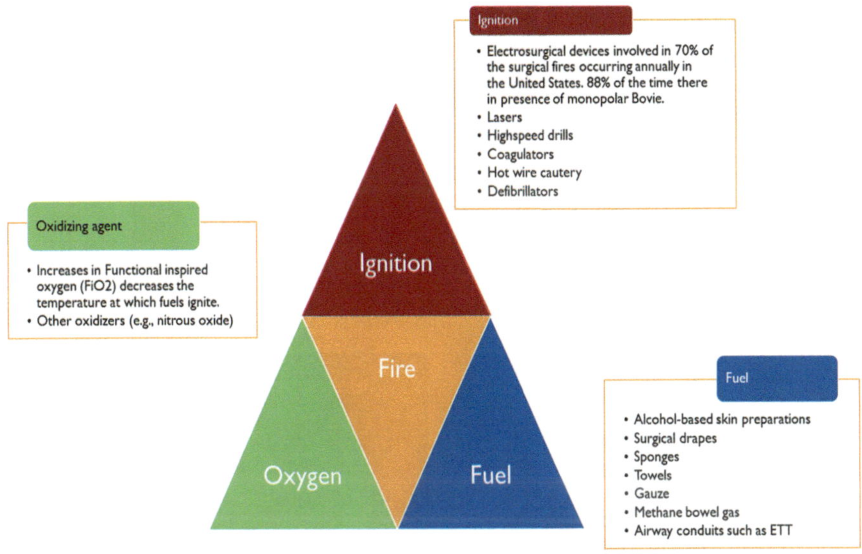

Fig. 9.4 The Fire Triangle illustration created by Anwar Alinani in MS PowerPoint [38, 39]

in all high-risk procedures during MAC, oxygen was administered via an open delivery system. In contrast, alcohol-containing prep solutions were present in only 15% of OR fires during MAC in this series [41, 42]. These findings underscore the critical role of supplemental oxygen delivered via open systems during MAC with electrocautery use, particularly in head and neck surgery, as a major contributing factor to OR fires leading to malpractice claims.

Looking at response efficiency during these episodes, analyses of the Joint Commission Sentinel Event database revealed that the primary contributors of operating room fires stem from failures in teamwork, communication, process design, staffing, and equipment. On the organizational level, key contributing factors included poor communication, lack of shared understanding among anesthesia and surgical team members before or during procedures, inadequate time-outs to assess fire risks or implement safety measures, insufficient competency in identifying or mitigating risks, overconfidence, complacency, or loss of situational awareness during surgery, equipment malfunctions or failures, and inadequate training or orientation on operating room equipment [16]. In light of these pitfalls and to work towards improved outcomes, anesthesiologists should practice the following:

- Exercise extreme caution with supplemental oxygen administration during MAC, especially in high fire risk procedures. Consider using compressed air instead of oxygen to prevent O2 buildup [41].

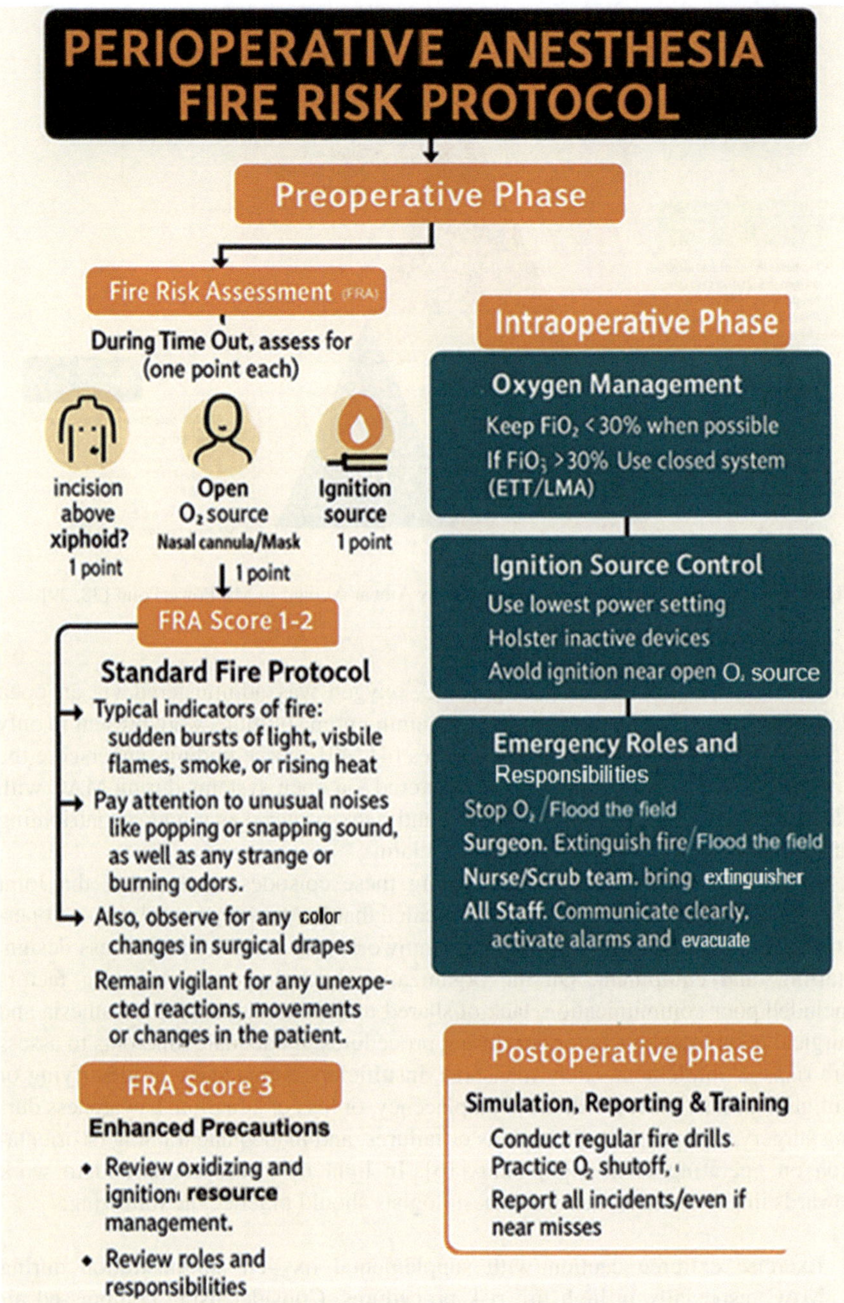

Fig. 9.5 Sample perioperative fire risk protocol. (Illustration compiled by Anwar Alinani from ASA practice advisory on operating room fires [28] and Joint commission sentinel event alert, 2023 [28])

- Minimizing oxygen concentrations when ignition sources are in use near the airway or face [35].
- Reinforce team communication regarding fire risk assessment and prevention strategies during the pre-surgical checklist and at key junctions intraoperatively [43].
- Emphasize the importance of using sealed airway devices (cuffed endotracheal tube or laryngeal mask airway) when deep sedation is required, or when the patient is oxygen-dependent during high-risk procedures [28, 32, 37].

9.4.4 Developing Fire Prevention and Response Protocols in a New Practice Setting

Establishing effective fire prevention and response protocols in a new healthcare setting requires a systematic and multidisciplinary approach. Anesthesiologists can contribute significantly to this process with the following steps.

- Anesthesiologists should be familiar with relevant national guidelines and recommendations from organizations such as Joint Commission International (JCI), American Society of Anesthesiologists (ASA), and Anesthesia Patient Safety Foundation (APSF), [40, 41]. These guidelines provide a foundation for developing local protocols, advocating for mandatory fire safety education and regular team training, including formal and periodic OR fire drills that simulate fire scenarios during dedicated educational time. Training should emphasize the fire triad and interplay of the elements that constitute it. Individual roles during a fire, the proper use of fire safety equipment and practicing critical maneuvers such as gas shut off from main supply, flooding the field, removing and re-introducing endotracheal airways, as well as patient evacuation should be practiced during these simulated environments.
- Having an anesthesiologist champion the implementation of a standardized preoperative fire risk assessment (FRA) score for every surgical procedure as part of the surgical pause or "time-out", is fundamental in generating an organized fire prevention and mitigation initiative [30, 34, 37, 40, 44].
- Collaboration with surgeons, nurses, technicians, and hospital administration is a crucial step to developing clear, concise, and easily visible protocols for fire prevention and management. These protocols should be posted in every OR and procedure area, and clearly outline pre-assigned tasks for each team member in the event of a fire [30, 44].
- Lastly, promoting a culture of open communication where all OR personnel feel comfortable raising concerns about fire safety is a must in this process. This includes establishing a transparent process for incident reporting and root cause analysis to identify systemic vulnerabilities and improve the quality of the response [28, 45].

References

1. Barash PG. Clinical anesthesia fundamentals. Place of publication not identified: Wolters Kluwer Health; 2015. 912 p.
2. Watt S, McAllister RK. Malignant hyperthermia. [Updated 2023 Aug 17]. In: StatPearls [Internet] [Internet]. Treasure Island (FL): StatPearls Publishing. Available from: https://www.ncbi.nlm.nih.gov/books/NBK430828/.
3. Centers for Medicare & Medicaid Services. Quality, safety & oversight – regulations, certification & compliance [Internet]. Available from: https://www.cms.gov/medicare/health-safety-standards/certification-compliance.
4. Centers for Medicare & Medicaid Services. State operations manual; Appendix A – survey protocol, regulations and interpretive guidelines for hospitals [Rev. 220] [Internet]. 2024. Available from: https://www.cms.gov/Regulations-and-Guidance/Guidance/Manuals/downloads/som107ap_a_hospitals.pdf.
5. Centers for Medicare & Medicaid Services. State operations manual; Appendix W – survey protocol, regulations and interpretive guidelines for critical access hospitals (CAHs) and swing-beds in CAHs [Rev. 200] [Internet]. 2020. Available from: https://www.cms.gov/Regulations-and-Guidance/Guidance/Manuals/downloads/som107ap_w_cah.pdf.
6. Centers for Medicare & Medicaid Services. State operations manual; Appendix L – guidance for surveyors: ambulatory surgical centers [Rev. 215] [Internet]. 2023. Available from: https://www.cms.gov/Regulations-and-Guidance/Guidance/Manuals/downloads/som107ap_l_ambulatory.pdf.
7. Malignant Hyperthermia Association of the United States (MHAUS). MHAUS recommendations [Internet]. 2012. Available from: https://www.mhaus.org/mhau001/assets/File/Recommendations/Recommendations%20with%20Table%20of%20Contents.pdf.
8. Malignant Hyperthermia Association of the United States (MHAUS). What should be on an MH cart? [Internet]. Available from: https://www.mhaus.org/healthcare-professionals/be-prepared/what-should-be-on-an-mh-cart/.
9. Ho PT, Carvalho B, Sun EC, Macario A, Riley ET. Cost-benefit analysis of maintaining a fully stocked malignant hyperthermia cart versus an initial dantrolene treatment dose for maternity units. Anesthesiology. 2018;129(2):249–59.
10. Aderibigbe T, Lang BH, Rosenberg H, Chen Q, Li G. Cost-effectiveness analysis of stocking dantrolene in ambulatory surgery centers for the treatment of malignant hyperthermia. Anesthesiology. 2014;120(6):1333–8.
11. Mahajan A, Song K, Derian A. Local anesthetic toxicity. [Updated 2022 Oct 3]. In: StatPearls [Internet] [Internet]. Treasure Island (FL): StatPearls Publishing. Available from: https://www.ncbi.nlm.nih.gov/books/NBK499964/.
12. Neal JM, Neal EJ, Weinberg GL. American Society of Regional Anesthesia and Pain Medicine Local Anesthetic Systemic Toxicity checklist: 2020 version. Reg Anesth Pain Med. 2021;46(1):81–2.
13. Brull SJ. Lipid emulsion for the treatment of local anesthetic toxicity: patient safety implications. Anesth Analg. 2008;106(5):1337–9.
14. Kosh MC, Miller AD, Michels JE. Intravenous lipid emulsion for treatment of local anesthetic toxicity. Ther Clin Risk Manag. 2010;6:449–51.
15. Paul RA, Beaman C, West DA, Duke GJ. COBRA: COde Blue Retrospective Audit in a metropolitan hospital. Intern Med J. 2023;53(5):745–52.
16. Nallamothu BK, Guetterman TC, Harrod M, Kellenberg JE, Lehrich JL, Kronick SL, et al. How do resuscitation teams at top-performing hospitals for in-hospital cardiac arrest succeed? A qualitative study. Circulation. 2018;138(2):154–63.
17. Factora F, Maheshwari K, Khanna S, Chahar P, Ritchey M, O'Hara J, et al. Effect of a rapid response team on the incidence of in-hospital mortality. Anesth Analg. 2022;135(3):595–604.
18. Semeraro F, Greif R, Böttiger BW, Burkart R, Cimpoesu D, Georgiou M, et al. European Resuscitation Council Guidelines 2021: systems saving lives. Resuscitation. 2021;161:80–97.

19. Soar J, Böttiger BW, Carli P, Couper K, Deakin CD, Djärv T, et al. European Resuscitation Council Guidelines 2021: adult advanced life support. Resuscitation. 2021;161:115–51.
20. Nolan JP, Ornato JP, Parr MJA, Perkins GD, Soar J. Resuscitation highlights in 2016. Resuscitation. 2017;114:A1–7.
21. Perkins GD, Graesner JT, Semeraro F, Olasveengen T, Soar J, Lott C, et al. European Resuscitation Council Guidelines 2021: executive summary. Resuscitation. 2021;161:1–60.
22. Lott C, Truhlář A, Alfonzo A, Barelli A, González-Salvado V, Hinkelbein J, et al. European Resuscitation Council Guidelines 2021: cardiac arrest in special circumstances. Resuscitation. 2021;161:152–219.
23. Dennis M, Zmudzki F, Burns B, Scott S, Gattas D, Reynolds C, et al. Cost effectiveness and quality of life analysis of extracorporeal cardiopulmonary resuscitation (ECPR) for refractory cardiac arrest. Resuscitation. 2019;139:49–56.
24. Nallamothu BK, Greif R, Anderson T, Atiq H, Couto TB, Considine J, et al. Ten steps toward improving in-hospital cardiac arrest quality of care and outcomes. Circ Cardiovasc Qual Outcomes. 2023;16(11):e010491.
25. Anderson TM, Secrest K, Krein SL, Schildhouse R, Guetterman TC, Harrod M, et al. Best practices for education and training of resuscitation teams for in-hospital cardiac arrest. Circ Cardiovasc Qual Outcomes. 2021;14(12):e008587.
26. Sundelin A, Stålman A, Djärv T. Effectiveness of ultra-rapid (20 min) high-frequency in-situ cardiac arrest simulations in a high-volume operating department – a tool for evaluating and implementing emergency routines. Resusc Plus. 2025;22:100887.
27. Kuschner CE, Becker LB. Recent advances in personalizing cardiac arrest resuscitation. F1000Res. 2019;8:F1000 Faculty Rev-915.
28. Apfelbaum JL, Caplan RA, Barker SJ, Connis RT, Cowles C, Ehrenwerth J, et al. Practice advisory for the prevention and management of operating room fires: an updated report by the American Society of Anesthesiologists Task Force on Operating Room Fires. Anesthesiology. 2013;118(2):271–90.
29. Anesthesia Patient Safety Foundation. Surgical fire injuries continue to occur: prevention may require more cautious use of oxygen [Internet]. apsf Newsletter. Available from: https://www.apsf.org/article/surgical-fire-injuries-continue-to-occur-prevention-may-require-more-cautious-use-of-oxygen/.
30. Kaye AD, Kolinsky D, Urman RD. Management of a fire in the operating room. J Anesth. 2014;28(2):279–87.
31. Remz M, Luria I, Gravenstein M, Rice SD, Morey TE, Gravenstein N, et al. Prevention of airway fires: do not overlook the expired oxygen concentration. Anesth Analg. 2013;117(5):1172–6.
32. Akhtar N, Ansar F, Baig MS, Abbas A. Airway fires during surgery: management and prevention. J Anaesthesiol Clin Pharmacol. 2016;32(1):109–11.
33. Lee JY, Park CB, Cho EJ, Kim CJ, Chea JS, Lee BH, et al. Airway fire injury during rigid bronchoscopy in a patient with a silicon stent -a case report. Korean J Anesthesiol. 2012;62(2):184–7.
34. Smith LP, Roy S. Operating room fires in otolaryngology: risk factors and prevention. Am J Otolaryngol. 2011;32(2):109–14.
35. Day AT, Rivera E, Farlow JL, Gourin CG, Nussenbaum B. Surgical fires in otolaryngology: a systematic and narrative review. Otolaryngol Head Neck Surg. 2018;158(4):598–616.
36. Roy S, Smith LP. What does it take to start an oropharyngeal fire? Oxygen requirements to start fires in the operating room. Int J Pediatr Otorhinolaryngol. 2011;75(2):227–30.
37. Eichhorn JH, Eisenkraft JB. Expired oxygen as the unappreciated issue in preventing airway fires: getting to "never". Anesth Analg. 2013;117(5):1042–4.
38. Jones TS, Black IH, Robinson TN, Jones EL. Operating room fires. Anesthesiology. 2019;130(3):492–501.
39. Overbey DM, Townsend NT, Chapman BC, Bennett DT, Foley LS, Rau AS, et al. Surgical energy-based device injuries and fatalities reported to the food and drug administration. J Am Coll Surg. 2015;221(1):197–205.e1.
40. Ehrenwerth J. Fire safety in the operating room [Internet]. UpToDate. 2024. Available from: https://www.uptodate.com/contents/fire-safety-in-the-operating-room.

41. Bhananker SM, Posner KL, Cheney FW, Caplan RA, Lee LA, Domino KB. Injury and liability associated with monitored anesthesia care: a closed claims analysis. Anesthesiology. 2006;104(2):228–34.
42. Mehta SP, Bhananker SM, Posner KL, Domino KB. Operating room fires: a closed claims analysis. Anesthesiology. 2013;118(5):1133–9.
43. Rinder CS. Fire safety in the operating room. Curr Opin Anaesthesiol. 2008;21(6):790–5.
44. Stewart MW, Bartley GB. Fires in the operating room: prepare and prevent. Ophthalmology. 2015;122(3):445–7.
45. Stormont G, Anand S, Deibert CM. Surgical fire safety. [Updated 2023 Jan 29]. In: StatPearls [Internet] [Internet]. Treasure Island (FL): StatPearls Publishing. Available from: https://www.ncbi.nlm.nih.gov/books/NBK544303/.

Perioperative Blood Management: The Anesthesiologist's Role in Safer Transfusion Practices

10

Ashley Yager, Sadaf Chaugle, Douglas Nguyen, and Ravi V. Joshi

10.1 Introduction

The transfusion of allogeneic whole blood or blood components remains a mainstay for the treatment of perioperative hemorrhage, anemia, and blood disorders in modern medicine. Based on data from America's Blood Centers (ABC) and Association of Blood Donor Professionals (ADRP) 2024 report on blood donation, approximately 16 million blood units or components were transfused in the year 2021 with about 10.7% transfused during surgery and an additional 16.1% transfused in the intensive care setting [1]. As a potentially life-saving treatment, neither whole blood nor its components have a true equivalent synthetic or pharmacological alternative, making the national blood product supply a critical resource that requires mindful conservation. Empirical use for questionable indications can lead to wasteful loss of a precious resource that is exceedingly difficult to replace despite the best efforts of blood donation programs and centers. In addition, although blood products are an essential part of patient management, transfusions have been independently associated with increased risk of morbidity and mortality in the perioperative setting [2–6]. Complications arising from unnecessary or excessive blood product administration include hemolytic and non-hemolytic transfusion reactions, transfusion-related acute lung injury (TRALI), transfusion-related cardiac overload (TACO), and transfusion-associated sepsis (TAS).

The growing evidence is that blood products are a mixed blessing, and judicious administration driven by clinical evidence, institutional guidelines, and expert-based consensus is highly recommended. In the past decade, institutional patient

A. Yager · S. Chaugle · D. Nguyen · R. V. Joshi (✉)
Division of Cardiothoracic and Vascular Anesthesiology, University of Texas Southwestern Medical Center (UTSW), Dallas, TX, USA

Department of Anesthesiology & Pain Management, University of Texas Southwestern Medical Center (UTSW), Dallas, TX, USA
e-mail: ravi.joshi@utsouthwestern.edu

G. Tewfik (ed.), *The Anesthesiologist as Perioperative Leader*,
https://doi.org/10.1007/978-3-032-18058-2_10

blood management (PBM) programs developed in order to address the issue of excess or unnecessary transfusion in the perioperative setting.

The chief three pillars of patient blood management include:

I. **Preoperative optimization of patient red cell mass and treatment of anemia**
II. **Intraoperative minimization of blood loss and transfusion of blood products**
III. **Tolerance of intraoperative and postoperative anemia**

A recent meta-analysis of 17 retrospective studies demonstrated that multidisciplinary patient blood management programs are highly effective in reducing blood transfusion rates by as much as 40% and show a measurable decrease in perioperative complications and mortality [7]. PBM programs are also cost-effective, producing institutional cost-savings due to several factors including the reduction in perioperative blood product usage, shorter length of hospital stays, and reduced complication rates. Based on the growing body of evidence for efficacy, PBM programs have been wholly endorsed by the World Health Organization (WHO) [8].

In this chapter, we will describe the most common and effective patient blood management interventions and therapies supported currently in the literature. The chapter is separated into preoperative, intraoperative, and postoperative PBM initiatives and interventions.

10.2 Multidisciplinary PBM Teams

There is great interest and motivation among hospital systems to implement patient blood management programs. The development of PBM programs has been shown to have impactful cost savings and more efficient conservation of blood product resources [9]. On a survey of cardiac anesthesiology practices, institutions that had a multidisciplinary PBM team were more likely to align with QCDR blood conservation initiatives than those without such teams [10]. Successful programs that implement recent advances in transfusion medicine and put consensus guidelines in practice require advocates from several disciplines including surgery, anesthesiology, critical care, hematology, transfusion medicine, and hospital administration. Barriers to implementation of PBM initiatives include knowledge gaps in blood conservation measures, lack of infrastructure, initial start-up cost (including time), and institutional acceptance [11].

10.3 Preoperative Approach to Anemia and Red Cell Optimization

10.3.1 Preoperative Anemia

Preoperative anemia is common in the surgical population, with a prevalence rate reported between 29.9% and 39.1% [12]. Identification and evaluation of preoperative anemia is an essential component for improving perioperative outcomes. Preoperative anemia has been associated with increased morbidity and mortality, prolonged hospital stays, and higher likelihood of postoperative complications [13] such as stroke, acute kidney injury, and infection [12]. In addition to affecting patient centered outcomes and resulting in higher rates of RBC transfusions, anemia has a significant burden to the healthcare system as a whole. Large claims analyses have demonstrated increased healthcare utilization and expenditures when anemia coexists with several major disorders. A 2005 study of approximately 2.3 million health plan members found that patients with a systemic disorder condition (CKD, solid-tumor cancers, HIV, RA, IBD, or congestive heart failure) who were also anemic had twice the average annualized costs of nonanemic patients with the same condition [14]. As such, the anesthesiologist has a key role to identify and lead interventions to minimize the risks that coincide with preoperative anemia. Diagnosis begins with screening. Due to the high prevalence of anemia in the general population, it is reasonable to preoperatively screen all patients undergoing major surgical procedures. The most used criteria for anemia are the WHO definitions (Hb <12.0 g/dL for women or <13.0 g/dL for men), though there has been a range of Hgb cutoff levels used in studies [15]. Screening may provide the opportunity to treat previously unrecognized anemia, particularly in cases at high risk for significant blood loss, and in patients who may not tolerate anemia. Patients should be identified and undergo workup early enough to allow sufficient time for any treatments to be successful. For example, at the University of Texas Southwestern Medical Center, treatment at least 4 weeks before surgery has been suggested as the optimal time runway for evaluation [16]. Urgent or emergent surgery requiring shorter time frames should not prevent evaluation.

Iron deficiency is the most common cause of anemia [17]. As such, all anemic patients should be screened for iron deficiency anemia, which is considered when ferritin is less than 30 mg/L. It is also reasonable to evaluate nonanemic surgical patients for iron deficiency who are undergoing planned surgery with expected large blood loss [18]. Typical lab studies are serum iron, total iron-binding capacity, transferrin saturation, and serum ferritin, as well as complete blood count. Diagnosis can be challenging in the chronically ill or patients in inflammatory states, as ferritin is an acute phase reactant and often elevated independent of iron status. If not iron deficient, additional multidisciplinary consultation with hematology disorder specialist may be warranted for anemia. Furthermore, other causes of anemia such as renal, hematologic, or nutritional deficiencies should be evaluated. One such example of a multidisciplinary anemia screening and referral protocol was demonstrated by the Duke Perioperative Enhancement Team (POET); below is their workflow for evaluation and treatment of iron deficiency in parturients (Fig. 10.1) [19].

10.3.2 Preoperative Red Cell Optimization

The goal of treatment of preoperative anemia is to restore Hgb levels to a normal range; the exact target depends on the clinical setting (i.e., patient factors and surgical factors). At UT Southwestern, we utilize a Hgb of 10 g/dL for the majority of surgical patients as a good threshold to consider therapy. We recommend initiating therapy at least 4 weeks prior to planned surgery to allow targeted anemia therapy to take effect. In practice, shorter time frames are common at the time of referral, although this should not preclude the initiation of treatment if possible. When choosing among different preoperative treatments for anemia, one should consider the type of surgery and potential blood loss, the target Hgb level, speed of correction of anemia versus urgency of surgery, and the possible side effects of therapy. Ultimately, this decision should be made jointly with a multidisciplinary team involving the preoperative provider, a hematology specialist, and the referring surgeon.

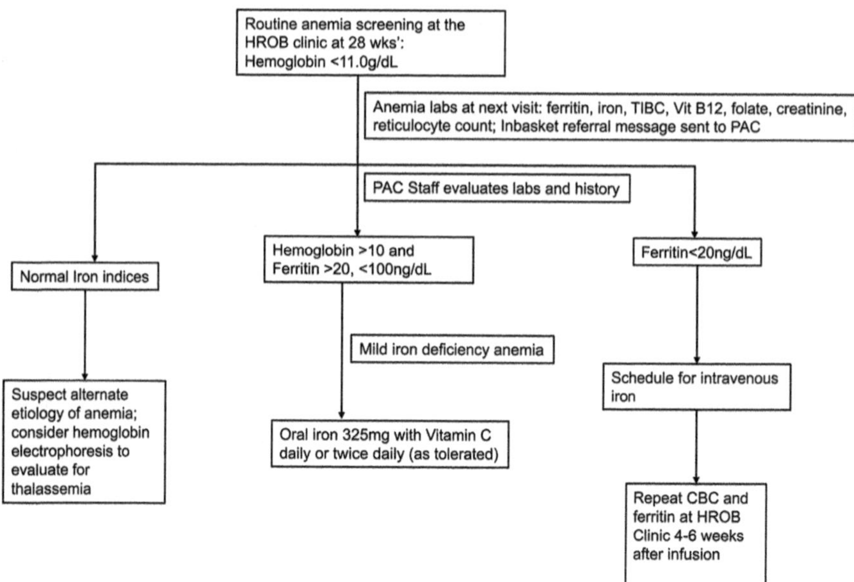

Fig. 10.1 Workflow for iron deficiency anemia. (Reprinted with permission from Gunn et al. [19])

10.3.3 Iron Therapy

Supplemental iron therapy is the primary recommended treatment for patients with iron deficiency anemia. Despite this, there is still uncertainty regarding the effectiveness and reliability of iron therapy in clinically important outcomes. Oral iron supplementation can be effective for mild-moderate iron deficiency anemia but requires 6 weeks to months for significant improvement of red cell count. Accordingly, it is best used for non-emergent surgeries that can be scheduled after therapeutic levels can be achieved. The feasibility of this form of therapy is limited greatly by its high frequency of side effects, noncompliance, unpredictable intestinal absorption, and long duration to therapeutic effect.

By comparison, a systematic review of preoperative IV iron therapy in patients undergoing major surgery found that IV iron significantly decreased perioperative blood transfusions and provided a modest increase in Hgb concentration that lasts greater than 4 weeks postoperatively when compared to placebo or oral iron [20]. Another review described patients receiving IV iron as having lower 30-day mortality, reduced blood transfusions, and lower risk of postoperative infection [21]. It is contraindicated in patients with allergy to iron and in septic patients with ongoing infections. Adverse reactions rates are low [22], with an estimated incidence of less than 1 in 250,000 administrations. These included dyspnea, hypotension, and anaphylaxis. In comparison, the estimated incidence of adverse reactions associated with blood transfusions is 1 in 21,413. Due to its rapid onset and more reliable pharmacodynamics, practitioners often choose IV iron over oral iron as first line for patients with preoperative iron deficiency anemia seen in pre-surgical testing. Patients require multiple infusions which are separated by 1-week intervals. Hgb increase is variable among patients as well as with different IV iron formulations which are dependent on patient insurance. The minimum time to improvement is 2 weeks, though optimal response time is usually 4 weeks. If anemia is severe, time to reach optimal levels of red blood cell mass may be prolonged. A formula published by Ganzoni et al. [23] can be used to calculate a patient's total body iron deficit to guide therapy dosing, though clinically, most infusion centers utilize weight and Hgb based manufacturer dosing tables instead. A sample preoperative iron therapy schedule is provided below (see Fig. 10.2).

10.3.4 Erythropoietin (EPO)

Anemia of chronic disease is characterized by a failure of erythropoietin concentrations to increase in response to reduced Hgb. Inflammatory modulators inhibit erythropoietin production and receptors leading to reduced erythropoiesis. As such, EPO was approved for treatment of preoperative anemia. It has also been demonstrated to work synergistically with iron supplementation. However, in 2007, a black box warning was issued based on evidence that therapy increased the risk of death and other adverse events, most notably venous thromboembolism (VTE) in patients with renal failure or cancer. Since then, several randomized clinical trials

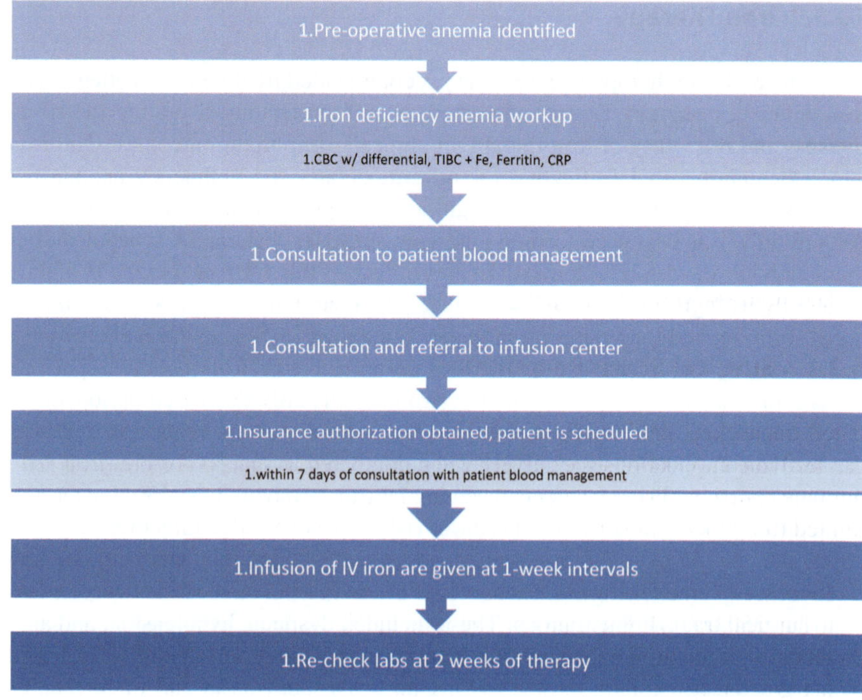

Fig. 10.2 Preoperative iron therapy schedule

(RCTs) and subsequent meta-analyses have demonstrated that EPO reduces the likelihood of RBC transfusion and increases Hgb concentration, without increasing the risk of thromboembolic events [24–26]. There is no consensus on standard dose or duration of erythropoiesis stimulating agent (ESA) treatment. If used, the treatment duration should be limited to the minimum required and IV iron therapy should be given concomitantly to minimize the risk of thrombocytosis. Furthermore, the risk of VTE and high cost poses a need for individualized risk assessment for each patient and has limited its widespread use.

10.3.5 The Anticoagulated Patient

Anticoagulated patients are increasingly more common with the advancement of coronary stents, heart valves, endovascular grafts, and more. Ideally, anticoagulation and anti-platelet agents that would result in excessive blood loss should be minimized. This discussion should be multidisciplinary with the anesthesiologist serving to facilitate discussions with the primary prescriber of therapy and the surgeon that weigh the benefit of continuing anti-thrombotic therapy and the risk of uncontrolled bleeding in the perioperative period. Several guidelines published by various societies exist for stratifying a patient's thrombotic risk, as well as when anti-thrombotic therapy can be discontinued. Additionally, guidelines such as those published by the American College of Cardiology entail an appendix of common procedures per specialty society with assigned bleeding risk for a given procedure (see Table 10.1). Special care should also be taken to consider the resumption of the anticoagulation in the recovery phase.

10.3.6 Special Populations

10.3.6.1 Hemophilia A & B

Preoperative considerations: Engage a hematologist early to coordinate the workup, they should write a detailed treatment plan outlining duration and dosage of hemostatic therapies to reach target factor levels needed for hemostasis. Patients should also be screened for the presence of inhibitors to factor VIII and IX as this may affect treatment. According to Nordic guidelines, Factor replacement therapy should target factor levels of 70–100 IU/dL immediately before surgery, with planned replacement therapy for 7–10 days after major surgery. Tranexamic acid (10 mg/kg IV) should be combined with factor replacement therapy during this period. The patient should have daily assessments of factor levels for 7–10 days following surgery. For minor surgery: factor level of 50 IU/dL is recommended with replacement therapy lasting 1–5 days depending on the procedure.

10.3.6.2 Thalassemia

Thalassemias are a heterogeneous group of autosomal recessive genetic disorders characterized by an absence or decreased synthesis of alpha or beta globin chains of hemoglobin. This aberrant hemoglobin leads to increased apoptosis and red blood cell turnover, with many patients presenting with chronic anemia requiring multiple transfusions over their lifetime. Cardiac failure is the primary cause of death in many patients with any form of thalassemia due to chronic iron overload. Typically, thalassemia minor is described as a carrier state where most patients are

Table 10.1 Preoperative recommendations for common anticoagulant classes

Anti-coagulant Class	Recommendation for Discontinuation
Vitamin K Inhibitors (e.g., Warfarin)	**Discontinue 5–7 days before surgery and bridge with low-molecular-weight heparin (LMWH) if high thrombotic risk.**
Direct Oral Anticoagulants (anti-Factor Xa) (e.g., Rivaroxaban, Apixaban, Edoxaban)	**Discontinue 2–3 days before surgery, longer for major surgeries or impaired renal function.**
Direct Thrombin Inhibitors (e.g., Dabigitran)	**Discontinue 3–5 days before surgery based on renal function**
Antiplatelet Agents (e.g., aspirin, clopidogrel)	**Discontinue 5–7 days before surgery, depending on bleeding risk and cardiovascular status.**

asymptomatic. Conversely, thalassemia major has more severe symptoms, involving multiple organ systems being iron overloaded resulting in hepatosplenomegaly, endocrine dysfunction, and osteoporosis. Diagnosis is suspected in patients with microcytic, hypochromic hemolytic anemia. Pretransfusion hemoglobin of 9.5–10 g/dL is commonly used as a transfusion threshold and chelation therapy is initiated after 10–12 transfusions with agents such as deferoxamine or deferasirox. Engaging hematology input for the perioperative period is advised.

10.3.6.3 Sickle Cell

Clinical assessment of their disease burden, frequency of transfusions, and thrombotic co-morbidities should be performed. The perioperative team may consider exchange transfusions to drop the levels of hemoglobin S to below 30%. Particular care should be taken to avoid conditions that promote sickling, including dehydration, hypoxia, hypercapnia, hypothermia. Transfusion thresholds to maintain hemoglobin levels above 10 g/dL have been recommended.

10.3.6.4 The Jehovah's Witness (JW) Patient

Healthcare professions must respect and care for the ethical and clinical considerations for patient's autonomy and the decision to decline blood products. While some exceptions may exist, such as fractionated products including albumin, clotting factors, or autologous blood, generally, blood products such as whole blood, red blood cells, platelets and plasma are unacceptable to certain patient populations. The practices for the administration and delivery of specific products should be carefully outlined with each patient prior to surgery and re-confirmed on the day of a procedure. Due to these limitations, preoperative optimization, as outlined above, are crucial to minimizing the risks to this patient population. It is also important to engage early in discussions so that surgical and patient goals align. As an example, below is the UT Southwestern Medical Center protocol once a Jehovah's Witness patient undergoing major surgery is identified (Fig. 10.3).

10.4 Intraoperative Minimization of Blood Loss and Transfusion of Blood Products

10.4.1 Physiology of Coagulation

Primary Hemostasis Understanding effective blood management in cardiac surgery begins with a comprehensive grasp of coagulation physiology (see Fig. 10.4). The coagulation process starts with primary hemostasis, where platelets are activated and adhere to damaged vessel walls through von Willebrand Factor (vWF) binding to exposed collagen via glycoprotein Ib (gpIb). Activated platelets undergo crucial conformational changes in their glycoprotein IIb-IIIa (gpIIb-IIIa) receptors, enabling fibrinogen binding and platelet aggregation [27].

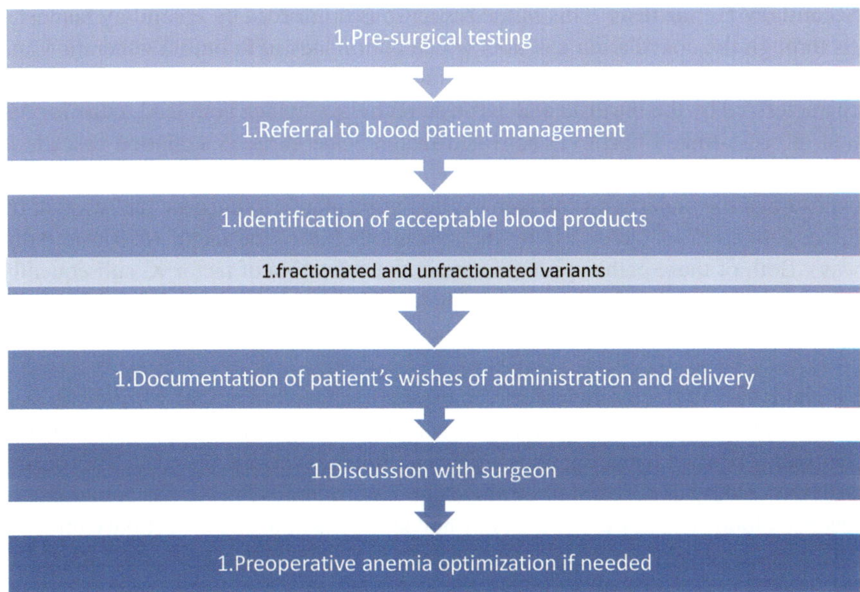

Fig. 10.3 Preoperative work-flow for special populations

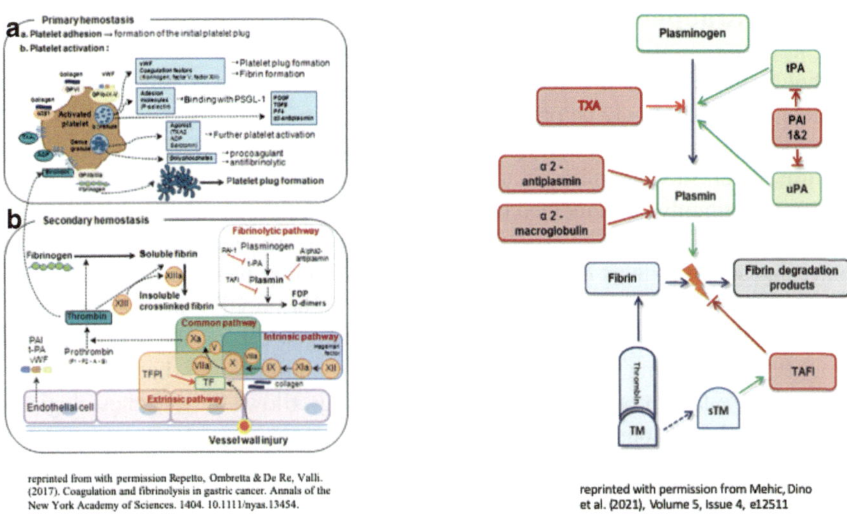

Fig. 10.4 Physiology of coagulation. Schematic of 1° hemostasis and 2° hemostasis (*left panel*) and fibrinolysis (*right panel*)

Secondary Hemostasis This initial response is reinforced by secondary hemostasis through the coagulation cascade, which culminates in thrombin generation and fibrin cross-linking. In turn, this encapsulates and strengthens the thrombus. It is characterized by the intrinsic and extrinsic pathways, which both lead to the formation of cross-linked fibrin via activated factors. The entire coagulation cascade is activated in two ways by either contact with damaged endothelium and subsequent exposure of the underlying collagen to circulating platelets (intrinsic pathway) or by direct activation of factor VII by the subendothelial tissue factor (extrinsic pathway). Both of these pathways culminate in the activation of factor X, subsequently producing thrombin, and an enzyme that converts fibrinogen to insoluble fibrin, which then determines the integrity of the clot [25].

Fibrinolysis The body maintains hemostatic balance through the fibrinolytic system, regulated by tissue plasminogen activator (tPA) and plasminogen activator inhibitor-1 (PAI-1), ensuring appropriate clot breakdown when needed. This occurs with the binding of tPA and plasminogen to C-terminal lysine residues, initiating a feedback loop. The key enzyme in fibrinolysis is plasmin, and the primary function is to degrade the fibrin polymers, generating fibrin degradation products, such as the D-dimer. Still, the rate of fibrinolysis is determined by the structural properties of the fibrin clots, and the thinner the fibrin fibers, the denser the clot [28].

10.4.2 Intraoperative Techniques

Although many of the following intraoperative techniques (particularly for cardiopulmonary bypass) may be primarily a surgical intervention, the anesthesiologist's role should be advocate for the use of these strategies where applicable. Specifically, the use of cell salvage, mini-circuits, ultrafiltration, and autologous priming protocols are commonly implemented by the surgeon or clinical cardiac perfusionist with input from anesthesiologist especially in voicing concerns about hemodynamic stability and volume status of the patient. In contrast, other procedures such as acute normovolemic hemodilution or therapies like antifibrinolytics and factor concentrates are direct interventions that the anesthesiologist can resolve to use in their practice for reducing allogeneic transfusions. In addition, the diagnostic use of point-of-care laboratories (e.g., viscoelastic testing) allows the anesthesiologist to make critical decisions guiding hemostasis management in real-time.

10.4.3 Cell Salvage

Modern blood conservation techniques have evolved significantly, with cell salvage remaining a cornerstone of effective management. Cell salvage essentially takes blood from the operative field and returns it back to the patient, and the red blood cells may be washed and centrifuged before being returned. Contemporary cell salvage systems wash the scavenged blood with 0.9% normal saline and return the blood with a hematocrit of 50–70%. Meta-analysis published in the 2010 Cochrane review demonstrated a relative risk reduction in allogenic blood transfusion of 23%, and that the outcomes were superior with washed as opposed to unwashed blood. Contemporary practice tends to be in favor of utilizing intraoperative cell salvage in cardiac surgery, with studies showing that some form of pump salvage and eventual reinfusion back into the patient is an effective way to decrease blood transfusion [29]. Use of cell salvage in patients with cancer or systemic infection is controversial but not absolutely contraindicated.

10.4.4 Acute Normovolemic Hemodilution (ANH)

Acute normovolemic hemodilution (ANH) is done by strategically removing a certain blood volume from the patient while hydrating the patient to maintain euvolemia, storing the blood with anticoagulants at room temperature, and giving it back to the patient during their surgery, typically after weaning from cardiopulmonary bypass. The benefits include decreased risk of reactions related to allogenic blood transfusions, preservation of the red blood cells from shearing forces related to cardiopulmonary bypass, and improving post-bypass coagulation by administering whole blood back to the patient that contains coagulation factors and platelets. Additionally, administering the whole blood after weaning from bypass helps prevent alterations that result in platelet consumption, activation of the complement system and the inflammatory cascade. One study in 2017 looked at 29 randomized controlled trials and found that the ANH group received less blood transfusions, and these patients also had statistically significant less total estimated blood loss [30]. Another study notes that ANH is effective in reducing allogenic blood transfusion when surgical blood loss exceeds 1 L or 20% of the patient's total blood volume. However, patient selection remains crucial, with specific contraindications for those with severe coronary artery disease or heart failure, which may limit its use in cardiac surgery patients [31]. This technique is often entirely performed either preoperatively or intraoperatively by the anesthetic team. The decision to perform ANH is a discussion between the anesthesiologist, surgeon, and the patient.

10.4.5 Blood Conservation on Cardiopulmonary Bypass

Cardiac surgery presents unique challenges and opportunities for blood conservation, specifically because cardiac surgeries tend to generate the greatest need for blood transfusions. In the 2010s, approximately 34% of all cardiac surgery patients required a transfusion. These transfusions are necessary due to coagulopathy, blood loss, and the hemodilution from pump priming. Additionally, the patients that are undergoing cardiac surgery often have anemia and coronary artery disease, which inherently increases the risk of complications [32]. The primary issue is the utilization of cardiopulmonary bypass and the disruption of normal hemostatic and inflammatory mechanisms that occur with extracorporeal circulation. Initiation of cardiopulmonary bypass requires systemic anticoagulation, preferably with heparin, and the exposure of non-native surfaces commonly activate fibrinolysis and consume platelets. In addition, 800 mL–1.2 L of crystalloid is used to prime the bypass circuit prior to initiation leading to significant hemodilution of the patient. This coupled with surgical blood loss invariably necessitates blood product administration in this surgical population. STS guidelines recommend a strict transfusion protocol for cardiac surgery patients with a hemoglobin of less than 7 g/dL, especially when the patient demonstrates hemodynamic instability. However, excessive and liberal thresholds for blood transfusions have been associated with substantially increased morbidity and mortality [33].

10.4.6 Retrograde Autologous Priming (RAP)

One popular conservation technique is Retrograde Autologous Priming (RAP), as it effectively reduces hemodilution during cardiopulmonary bypass (CPB) initiation. Patient blood is drained retrograde into both arterial and venous limbs of the bypass circuit to displace pump priming volume which is emptied into an external container. Recent studies demonstrate that RAP decreases postoperative transfusion requirements and is associated with a shorter length of stay but does not have a statistically significant mortality benefit [34].

10.4.7 Minimal Extracorporeal Circulation (MECC)

Another intervention is the use of "mini-bypass" circuits, or minimal extracorporeal circulation (MECC), featuring closed systems with reduced prime volumes and biocompatible surfaces. MECC has been shown to decrease rates of systemic inflammation by limiting the blood-air interface, decreased length of tubing (about half the standard bypass circuit, therefore decreasing rates of hemodilution), and complete heparin coating of the circuit. The significant difference is that MECC lacks a venous reservoir, and the reservoir is the patient themselves. Meta-analyses consistently indicate a reduced inflammatory response and lower transfusion requirements compared to conventional CPB circuits [35].

10.4.8 Modified Ultrafiltration

Lastly, hemoconcentration techniques, particularly modified ultrafiltration, have been shown to be effective in removing excess fluid and inflammatory mediators. This results in increased end-hematocrit, with the greatest benefits seen with ultrafiltrate volumes up to 2.5 L. However, with ultrafiltration, there is decreased urine output, and with excessive fluid removal, there may be in increased incidence of acute kidney injury [36].

10.4.9 Factor and Fibrinogen Concentrates

The pharmacological approach to blood management has seen significant advancement as well. Prothrombin complex concentrates (PCCs) have emerged as effective alternatives to fresh frozen plasma (FFP), particularly for urgent reversal of vitamin K antagonists, with current guidelines supporting their use for major bleeding in patients on vitamin K antagonists (Class I, Level B evidence). Fibrinogen concentrates have demonstrated superior efficacy compared to cryoprecipitate, offering faster preparation time and standardized dosing, with recommendations targeting fibrinogen levels above 200 mg/dL during active bleeding.

In 2019, the Society of Cardiovascular Anesthesiologists (SCA) published an article highlighting management of perioperative bleeding and hemostasis particularly in cardiac surgery patients. They recognized that bleeding post-cardiac surgery is a serious complication that results in increased morbidity and mortality, and that transfusion rates were provider dependent [35]. There is significant evidence to suggest that allogenic blood transfusions are associated with infections, transfusion reactions, atrial fibrillation, respiratory issues, acute kidney injury, and overall mortality, and is also directly proportional to the number of units transfused. There is a thought, however, that adopting point of care (POC) testing and treatment algorithms routinely may decrease transfusions to some degree.

Their recommended management begins with preoperative optimization with iron therapy and erythropoietin in some select cases. Intraoperatively, for patients with heparin resistance, as opposed to giving large doses of heparin to achieve an adequate activated clotting time (ACT) for going on bypass, it is recommended to administer antithrombin III (ATIII), which can restore antithrombin levels, improve the sensitivity of heparin, and establish the level of anticoagulation needed to safely go on full CPB. Although fresh frozen plasma can be used for management of heparin resistance, use of ATIII is preferred. As mentioned above, strategies to minimize hemodilution are strongly recommended to decrease rate of postoperative transfusions. For patients on P2Y12 inhibitors, POC platelet function testing can inform providers regarding overall platelet function and possible delay of surgery until the drug effects are no longer seen [37].

According to the a 2021 subgroup analysis of the FIBRES trial published in 2019, FFP is administered to approximately 15% of cardiac surgery patients in the United States for bleeding patients with coagulation factor deficiencies. These factor deficiencies occur in large part due to the potential drop of 40–50% in coagulation factor levels associated with CPB. However, administration of FFP is associated with hemodilution and subsequent RBC transfusion, as well as higher rates of transfusion-associated cardiac overload (TACO) and transfusion-related acute lung injury (TRALI), which are the two most common causes of death related to transfusion. Therefore, administration of FFP versus PCC, PCC has been shown to be superior in CPB-related coagulopathy and subsequently leads to decreased postoperative transfusions. PCCs come in either three- or four-factor formulations, with the latter containing factor VII as the fourth factor. They also contain a small amount of an anticoagulant to decrease the risk of excessive coagulation [38].

The 2021 subgroup study randomized patients with similar comorbidity profiles to either the FFP or PCC group and compared the results. Between the two groups, there was statistically different amount of overall RBC transfusions (87% in the FFP group to 61% in the PCC group) and platelet transfusions (93% to 81%). There was also a statistically significant lower rate of acute kidney injury within the first 7 days in the PCC group (19–29% in the FFP group). Overall, this study aimed to further examine the use of FFP versus PCC in cardiac surgery, and the results were promising in favor of PCC use. The results suggested a dose between 1000 and 2000 IUs as an effective dose for management of coagulopathy [38].

More recently, in 2025, the FARES-II (Factor Replacement in Surgery-II) trial was published, aiming to further evaluate the efficacy of PCC over FFP for coagulopathic bleeding, specifically in cardiac surgery patients. PCCs are human factor derived, purified, pathogen-reduced, and can be stored at room temperature. Several advantages include a lower total infusion volume for reconstitution, resulting in less hemodilution. Patients were again randomized to either FFP or PCC if they had at least moderate bleeding and had an international normalized ratio (INR) of greater than 1.5. The primary outcome in this study was the hemostatic response. The PCC group demonstrated a higher hemostatic effectiveness and a shorter time for drug administration. Additionally, the FFP group was shown to have higher rates of AKI, increased chest tube outputs, and more overall serious adverse events. The rate of thromboembolic events was similar in the two groups despite PCC having superior hemostatic efficacy. This study recommended a slightly higher dosage of PCC at 25 IU/kg (with a maximum dose of 50 IU/kg if needed), compared to 15 IU/kg that had been used in the past. Certain patients with a high risk of thromboembolism were excluded from this study, however, including those with a thrombotic event in the past 3 months, patients with thoracoabdominal aortic aneurysms, and patients with ventricular assist devices. The biggest conclusion drawn from this study is the superiority of PCC for hemostatic efficacy and overall safety advantages in the setting of coagulation factor deficiency [39].

10.4.10 Antifibrinolytic Therapy

Antifibrinolytic therapy has robust supporting evidence and is commonly used during cardiac surgeries with CPB to reduce post-bypass bleeding and transfusion requirements. Two of the most used agents are epsilon aminocaproic acid and tranexamic acid (TXA), which are both lysine analogs. A third product, aprotinin, is highly effective however was withdrawn from the US market a few years ago due to safety concerns and studies demonstrating increased mortality [40]. All transfusion guidelines support the use of antifibrinolytics in patients undergoing cardiac surgery with CPB due to a significantly decreased risk of reoperation due to bleeding and decreased transfusion requirements [35]. Both aminocaproic acid and TXA work by preventing excessive plasmin formation by binding to the lysine binding site on plasminogen, preventing fibrin from binding to it, which essentially inhibits the tPA-induced fibrinolysis. Dosing can vary to some degree, but typically TXA is given as a 10 mg/kg bolus followed by a 1–2 mg/kg bolus on CPB, and a continuous infusion of 1 mg/kg/h. Aminocaproic acid can be given as a bolus of 100 mg/kg, 5 mg/kg on CPB, and an infusion of 30 mg/kg/h. [41] Antifibrinolytic therapy has also shown efficacy in massive trauma, neurosurgical trauma, and OB hemorrhage. The CRASH-2 RCT demonstrated the use of 1 g TXA bolus followed by 1 g over an 8-h infusion reduces mortality without an increase in thrombotic events in a variety of major traumas [42]. More recent meta-analyses have found a decrease in blood products but have not found the mortality benefit [43]. The follow-up CRASH-3 revealed that there is a mortality benefit to administer TXA (1 g in 10 min bolus, 1 g infusion over 8-h) in patients with mild-moderate head-injury but not patients with severe traumatic brain injury [10]. In obstetric hemorrhage, early administration of TXA (1 g bolus, and second 1 g bolus if continued bleeding within 24 h) reduced mortality from bleeding without increase vascular complications [44].

10.4.11 Viscoelastic Testing (VET) and Transfusion Algorithms

Laboratory-based transfusion management has been revolutionized by viscoelastic testing platforms. Thromboelastography (TEG) provides comprehensive assessment of clot formation, clot strength, and speed of lysis, with utility in detecting hyperfibrinolysis. Rotational Thromboelastometry (ROTEM) offers faster results than TEG through multiple concurrent channels and better differentiation of specific coagulation factor deficiencies, while enhancing detection of fibrinogen contribution to clot strength. The newer Quantra technology, utilizing sonic estimation of elasticity via resonance, provides faster time to results compared to traditional platforms and features automated interpretation that reduces operator variability. With regards to coagulation monitoring, the use of viscoelastic testing with either thromboelastography (TEG) or rotational thromboelastometry (ROTEM) has been associated with decreased transfusion requirements and overall improved patient outcomes (see Fig. 10.5, left panel). Evidence strongly supports the implementation of algorithm-based transfusion protocols that incorporate viscoelastic testing [35]. Unfortunately, the use of laboratory-based algorithms has been limited, even among academic cardiac centers in the United States [46]. These algorithms have demonstrated a significant reduction in blood product utilization, decreased transfusion-associated costs, and improved patient outcomes including reduced mortality. Effective protocols typically include baseline viscoelastic testing after heparin reversal, with specific trigger points for various interventions: platelet transfusion based on low MCF/MA in EXTEM/FIBTEM comparison, fibrinogen replacement guided by low FIBTEM A10, and factor concentrate administration determined by prolonged CT/R time, with repeat testing following interventions to assess response. A sample algorithm from the Society of Cardiovascular Anesthesiology is presented in Fig. 10.5 (right panel). Management of hemorrhage in cardiac surgery should be individualized and goal directed, and studies have shown that the use of POC algorithms, such as the ones below, have been shown to decrease blood transfusion rates, decrease incidence of thrombotic events, and decrease overall hospital costs [45].

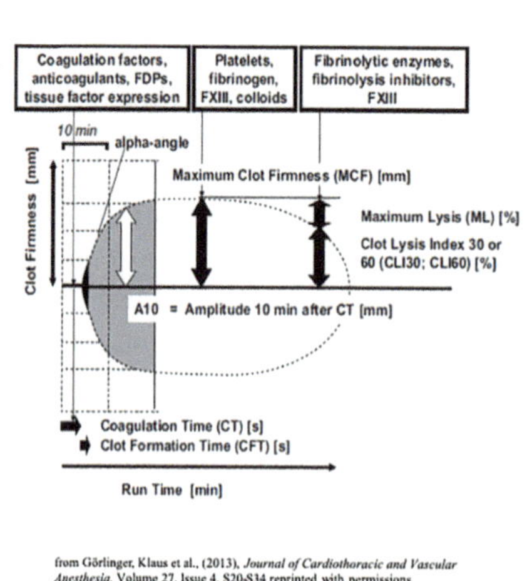

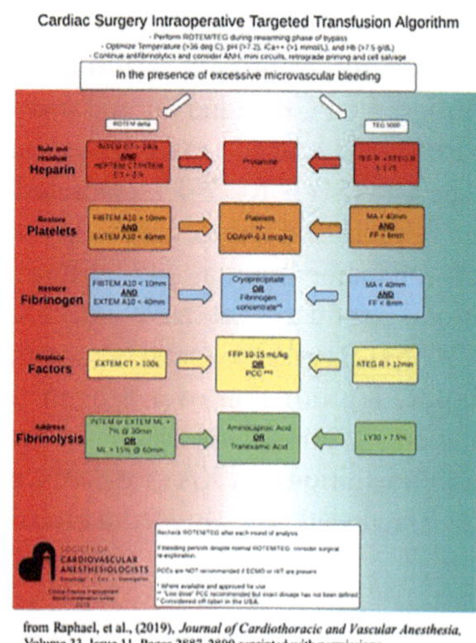

Fig. 10.5 Thromboelastography and elements of ROTEM analysis (*left panel*) from Gorlinger et al. [45] and Society of Cardiovascular Anesthesiology recommended transfusion algorithm (*right panel*) from Raphael et al. [37]

10.5 Tolerance of Anemia and Postoperative Interventions

10.5.1 Transfusion Triggers in the OR and ICU

Postoperative anemia is very common and can be seen in up to 90% of patients who have undergone a major surgery [47]. When considering postoperative transfusion, the provider needs to consider risk to the patient for both giving and withholding the transfusion. Red blood cell transfusions are given to approximately 25 percent of critically ill patients in the United States which leads to roughly 1.8 million transfusions annually [48]. In many institutions, cutoffs of 7 or 8 grams per deciliter (g/dL) have been frequently utilized. Although blood transfusion improves oxygen delivery and therefore can reduce the risk of ischemia, it is not without risks. As mentioned above, transfusion leads to increased risk of volume overload and heart failure, transfusion-related acute lung injury, transmission of infectious disease, transfusion reaction, or effects of increased blood viscosity. In addition, perioperative transfusions have been linked to increased risk of recurrence in colorectal cancer. Multiple studies have shown a relationship between blood transfusion and cardiac, pulmonary, renal, neurological, and wound complications though further investigation needs to be held regarding the contribution of secondary factors [42]. Another consideration is the cost involved in transfusing blood. An evaluation of four hospitals looking at cost of transfusion in the surgical population determined that $522–$1183 were required per red blood cell unit [49]. The effect on blood bank supplies also needs to be considered, especially now while the gap between supply and demand continues to increase.

The Transfusion Requirements in Critical Care (TRICC) trial was one of the seminal studies in transfusion with 838 patients comparing liberal vs restrictive transfusion strategies with hemoglobin <7 g/dL (goal 7.0–9.0 g/dL) being used for the restrictive group and hemoglobin <10 g/dL (goal 10.0–12.0 g/dL) being used for the liberal group. No significant difference was found when comparing all-cause mortality at 30 days; however, the restrictive group did show lower rates of mortality in patients age less than 55 and those that were less acutely ill but not in those with significant cardiac disease. This led them to the conclusion that, with the exception of those patients with significant cardiac disease, the restrictive strategy is at least as effective as the liberal in critically ill patients [50] (Hebert).

10.5.2 Transfusion Triggers in Surgery

In the same vein as the TRICC trial, avoidance of unnecessary transfusions during surgery and tolerance of lower patient hemoglobin concentrations is a key intervention in patient blood management. The question remains what hemoglobin level is acceptable for adequate oxygen deliver and perfusion in the surgical patient. The TRICS III trial looked at this liberal vs. restrictive transfusion triggers in cardiac surgery, an often critically ill population. A total of 5243 Patients were randomized to either a hemoglobin level of <7.5 g/dL or <9.5 g/dL as restrictive and liberal transfusion triggers, respectively. The results looked at death, myocardial infarction, stroke, or acute renal failure as primary outcomes. Results from TRICS III demonstrated that a restrictive transfusion strategy using a <7.5 g/dL trigger was non-inferior to more liberal transfusion strategies.

As part of the Myocardial Ischemia and Transfusion (MINT) trial randomized 3504 patients to either restrictive or liberal transfusion strategies in patients with myocardial infarction. In the restrictive group, transfusion was allowed for hemoglobin <8 g/dL and recommended with hemoglobin <7 g/dL or in patients with anginal symptoms that could not be controlled with medication. The cutoff for transfusion in the liberal group was a hemoglobin <10 g/dL. They concluded that the risk of recurrent myocardial infarction or death at 30 days was not significantly reduced with the liberal transfusion strategy; however, a noted trend toward clinical benefit may bring into question the non-inferiority of restrictive transfusion strategies [51].

While uncertainty still exists in certain subgroups, overall, there is now strong evidence showing that a restrictive strategy is safe and may lead to a reduction in the number of patients receiving red cells by 41%. This data encompasses a range of clinical settings with data studied by 48 randomized trials that analyzed over 20,000 patients [52]. Other meta-analyses comparing liberal vs restrictive transfusion strategies in a broad list of scenarios also confirm restrictive transfusion strategies do not have a negative impact on morbidity and mortality [42].

10.5.3 Transfusion Strategies in Critically Ill Patients

There are steps that can be considered when assessing transfusion in the ICU setting. When appropriate, reassessment after a single unit should take place prior to administration of additional blood products. This can help avoid unnecessary transfusion. There was a noted decrease in red blood cell units transfused by 50% when units were transfused one at a time with hemoglobin measurements checked prior to subsequent transfusion [26]. In order to increase a patient's tolerance of anemia, providers can focus on optimizing oxygenation and hemodynamics. Additional factors such as central venous oxygenation, acidosis, lactate levels, hemodynamics, and electrocardiogram changes can be used as secondary factors when considering transfusion, although there has not been a proven impact on clinical outcome [29].

10.5.4 Transfusion Algorithms and Viscoelastic Testing

Transfusion algorithms can be used in both the intraoperative setting as well as in the intensive care setting (Fig. 10.6). Modifications would need to be considered on an institutional basis to accommodate available laboratory analysis, blood products, and factor concentrates. Algorithms can be used to focus on specific factor deficiencies in a targeted manner (see Fig. 10.6) [53]. Viscoelastic testing (VET) can be used postoperatively in the intensive care unit with benefits similar to the operating room. VET algorithms will allow the direct targeting of therapy for intraoperative bleeding. This can reduce unnecessary transfusions seen in unguided or empirical treatment of hemorrhage. Improved turnaround time is another benefit of VET, as current point of care (POC) devices can result in an answer in as little as 20 min. VET provides the underlying mechanism of bleeding, directing the type of transfusion therapy (PRBCs, fresh frozen plasma, platelets, and cryoprecipitate) as well as the need for factor concentrates, antifibrinolytics, or protamine.

10.5.5 Massive Transfusion and Massive Transfusion Protocols (MTPs)

Massive bleeding can occur in the emergency room, intraoperatively, in the labor-delivery suite, or in the intensive care unit. In the case of severe hemorrhage, the introduction of massive transfusion protocols (MTP) has helped in the management of massive bleeding by early administration of blood products although outcomes data is lacking. In the past, empirical administration of blood products often led to worsening outcomes due to the imbalance of blood components (FFP vs. PRBCs) and the targeting of higher blood pressures. Unbalanced transfusions often lead to dilutional coagulopathy resulting in poor hemostasis. Other immediate complications include transfusion-associated circulatory overload (TACO), citrate toxicity, hyperkalemia, acidosis, and hypothermia. Later-stage complications include transfusion-related acute lung injury (TRALI), sepsis, and thrombotic

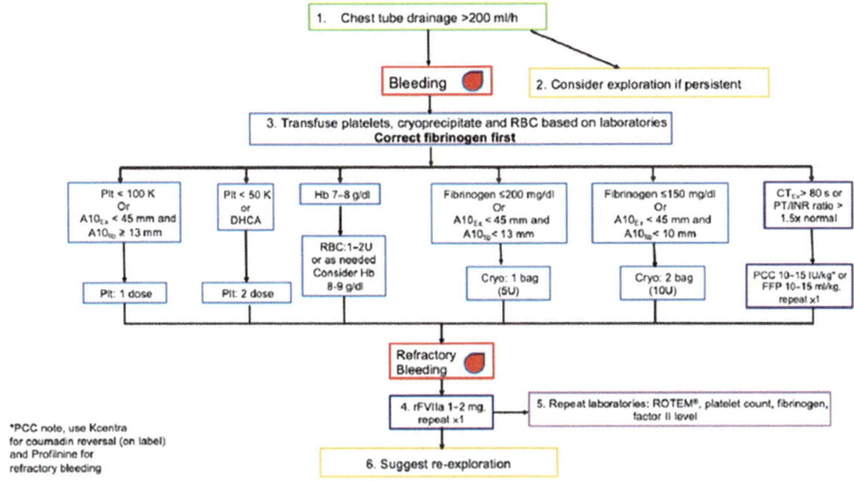

Fig. 10.6 Sample transfusion ICU algorithm from Hashmi et al. [53]

complications [54]. Massive transfusion protocols require (1) standard indications for massive transfusion, (2) rapid deployment of blood products, (3) and a protocol for fixed ratio transfusion. Various definitions for what is considered "massive bleeding/hemorrhage" exist and often differ by institution. Several of common definitions suggested for massive hemorrhage in multiple studies have been reviewed by Patil and Shetmahajan [54] including [48]:

- Replacement of one entire blood volume per 24 h
- Transfusion of >10 units of packed red blood cells (PRBCs) per 24 h
- Transfusion of >20 units of PRBCs per 24 h
- Transfusion of >4 units of PRBCs in 1 h
- Replacement of 50% of total blood volume (TBV) in 3 h.

MTPs require coordination with the blood bank and transfusion medicine to have specific units of blood products (PRBC, FFP, platelets) packaged together for emergency use. Current recommendations now include a fixed ratio of blood products, and although there is much debate on the optimal ratio; nonetheless, 1:1:1 PRBC to FFP to platelets is the most common ratio [55–57].

10.5.6 Reduce Blood Sampling/Testing

One significant cause of anemia in the intensive care setting is iatrogenic and associated with phlebotomy. Assessing the necessity of each blood draw prior to ordering can help decrease blood loss from lab collection. As soon as labs can be safely decreased in frequency, standing orders should be updated and labs should be drawn with the smallest possible volume for reliable results. While two milliliters may not seem significant in the course of a patient's recovery, when this is multiplied by several tubes collected at frequent regular intervals, this volume rapidly increases. The cumulative median blood volume from phlebotomy was found to be 454 mL in cardiac surgery and increased with the length of stay. One study looked at transitioning to pediatric blood tubes from adult sized tubes and found a 47% reduction in blood loss associated with lab testing however cost and logistics need to be considered [58, 59].

10.5.7 Blood Sampling with Closed Loop Systems

In addition to decreasing unnecessary labs, utilizing a closed loop system can help to prevent blood loss during repeat blood draws. Blood waste associated with an open system is inevitable given the need to utilize a waste syringe to rid saline. Though the amount may be small, with repeated blood draws, small volume blood loss can contribute to significant anemia potentially requiring need for additional blood transfusion.

10.5.8 Alternative Noninvasive Physiologist Monitors

Despite smooth placement, there is still blood loss associated with invasive monitoring. When the situation is appropriate, noninvasive monitoring can aid in decreasing the blood loss from placement and line associated hemorrhage. It has also been found that patients with invasive arterial access in the intensive care unit were subject to more blood draws even with similar risk factors for mortality [47].

10.5.9 The Role of the Anesthesiologist as the Perioperative Physician in PBM

Patient blood management is essential in the perioperative care of the surgical patient. Multidisciplinary PBM programs have shown reductions in the unnecessary administration of blood products leading to cost savings and reduction in complication rates. In addition to understanding the risks and benefits of blood transfusion, as the perioperative physician, the anesthesiologist is poised more than any other specialty to advocate, coordinate, and implement PBM strategies to reduce blood product wastage. Preoperatively, the anesthesiologist can engage in many facets of PBM practices including preoperative diagnosis of anemia via the preoperative clinic, facilitation of preoperative anemia therapy, and the optimization of care for special populations (e.g., Jehovah's Witness patients) all in coordination with other services such as surgery and transfusion medicine. In the operating room and intensive care unit, the anesthesiologist utilizes clinical judgment in conjunction with the use of viscoelastic testing and laboratory-guided algorithms, lower perioperative transfusion triggers, and alternative therapies such as factor concentrates, all to reduce blood product administration while preserving adequate hemostasis. The perioperative physician must be intimately involved in evaluating success of PBM policies through constant audit and feedback as well as data-driven clinical metrics including mortality outcomes and cost savings. Finally, anesthesiologists should be champions in their respective institutions for promoting perioperative blood conservation through education and research.

10.6 Conclusion

Although life-saving in many instances, unnecessary blood product transfusions can lead to increased mortality and morbidity in our surgical patient population. Prudent and thoughtful transfusion practices have the potential for improving surgical outcomes, reducing waste, and provide tangible cost-savings. In this chapter, we have discussed the ever-expanding field of perioperative patient blood management (PBM) including the preoperative, intraoperative, and postoperative strategies to reduce blood product usage in various perioperative and surgical settings. As primary administrator of blood products in the perioperative setting, the anesthesiologist can take a leading role in promoting institution-wide blood conservation practices.

References

1. America's Blood Centers and ADRP: Association of Blood Donor Professionals. U.S. blood donation: statistics and pubic messaging guide. January 2024 version 2.0. https://americasblood.org/wp-content/uploads/2024/08/U.S.-Blood-Donation-Statistics-and-Public-Messaging-Guide-Jan.-2024-v-2.1-FINAL.pdf.
2. Morris FJD, Fung YL, Craswell A, Chew MS. Outcomes following perioperative red blood cell transfusion in patients undergoing elective major abdominal surgery: a systematic review and meta-analysis. Br J Anaesth. 2023;131(6):1002–13. https://doi.org/10.1016/j.bja.2023.08.032. Epub 2023 Sep 21
3. Murphy GJ, Reeves BC, Rogers CA, Rizvi SI, Culliford L, Angelini GD. Increased mortality, postoperative morbidity, and cost after erythrocytes transfusion in patients having cardiac surgery. Circulation. 2007;116:2544–52.
4. Glance LG, Dick AW, Mukamel DB, et al. Association between intraoperative blood transfusion and mortality and morbidity in patients undergoing noncardiac surgery. Anaesthesiology. 2011;114:283–92.
5. Malone DL, Dunne J, Tracy JK, Putnam AT, Scalea TM, Napolitano LM. Blood transfusion, independent of shock severity, is associated with worse outcome in trauma. J Trauma. 2003;54:898–905.
6. Corwin HL, Gettinger A, Pearl RG, et al. The CRIT Study: anemia and blood transfusion in the critically ill-current clinical practice in the United States. Crit Care Med. 2004;32:39–52.
7. Althoff FC, Neb H, Herrmann E, Trentino KM, Vernich L, Füllenbach C, Freedman J, Waters JH, Farmer S, Leahy MF, Zacharowski K, Meybohm P, Choorapoikayil S. Multimodal patient blood management program based on a three-pillar strategy: a systematic review and meta-analysis. Ann Surg. 2019;269(5):794–804. https://doi.org/10.1097/SLA.0000000000003095.

8. Bolliger D, Buser A, Tanaka KA. Outcomes, cost-effectiveness, and ethics in patient blood management. Curr Opin Anaesthesiol. 2025;38(2):151–6. https://doi.org/10.1097/ACO.0000000000001466. Epub 2025 Feb 12
9. Meybohm P, Richards T, Isbister J, et al. Patient blood management bundles to facilitate implementation. Transfus Med Rev. 2017;31:62–71.
10. CRASH-3 Trial Collaborators. Effects of tranexamic acid on death, disability, vascular occlusive events and other morbidities in patients with acute traumatic brain injury (CRASH-3): a randomised, placebo-controlled trial. Lancet. 2019;394(10210):1713–23. https://doi.org/10.1016/S0140-6736(19)32233-0. Epub 2019 Oct 14. Erratum in: Lancet. 2019 Nov 9;394(10210):1712. https://doi.org/10.1016/S0140-6736(19)32641-8. PMID: 31623894; PMCID: PMC6853170.
11. Kwak J, Wilkey AL, Abdalla M, Joshi R, Roman PEF, Greilich PE. Perioperative blood conservation: guidelines to practice. Adv Anesth. 2019;37:1–34. https://doi.org/10.1016/j.aan.2019.08.011. Epub 2019 Sep 27
12. Fowler AJ, Ahmad T, Phull MK, Allard S, Gillies MA, Pearse RM. Meta-analysis of the association between preoperative anaemia and mortality after surgery. J Br Surg. 2015;102(11):1314–24.
13. Muñoz M, Gómez-Ramírez S, Campos A, Ruiz J, Liumbruno GM. Pre-operative anaemia: prevalence, consequences and approaches to management. Blood Transfus. 2015;13(3):370.
14. Smith RE Jr. The clinical and economic burden of anemia. Am J Manag Care. 2010;16 Suppl Issues:S59–66.
15. Pasricha SR, Colman K, Centeno-Tablante E, Garcia-Casal MN, Peña-Rosas JP. Revisiting WHO haemoglobin thresholds to define anaemia in clinical medicine and public health. Lancet Haematol. 2018;5(2):e60–2.
16. Geisser P, Burkhardt S. The pharmacokinetics and pharmacodynamics of iron preparations. Pharmaceutics. 2011;3:12–33.
17. Muñoz M, Laso-Morales MJ, Gómez-Ramírez S, Cadellas M, Núñez-Matas MJ, García-Erce JA. Pre-operative haemoglobin levels and iron status in a large multicentre cohort of patients undergoing major elective surgery. Anaesthesia. 2017;72(7):826–34.
18. Al-Naseem A, Sallam A, Choudhury S, Thachil J. Iron deficiency without anaemia: a diagnosis that matters. Clin Med. 2021;21(2):107–13.
19. Guinn NR, et al. How do I develop a process to effectively treat parturients with iron deficiency anemia? Transfusion. 2020;60(11):2476–81. https://doi.org/10.1111/trf.15930.
20. Elhenawy AM, Meyer SR, Bagshaw SM, MacArthur RG, Carroll LJ. Role of preoperative intravenous iron therapy to correct anemia before major surgery: a systematic review and meta-analysis. Syst Rev. 2021;10:1–4.
21. Schack A, Berkfors AA, Ekeloef S, Gögenur I, Burcharth J. The effect of perioperative iron therapy in acute major non-cardiac surgery on allogenic blood transfusion and postoperative haemoglobin levels: a systematic review and meta-analysis. World J Surg. 2019;43:1677–91.
22. Chertow GM, Mason PD, Vaage-Nilsen O, Ahlmen J. Update on adverse drug events associated with parenteral iron. Nephrol Dial Transplant. 2006;21(2):378–82.
23. Ganzoni AM. Eisen-Dextran intravenös: therapeutische und experimentelle Möglichkeiten [Intravenous iron-dextran: therapeutic and experimental possibilities]. Schweiz Med Wochenschr. 1970;100(7):301–3.
24. Cho BC, Serini J, Zorrilla-Vaca A, Scott MJ, Gehrie EA, Frank SM, Grant MC. Impact of preoperative erythropoietin on allogeneic blood transfusions in surgical patients: results from a systematic review and meta-analysis. Anesth Analg. 2019;128(5):981–92.
25. Kei T, Mistry N, Curley G, Pavenski K, Shehata N, Tanzini RM, Gauthier MF, Thorpe K, Schweizer TA, Ward S, Mazer CD. Efficacy and safety of erythropoietin and iron therapy to reduce red blood cell transfusion in surgical patients: a systematic review and meta-analysis. Can J Anesth. 2019;66(6):716–31.
26. Kaufner L, von Heymann C, Henkelmann A, Pace NL, Weibel S, Kranke P, Meerpohl JJ, Gill R. Erythropoietin plus iron versus control treatment including placebo or iron for

preoperative anaemic adults undergoing non-cardiac surgery. Cochrane Database Syst Rev. 2020;8(8):CD012451.

27. Repetto O, De Re V. Coagulation and fibrinolysis in gastric cancer. Ann N Y Acad Sci. 2017;1404. https://doi.org/10.1111/nyas.13454.
28. Mehic D, et al. Fibrinolysis and bleeding of unknown cause. Res Pract Thromb Haemost. 2021;5(4):e12511.
29. Baker RA, Merry AF. Cell salvage is beneficial for all cardiac surgical patients: arguments for and against. J Extra Corpor Technol. 2012;44(1):P38–41. PMID: 22730871; PMCID: PMC4557446
30. Barile L, et al. Acute normovolemic hemodilution reduces allogeneic red blood cell transfusion in cardiac surgery: a systematic review and meta-analysis of randomized trials. Anesth Analg. 2017;124(3):743–52. https://doi.org/10.1213/ANE.0000000000001609.
31. Zhou X, Zhang C, Wang Y, Yu L, Yan M. Preoperative acute normovolemic hemodilution for minimizing allogeneic blood transfusion: a meta-analysis. Anesth Analg. 2015;121(6):1443–55. https://doi.org/10.1213/ANE.0000000000001010.
32. Arias-Morales CE, Stoicea N, Gonzalez-Zacarias AA, Slawski D, Bhandary SP, Saranteas T, Kaminiotis E, Papadimos TJ. Revisiting blood transfusion and predictors of outcome in cardiac surgery patients: a concise perspective. F1000Res. 2017;6:F1000 Faculty Rev-168. https://doi.org/10.12688/f1000research.10085.1. PMID: 28299184; PMCID: PMC5321117
33. Patel NN, et al. Indications for red blood cell transfusion in cardiac surgery: a systematic review and meta-analysis. Lancet Haematol. 2015;2(12):e543–53.
34. Gupta S, McEwen C, Basha A, Panchal P, Eqbal A, Nicole W, Belley-Cote EP, Whitlock R. Retrograde autologous priming in cardiac surgery: a systematic review and meta-analysis. Eur J Cardiothorac Surg. 2021;60(6):1245–56.
35. Baikoussis NG, Papakonstantinou NA, Apostolakis E. The "benefits" of the mini-extracorporeal circulation in the minimal invasive cardiac surgery era. J Cardiol. 2014;63(6):391–6. ISSN 0914-5087.
36. Mongero L, Stammers A, Tesdahl E, Stasko A, Weinstein S. The effect of ultrafiltration on end-cardiopulmonary bypass hematocrit during cardiac surgery. Perfusion. 2018;33(5):367–74. https://doi.org/10.1177/0267659117747046.
37. Jacob Raphael C, Mazer D, Subramani S, Schroeder A, Abdalla M, Ferreira R, Roman PE, Patel N, Welsby I, Greilich PE, et al. Society of Cardiovascular Anesthesiologists clinical practice improvement advisory for management of perioperative bleeding and hemostasis in cardiac surgery patients. J Cardiothorac Vasc Anesth. 2019;33(11):2887–99. ISSN 1053-0770.
38. Bartoszko J, Callum J, Karkouti K, FIBRES Study Investigators. The association of prothrombin complex concentrates with postoperative outcomes in cardiac surgery: an observational substudy of the FIBRES randomized controlled trial. Can J Anaesth. 2021;68(12):1789–801. https://doi.org/10.1007/s12630-021-02100-4. Epub 2021 Sep 14. Erratum in: Can J Anaesth. 1848–1849. https://doi.org/10.1007/s12630-021-02123-x. PMID: 34523108; PMCID: PMC8563600.
39. Karkouti K, Callum JL, Bartoszko J, et al. Prothrombin complex concentrate vs frozen plasma for coagulopathic bleeding in cardiac surgery: the FARES-II multicenter randomized clinical trial. JAMA. 2025. https://doi.org/10.1001/jama.2025.3501.
40. Aggarwal NK, Subramanian A. Antifibrinolytics and cardiac surgery: the past, the present, and the future. Ann Card Anaesth. 2020;23(2):193–9. https://doi.org/10.4103/aca.ACA_205_18. PMID: 32275035; PMCID: PMC7336973.
41. Fergusson D, Herbert P. A comparison of aprotinin and lysine analogues in high-risk cardiac surgery. N Engl J Med. 2008;358(22):2319–31.
42. CRASH-2 Trial Collaborators, Shakur H, Roberts I, Bautista R, Caballero J, Coats T, Dewan Y, El-Sayed H, Gogichaishvili T, Gupta S, Herrera J, Hunt B, Iribhogbe P, Izurieta M, Khamis H, Komolafe E, Marrero MA, Mejía-Mantilla J, Miranda J, Morales C, Olaomi O, Olldashi F, Perel P, Peto R, Ramana PV, Ravi RR, Yutthakasemsunt S. Effects of tranexamic acid on death, vascular occlusive events, and blood transfusion in trauma patients with significant haemorrhage

(CRASH-2): a randomised, placebo-controlled trial. Lancet. 2010;376(9734):23–32. https://doi.org/10.1016/S0140-6736(10)60835-5. Epub 2010 Jun 14.
43. Lawati KA, Sharif S, Maqbali SA, et al. Efficacy and safety of tranexamic acid in acute traumatic brain injury: a systematic review and meta-analysis of randomized-controlled trials. Intensive Care Med. 2021;47:14–27. https://doi.org/10.1007/s00134-020-06279-w.
44. WOMAN Trial Collaborators. Effect of early tranexamic acid administration on mortality, hysterectomy, and other morbidities in women with post-partum haemorrhage (WOMAN): an international, randomised, double-blind, placebo-controlled trial. Lancet. 2017;389(10084):2105–16. https://doi.org/10.1016/S0140-6736(17)30638-4. Epub 2017 Apr 26. Erratum in: Lancet. 2017 May 27;389(10084):2104. https://doi.org/10.1016/S0140-6736(17)31220-5. PMID: 28456509; PMCID: PMC5446563.
45. Görlinger K, et al. Management of hemorrhage in cardiothoracic surgery. J Cardiothorac Vasc Anesth. 2013;27(4):S20–34.
46. Joshi RV, Wilkey AL, Blackwell JM, Kwak J, Raphael J, Shore-Lesserson L, Greilich PE. Blood conservation and hemostasis in cardiac surgery: a survey of practice variation and adoption of evidence-based guidelines. Anesth Analg. 2021;133(1):104–14. https://doi.org/10.1213/ANE.0000000000005553.
47. Desai N, Schofield N, Richards T. Perioperative patient blood management to improve outcomes. Anesth Analg. 2018;127(5):1211–20. https://doi.org/10.1213/ANE.0000000000002549.
48. Coz Yataco AO, Soghier I, Hébert PC, Belley-Cote E, Disselkamp M, Flynn D, Halvorson K, Iaccarino JM, Lim W, Lindenmeyer CC, Miller PJ, O'Neil K, Pendleton KM, Vande Vusse L, Ouellette DR. Red blood cell transfusion in critically ill adults: an American College of Chest Physicians clinical practice guideline. Chest. 2025;167(2):477–89. https://doi.org/10.1016/j.chest.2024.09.016. Epub 2024 Sep 26. PMID: 39341492; PMCID: PMC11867898.
49. Shander A, Hofmann A, Ozawa S, Theusinger OM, Gombotz H, Spahn DR. Activity-based costs of blood transfusions in surgical patients at four hospitals. Transfusion. 2010;50:753–65.
50. Hébert PC, Wells G, Blajchman MA, Marshall J, Martin C, Pagliarello G, Tweeddale M, Schweitzer I, Yetisir E. A multicenter, randomized, controlled clinical trial of transfusion requirements in critical care. Transfusion Requirements in Critical Care Investigators, Canadian Critical Care Trials Group. N Engl J Med. 1999;340(6):409–17.
51. Carson JL, Brooks MM, Hébert PC, Goodman SG, Bertolet M, Glynn SA, Chaitman BR, Simon T, Lopes RD, Goldsweig AM, DeFilippis AP, Abbott JD, Potter BJ, Carrier FM, Rao SV, Cooper HA, Ghafghazi S, Fergusson DA, Kostis WJ, Noveck H, Kim S, Tessalee M, Ducrocq G, de Barros E, Silva PGM, Triulzi DJ, Alsweiler C, Menegus MA, Neary JD, Uhl L, Strom JB, Fordyce CB, Ferrari E, Silvain J, Wood FO, Daneault B, Polonsky TS, Senaratne M, Puymirat E, Bouleti C, Lattuca B, White HD, Kelsey SF, Steg PG, Alexander JH, MINT Investigators. Restrictive or liberal transfusion strategy in myocardial infarction and anemia. N Engl J Med. 2023;389(26):2446–56. https://doi.org/10.1056/NEJMoa2307983. Epub 2023 Nov 11. PMID: 37952133; PMCID: PMC10837004
52. Shah A, Klein AA, Agarwal S, Lindley A, Ahmed A, Dowling K, Jackson E, Das S, Raviraj D, Collis R, Sharrock A, Stanworth SJ, Moor P. Association of Anaesthetists guidelines: the use of blood components and their alternatives. Anaesthesia. 2025;80(4):425–47. https://doi.org/10.1111/anae.16542. Epub 2025 Jan 9. PMID: 39781579; PMCID: PMC11885198
53. Hashmi NK, Ghadimi K, Srinivasan AJ, Li YJ, Raiff RD, Gaca JG, Root AG, Barac YD, Ortel TL, Levy JH, Welsby IJ. Three-factor prothrombin complex concentrates for refractory bleeding after cardiovascular surgery within an algorithmic approach to haemostasis. Vox Sang. 2019;114(4):374–85. https://doi.org/10.1111/vox.12774. Epub 2019 Apr 2. PMID: 30937927; PMCID: PMC6525021
54. Patil V, Shetmahajan M. Massive transfusion and massive transfusion protocol. Indian J Anaesth. 2014;58(5):590–5. https://doi.org/10.4103/0019-5049.144662. PMID: 25535421; PMCID: PMC4260305.
55. Hess JR, Holcomb JB, Hoyt DB. Damage control resuscitation: the need for specific blood products to treat the coagulopathy of trauma. Transfusion. 2006;46(5):685–6. https://doi.org/10.1111/j.1537-2995.2006.00816.x.

56. Holcomb JB, Tilley BC, Baraniuk S, et al. Transfusion of plasma, platelets, and red blood cells in a 1:1:1 vs a 1:1:2 ratio and mortality in patients with severe trauma: the PROPPR randomized clinical trial. JAMA. 2015;313(5):471–82. https://doi.org/10.1001/jama.2015.12.
57. Vlaar APJ, Dionne JC, de Bruin S, Wijnberge M, Raasveld SJ, van Baarle FEHP, Antonelli M, Aubron C, Duranteau J, Juffermans NP, Meier J, Murphy GJ, Abbasciano R, Müller MCA, Lance M, Nielsen ND, Schöchl H, Hunt BJ, Cecconi M, Oczkowski S. Transfusion strategies in bleeding critically ill adults: a clinical practice guideline from the European Society of Intensive Care Medicine. Intensive Care Med. 2021;47(12):1368–92. https://doi.org/10.1007/s00134-021-06531-x. Epub 2021 Oct 22. PMID: 34677620; PMCID: PMC8532090.
58. Smoller BR, Kruskall MS, Horowitz GL. Reducing adult phlebotomy blood loss with the use of pediatric-sized blood collection tubes. Am J Clin Pathol. 1989;91(6):701–3. https://doi.org/10.1093/ajcp/91.6.701.
59. Fischer DP, Zacharowski KD, Meybohm P. Savoring every drop – vampire or mosquito? Crit Care. 2014;18(3):306. https://doi.org/10.1186/cc13884. PMID: 25032998; PMCID: PMC4056661.

Surgical Site Infection Prophylaxis

11

Eric Reilly and Jazmine Skala-Wade

11.1 Introduction

A major component of healthcare associated infections (HAI) is surgical site infections (SSI). Surgical site infections occur at the surgical site within 30 days of surgery and are estimated to affect 2–3% of all surgical patients [2]. An SSI can pose numerous dangers to patients such as delayed surgical recovery, prolonged hospitalization, re-admission, organ dysfunction, and even death. Beyond physical patient impacts, SSIs pose numerous economic burdens to both patients and healthcare systems. Thankfully, many measures can be taken to help prevent and treat SSIs—and such initiatives are often created, led, and implemented by anesthesiologists. Despite fiscal, institutional, and administrative barriers, anesthesiologists remain invaluable champions in patient safety and SSI prevention.

11.2 Patient Impact

Any hospital visit can be a harrowing and vulnerable time for patients and their families; the addition of a surgical encounter serves to heighten associated fear and anxiety. If such occurrences are compounded with an untimely SSI, then patients suffer greatly. The Centers for Disease Control and Prevention (CDC) estimates there are roughly 500,000 SSIs annually, and that SSIs increase hospital lengths of stay by an average of 9.7 days [1, 3]. Those affected cases represent patients who faced a life-threatening—and possibly preventable—complication in their care. As with any health condition, one disease state (such as an SSI) can precipitate other associated maladies. Mild surgical site infections can lead to pain and fatigue, but more severe cases may lead to sepsis, cardiovascular instability, pulmonary

E. Reilly (✉) · J. Skala-Wade
Department of Anesthesiology & Pain Medicine, Corewell Health William Beaumont University Hospital, Royal Oak, MI, USA

G. Tewfik (ed.), *The Anesthesiologist as Perioperative Leader*,
https://doi.org/10.1007/978-3-032-18058-2_11

compromise, loss of limbs, permanent organ damage, or even death. Of note, SSIs are associated with up to an 11-fold increased risk for death and research suggests nearly 75% of SSI-associated deaths are caused directly by the SSI [12, 13]. Aside from their physical assaults, SSIs can also subject patients to emotional distress such as feelings of fear, insecurity, isolation, and dependency [2].

11.3 Economic Impact

Adding to the physical and emotional toll, SSIs also cause huge financial burdens on patients, families and the healthcare system. SSIs can lead to prolonged hospital stays, ICU admissions, additional treatments, and allocation of numerous other healthcare resources. Such occurrences are expensive, and it is estimated that SSIs cost US healthcare systems $3.5 to $10 billion annually [4]. A 3-year study out of The Johns Hopkins Health System suggests a profit loss of $22,239 per SSI [5]. Beyond healthcare systems, estimates suggest SSIs cost a patient $3382 out-of-pocket within the 8 weeks of their discharge [3]. Cost is already a huge barrier for individuals seeking medical care. Such occurrences—where patients are staying in the hospital longer, using more healthcare resources, and owing more in personal expenses—congest an already crowded system, and further dissuade individuals from seeking the care they need.

11.4 Anesthesiologist-Led Initiatives

The physical, emotional, and economic impacts of SSIs are broad and destructive. Nonetheless, it is important to consider that estimates suggest 60% of SSI's are preventable [4]. It requires dedicated staff to accurately understand, measure, and act through coordinated efforts to help achieve such prevention. Anesthesiologists—the perioperative leaders—often find themselves in a position to take on such tasks. Many factors influencing SSIs are intertwined with an anesthesiologist's role, ensuring that perioperative physicians must play a crucial role in a robust program to prevent surgical site infections.

11.5 Checklists

Perioperative checklists—such as the World Health Organization's (WHO) surgical safety checklist—consisting of the sign-in, time-out, and sign-out—are widely used to help confirm key elements such as the correct patient, correct surgical site, and correct staff. Similarly, the surgical patient safety system (SURPASS) checklist was co-developed by an anesthesiologist and is successfully utilized globally [23]. These checklists require collaborative communication between surgeons, anesthesiologists, and other OR staff to help reduce surgical errors and adverse perioperative events. Some of the factors addressed in these checklists—such as antibiotic prophylaxis, sterile equipment, temperature goals, glycemic control, fluid management, and analgesic plans—are the responsibility of the anesthesiologist and play a major role in helping prevent SSIs along with other adverse events.

11.6 Antibiotic Prophylaxis

It is not uncommon for a surgical wound to be contaminated from a patient's inherent skin and organ flora. Yet, the evolution from contamination to an infection is the process worth eliminating, or severely inhibiting. Most surgical procedures constitute an indication for perioperative antibiotics, but the timing, route, and frequency can be complex and must be individualized for each patient. There is evidence to suggest the best person to coordinate and optimize such antibiotic therapy is a patient's own anesthesiologist.

A crucial first step to reducing SSIs is identifying which patients and procedures require antibiotic prophylaxis. Knowledge and training in the pharmacokinetics, indications, side effect profiles, weight-based dosing, and other factors give anesthesiologists unique expertise in understanding surgical antibiotic prophylaxis. As such, algorithms have been extensively studied, authored, and implemented by anesthesiologists as evidenced via numerous institutional, national, and international guidelines [10, 11].

After identifying a need for prophylaxis, the next barrier is implementation of a policy. A 2006 study at the Baystate Medical Center outlined anesthesiologists as the individuals most likely to accomplish successful perioperative antibiotic administration. By adjusting protocol to place anesthesiologists in charge of antibiotic administration, the center recorded significant (0.4% to 2.4%) decreases in SSIs, depending on the type of case. As an extrapolation of their results, the center is presumed to have saved $328,295 and 292 days of hospitalization over the course of a year as a result of their protocol change [6]. Those savings are directly correlated to the leadership and involvement of anesthesiologists in the center's new protocols..

After implementation, it is imperative to analyze and adapt to unforeseen barriers in policy adherence. In a 2023 study out of Emory, which was co-authored by an anesthesiologist, the department created a novel antibiotic compliance feedback tool. This quality improvement tool tracked antibiotic administrations, SSIs, and provided personalized feedback to members of the surgical and anesthesia care teams. Ultimately, implementation of the feedback tool allowed individuals to recognize and adjust their practices, which subsequently led to a 10.3% increase in antibiotic compliance and 0.9% decrease in SSIs [7]. Similar data collection and feedback groups, such as the Multicenter Perioperative Outcomes Group (MPOG), are run by anesthesiologists and help improve patient safety across the nation.

Through identification of SSIs, scientific measurement of appropriate antibiotic prophylaxis practices, implementation of policy revisions, and creating feedback mechanisms—anesthesiologists are helping lead the way for meaningful SSI reduction through antibiotic prophylaxis.

11.7 Hand Hygiene and Personal Protective Equipment

Anesthesiologists have extensive direct patient contact perioperatively. The preoperative physical exam, regional anesthesia procedures, intubations, invasive line placement, patient positioning, bed transfers, and numerous other instances involve direct physical touch. Such occurrences are inevitable opportunities for pathogen spread and contamination. Anticipating and reducing these chances for contamination, such as through hand hygiene and utilizing personal protective equipment (PPE), is crucial to an anesthesiologist's practice in reducing SSIs. Furthermore, this knowledge helps anesthesiologists recognize and prevent similar contamination events between patients and other healthcare providers

In an effort to prioritize patient safety, anesthesiologists at the University of Colorado authored a review article which outlines the importance of hand hygiene, workplace cleanliness, and patient decolonization to help reduce perioperative infections. They even published evidence-based guidelines by which other departments can follow suit to help further reduce infection burdens [14]. Similarly, the Department of Anesthesiology from the University of Iowa showed how proper hand hygiene practices among anesthesia providers can greatly reduce the incidence of pathogen transmission and development of SSIs [15]. That same anesthesiology department even made great strides in determining how some pathogens, like methicillin-resistant staphylococcus aureus (MRSA), are spread and controlled intraoperatively [16].

While imperative for reducing SSIs, many of these anesthesiologist-led initiatives are utilized and extrapolated for reducing HAIs as a whole. Many MRSA and COVID-19 precautions have been developed both directly and indirectly by the groundwork of anesthesiologists promoting hand hygiene and PPE—which has undoubtedly saved countless lives [17, 18].

11.8 Thermoregulation

A patient's body temperature can influence their immune system. Hypothermia is a known culprit of impairing leukocyte function, and may attenuate antibody and cytokine production, ultimately increasing risks of SSI development [8]. Operating rooms are often kept frigid, and many anesthesia medications promote heat loss through peripheral vasodilation and inhibition of a body's inherent thermoregulatory responses. As such, anesthesiologists are extensively trained in the various forms of heat loss and how to best prevent such occurrences. Numerous anesthesiologists have even contributed to standardized guidelines, and policy revisions for addressing and preventing perioperative hypothermia [42, 43]. In addition to preventing SSIs, an anesthesiologist's role in maintaining normothermia helps reduce a patient's length of hospitalization, which can indirectly help prevent additional inpatient complications and unnecessary healthcare resource utilization [9].

11.9 Regional Anesthesia

Surgical site infections are identified in the period following a surgery. A surgery is typically defined as a method of treatment which encompasses manual or instrumental means—often involving an incision or penetration of tissues. Therefore, needle-based regional procedures by anesthesiologists—such peripheral nerve blocks, fascial plane blocks, intrathecal injections, and epidural catheter placements—may be viewed as a minor form of surgery. Regional anesthesia techniques are commonly used perioperatively, involve invasive tissue disruption, and require appropriate consideration for helping reduce surgical site infections.

In January of 2025, the American Society of Regional Anesthesia and Pain Medicine (ASRA Pain Medicine) published a comprehensive risk mitigation guideline to help appropriately reduce, diagnose, and treat infectious complications of regional anesthetic techniques, as well as other acute and chronic pain interventions. It is an evidence-based guideline which serves to help reduce risk of SSIs and HAIs. Over a dozen anesthesiologists contributed as authors to the guidelines. Some of the proposed methods include hand washing techniques, sterile site preparation, and protocols for the timing and appropriateness of certain procedures [19].

Surgical volume is expected to expand precipitously in the next decade, with some estimates anticipating a 21% increase in surgical cases performed at ambulatory surgery centers by 2034 [20]. Greater surgical volume leads to a greater utilization of regional anesthesia, and an overall increased potential for SSIs. The goal of expanded surgical services should include a reduction of surgical complication rates, in order to ensure access and demand is met by safety and equity. Patient safety and reduction of complications—such as SSIs—is prioritized by the individuals who anticipate, treat, and avoid disastrous variables. Those individuals, time and time again, are anesthesiologists. Undoubtedly, anesthesiologist involvement will remain crucial in safely reducing SSIs as surgical volume and regional anesthesia encounters increase in the future.

11.10 Inspired Gas Concentration

Most anesthetic patient encounters involve the administration and monitoring of inspired gases such as oxygen, medical air, and volatile anesthetics. Sometimes overlooked, even a simple nasal cannula supplying oxygen can be a crucial consideration in patient outcomes and development of SSIs.

In 2005, an anesthesiologist-led study published in JAMA showed that colorectal surgery patients receiving a higher percentage of inspired oxygen perioperatively had a 39% lower incidence of SSIs [21]. While still a topic of debate, numerous other studies have concluded similar results; therefore, thoughtful consideration should be given to inspired gas concentrations when aiming to reduce SSIs [22]. As the individuals best trained in the pharmacokinetics and mechanics of inspired gas flows, anesthesiologists remain paramount in optimizing gas concentrations in order to promote positive outcomes.

11.11 Glycemic Control

Hyperglycemia is considered one of the strongest independent risk factors for developing SSIs, and is not only seen in diabetic patients [26]. About 15% of patients undergoing surgery have a diagnosis of diabetes and are high risk for hyperglycemia, but one anesthesiologist authored study found that even 14.7% of non-diabetic patients experience intraoperative hyperglycemia [24, 25]. These occurrences may be due to multiple variables including patient co-morbidities and medication side effects.

A major responsibility of anesthesiologists is glycemic control. As such, numerous anesthesiologists and anesthesiologist groups, such as the Society for Ambulatory Anesthesia (SAMBA) have published guidelines and protocols to assist in diagnosing and treating perioperative hyperglycemia [27]. One study—co-authored by an anesthesiologist—implemented comprehensive preoperative, intraoperative, and postoperative glycemic control initiatives at their institution, which resulted in a two-fold reduction in SSI incidence. Such interventions included preoperative testing and triage, standardization of perioperative insulin choices, and postoperative communication with patients' respective primary care providers [28].

Strong dedication to positive patient outcomes and deep understanding of the science behind glucose management are factors which make anesthesiologists uniquely equipped to tackle hyperglycemia, and ultimately SSIs..

11.12 Fluid Management and Blood Transfusions

Numerous publications—many authored by anesthesiologists—demonstrate the important role for intraoperative fluid management, and specifically goal-directed fluid therapy, in helping prevent SSIs [29, 30]. Importantly, not all intravenous fluids are the same. It requires expertise to delineate when a patient may or may not need infusions of saline, lactated ringers, plasmalyte, albumin, blood products, or any of the numerous options.

Furthermore, blood products are of particular concern, as their transfusion can be a major risk factor for SSIs. Anesthesiologists may interpret dozens of labs, images, and other variables to decide if and when it may be appropriate to initiate a transfusion of blood products. As such, anesthesiologists have made great contributions to developing guidelines to help optimize and safely reduce perioperative blood transfusions. For example, an anesthesiologist at Johns Hopkins healthcare system helped implement a novel electronic blood release system, while simultaneously updating blood ordering guidelines. These changes led to a safe decrease in unnecessary transfusions by 27%, and a six-figure cost reduction for surgical patients during the study period, not accounting for additional potential savings from SSI reductions [31]. From a global standpoint, numerous anesthesiologists contributed to the World Society of Emergency Surgery (WSES) and American Association for the Surgery of Trauma (AAST) joint guidelines to outline strategies to reduce transfusions, a highly regarded resource for clinicians worldwide [32].

As with any treatment, the ability to prescribe comes quick. However, the ability to anticipate and evade detrimental scenarios—while also avoiding unnecessary treatments—is a skillset mastered by anesthesiologists. This is commonly reflected in their approach to fluid therapy and blood transfusions. Such prowess protects patients through multiple avenues, including decreased risks of SSIs.

11.13 Opioid Induced Immunosuppression

Despite multimodal analgesia efforts, opioid therapy remains effective and widely utilized for perioperative pain. Opioids, while effective analgesics, have commonly recognized side effects such as bradypnea, constipation, urinary retention, nausea, and mental status changes. However, a lesser-known side effect is the potential for immunosuppression and subsequent SSIs.

The exact mechanism of opioid induced immunosuppression is inconclusive, yet the incidental data is often clear. According to a 2020 multicenter study, patients with opioid use disorder are at a 1% to 4% increased risk of SSIs after orthopedic procedures [33]. Similarly, researchers have shown that preoperative opioid use is significantly associated with increased SSIs in both ventral hernia repair and lumbar fusion patients [34, 35]. Even in the intensive care unit (ICU)—where many anesthesiologists round and practice—opioids are associated with increased risks of infection and all-cause mortality [36, 37].

Beginning in the first year of medical school and extending through their entire career, anesthesiologists extensively study the pharmacokinetics, indications, side effects, and alternative options for opioid therapy. Collectively, anesthesiologists have made great contributions at both institutional and global levels through publishing of opioid reduction guidelines, and creating opioid-sparing anesthesia techniques [38, 39]. These efforts not only enhance patient safety but also represent an overall cost savings [40]. In the OR, pain clinics, and ICU—anesthesiologists remain vigilant in opioid stewardship, which inherently helps reduce the incidence of SSIs.

11.14 Barriers and Anesthesiologists as the Solution

Despite evidence for prevention methodology, numerous barriers exist to reducing SSIs. New protocols, even when appropriate, are often difficult to implement due to complexity, poor communication, aversion to change, lack of leadership, and an incapacity to provide reflective evaluation. In this realm, anesthesiologists are uniquely capable of executing such efforts.

As discussed, anesthesiologists have already created and implemented countless protocols to help reduce SSIs throughout healthcare. This is a reflection of the skills anesthesiologists use every day through patient care and interaction with surgical staff. An anesthesiologist has inherent clinical responsibilities of anticipating barriers, assessing readiness, team-based communication, adaptiveness, sharing knowledge, organization, plan implementation, and quality monitoring. These exact qualities are endorsed in the Expert Recommendations for Implementing Change (ERIC) strategies for enacting SSI protocols in the face of institutional barriers [41]. A 2023 federally funded cohort even concluded that certain interpersonal and professional skills were most consistent with successful SSI protocol implementation; these skills are possessed and demonstrated prominently by anesthesiologists.

11.15 Conclusion

Surgical site infections are detrimental to both patient safety and healthcare spending. They represent a problem for which anesthesiologists often serve as a solution. Through both academic and clinical means—ranging from data collection and protocol creation, to perioperative glycemic control and opioid stewardship—anesthesiologists lead the way in SSI reduction. As healthcare practices and surgical volume continue to expand in the future, anesthesiologists will remain pivotal in helping reduce SSIs, prioritizing patient safety, and leading by example.

References

1. Centers for Disease Control and Prevention. Surgical site infection (SSI) event. Atlanta: CDC; 2024. [cited 2025 February 17]. Available from: https://www.cdc.gov/nhsn/pdfs/pscmanual/9pscssicurrent.pdf
2. Andersson AE, Bergh I, Karlsson J, Nilsson K. Patients' experiences of acquiring a deep surgical site infection: an interview study. Am J Infect Control. 2010;38(9):711–7. https://doi.org/10.1016/j.ajic.2010.03.017. PMID: 21034980
3. Perencevich EN, Sands KE, Cosgrove SE, Guadagnoli E, Meara E, Platt R. Health and economic impact of surgical site infections diagnosed after hospital discharge. Emerg Infect Dis. 2003;9(2):196–203. https://doi.org/10.3201/eid0902.020232.
4. Ban KA, Minei JP, Laronga C, Harbrecht BG, Jensen EH, Fry DE, Itani KMF, Dellinger PE, Ko CY, Duane TM. American College of Surgeons and Surgical Infection Society: Surgical Site Infection Guidelines, 2016 Update. J Am Coll Surg. 2017;224(1):59–74. https://doi.org/10.1016/j.jamcollsurg.2016.10.029.
5. Shepard J, Ward W, Milstone A, et al. Financial impact of surgical site infections on hospitals: the hospital management perspective. JAMA Surg. 2013;148(10):907–14. https://doi.org/10.1001/jamasurg.2013.2246.
6. Kanter G, Connelly NR, Fitzgerald J. A system and process redesign to improve perioperative antibiotic administration. Anesth Analg. 2006;103(6):1517–21. https://doi.org/10.1213/01.ane.0000221442.30952.83.
7. Codner JA, Falconer EA, Mlaver E, Zeidan RH, Sharma J, Lynde GC. A self-sustaining antibiotic prophylaxis program to reduce surgical site infections. Surg Infect. 2023;24(8):716–24. https://doi.org/10.1089/sur.2023.111. Epub 2023 Oct 13. PMID: 37831935
8. Kumar S, Wong PF, Melling AC, Leaper DJ. Effects of perioperative hypothermia and warming in surgical practice. Int Wound J. 2005;2:193–204.
9. Kurz A, Sessler DI, Lenhardt R. Perioperative normothermia to reduce the incidence of surgical-wound infection and shorten hospitalization. Study of wound infection and temperature group. N Engl J Med. 1996;334(19):1209–15. https://doi.org/10.1056/NEJM199605093341901. PMID: 8606715

10. Cheng EY, Nimphius N, Hennen CR. Antibiotic therapy and the anesthesiologist. J Clin Anesth. 1995;7(5):425–39, ISSN 0952-8180,. https://doi.org/10.1016/0952-8180(95)00034-F.
11. Eckmann C, Aghdassi SJS, Brinkmann A, Pletz M, Rademacher J. Perioperative antibiotic prophylaxis—indications and modalities for the prevention of postoperative wound infection. Dtsch Arztebl Int. 2024;121(7):233–42. https://doi.org/10.3238/arztebl.m2024.0037. PMID: 38440828; PMCID: PMC11539872
12. Ban KA, Minei JP, Laronga C, Harbrecht BG, Jensen EH, Fry DE, et al. American College of Surgeons and surgical infection society: surgical site infection guidelines, 2016 update. J Am Coll Surg. 2017;224(1):59–74. https://doi.org/10.1016/j.jamcollsurg.2016.10.029.
13. Zimlichman E, Henderson D, Tamir O, Franz C, Song P, Yamin CK, et al. Health care-associated infections: a meta-analysis of costs and financial impact on the US health care system. JAMA Intern Med. 2013;173(22):2039–46. https://doi.org/10.1001/jamainternmed.2013.9763.
14. Simmons CG, Hennigan AW, Loyd JM, Loftus RW, Sharma A. Patient safety in anesthesia: hand hygiene and perioperative infection control. Curr Anesthesiol Rep. 2022;12(4):493–500. https://doi.org/10.1007/s40140-022-00545-x. Epub 2022 Nov 3. PMID: 36345323; PMCID: PMC9631600
15. Loftus RW. Infection control in the operating room: is it more than a clean dish? Curr Opin Anaesthesiol. 2016;29(2):192–7. https://doi.org/10.1097/ACO.0000000000000300. PMID: 26765978
16. Loftus RW, Dexter F, Robinson ADM. Methicillin-resistant Staphylococcus aureus has greater risk of transmission in the operating room than methicillin-sensitive S aureus. Am J Infect Control. 2018;46(5):520–5. https://doi.org/10.1016/j.ajic.2017.11.002. Epub 2018 Jan 4. PMID: 29307750
17. Sharma A, Fernandez PG, Rowlands JP, Koff MD, Loftus RW. Perioperative infection transmission: the role of the anesthesia provider in infection control and healthcare-associated infections. Curr Anesthesiol Rep. 2020;10(3):233–41. https://doi.org/10.1007/s40140-020-00403-8. Epub 2020 Jul 17. PMID: 32837343; PMCID: PMC7366489
18. Odor PM, Neun M, Bampoe S, Clark S, Heaton D, Hoogenboom EM, Patel A, Brown M, Kamming D. Anaesthesia and COVID-19: infection control. Br J Anaesth. 2020;125(1):16–24. https://doi.org/10.1016/j.bja.2020.03.025. Epub 2020 Apr 8. PMID: 32307115; PMCID: PMC7142687
19. Provenzano DA, Hanes M, Hunt C, et al. ASRA pain medicine consensus practice infection control guidelines for regional anesthesia and pain medicine. Reg Anesth Pain Med. Online First:. 2025; https://doi.org/10.1136/rapm-2024-105651.
20. SG2. 2024 annual report projects high growth in ASC volume. ASC Focus. 2024 [cited 2025 Mar 12]. Available from: https://www.ascfocus.org/ascfocus/content/articles-content/articles/2024/digital-debut/sg2-2024-annual-report-projects-high-growth-in-asc-volume
21. Belda FJ, Aguilera L, García de la Asunción J, et al. Supplemental perioperative oxygen and the risk of surgical wound infection: a randomized controlled trial. JAMA. 2005;294(16):2035–42. https://doi.org/10.1001/jama.294.16.2035.
22. Anderson DJ. Prevention of surgical site infection: beyond SCIP. AORN J. 2014;99(2):315–9. https://doi.org/10.1016/j.aorn.2013.11.007. PMID: 24472594; PMCID: PMC3947534
23. de Vries EN, Dijkstra L, Smorenburg SM, Meijer RP, Boermeester MA. The SURgical PAtient safety system (SURPASS) checklist optimizes timing of antibiotic prophylaxis. Patient Saf Surg. 2010;4(1):6. https://doi.org/10.1186/1754-9493-4-6. PMID: 20388204; PMCID: PMC2867812
24. Drayton DJ, Birch RJ, D'Souza-Ferrer C, Ayres M, Howell SJ, Ajjan RA. Diabetes mellitus and perioperative outcomes: a scoping review of the literature. Br J Anaesth. 2022;128(5):817–28. https://doi.org/10.1016/j.bja.2022.02.013. Epub 2022 Mar 14. PMID: 35300865; PMCID: PMC9131255
25. Sermkasemsin V, Rungreungvanich M, Apinyachon W, Sangasilpa I, Srichot W, Pisitsak C. Incidence and risk factors of intraoperative hyperglycemia in non-diabetic patients: a prospective observational study. BMC Anesthesiol. 2022;22(1):287. https://doi.org/10.1186/s12871-022-01829-9. PMID: 36088294; PMCID: PMC9463729

26. Ata A, Lee J, Bestle SL, Desemone J, Stain SC. Postoperative hyperglycemia and surgical site infection in general surgery patients. Arch Surg. 2010;145(9):858–64. https://doi.org/10.1001/archsurg.2010.179.
27. Rajan N, Duggan EW, Abdelmalak BB, Butz S, Rodriguez LV, Vann MA, Joshi GP. Society for Ambulatory Anesthesia updated consensus statement on perioperative blood glucose management in adult patients with diabetes mellitus undergoing ambulatory surgery. Anesth Analg. 2024;139(3):459–77. https://doi.org/10.1213/ANE.0000000000006791. Epub 2024 Mar 22. PMID: 38517760
28. Hopkins L, Brown-Broderick J, Hearn J, Malcolm J, Chan J, Hicks-Boucher W, De Sousa F, Walker MC, Gagné S. Implementation of a referral to discharge glycemic control initiative for reduction of surgical site infections in gynecologic oncology patients. Gynecol Oncol. 2017;146(2):228–33. https://doi.org/10.1016/j.ygyno.2017.05.021. Epub 2017 May 20. PMID: 28532856
29. Yuan J, Sun Y, Pan C, Li T. Goal-directed fluid therapy for reducing risk of surgical site infections following abdominal surgery—a systematic review and meta-analysis of randomized controlled trials. Int J Surg. 2017;39:74–87. https://doi.org/10.1016/j.ijsu.2017.01.081. Epub 2017 Jan 23. PMID: 28126672
30. Gundersen SK, Meyhoff CS, Wetterslev J, Rasmussen LS, Jørgensen LN. The impact of intraoperative fluid therapy and body temperature on surgical site infection—re-assessment of a randomized trial. Chirurgia (Bucur). 2018;113(4):516–23. https://doi.org/10.21614/chirurgia.113.4.516. PMID: 30183582
31. Frank SM, Oleyar MJ, Ness PM, Tobian AA. Reducing unnecessary preoperative blood orders and costs by implementing an updated institution-specific maximum surgical blood order schedule and a remote electronic blood release system. Anesthesiology. 2014;121(3):501–9. https://doi.org/10.1097/ALN.0000000000000338. PMID: 24932853; PMCID: PMC4165815
32. Coccolini F, Shander A, Ceresoli M, Moore E, Tian B, Parini D, Sartelli M, Sakakushev B, Doklestich K, Abu-Zidan F, Horer T, Shelat V, Hardcastle T, Bignami E, Kirkpatrick A, Weber D, Kryvoruchko I, Leppaniemi A, Tan E, Kessel B, Isik A, Cremonini C, Forfori F, Ghiadoni L, Chiarugi M, Ball C, Ottolino P, Hecker A, Mariani D, Melai E, Malbrain M, Agostini V, Podda M, Picetti E, Kluger Y, Rizoli S, Litvin A, Maier R, Beka SG, De Simone B, Bala M, Perez AM, Ordonez C, Bodnaruk Z, Cui Y, Calatayud AP, de Angelis N, Amico F, Pikoulis E, Damaskos D, Coimbra R, Chirica M, Biffl WL, Catena F. Strategies to prevent blood loss and reduce transfusion in emergency general surgery, WSES-AAST consensus paper. World J Emerg Surg. 2024;19(1):26. https://doi.org/10.1186/s13017-024-00554-7. PMID: 39010099; PMCID: PMC11251377
33. Sodhi N, Anis HK, Acuña AJ, Vakharia RM, Gold PA, Garbarino LJ, Mahmood BM, Ehiorobo JO, Grossman EL, Higuera CA, Roche MW, Mont MA. Opioid use disorder is associated with an increased risk of infection after Total joint arthroplasty: a large database study. Clin Orthop Relat Res. 2020;478(8):1752–9. https://doi.org/10.1097/CORR.0000000000001390. PMID: 32662956; PMCID: PMC7371033
34. Pirkle S, Reddy S, Bhattacharjee S, Shi LL, Lee MJ. Chronic opioid use is associated with surgical site infection after lumbar fusion. Spine (Phila Pa 1976). 2020;45(12):837–42. https://doi.org/10.1097/BRS.0000000000003405. PMID: 32032322
35. Hassan Z, Nisiewicz MJ, Ueland W, Plymale MA, Plymale MC, Davenport DL, Totten CF, Roth JS. Preoperative opioid use and incidence of surgical site infection after repair of ventral and incisional hernias. Surgery. 2020;168(5):921–5. https://doi.org/10.1016/j.surg.2020.05.048. Epub 2020 Jul 18. PMID: 32690335
36. Bissell BD, Sturgill JL, Bruno MEC, Lewis ED, Starr ME. Assessment of opioid-induced immunomodulation in experimental and clinical sepsis. Crit Care Explor. 2023;5(1):e0849. https://doi.org/10.1097/CCE.0000000000000849. PMID: 36699245; PMCID: PMC9848529
37. Zhang R, Meng J, Lian Q, Chen X, Bauman B, Chu H, Segura B, Roy S. Prescription opioids are associated with higher mortality in patients diagnosed with sepsis: a retrospective cohort study using electronic health records. PLoS One. 2018;13(1):e0190362. https://doi.org/10.1371/journal.pone.0190362. PMID: 29293575; PMCID: PMC5749778

38. Soffin EM, Lee BH, Kumar KK, Wu CL. The prescription opioid crisis: role of the anaesthesiologist in reducing opioid use and misuse. Br J Anaesth. 2019;122(6):e198–208. https://doi.org/10.1016/j.bja.2018.11.019. Epub 2018 Dec 28. PMID: 30915988; PMCID: PMC8176648
39. Evrard E, Motamed C, Pagès A, Bordenave L. Opioid reduced anesthesia in major oncologic Cervicofacial surgery: a retrospective study. J Clin Med. 2023;12(3):904. https://doi.org/10.3390/jcm12030904. PMID: 36769551; PMCID: PMC9917718
40. Gray CF, Smith C, Zasimovich Y, Tighe PJ. Economic considerations of acute pain medicine programs. Tech Orthop. 2017;32(4):217–25. https://doi.org/10.1097/BTO.0000000000000241. PMID: 29403150; PMCID: PMC5796771
41. Dukes KC, Reisinger HS, Schweizer M, Ward MA, Chapin L, Ryken TC, Perl TM, Herwaldt LA. Examining barriers to implementing a surgical-site infection bundle. Infect Control Hosp Epidemiol. 2024;45(1):13–20. https://doi.org/10.1017/ice.2023.114. Epub 2023 Jul 26. PMID: 37493031; PMCID: PMC10782202
42. Forstot RM. The etiology and management of inadvertent perioperative hypothermia. J Clin Anesth. 1995;7(8):657–74. https://doi.org/10.1016/0952-8180(95)00099-2. PMID: 8747566
43. Rauch S, Miller C, Bräuer A, Wallner B, Bock M, Paal P. Perioperative hypothermia-a narrative review. Int J Environ Res Public Health. 2021;18(16):8749. https://doi.org/10.3390/ijerph18168749. PMID: 34444504; PMCID: PMC8394549

Venous Thromboembolism Prevention: The Role of Anesthesiologists

12

Sharon Sun and Shelby Badani

12.1 Background

Venous thromboembolism (VTE) is a broad term that encompasses deep vein thrombosis (DVT) and pulmonary embolism (PE). DVT refers specifically to a blood clot that forms in the deep veins, most commonly in the legs. Studies estimate that one-quarter to one-half of patients undergoing surgery who do not receive any prophylaxis will develop DVT postoperatively. [1, 2]. Given the high rates of morbidity and mortality associated with VTE, it is important for the anesthesiologist to understand and aid in the prevention of VTE in the postoperative patient population. Additionally, anesthesiologists may modify aspects of the anesthetic plan to reduce risk of VTE.

12.1.1 Epidemiology and Prevalence

The estimated incidence of asymptomatic VTE and pulmonary embolism varies widely due to the lack of routine screening and based on the population and diagnostic methods used. While exact numbers are elusive, the CDC estimates that as many as 900,000 people may be afflicted each year and that approximately 60,000 to 100,000 Americans die from VTE annually [3]. The highest risks are seen in individuals with hypercoagulable states such as malignancy or those undergoing major orthopedic or trauma surgeries. The estimated risk of calf-vein thrombosis ranges from 40 to 80%, proximal vein thrombosis 10–20% and clinical pulmonary embolism from 4 to 10%. These estimates are drastically increased compared to the

S. Sun
Robert Wood Johnson Hospital, New Brunswick, NJ, USA

S. Badani (✉)
Department of Anesthesiology, New York-Presbyterian/Weill Cornell Medicine, New York, NY, USA

G. Tewfik (ed.), *The Anesthesiologist as Perioperative Leader*,
https://doi.org/10.1007/978-3-032-18058-2_12

lowest risk category of patients younger than 40 undergoing minor surgery with no additional risk factors, where the estimated incidence of proximal vein thrombosis is 0.4% and clinical pulmonary embolism is 0.2% [4]. The precise number of VTEs associated with surgery and anesthesia is unknown, but estimated at 20–30% [5]. Development of symptomatic VTE can more than double the risk of death [6].

12.1.2 Associated Cost of VTE

In addition to the clinical toll VTE takes, there exists a significant financial burden to the individual patient as well as the healthcare system. The average median annual cost of a DVT, PE, or post-thrombotic syndrome event ranges from $12,000 to $20,000 per individual. With its widespread incidence, the estimated cost totals approximately $7–10 billion a year. [7–9].

12.2 Pathophysiology of DVT

12.2.1 Pathogenesis

Classically, Virchow's triad highlights three main factors that contribute to the development of thrombosis: venous stasis (impaired blood flow), endothelial injury (damage to the blood vessel lining), and hypercoagulability (increased blood clotting tendency). While the exact pathophysiology of VTE is unknown, clots tend to form in a venous valve or areas of reduced flow. In these low flow areas, thrombi develop, forming fibrin, red blood cell and platelet neutrophil-rich Lines of Zahn. Fresh venous blood increases aggregation of fibrin-platelet material and increases the size of the thrombus. Lack of continuous and pulsatile flow further exacerbates thrombus formation by allowing for the accumulation of thrombin in venous valve pockets. Venous valves typically express higher levels of anticoagulant like thrombomodulin and anti-protein C receptor and lower levels of procoagulant factors such as tissue factor (TF) and vWF; additionally, hypoxia in valves due to venous stasis in the surgical state increases thrombosis. [5] The subsequent post-surgical inflammation that occurs in the hours to days following surgery has also been implicated in the pathogenesis of VTE through upregulation of proinflammatory cytokines, triggering neutrophil extracellular traps (NETs), endothelial dysfunction and platelet activation and aggregation. [10] All these mechanisms are theorized to contribute to VTE formation perioperatively.

12.2.2 Risk Factors

Identifying risk factors based on patient history and type of surgery are essential in identifying the most appropriate prophylaxis regimen for each patient. Commonly identified risk factors include age, prior VTE, immobility and cancer. Additional risk factors include hypercoagulable states such as Factor V Leiden, pregnancy, oral contraceptives and antiphospholipid antibody syndrome.

Surgery type has been shown to be important in stratifying patients at high VTE risk. Trauma and orthopedic surgery patients are at highest risk for VTEs with estimated risk at 8.7% and 1–5%, respectively. Cardiac surgery is moderate risk with risk of symptomatic VTE between 0.5% and 3.0% with other estimates placing risk for this cohort three times higher than the general surgery population. Other surgeries including general surgery, urologic surgery, gynecologic, ENT and plastic surgery have highly variable rates of VTE ranging from 0.3% to as high as 15.7%, though this is confounded by patients with cancer undergoing surgery [7].

Multiple scoring systems exist to help risk-stratify patients at risk for VTE. The most widely recommended for use in surgical populations is the Caprini score (Table 12.1) [11]. This scoring system identifies 20 risk factors that categorize patients as low, medium, or high risk of developing VTE. The scoring system has been validated in multiple surgical populations including general, urologic, orthopedic, gynecologic, ENT, and vascular surgeries. [12]. Recommendations based on Caprini score are used to determine the appropriate prophylactic regimen. For minimal risk (score 0) patients, only early frequent ambulation is recommended with

Table 12.1 Caprini Score used to assess post-surgical patients for risk of VTE. Patients are scored based on these risk factors and assigned a total score to stratify them into risk categories: low risk (0–1), moderate risk (2), high risk (3), and highest risk (≥5) [12]

Risk factor	Points
Age 41–60 years	1
Age 61–74 years	2
Age ≥75 years	3
Minor surgery (<45 min)	1
Major surgery (>45 min)	2
BMI ≥30 kg/m^2	1
Swollen legs	1
Varicose veins	1
History of unexplained/recurrent miscarriage	1
Hormonal therapy (OCP/HRT)	1
Pregnancy or postpartum	1
Sepsis (<1 month)	1
Serious lung disease (e.g., pneumonia)	1
Bed rest >72 h	2
Active malignancy	2
History of DVT/PE	3
Family history of VTE	3
Stroke (<1 month)	5
Multiple trauma	5
Elective lower extremity arthroplasty	5
Hip, pelvis, or leg fracture	5
Acute spinal cord injury (<1 month)	5
Central venous access	2
Congestive heart failure	1
Inflammatory bowel disease	1
Nephrotic syndrome	1
COVID-19 infection (hospitalized)	

mechanical prophylaxis to be added at the discretion of the surgical team. For low [1–2] or moderate [3–4] risk, either pneumatic compression devices (PCDs) and/or graduated compression stockings (GCS) are recommended. For high [5–6, 7–8] or highest risk patients [9], combination mechanical and pharmacologic prophylaxis is recommended, specifically PCDs in combination with either low molecular weight heparin or low dose heparin. Patients at high risk of bleeding should receive mechanical prophylaxis until risk of bleeding is reduced [7]. The Caprini score has since been updated to include newer risk factors such as central venous access and history of inflammatory bowel disease.

Other scoring systems for VTE risk stratification tools include the PADUA score and IMPROVE score (Tables 12.2 and 12.3). While not specific to postoperative patients, the PADUA score studied hospitalized patients for risk of VTE with a score of ≥4 being high risk for VTE. Patients with a score of ≥4 without thromboprophylaxis had a significantly higher rate of VTE complications than patients scoring <4. Therefore, it is recommended that patients with a PADUA score of ≥4 receive pharmacologic prophylaxis; for patients with a score of <4, pharmacologic prophylaxis is not indicated and mechanical prophylaxis should be considered. The frequency of VTE complications in patients who received adequate thromboprophylaxis was significantly lower than in the group that did not. [13]

The IMPROVE score is a tool also used to stratify hospitalized patients for VTE risk and was recently updated to the IMPROVEDD score with the incorporation of a D-dimer. This scoring system was designed to assess 3-month VTE risk. A patient with a score of ≥2 has a 1.0% chance of developing a VTE within 3 months and is recommended for initiation of appropriate pharmacological or mechanical prophylaxis. A score of <2 suggests pharmacologic thrombophylaxis is not warranted and early ambulation with or without mechanical prophylaxis may be most appropriate [14, 15]. The IMPROVE bleeding tool expands upon the IMPROVE score by identifying risk factors that increase a patient's risk of bleeding. A score of ≥7 is considered a high bleeding risk. [16] The combination of these scoring scales can be used to weigh the risk-benefit of initiating pharmacologic prophylaxis versus a patient's risk for bleeding.

Table 12.2 The PADUA score to assess hospitalized patients for risk of VTE. A score of ≥4 suggests a high risk of VTE [13, 16]

Risk Factor	Points
Active cancer	3
Previous VTE (DVT or PE)	3
Reduced mobility (≥3 days)	3
Known thrombophilic condition	3
Recent (≤1 month) trauma/surgery	2
Age ≥70 years	1
Heart and/or respiratory failure	1
Acute myocardial infarction/stroke	1
Acute infection and/or rheumatologic disorder	1
Obesity (BMI ≥30 kg/m^2)	1
Ongoing hormonal treatment	

Table 12.3 The IMPROVEDD score for VTE risk in assessment of hospitalized patients [14]

Risk factor	Points
Previous VTE	3
Known thrombophilia	2
Current cancer	2
Immobilization ≥7 days	1
ICU/CCU admission	1
Lower limb paralysis	1
Age >60 years	1
D-dimer >2x ULN	2

All these scoring tools have been well-validated and provide a useful framework for determining which patients would be most appropriate for prophylaxis. [17]

12.3 Prevention Strategies

Prevention of VTE postoperatively is essential for reducing morbidity and mortality. Various methods have been shown to be effective in reducing VTE, including low molecular weight heparin (LMWH), unfractionated heparin (UFH), and direct oral anticoagulants (DOACs), which function by inhibiting different aspects of the coagulation cascade. Mechanical prophylaxis, such as intermittent pneumatic compression devices (IPCs) or graduated compression stockings (GCS), enhances blood circulation and reduces venous stasis, particularly in patients at high risk of bleeding and in whom anticoagulation should be avoided. Encouraging early mobilization and utilizing risk assessment models helps identify at-risk patients and tailors the prophylactic regimen to individual patient and specific surgical needs. Society-specific guidelines should be followed in the case of surgeries at higher risk of bleeding (e.g., ophthalmology, neurosurgery) and surgeries with higher risk of VTE (e.g., orthopedic, trauma).

12.3.1 Pharmacological Prophylaxis

Pharmacological prophylaxis, when used appropriately, is highly effective for preventing the development of VTE.

12.3.1.1 Low Molecular Weight Heparin

LMWH (e.g., enoxaparin and dalteparin) activates antithrombin III (AT III), thereby inhibiting factor Xa and the subsequent conversion of prothrombin (factor II) to thrombin (factor IIa). This inhibition of the common pathway results in decreased conversion of fibrinogen into fibrin for clot formation. Due to its predictable pharmacokinetics and reduced propensity for nonspecific protein binding, LMWH exhibits a more favorable therapeutic index compared to unfractionated heparin

(UFH). LMWH is administered as a subcutaneous injection and is typically dosed every 12 or 24 h for prophylaxis.

12.3.1.2 Unfractionated Heparin

UFH binds to AT III, leading to inhibition of factor Xa and IIa, resulting in the inhibition of thrombin (factor IIa). UFH has a faster onset of action and shorter half-life but a less predictable pharmacokinetic profile. UFH is administered as a subcutaneous injection, typically every 8 or 12 h, for prophylactic dosing. Patients receiving UFH are at higher risk of developing heparin-induced thrombocytopenia (HIT), a serious complication resulting in both thrombocytopenia and thrombosis. Heparin can be reversed using protamine.

12.3.1.3 Direct Oral Anticoagulants

DOACs are a class of anticoagulants that selectively target specific coagulation factors. Factor Xa inhibitors (e.g., rivaroxaban, apixaban, edoxaban) bind directly to the active site of factor Xa. Direct thrombin inhibitors (e.g., dabigatran) interact with thrombin's active site, directly inhibiting its capacity to convert fibrinogen to fibrin. One major advantage is the lack of routine laboratory monitoring and relative ease of PO administration [18]. Idarucizumab is approved for reversal of dabigatran. Andexanet alfa is approved for reversal of apixaban and rivaroxaban. Prothrombin complex concentrate (PCC) can be used if neither medication is available.

12.3.1.4 Vitamin K Antagonists

Vitamin K antagonists (e.g. warfarin), function by inhibiting the enzyme vitamin K epoxide reductase complex 1. This inhibition depletes the reduced form of vitamin K, an essential cofactor for the γ-carboxylation of glutamic acid residues on clotting factors II, VII, IX, and X, as well as anticoagulant proteins C and S. Route of administration is PO but patients require frequent monitoring of INR, which can be challenging for patient adherence. Titration to target INR level may take several days. Reversal for surgical indication can be achieved with Vitamin K, fresh frozen plasma (FFP) or prothrombin complex concentrate (PCC).

12.3.1.5 Aspirin

Aspirin (ASA) does not act directly on the coagulation cascade. ASA is an antiplatelet agent that irreversibly inhibits cyclooxygenase-1 (COX-1), an enzyme responsible for the synthesis of thromboxane A2, a key mediator of platelet aggregation and vasoconstriction. By blocking its production, aspirin reduces platelet activation and aggregation, thereby lowering the risk of clot formation. Due to its irreversible inhibition, there is no direct reversal agent available. However, administration of platelets and desmopressin (DDAVP) can help promote platelet aggregation to reduce bleeding. Use of ASA has not been shown to be superior to other pharmacologic agents such as LMWH or UFH though it is still commonly used in extended prophylaxis regimens following elective joint replacement in orthopedic surgery [19–22]

12.3.2 Mechanical Prophylaxis

Mechanical prophylaxis offers a method of VTE prophylaxis in patients either as an adjunct to patients already receiving pharmacologic prophylaxis or as the primary method of VTE prophylaxis in patients who are at high risk of bleeding. Intermittent pneumatic compression (IPC) generates a predetermined cycle of pressure that produces a pulse of blood that travels proximally. Graduated compression stockings (GCS) apply constant pressure to the limb to reduce venous caliber and prevent stasis of blood. Efficacy of GCS in preventing VTE is well-supported in the literature [21]. A systematic review comparing the two has yielded mostly no difference with some weak studies favoring IPC performance. [22] Research into the effectiveness of intermittent pneumatic compression devices (IPCs) alone has also yielded positive results. In a large randomized controlled trial of patients in the intensive care unit receiving IPCs and pharmacologic prophylaxis such as UFH or LMWH versus control, there was no significant difference in development of lower extremity VTEs between the groups. [23] A meta-analysis of randomized control trials (RCTs) on the effectiveness of IPCs in VTE prevention found that there was a significant effect in preventing PEs when compared to no prophylaxis. IPCs also demonstrated reduced bleeding risk when compared to groups with combined pharmacologic prophylaxis [24]. However, findings on whether IPCs and thromboprophylaxis versus thromboprophylaxis alone are more effective are mixed [25].

12.3.3 Other Strategies

12.3.3.1 Ambulation

Ambulation is commonly recommended in enhanced recovery after surgery (ERAS) protocols to prevent VTE due to the theory that venous stasis increases risk of clot formation. However, there is no evidence that ambulation alone is adequate to prevent VTE [26]. Early ambulation should still be encouraged along with other methods of VTE prophylaxis.

12.3.3.2 Regional Anesthesia

Despite early studies suggesting a benefit to regional anesthesia over general anesthesia with regard to VTE occurrence, this benefit did not persist after the introduction of more routine mechanical and chemoprophylaxis use perioperatively [27–29]. However, several studies show that spinal and epidural anesthesia have facilitated earlier mobilization compared to patients receiving general anesthesia [30, 31]. In addition, patients under epidural anesthesia have been shown to have increased velocity of blood flow in lower extremity veins during surgery. [32] Patients receiving epidural anesthesia have not been found to have higher rates of VTE though epidurals alone have not been shown to be effective in the prevention of VTE [33, 34]. The evidence alone is not strong enough to support use of regional anesthesia solely based on VTE reduction. The decision to proceed with regional and/or general anesthesia must be made on a case-by-case basis.

12.3.3.3 IVC Filters

Inferior vena cava (IVC) filters are mechanical devices designed to capture DVTs from the lower extremities before they embolize to the lungs, resulting in a PE. Indications primarily include patients with contraindications to therapeutic anticoagulation or recurrent VTE despite therapeutic anticoagulation. IVC filters are available in both permanent and retrievable models, with the latter being preferred for temporary risk mitigation, allowing for removal once the patient's embolic risk has decreased. However, long-term placement has been associated with complications such as filter thrombosis, migration, caval wall penetration, and, ironically, an increased likelihood of deep vein thrombosis (DVT). There is a lack of strong evidence to support the efficacy of IVC filter placement in VTE reduction [35].

12.3.4 Summary Recommendations

Much research has been done on the efficacy of various prophylactic regimens. Pharmacologic prophylaxis is typically recommended after most types of major surgery including cardiac surgery. However, specific choice in pharmacologic agent leads to different results due in part due to the breadth of surgical types, patient populations studied, duration of regimen and difference in measured outcome of symptomatic versus asymptomatic VTE. [36, 37, 38]. Several leading organizations, including the American College of Chest Physicians (ACCP) and the American Society of Hematology (ASH), have published guidelines outlining best recommendations based on available evidence.

The ACCP guidelines (2012) emphasize a risk-based approach to thromboprophylaxis. Separate guidelines for orthopedic and nonorthopedic surgical patients were released. For total hip arthroplasty (THA), total knee arthroplasty (TKA), and hip fracture surgery (HFS), LMWH is the preferred agent, though other anticoagulants such as UFH, DOACS, vitamin K antagonists and ASA are also included as alternative options. Extended thromboprophylaxis for up to 35 days rather than 10–14 days is recommended in orthopedic patients, particularly those with additional risk factors. In nonorthopedic surgical patients, the ACCP stratifies prophylaxis based on Caprini risk scores. However, some of these recommendations are controversial as a large meta-analysis found benefit for chemoprophylaxis only in patients with Caprini scores > = 7. [39]

Extended prophylaxis of 4 weeks is advised for patients undergoing abdominal or pelvic cancer surgery. IVC filters are not recommended in either population [11, 40, 41].

The ASH guidelines (2019) recommend DOACs over LMWH in orthopedic patients. In patients undergoing major general surgery, they recommend pharmacologic prophylaxis with a weak recommendation for LMWH or UFH as the agent of choice with extended prophylaxis for at least 3 weeks. Interestingly, they provide a weak recommendation for use of pharmacologic prophylaxis in cardiac, major vascular, major gynecological and trauma surgery and recommend against pharmacologic prophylaxis in the neurosurgical, laparoscopic cholecystectomy and urologic surgery populations. The ASH emphasizes a combined pharmacologic and mechanical approach with a stronger recommendation for ICD over GCS for patients receiving mechanical prophylaxis [42].

Timing of initiation has been debated but generally it is recommended to begin prophylaxis between 6 and 24 h postoperatively [43–45]. Ultimately the best VTE prophylaxis regimen is individualized to specific patient factors. Physicians should refer to the most updated societal guidelines in developing an appropriate strategy.

12.4 Special Populations

12.4.1 Patients with Prior or Existing DVTs

Patients who are already on anticoagulation or antiplatelet agents for any reason including coronary stents, prosthetic valves, VTE or PE should hold these medications before surgery according to instructions from their surgeon, anesthesiologist, and/or subspecialists such as cardiology or hematology based on a risk–benefit discussion weighing risk of VTE versus postoperative bleeding risk. Discussion should also include when to resume therapeutic anticoagulation which is higher than prophylactic dosing and can be used in place of the standard VTE prophylaxis regimen. Therapeutic anticoagulation should not be resumed while the patient has an epidural in place per the most recent American Society of Regional Anesthesia (ASRA) guidelines (2025). [17]

12.4.2 Cancer Patients

Cancer patients represent a unique population undergoing surgery given their hypercoagulable state. The ASCO guidelines (2023) recommend LMWH as the first-line option for pharmacologic prophylaxis. However, emerging evidence supports DOACs (rivaroxaban and apixaban) as alternative options for extended prophylaxis, though this recommendation is classified as weak due to limited trial data. The ASCO guidelines also advocate for prophylaxis in hospitalized cancer patients with reduced mobility and recommend at least 7–10 days of thromboprophylaxis following major cancer surgery, with extended prophylaxis for up to 4 weeks in high-risk individuals (e.g., obesity, immobility, or prior VTE history). [46]

12.5 Conclusion

Effective prevention of venous thromboembolism (VTE) in surgical patients depends upon individualized prophylactic strategies carefully selected according to each patient's unique risk factors, surgical context, potential for bleeding complications and in the case of extended prophylaxis, patient preference and adherence [47]. Selecting suitable prophylactic methods—including pharmacological and mechanical approaches—requires thoughtful evaluation to balance efficacy and safety, minimizing the risk of complications such as pulmonary embolism or bleeding. Anesthesiologists play an essential role in this tailored approach, collaborating closely with surgical teams and other healthcare providers to implement and manage perioperative protocols, thereby significantly improving patient outcomes and reducing overall morbidity and mortality associated with postoperative thrombotic events.

Caprini Score—self-generated from score elements mentioned in reference 12
PADUA Score—self-generated from score elements mentioned in reference 13, 16
IMPROVE Score—self generated from elements mentioned in reference 14

References

1. ANZ Journal of Surgery – 2004 – Edmonds – Evidence-based risk factors for postoperative deep vein thrombosis.pdf.
2. Flanders SA, Greene MT, Grant P, Kaatz S, Paje D, Lee B, et al. Hospital performance for pharmacologic venous thromboembolism prophylaxis and rate of venous thromboembolism: a cohort study. JAMA Intern Med. 2014;174(10):1577.
3. Center for Disease Control. Data and statistics on venous thromboembolism [Internet]. 2025 [cited 2025 Mar 10]. Available from: https://www.cdc.gov/blood-clots/data-research/facts-stats/index.html.
4. De Wet CJ, Pearl RG. Postoperative thrombotic complications. Anesthesiol Clin N Am. 1999;17(4):895–922.
5. Gordon RJ, Lombard FW. Perioperative venous thromboembolism: a review. Anesth Analg. 2017;125(2):403–12.
6. Gangireddy C, Rectenwald JR, Upchurch GR, Wakefield TW, Khuri S, Henderson WG, et al. Risk factors and clinical impact of postoperative symptomatic venous thromboembolism. J Vasc Surg. 2007;45(2):335–342.e1.
7. Bartlett MA, Mauck KF, Stephenson CR, Ganesh R, Daniels PR. Perioperative venous thromboembolism prophylaxis. Mayo Clin Proc. 2020 Dec;95(12):2775–98.
8. Grosse SD, Nelson RE, Nyarko KA, Richardson LC, Raskob GE. The economic burden of incident venous thromboembolism in the United States: a review of estimated attributable healthcare costs. Thromb Res. 2016 Jan;137:3–10.
9. MacDougall DA, Feliu AL, Boccuzzi SJ, Lin J. Economic burden of deep-vein thrombosis, pulmonary embolism, and post-thrombotic syndrome. Am J Health Syst Pharm. 2006;63(20_Supplement_6):S5–15.
10. Albayati M, Grover S, Saha P, Lwaleed B, Modarai B, Smith A. Postsurgical inflammation as a causative mechanism of venous thromboembolism. Semin Thromb Hemost. 2015;41(06):615–20.
11. Gould MK, Garcia DA, Wren SM, Karanicolas PJ, Arcelus JI, Heit JA, et al. Prevention of VTE in nonorthopedic surgical patients. Chest. 2012;141(2):e227S–77S.
12. Caprini JA. Risk assessment as a guide to thrombosis prophylaxis. Curr Opin Pulm Med. 2010;16(5):448–52.
13. Barbar S, Noventa F, Rossetto V, Ferrari A, Brandolin B, Perlati M, et al. A risk assessment model for the identification of hospitalized medical patients at risk for venous thromboembolism: the Padua prediction score. J Thromb Haemost. 2010;8(11):2450–7.

14. Gibson C, Spyropoulos A, Cohen A, Hull R, Goldhaber S, Yusen R, et al. The IMPROVEDD VTE risk score: incorporation of D-Dimer into the IMPROVE score to improve venous thromboembolism risk stratification. TH Open. 2017;01(01):e56–65.
15. Spyropoulos AC, Anderson FA, FitzGerald G, Decousus H, Pini M, Chong BH, et al. Predictive and associative models to identify hospitalized medical patients at risk for VTE. Chest. 2011;140(3):706–14.
16. Decousus H, Tapson VF, Bergmann JF, Chong BH, Froehlich JB, Kakkar AK, et al. Factors at admission associated with bleeding risk in medical patients. Chest. 2011 Jan;139(1):69–79.
17. Kopp SL, Vandermeulen E, McBane RD, Perlas A, Leffert L, Horlocker T. Regional anesthesia in the patient receiving antithrombotic or thrombolytic therapy: American Society of Regional Anesthesia and Pain Medicine Evidence-Based Guidelines 5th ed.. Reg Anesth Pain Med. 2025.;rapm-2024-105766.
18. Burnett AE, Mahan CE, Vazquez SR, Oertel LB, Garcia DA, Ansell J. Guidance for the practical management of the direct oral anticoagulants (DOACs) in VTE treatment. J Thromb Thrombolysis. 2016;41(1):206–32.
19. Anderson DR, Dunbar MJ, Bohm ER, Belzile E, Kahn SR, Zukor D, et al. Aspirin versus low-molecular-weight heparin for extended venous thromboembolism prophylaxis after total hip arthroplasty: a randomized trial. Ann Intern Med. 2013;158(11):800.
20. CRISTAL Study Group, Sidhu VS, Kelly TL, Pratt N, Graves SE, Buchbinder R, et al. Effect of Aspirin vs Enoxaparin on symptomatic venous thromboembolism in patients undergoing hip or knee arthroplasty: the CRISTAL randomized trial. JAMA. 2022;328(8):719.
21. Amaragiri SV, Lees T. Elastic compression stockings for prevention of deep vein thrombosis. In: The Cochrane Collaboration, editor. Cochrane database of systematic reviews [Internet]. Chichester: Wiley; 2000. p. CD001484. [cited 2025 Mar 13]. Available from: https://doi.wiley.com/10.1002/14651858.CD001484.
22. Morris RJ, Woodcock JP. Intermittent pneumatic compression or graduated compression stockings for deep vein thrombosis prophylaxis?: A systematic review of direct clinical comparisons. Ann Surg. 2010;251(3):393–6.
23. Arabi YM, Al-Hameed F, Burns KEA, Mehta S, Alsolamy SJ, Alshahrani MS, et al. Adjunctive intermittent pneumatic compression for venous thromboprophylaxis. N Engl J Med. 2019;380(14):1305–15.
24. Kim NY, Ryu S, Kim YH. Effects of intermittent pneumatic compression devices interventions to prevent deep vein thrombosis in surgical patients: a systematic review and meta-analysis of randomized controlled trials. Serra R, editor. PLOS One. 2024;19(7):e0307602.
25. Ho KM, Tan JA. Stratified meta-analysis of intermittent pneumatic compression of the lower limbs to prevent venous thromboembolism in hospitalized patients. Circulation. 2013;128(9):1003–20.
26. Lau BD, Murphy P, Nastasi AJ, Seal S, Kraus PS, Hobson DB, et al. Effectiveness of ambulation to prevent venous thromboembolism in patients admitted to hospital: a systematic review. CMAJ Open. 2020;8(4):E832–43.
27. Prins MH, Hirsh J. A comparison of general anesthesia and regional anesthesia as a risk factor for deep vein thrombosis following hip surgery: a critical review. Thromb Haemost. 1990;64(04):497–500.
28. Macfarlane AJR, Prasad GA, Chan VWS, Brull R. Does regional anaesthesia improve outcome after total hip arthroplasty? A systematic review. Br J Anaesth. 2009;103(3):335–45.
29. Gulur P, Nishimori M, Ballantyne JC. Regional anaesthesia versus general anaesthesia, morbidity and mortality. Best Pract Res Clin Anaesthesiol. 2006;20(2):249–63.
30. Thurm M, Hultin M, Johansson G, Dahlin BI, Winsö O, Ljungberg B. Spinal anaesthesia with clonidine: pain relief and earlier mobilisation after open nephrectomy – a randomised clinical trial. J Int Med Res. 2022;50(9):03000605221126883.
31. Ezhevskaya AA, Mlyavykh SG, Anderson DG. Effects of continuous epidural anesthesia and postoperative epidural analgesia on pain management and stress response in patients undergoing major spinal surgery. Spine. 2013;38(15):1324–30.

32. Delis K, Knaggs A, Mason P, Macleod K. Effects of epidural-and-general anesthesia combined versus general anesthesia alone on the venous hemodynamics of the lower limb: a randomized study. Thromb Haemost. 2004;92(11):1003–11.
33. Caruso JD, Elster EA, Rodriguez CJ. Epidural placement does not result in an increased incidence of venous thromboembolism in combat-wounded patients. J Trauma Acute Care Surg. 2014 Jul;77(1):61–6.
34. Manguso N, Hong J, Shouhed D, Popelka S, Amersi F, Hemaya E, et al. The impact of epidural analgesia on the rate of thromboembolism without chemical thromboprophylaxis in major oncologic surgery. Am Surg. 2018;84(6):851–5.
35. Visconti L, Celi A, Carrozzi L, Tinelli C, Crocetti L, Daviddi F, et al. Inferior vena cava filters: concept review and summary of current guidelines. Vascul Pharmacol. 2024 Jun;155:107375.
36. Steele KE, Canner J, Prokopowicz G, Verde F, Beselman A, Wyse R, et al. The EFFORT trial: preoperative enoxaparin versus postoperative fondaparinux for thromboprophylaxis in bariatric surgical patients: a randomized double-blind pilot trial. Surg Obes Relat Dis. 2015 May;11(3):672–83.
37. Strebel N, Prins M, Agnelli G, Büller HR. Preoperative or postoperative start of prophylaxis for venous thromboembolism with low-molecular-weight heparin in elective hip surgery? Arch Intern Med. 2002;162(13):1451.
38. Becattini C, Pace U, Pirozzi F, Donini A, Avruscio G, Rondelli F, et al. Rivaroxaban vs placebo for extended antithrombotic prophylaxis after laparoscopic surgery for colorectal cancer. Blood. 2022;140(8):900–8.
39. Pannucci CJ, Swistun L, MacDonald JK, Henke PK, Brooke BS. Individualized venous thromboembolism risk stratification using the 2005 Caprini score to identify the benefits and harms of chemoprophylaxis in surgical patients: a meta-analysis. Ann Surg. 2017 Jun;265(6):1094–103.
40. Falck-Ytter Y, Francis CW, Johanson NA, Curley C, Dahl OE, Schulman S, et al. Prevention of VTE in orthopedic surgery patients. Chest. 2012;141(2):e278S–325S.
41. Lieberman JR, Bell JA. Venous thromboembolic prophylaxis after total hip and knee arthroplasty. J Bone Jt Surg. 2021;103(16):1556–64.
42. Anderson DR, Morgano GP, Bennett C, Dentali F, Francis CW, Garcia DA, et al. American Society of Hematology 2019 guidelines for management of venous thromboembolism: prevention of venous thromboembolism in surgical hospitalized patients. Blood Adv. 2019;3(23):3898–944.
43. Paikin JS, Hirsh J, Chan NC, Ginsberg JS, Weitz JI, Eikelboom JW. Timing the first postoperative dose of anticoagulants. CHEST. 2015;148(3):587–95.
44. PROTECTinG investigators, VERITAS Collaborative. Postoperative timing of chemoprophylaxis and its impact on thromboembolism and bleeding following major abdominal surgery: a multicenter cohort study. World J Surg. 2023;47(5):1174–83.
45. Raskob GE, Hirsh J. Controversies in timing of the first dose of anticoagulant prophylaxis against venous thromboembolism after major orthopedic surgery. Chest. 2003 Dec;124(6):379S–85S.
46. Key NS, Khorana AA, Kuderer NM, Bohlke K, Lee AYY, Arcelus JI, et al. Venous thromboembolism prophylaxis and treatment in patients with cancer: ASCO guideline update. J Clin Oncol. 2023;41(16):3063–71.
47. MacLean S, Mulla S, Akl EA, Jankowski M, Vandvik PO, Ebrahim S, et al. Patient values and preferences in decision making for antithrombotic therapy: a systematic review. Chest. 2012;141(2):e1S–e23S.

Supply Chain and Fundamentals of Procuring Anesthesia Supplies

13

Jordan Zunder, Matthew Zemel, Cole Crosby, and Rajen Nathwani

13.1 Introduction to Supply Chain in Healthcare

According to the Council of Supply Chain Management Professionals, supply chain management involves the "planning and management of all activities involved in sourcing, procurement, conversion, and all logistics management activities" [1]. In healthcare, this process is particularly crucial for sourcing, storing, and delivering medical products to ensure timely, cost-effective, and reliable access to essential patient care supplies. The anesthesia supply chain is especially critical due to the direct impact of its drugs and equipment on patient safety and surgical outcomes [2].

The perioperative healthcare supply chain involves multiple stakeholders. At the highest level, regulatory bodies like the Food and Drug Administration (FDA) and the World Health Organization (WHO) ensure products meet strict safety and quality standards. Manufacturers and suppliers develop and produce these products, while distributors and intermediaries, such as Group Purchasing Organizations (GPOs), handle their logistics and availability [3]. Ultimately, healthcare providers—including anesthesiologists—are the end-users who depend on a steady supply of high-quality drugs and equipment to deliver safe, effective care [4].

J. Zunder (✉)
Department of Anesthesiology and Pain Medicine, University of Ottawa, The Ottawa Hospital, Ottawa, ON, Canada
e-mail: jzunder@toh.ca

M. Zemel
Seattle Children's Hospital, Seattle, WA, USA

C. Crosby
Harborview Medical Center, University of Washington Anesthesiology and Pain Medicine, Seattle, WA, USA

R. Nathwani
Department of Anesthesiology and Pain Medicine, University of Washington, Seattle, WA, USA

G. Tewfik (ed.), *The Anesthesiologist as Perioperative Leader*,
https://doi.org/10.1007/978-3-032-18058-2_13

Healthcare supply chains face unique challenges compared to other industries. They are burdened by strict regulatory requirements that may complicate procurement and distribution. Anesthesia supply chains are especially vulnerable to disruptions from manufacturing delays or drug shortages, which can lead to delays in the ability to provide patients with timely and safe care [5]. Drug shortages, for example, can force clinicians to use unfamiliar alternatives, increasing the risk of medication errors. Hospitals also face internal logistical complexities and must manage potentially high costs and persistent budget constraints [6] while maintaining high-quality care. Additionally, the short shelf-life and specific storage requirements for many anesthetic products necessitate careful inventory management to prevent waste and ensure appropriate access.

Anesthesia supplies are a broad category that includes essential drugs (e.g., local anesthetics, opioids, neuromuscular blockers), airway management devices (e.g., laryngoscopes, endotracheal tubes), monitoring equipment (e.g. non-invasive blood pressure cuffs, disposable EKG leads), and single-use consumables (e.g., intravenous cannulas, central lines and arterial lines). The immediate availability of these items is critical to prevent surgical delays or cancelations and maintain patient safety [7]. An efficient and resilient supply chain is vital for avoiding shortages that can lead to rationing, using suboptimal alternatives, and increasing the risk of adverse patient events [8]. Maintaining a stable supply chain is not only essential for patient care but is also financially beneficial, as it reduces unexpected expenses from emergency procurement and optimizes resource allocation [9]. As primary end-users, anesthesiologists play a crucial role in advocating for a well-structured supply chain to ensure the availability of essential resources and to improve patient outcomes.

13.2 Key Components of Anesthesia Supply Chain

The anesthesia supply chain encompasses several key components: manufacturers and suppliers, distributors, and end-users.

Manufacturers and suppliers include both global and regional entities producing anesthesia drugs, equipment, and consumables. Global suppliers may provide brand-name products, while regional suppliers may instead choose to focus on generic alternatives, which are critical for cost containment and access, especially in low-resource settings [10]. The choice between brand and generic products impacts both cost and availability, with generics often preferred for routine agents due to their lower price and comparable efficacy [11]. Diversification of suppliers and transparency in sourcing are essential strategies to mitigate supply chain shocks and shortages, as highlighted during crises such as the COVID-19 pandemic [12].

Distributors serve as key intermediaries, purchasing from wholesalers or directly from manufacturers and managing the logistics of transportation and warehousing to ensure a steady, reliable supply of products to healthcare facilities [4]. Through just-in-time (JIT) delivery (see below) and perpetual inventory systems, distributors help optimize stock levels and reduce waste [9].

Hospitals often partner with GPOs, organizations formed as a strategy to leverage the combined buying power of multiple healthcare organizations to negotiate better prices and terms with vendors. This centralized procurement model is meant to reduce cost and streamline purchasing for the end user. However, many GPOs are now very large businesses (e.g., Vizient controls over 450,000 staffed beds in the USA [13]) and come with additional infrastructure costs. These issues regarding scale have made negotiating directly with manufacturers very difficult. While GPOs offer pre-negotiated contracts, hospitals must balance cost savings with clinical needs. This requires close collaboration between clinical staff and the supply chain team to ensure that purchasing decisions are both financially prudent and clinically sound. Ultimately, GPOs are vital for helping healthcare organizations manage rising costs, mitigate shortages, and standardize procurement practices.

End-users of healthcare supply chains include hospitals, clinics, and outpatient facilities. These organizations are responsible for the final procurement and utilization of anesthesia supplies. Clinical collaboration in procurement—by involving anesthesiologists in preference list updates and supply selection—improves efficiency, safety, and cost-effectiveness. Lean Six Sigma and intelligent management systems are design methodologies that have demonstrated improvements in supply chain quality [14], reducing errors and enhancing workflow [15].

The Biomedical Engineering (BioMed) department in hospitals or healthcare facilities is critical for maintaining and ensuring the safety of medical equipment in a hospital. BioMed teams manage the entire lifecycle of devices, from initial evaluation to repair and preventive maintenance. Effective communication from clinicians is essential for reporting malfunctions and ensuring timely service requests. BioMed also plays a key role during the value analysis process for new equipment, assessing compatibility and safety standards before it is integrated. By partnering effectively with BioMed, healthcare organizations and physician anesthesiologists enhance patient safety and reinforce operational reliability.

13.3 Demand Forecasting and Planning

Demand forecasting and planning for anesthesia equipment relies on integrating historical usage data, robust inventory management, and advanced data-driven decision-making.

Analyzing historical usage involves tracking trends in anesthesia drugs and supplies, which are closely linked to surgical case volumes and types. Usage patterns often incorporate elective versus emergency surgery rates, with notable impacts from seasonal variations and holidays, as demonstrated by time series analyses that reveal predictable fluctuations in surgical demand and supply needs [16]. Longitudinal data from anesthesia departments show that while population changes may not reliably predict local anesthesia workload, historical case volumes and procedural data are highly correlated with supply requirements and should be modeled for planning [17, 18].

Inventory management strategies include JIT inventory [19] and safety stock approaches. JIT aims to minimize on-hand inventory by synchronizing supply deliveries with scheduled procedures, reducing waste and costs but increasing vulnerability to supply chain disruptions [20]. Safety stock, in contrast, maintains buffer inventory to mitigate shortages, especially for critical or high-turnover items. Inventory turnover ratios—calculated as the frequency with which inventory is replaced—are key metrics; higher turnover indicates efficient inventory use but may risk stockouts if not balanced with adequate safety stock [9].

Data-driven decision-making leverages software and technology, such as electronic health record (EHR) dashboards and mobile apps, to forecast demand and optimize supply chain operations. These tools incorporate patient volume, procedural data, and real-time supply metrics, enabling dynamic adjustments to procurement and inventory levels [7]. Machine learning and statistical models further enhance forecasting accuracy, supporting both short-term operational and long-term strategic planning for anesthesia equipment and supplies [21].

13.4 Procurement Fundamentals

The procurement cycle for anesthesia equipment aims to match equipment supply to demand, thereby maintaining operational efficiency. Vendor selection and contract negotiations are crucial steps where multidisciplinary teams evaluate suppliers based on technical specifications, cost, reliability, and clinical input [22]. GPOs and formal tender processes are commonly used to leverage pricing and ensure quality, with contracts specifying terms, service, and expected lead times [23]. Purchase order placement is then executed, with attention to lead times that can vary depending on equipment complexity and supplier location: e.g., changing anesthesia machines for a department may require several months of lead time.

Sourcing and vendor management require establishing reliable vendor relationships through systematic evaluation of suppliers. Criteria include cost-effectiveness, product quality, regulatory compliance, and delivery reliability [24]. GPOs work closely to align with clinician preferences while excluding those with conflicts of interest. Multi-criteria decision-making frameworks, such as those incorporating technical, financial, and general criteria, are increasingly used to rank and select vendors under uncertainty, supporting robust procurement decisions. Ongoing vendor performance monitoring and periodic re-evaluation are essential to maintain supply chain resilience and adapt to market changes.

Regulatory and compliance considerations are critical. In the USA, anesthesia equipment and drugs must comply with FDA guidelines, which mandate risk-based classification, premarket approval for high-risk devices, and adherence to rigorous manufacturing practices [25]. The fact that some technology is not FDA approved (such as Target controlled infusion [TCI] pumps for total intravenous anesthesia, or automated End Tidal MAC control for vapor anesthesia) does mean that these are not available for use in the US. Drug availability is also affected by the FDA (e.g., diamorphine is not available for medical use in the US). Safety standards are set by organizations such as the International Electrotechnical Commission (IEC) and the Organization for International Standardization (ISO), and compliance is required for both domestic and imported products [26]. Import and export regulations further govern anesthesia drug movement, ensuring products meet safety, labeling, and performance standards before market entry.

Value chain analysis is a process that evaluates all the activities that bring a product from the manufacturer to the clinician. Anesthesiologists must understand this process to advocate for reliable and cost-effective equipment. A key part of this is value analysis, where multidisciplinary committees consisting of anesthesia clinicians who are equipment champions, anesthesia technicians, biomedical engineers and the finance management assess new equipment requests. These committees evaluate a product's clinical benefits alongside its cost-effectiveness, supply chain impact, and contract terms. This ensures that new equipment, such as a video laryngoscope, is not only safe and beneficial for patients but also aligns with the hospital's operational and financial goals.

13.5 Challenges in Anesthesia Supply Procurement

Key challenges in anesthesia supply procurement include supply chain disruptions, backorders and stockouts, cost management, management of perishable items, and product expiration dates.

Supply chain disruptions—such as those caused by pandemics, geopolitical instability, and manufacturing delays—have led to critical shortages of anesthesia drugs and equipment. The American Society of Anesthesiologists notes that shortages of essential anesthetics (e.g., lidocaine, bupivacaine) have persisted for over a decade, with the COVID-19 pandemic exacerbating these issues and increasing the risk of medication errors due to unfamiliar alternatives [27]. The American College of Physicians highlights that disruptions arise from manufacturing problems, market concentration, and global events, resulting in negative patient outcomes and increased burden on clinicians [28]. For example, the damage caused by Hurricane Helene in September 2024 to the Baxter intravenous fluid manufacture facility caused widespread disruption to patient management in the USA and required emergency contingency plans to be implemented quickly. Dual sourcing and proactive inventory management are recommended to mitigate these risks [29].

Backorders and stockouts directly impact patient care by delaying procedures, forcing use of less effective or unfamiliar drugs, and increasing the risk of adverse events and medication errors. Stockouts can lead to undertreatment, treatment delays, and increased stress for both patients and providers [30]. Having a transparent vendor relationship to have backup second- or third-line items from alternative manufacturers can help mitigate equipment shortages and maintain patient safety and operational resilience [12].

Cost management is challenged by price volatility and the need to balance quality and cost. This is especially true in pharmaceuticals, where generic versus on-patent drug use can significantly affect the cost. Procurement decisions must consider not only acquisition costs but also reliability and clinical efficacy. Overemphasis on lowest price can compromise supply reliability and quality, while price spikes during shortages strain budgets [31]. Pharmacoeconomic evaluations and collaborative clinical input are essential for rational decision-making [32].

Management of perishable items and expiration dates are critical for anesthesia drugs, many of which are temperature sensitive. The American Society of Health-System Pharmacists and FDA guidelines require strict adherence to storage conditions to maintain drug potency and safety [33]. Failure to manage shelf-life and storage can result in drug degradation, loss of efficacy, and increased waste, especially for agents like midazolam and atropine, which degrade rapidly at high temperatures. This is especially true for blood products which fall under the governance structure of the FDA and the Association for the Advancement of Blood and Biotherapies (AABB). Managing supply chains in extreme climates, during military operations or when working in resource limited settings or disaster zones can be particularly challenging [34]. Barcode or RFID equipment monitoring systems (see below) and checklists may help to keep track of equipment expiration dates.

13.6 Quality Assurance and Risk Management

Quality assurance in anesthesia equipment procurement ensures product quality through certification, testing, and verification. As mentioned earlier, regulation oversight by agencies such as the FDA and European Commission mandates risk-based classification and premarket approval for anesthesia devices, with compliance to international standards (IEC, ISO) required for market entry. Trialing equipment within the department by a group of clinicians with an interest in equipment procurement alongside the Biomed department enables the anesthesia department to procure a quality product that will fit the requirements of their clinicians. Daily checking of equipment prior to use (such as anesthesia circuit and machine checks [35] and endotracheal tube cuff pressure testing) maintains patient safety. Routine servicing and post-servicing verification are also critical to prevent equipment malfunction and ensure ongoing reliability [36].

Monitoring product recalls and adverse event reports are key for post-market surveillance. National systems such as the UK National Reporting and Learning System collect incident data, enabling rapid identification and response to equipment failures and user errors. GPOs and manufacturers have a responsibility to monitor for product recall and inform departments of equipment problems. Analysis of critical incident reports reveals that both device faults and operator unfamiliarity contribute to adverse events, underscoring the need for continuous vigilance and organizational readiness to manage equipment-related risks [37].

Risk mitigation strategies include diversifying suppliers to reduce dependency and enhance supply chain resilience, especially during crises or disruptions. Contingency planning for critical anesthesia items involves maintaining safety stock, establishing alternative sourcing, and implementing emergency procurement protocols to ensure uninterrupted patient care [12]. The use of checklists, staff training, and accreditation further support process reliability and risk reduction [38].

13.7 Technology and Innovation in Supply Chain Management

Supply chain management for anesthesia equipment has been significantly advanced by technology. Specialized software platforms now streamline procurement and automate inventory updates, directly linking utilization data to purchasing. Intelligent systems, like smart drug cabinets and logistics robots, have enhanced efficiency and inventory accuracy in anesthesiology departments [39]. Mobile applications further enable real-time tracking of supply shortages, allowing for rapid response and data-driven improvements [7].

Automation and analytics are increasingly central to modern supply chains. Artificial intelligence (AI) [40] and machine learning (ML) algorithms analyze historical usage and patient data to predict demand for anesthesia supplies, optimize resource allocation, and reduce stockouts with greater precision [41]. Blockchain technology enhances transparency and traceability by providing a secure, decentralized record of medical products, which helps prevent counterfeiting [42]. Additionally, GPOs use innovative technology and algorithms to analyze pricing, purchasing, and usage data, allowing health systems to compare their practices with others and drive fair negotiations.

Standardization is a key strategy for optimizing hospital supply chains. This often involves a consortium of clinicians deciding to use a single vendor across multiple sites. This strategy aims to achieve four goals: securing best-in-class products, ensuring optimized clinical practice, reducing waste, and increasing buying power. For instance, some institutions give a portion of the money saved through standardization back to the clinicians who make these supply decisions, creating a direct incentive for efficiency and allowing for the continued pursuit of high-quality products.

Advanced item-level tracking technologies are vital for inventory management. Radio-frequency identification (RFID) and barcoding are widely used to improve accuracy. RFID systems allow for rapid, non-contact scanning of items, reducing labor and restocking errors compared to slower, operator-dependent barcoding [43]. RFID enables real-time tracking of supplies, automates expiration monitoring, and ensures accurate product assignment to patients.

Beyond technology, vendor training is a crucial strategy. Vendors provide education and training on purchased products, helping clinicians ensure optimal usage. This ties directly back to the principles of optimized clinical practice and reduced waste, ultimately streamlining the supply chain and increasing the institution's purchasing power.

13.8 Sustainability and Ethical Sourcing

Healthcare organizations are increasingly focused on green initiatives to reduce their environmental footprint. This often involves a collaborative approach with vendors to source and purchase sustainable products. Before adoption, these products undergo a rigorous, evidence-based evaluation to ensure they are clinically effective and cost-efficient. The overall goal toward sustainability is to show that the benefits of green initiatives outweigh their costs.

A significant part of this effort is managing the end-of-life for medical equipment. Rather than simply discarding old devices, hospitals can recycle them by selling them back to vendors, disassembling them for parts, or donating them to resource poor settings. These practices, while variable across institutions, are essential for a circular economy.

Anesthesia is a focus area for sustainability [44]. Single-use supplies, common in perioperative care, have a high carbon footprint [45]. Life cycle assessments show that reusable alternatives can significantly reduce emissions, especially when sterilization processes use low-carbon energy. The European Society of Anesthesiology and Intensive Care advocates for a "5R" approach: reduce, reuse, recycle, rethink, and research [46]. This includes strategies like optimizing inventory to reduce waste, favoring anesthetics with lower global warming potential [47], and implementing robust recycling and reprocessing programs [48].

Ethical purchasing is a subjective yet crucial aspect of supply chain management. It involves a healthcare organization's commitment to using suppliers who align with their ethical principles, such as supporting fair labor practices, sourcing from conflict-free regions and sustainable manufacturing practices [49].

Many hospitals reserve a part of their purchasing volume for local or smaller vendors to support their communities. This practice, while variable, is a key component of an ethical sourcing strategy. Audits and certifications are used to ensure that suppliers adhere to international labor standards and transparent manufacturing practices. By integrating ethical considerations, hospitals not only improve their supply chain but also uphold their moral obligation to promote health equity and social responsibility on a global scale.

13.9 Conclusion

A well-functioning anesthesia supply chain is vital for safe and effective patient care. Physician anesthesiologists collaborate with hospital administrators and supply chain professionals to ensure adequate stock levels, anticipate potential shortages, and advocate for efficient procurement strategies. Understanding these logistics helps enhance patient safety, reduce costs, and improve overall healthcare efficiency. Future use of AI and modern "green" manufacturing technologies should enhance efficiencies and environmental impact of anesthesia equipment.

References

1. Council of Supply Chain Management Professionals. SCM definitions and glossary of terms. Cscmporg; 2019. Available from: cscmp.org/CSCMP/Educate/SCM_Definitions_and_Glossary_of_Terms.aspx.
2. Tewfik G, Paschall SM, Stillman J. How leadership and process ownership can affect anesthesiology supply chain considerations. ASA Monit. 2023;87:25–6.
3. Katsaliaki K, Kumar S, Belani KG. Supply chain principles–a primer for anesthesiologists. ASA Monit. 2023;87(6):21–3.
4. Mehtsun WT, Hyland CJ, Offodile AC. Adopting a circular economy for surgical care to address supply chain shocks and climate change. JAMA Health Forum. 2023;4(11):e233497. https://doi.org/10.1001/jamahealthforum.2023.3497.
5. De Oliveira GS, Theilken LS, McCarthy RJ. Shortage of perioperative drugs: implications for anesthesia practice and patient safety. Anesth Analg. 2011;113(6):1429–35. https://doi.org/10.1213/ANE.0b013e31821f23ef.
6. Landry S, Beaulieu M. The challenges of hospital supply chain management, from central stores to nursing units. In: Handbook of healthcare operations management: methods and applications. New York, NY: Springer; 2013. p. 465–82.
7. Matava CT, Magbitang J, Choi S, Bhatia S, Tan M. A novel open-source novel app improves anesthesia operating room equipment supply. J Med Syst. 2018;42(9):167. https://doi.org/10.1007/s10916-018-1026-2.
8. Phuong JM, Penm J, Chaar B, Oldfield LD, Moles R. The impacts of medication shortages on patient outcomes: a scoping review. PLoS One. 2019;14(5):e0215837.
9. Park KW, Dickerson C. Can efficient supply management in the operating room save millions? Curr Opin Anaesthesiol. 2009;22(2):242–8. https://doi.org/10.1097/ACO.0b013e32832798ef.
10. Khan FA, Merry AF. Improving anesthesia safety in low-resource settings. Anesth Analg. 2018;126(4):1312–20. https://doi.org/10.1213/ANE.0000000000002728.
11. Jelacic S, Craddick K, Nair BG, et al. Relative costs of anesthesiologist prepared, hospital pharmacy prepared and outsourced anesthesia drugs. J Clin Anesth. 2017;36:178–83. https://doi.org/10.1016/j.jclinane.2016.10.015.
12. Okeagu CN, Reed DS, Sun L, et al. Principles of supply chain management in the time of crisis. Best Pract Res Clin Anaesthesiol. 2021;35(3):369–76. https://doi.org/10.1016/j.bpa.2020.11.007.
13. Definitive Healthcare. The 10 GPOs ranked by staffed bed count. Definitivehccom [cited 2025 Sep 27]. Available from: https://www.definitivehc.com
14. O'Mahony L, McCarthy K, O'Donoghue J, et al. Using lean six sigma to redesign the supply chain to the operating room department of a private hospital to reduce associated costs and release nursing time to care. Int J Environ Res Public Health. 2021;18(21):11011. https://doi.org/10.3390/ijerph182111011.
15. Roberts RJ, Wilson AE, Quezado Z. Using lean six sigma methodology to improve quality of the anesthesia supply chain in a pediatric hospital. Anesth Analg. 2017;124(3):922–4. https://doi.org/10.1213/ANE.0000000000001621.
16. Moore IC, Strum DP, Vargas LG, Thomson DJ. Observations on surgical demand time series: detection and resolution of holiday variance. Anesthesiology. 2008;109(3):408–16. https://doi.org/10.1097/ALN.0b013e318182a955.
17. Masursky D, Dexter F, O'Leary CE, Applegeet C, Nussmeier NA. Long-term forecasting of anesthesia workload in operating rooms from changes in a hospital's local population can be inaccurate. Anesth Analg. 2008;106(4):1223–31, table of contents. https://doi.org/10.1213/ane.0b013e318167906c.
18. Kane AD, Soar J, Armstrong RA, et al. Patient characteristics, anaesthetic workload and techniques in the UK: an analysis from the 7th National Audit Project (NAP7) activity survey. Anaesthesia. 2023;78(6):701–11. https://doi.org/10.1111/anae.15989.

19. Balkhi B, Alshahrani A, Khan A. Just-in-time approach in healthcare inventory management: does it really work? Saudi Pharm J. 2022;30(12):1830–5. https://doi.org/10.1016/j.jsps.2022.10.013.
20. Epstein RH, Dexter F. Economic analysis of linking operating room scheduling and hospital material management information systems for just-in-time inventory control. Anesth Analg. 2000;91(2):337–43. https://doi.org/10.1097/00000539-200008000-00019.
21. Illescas A, Zhong H, Cozowicz C, et al. Health services research in anesthesia: a brief overview of common methodologies. Anesth Analg. 2022;134(3):540–7. https://doi.org/10.1213/ANE.0000000000005884.
22. Hinrichs-Krapels S, Ditewig B, Boulding H, et al. Purchasing high-cost medical devices and equipment in hospitals: a systematic review. BMJ Open. 2022;12(9):e057516. https://doi.org/10.1136/bmjopen-2021-057516.
23. Miller FA, Lehoux P, Peacock S, et al. How procurement judges the value of medical technologies: a review of healthcare tenders. Int J Technol Assess Health Care. 2019;35(1):50–5. https://doi.org/10.1017/S0266462318003756.
24. Saleh N, Gaber MN, Eldosoky MA, Soliman AM. Vendor evaluation platform for acquisition of medical equipment based on multi-criteria decision-making approach. Sci Rep. 2023;13(1):12746. https://doi.org/10.1038/s41598-023-38902-3.
25. Darrow JJ, Avorn J, Kesselheim AS. FDA regulation and approval of medical devices: 1976–2020. JAMA. 2021;326(5):420–32. https://doi.org/10.1001/jama.2021.11171.
26. Dain SL. Anesthesia standards for facilities and equipment. Can J Anaesth. 2001;48(1):41–7. https://doi.org/10.1007/BF03019813.
27. American Society of Anesthesiologists. Statement on neuraxial medication shortage and alternatives. 2023.
28. Serchen J, Hilden D, Silberger JR. Bolstering the medication supply chain and ameliorating medication shortages: a position paper from the American College of Physicians. Ann Intern Med. 2025; https://doi.org/10.7326/ANNALS-25-00607.
29. Tosh PK, Feldman H, Christian MD, et al. Business and continuity of operations: care of the critically ill and injured during pandemics and disasters: CHEST consensus statement. Chest. 2014;146(4 Suppl):e103S–17S. https://doi.org/10.1378/chest.14-0739.
30. Aronson JK, Heneghan C, Ferner RE. Drug shortages. Part 1. Definitions and harms. Br J Clin Pharmacol. 2023;89(10):2950–6. https://doi.org/10.1111/bcp.15842.
31. Rinehardt EK, Sivarajan M. Costs and wastes in anesthesia care. Curr Opin Anaesthesiol. 2012;25(2):221–5. https://doi.org/10.1097/ACO.0b013e32834f00ec.
32. Suttner S, Kumle B, Boldt J. Pharmacoeconomic considerations in anaesthetic use. Expert Opin Pharmacother. 2002;3(9):1267–72. https://doi.org/10.1517/14656566.3.9.1267.
33. Orth LE, Ellingson AS, Azimi SF, et al. Allowable room temperature excursions for refrigerated medications: a 20-year review. Am J Health Syst Pharm. 2022;79(15):1296–300. https://doi.org/10.1093/ajhp/zxac118.
34. Armenian P, Campagne D, Stroh G, et al. Hot and cold drugs: National Park Service medication stability at the extremes of temperature. Prehosp Emerg Care. 2017;21(3):378–85. https://doi.org/10.1080/10903127.2016.1258098.
35. Hartle A, Anderson E, Bythell V, et al. Checking anaesthetic equipment 2012: association of anaesthetists of Great Britain and Ireland. Anaesthesia. 2012;67(6):660–8. https://doi.org/10.1111/j.1365-2044.2012.07163.x.
36. McIntyre JW. Anesthesia equipment malfunction: origins and clinical recognition. Can Med Assoc J. 1979;120(8):931–4.
37. Cassidy CJ, Smith A, Arnot-Smith J. Critical incident reports concerning anaesthetic equipment: analysis of the UK National Reporting and Learning System (NRLS) data from 2006–2008*. Anaesthesia. 2011;66(10):879–88. https://doi.org/10.1111/j.1365-2044.2011.06826.x.
38. Sweeney N, Owen H, Fronsko R, Hurlow E. An audit of level two and level three checks of anaesthesia delivery systems performed at three hospitals in South Australia. Anaesth Intensive Care. 2012;40(6):1040–5. https://doi.org/10.1177/0310057X1204000617.

39. Liu J, Xing LM, Shi X. Application of intelligent management mode for drugs and consumables in anesthesiology department. Eur Rev Med Pharmacol Sci. 2022;26(14):5053–62. https://doi.org/10.26355/eurrev_202207_29291.
40. Bellini V, Russo M, Domenichetti T, et al. Artificial intelligence in operating room management. J Med Syst. 2024;48(1):19. https://doi.org/10.1007/s10916-024-02038-2.
41. Younis H, Wuni IY. Application of industry 4.0 enablers in supply chain management: scientometric analysis and critical review. Heliyon. 2023;9(11):e21292. https://doi.org/10.1016/j.heliyon.2023.e21292.
42. Moosavi J, Naeni LM, Fathollahi-Fard AM, Fiore U. Blockchain in supply chain management: a review, bibliometric, and network analysis. Environ Sci Pollut Res Int. 2021; https://doi.org/10.1007/s11356-021-13094-3.
43. Wilke C, Bowden A, Sanders T, Nickman NA, Ashmead P. Implementation of radio-frequency identification technology to optimize medication inventory management in the intraoperative setting. Am J Health Syst Pharm. 2023;80(6):384–9. https://doi.org/10.1093/ajhp/zxac367.
44. Van Norman GA, Jackson S. The anesthesiologist and global climate change: an ethical obligation to act. Curr Opin Anaesthesiol. 2020;33(4):577–83. https://doi.org/10.1097/ACO.0000000000000887.
45. McGain F, Story D, Lim T, McAlister S. Financial and environmental costs of reusable and single-use anaesthetic equipment. Br J Anaesth. 2017;118(6):862–9. https://doi.org/10.1093/bja/aex098.
46. Gonzalez-Pizarro P, Brazzi L, Koch S, et al. European Society of Anaesthesiology and Intensive Care consensus document on sustainability: 4 scopes to achieve a more sustainable practice. Eur J Anaesthesiol. 2024;41(4):260–77. https://doi.org/10.1097/EJA.0000000000001942.
47. McGain F, Muret J, Lawson C, Sherman JD. Environmental sustainability in anaesthesia and critical care. Br J Anaesth. 2020;125(5):680–92. https://doi.org/10.1016/j.bja.2020.06.055.
48. Gasciauskaite G, Lunkiewicz J, Tucci M, et al. Environmental and economic impact of sustainable anaesthesia interventions: a single-centre retrospective observational study. Br J Anaesth. 2024;133(6):1449–58. https://doi.org/10.1016/j.bja.2023.11.049.
49. Trueba ML, Bhutta MF, Shahvisi A. Instruments of health and harm: how the procurement of healthcare goods contributes to global health inequality. J Med Ethics. 2020:medethics-2020-106286. https://doi.org/10.1136/medethics-2020-106286.

14 Medication and Formulary Management: The Hidden Value of Anesthesiologists

Gary Haynes

Hospitals in the USA are in a crisis.

Between 2010 and 2023, 300 hospitals closed and 192 opened resulting in a net closure of 108 [1]. One estimate suggests more than half of all rural hospitals are operating with financial deficits and potentially more than four hundred hospitals are at risk of closing or will need to merge into larger hospital systems in the next year [2].

Hospitals are struggling following the economically disastrous COVID-19 pandemic, given the sustained and increasing cost of caring for patients. Within hospitals, anesthesiologists have a unique role in delivering the clinical care that makes surgery and diagnostic procedures possible. When anesthesiologists focus only on clinical care, they limit their potential contributions to the hospital. Anesthesiologists' scientific and practical understanding of pharmacology, coupled with the experience of caring for every type of patient, gives the anesthesiologist a unique perspective on drugs and the hospital environment. This clinical experience provides opportunities for anesthesiologists to contribute to hospital success that goes beyond providing anesthesia care. Seizing opportunities to engage with hospital pharmacies and leveraging that relationship can enhance the standing of anesthesia groups with hospital leadership while improving patient care and safety. Failing to develop good working relationships with the hospital pharmacy may be more than a missed opportunity; it may cast the anesthesia department in a negative light and jeopardize their standing with hospital leadership.

G. Haynes (✉)
Tulane University, New Orleans, LA, USA
e-mail: ghaynes@tulane.edu

G. Tewfik (ed.), *The Anesthesiologist as Perioperative Leader*,
https://doi.org/10.1007/978-3-032-18058-2_14

14.1 The Hospital Pharmacy Environment

Hospital expenses fall into two categories: labor and non-labor expense. Beginning in 2020 with the COVID-19 pandemic, workforce shortages have resulted in an increasing need to contract nurses and physicians for short-term assignments, increasing labor costs dramatically. Drug costs are a major non-labor cost for hospitals. In recent years, drug prices have increased dramatically, coinciding with the end of the pandemic. Drug companies are constantly introducing new drugs to take the place of older medications, and these new drugs are more expensive. The costs associated with newly introduced drugs may even run as high as hundreds of thousands of dollars annually. However, the drug companies are not limiting price increases is to new medications as prices on commonly used older drug have also increased [3].

In hospital organizations, the pharmacy has specialized purchasing requirements and often exists within the materials management section. For financial accounting, pharmacy services usually function as a department with an annual budget. Pharmacy leadership is responsible for adhering to budget goals and reports to the hospital administration. Their responsibility is to the institution's Chief Financial Officer, who is, in turn, responsible for controlling expenses and receiving revenue generated from charges for drugs used in the hospital [4].

This organizational structure positions hospital pharmacy services in a financial silo, separate from the hospital areas that anesthesiologists know intimately, including the operating room, PACU, and non-OR anesthetizing locations. The hospital pharmacy must serve all areas of the hospital, and anesthesia and the OR compete for the attention of pharmacy services with hospital units. This arrangement is a potential source of conflict and misunderstanding. The potential for differences and misunderstanding can affect all medical staff members- not just anesthesiologists- particularly when the medical staff makes requests to add new medications to the formulary.

In US hospitals the average cost for materials and supplies needed to deliver care is 2.81% of hospital budgets, a large part of which is the cost of drugs [5]. Hospital pharmacy budgets vary by region and depend on size and the complexity of care delivered. Medications used in patient care account for most of the pharmacy budget, but hospital pharmacies are also responsible for acquiring all intravenous fluids, biologicals, and nonpharmacologic agents used in diagnostic procedures. Most anesthesia drugs are inexpensive; however, anesthesiologists should understand that their clinical practice decisions on the use of IV fluids and a few drugs account for about 15% of the top drug expenditures [6] (Table 14.1).

Table 14.1 Top 25 drugs by expenditures in nonfederal hospitals in 2024. (Modified from [6])

Drug	2024 expenditure ($ thousands)	Percent change From 2023
Pembrolizumab (Keytruda)	1,468,475	12.5
Immune globulin	1,040,191	6.4
Sugammadex (Bridion)	756,282	18.9
Daratumumab/hyaluronidase (Darzalex Faspro)	707,513	23.9
Bictegravir/emtricitabine/tenofovir alafenaminde (Biktarvy)	701,668	10.0
Remdesivir (Velkury)	642,653	−12.0
Nivolumab (Opdivo)	555,420	3.3
Inactivated influenza virus vaccine	529,663	−4.5
Antithymocyte immunoglobulin (Thymoglobulin)	522,425	8.6
Pneumococcal conjugate vaccine	509,005	−14.3
Sodium intravenous solutions	507,739	6.6
Denosumab (Prolia)	455,068	8.3
Rituximab (Rituxan)	452,083	−4.8
Alteplase (Activase)	440,820	−7.2
Natalizumab (Tysabri)	431,020	−15.2
Tenecteplase (TNKase)	401,119	28.6
Ocrelizumab (Ocrevus)	396,734	−12.5
Iohexol (Omnipaque)	384,195	6.5
Albumin	361,155	17.2
SARS-CoV-2 mRNA vaccine	341,132	18.2
Factor II/factor IX/factor VII/factor X/protein C/protein S	320,295	−2.0
Iopamidol (Isovue)	317,139	4.7
Durvbalumab (Imfinzi)	315,438	26.2
Pegfilgrastim (Neulasta)	303,083	4.5
Bupivacaine (Marcaine, Posimir)	291,645	−6.0

14.2 Hospital Pharmacy Management and Function

Hospital pharmacists maintain a formulary—once just a list of the drugs used in the hospital. The importance of the hospital formulary grew in the 1950s and 1960s when the business operation of hospitals became more sophisticated. Now the hospital formulary is a database of all drugs maintained in the hospital plus pharmacological information, decision support tools, instructional policies on how to use of each drug and associated products. Maintaining a hospital formulary is a continual process where the need to control costs is ever present. The Centers for Medicare and Medicaid Services require that hospitals maintain a formulary to receive payments.

Maintaining the hospital formulary and a steady supply of medications has been challenging. Hospital pharmacists acquire drugs from a supply chain that may not be dependable. Drug shortages have been a problem in the USA over the past 25 years, and it has been an increasing problem in the past 15 years [7]. Shortages are unpredictable since pharmaceutical companies manufacture many drugs outside the United States. Disruptions in the drug supply chain result from manufacturing, political, economic, distribution and regulatory issues, in addition to voluntary recalls and interruptions from natural disasters. When shortages involve anesthetic drugs or intravenous fluids, coordination between the anesthesia department and hospital pharmacy is essential to managing the crisis [8].

14.2.1 The Formulary

Hospital formularies reflect the activity and needs of the medical staff. Medication additions to the formulary often originate with requests from the medical staff. A potential source of friction between the medical staff and the hospital pharmacy occurs because physicians requesting adding new drugs bear no direct responsibility for their cost while hospital pharmacists are accountable to stay within their annual budget. Anesthesiologists who recognize the pharmacists' concerns can use this as an opportunity for demonstrating value to the hospital by presenting sound arguments based on published literature. Further, developing institutional guidelines for the use of a new drug, and including the hospital pharmacy staff when educating the anesthesia clinical staff on the use of all drugs, can overcome resistance and build rapport.

Anesthesiologists need both equipment and drugs to deliver care. With anesthetic drugs, anesthesiologists are dependent on hospital pharmacists for maintaining drug inventories at multiple points of care locations. The hospital pharmacy must have accurate, up-to-date documentation of drug administration to patients to maintain inventories and accurately charge for drugs used in anesthesia. They also expect anesthesiologists to maintain control of all drugs and avoid diversion of Schedule II drugs. These requirements mean anesthesiologists and hospital pharmacists are mutually dependent on each other to meet the fiscal interests of the hospital and not run afoul of the federal Drug Enforcement Agency (DEA).

14.3 Anesthesia and the Hospital Pharmacy

Anesthesiologists have historically practiced individually or as private or academic groups. In those situations, anesthesiologists were independent of the hospital, and consequently anesthesiologists viewed the hospital pharmacy only as a hospital service. The relationship has changed as anesthesia groups became financially dependent on hospitals, in many instances employed by hospitals. Hospital administrators now regard clinical anesthesia departments as an integral part of perioperative services. In return for financial support, hospital administrators expect anesthesiologists to contribute to institutional financial success through productive collaboration between departments, with pharmacy services being one of the most cost-sensitive.

Anesthesiologists may still view the hospital pharmacy as just delivering drugs to support their work, but the hospital pharmacists also regard anesthesia as a department responsible for adhering to institutional policies. Hospital administrators expect cooperation between departments to enhance productivity, reduce risk, and contribute to profitability. Anesthesiologists' education has rarely, if ever, prepared them for this expectation and collaborative relationship. Successful anesthesia practices will recognize this is a gap to overcome and that productive synergy with the hospital pharmacy is one way of demonstrating value in a large organization.

When approached professionally and in a spirit of cooperation, the relationship with the hospital pharmacy can be beneficial and productive. Failing to recognize this opportunity can produce points of friction and cast anesthesiologists in a negative light. Identifying individual anesthesia and pharmacy requirements as opportunities for collaboration, and restating them as projects with attainable goals, can provide ways to demonstrate institutional value and yield benefits for anesthesia groups.

14.3.1 Medication Safety

Diversion of drugs from patient use is a critical problem and consideration in healthcare. While drug diversion is not the only medication safety issue for anesthesiologists but it has also attracted considerable attention for decades. Immediate and easy access to controlled medications is a main contributor to the problem.

The Controlled Substances Act of 1970 created five categories of drugs according based on their medical utility and potential for abuse and dependence [9]. The concern about drug diversion and anesthesia professionals primarily centers on Schedule II drugs, which includes opiates and benzodiazepines. Diversion of non-Schedule II drugs like propofol, ketamine, gabapentin, and pregabalin is also a concern. Inhalational agents, including nitrous oxide, also have abuse potential [10].

Medication diversion puts patients at risk and creates serious jeopardy for anesthesia professionals and the institution. Drug diversion is possible in all perioperative locations and may involve both clinical and non-clinical personnel. While this has been a problem for decades, there is a suggestion the problem has become worse since the opioid epidemic [11].

There are multiple points in the internal supply chain where diversion of drugs from patient care may occur [12]. While hospital pharmacists are responsible for the overall process, the preparation and waste of controlled medications are processes shared by both pharmacy services and anesthesia (Table 14.2).

These areas of joint responsibility provide opportunities for collaboration. Fitzsimmons, et al. outline educational programs, drug surveillance, drug waste management, and diversion prevention programs as actions that can prevent drug

Table 14.2 Points of vulnerability in drug diversion. (Modified from [12])

	Pharmacy services	OR/NORA/Anesthesia
Procurement	Unauthorized orders Removing packing slips	
Storage	Replacement of drug	
Preparation	Product switch Drug dilution Removing small volume Harvesting waste "Accidental" damage	Theft Drug dilution Saline substitution Obtaining other credentials Taking unsecured drugs
Prescribing	Verbal orders	
Administration		Not administering drug
Documentation		Falsifying drug administration
Wastage	Diversion of expired drugs Retaining unused drugs Falsifying drug wastage	Switching substances Removal from waste containers Removal of waste containers Collaboration between providers

diversion [12]. Each area is an opportunity for the anesthesia department to participate and lead in preventing drug diversion. Additionally, anesthesiologists have responsibility for educational programs within their department. Leading interdisciplinary programs with all OR staff about diversion is a leadership and OR team building program opportunity. Anesthesiologists' participation strengthens institutional policies on employee drug screening, diversion prevention, and institutional controlled substance monitoring.

14.3.2 Drug Management

Protocols for anesthesia drug administration based on established evidence are necessary for improving outcomes and patient safety in the OR. Clinical protocols emphasizing the appropriate use and delivery of drugs improves patient safety, primarily because it reduces medication errors [13]. Protocols for the anesthetic conduct of complex cases are extremely helpful by improving communication and standardizing case management for improved patient care. Involving hospital pharmacists when developing anesthesia drug protocols incorporates their expertise and facilitates their work in providing their support in the OR. Implementation of protocols in cardiac surgery, solid organ transplants, and enhanced recovery after surgery (ERAS) protocols are prime examples. The desired outcome is having the right drug at the right place, at the right time, and administered safely to every patient.

Having a collaborative relationship with the hospital pharmacy is always helpful when requesting the addition of new anesthetic drugs to the formulary. In recent years anesthesiologists have embraced intravenous acetaminophen, liposomal bupivacaine, and sugammadex but many institutions resisted adding these drugs to the formulary because of cost considerations. Drug cost is always a consideration with new formulary requests, but departments that have an established reputation for responsible drug management will find it easier to gain acceptance with new requests.

14.3.3 Drug Preparation—Dilutions and Compounding

The U.S. Pharmacopeia (USP) is an independent, scientific, non-profit organization that sets the standards for medication compounding and drug dilution. Compounding and drug dilution standards are complicated. Compounding involves mixing or remixing drugs to meet the needs of individual patients when the usual form, or concentration, is not appropriate. Examples include modifying oral medications for topical application, or developing alternatives when patients are allergic to a solvent or stabilizer. Diluting involves preparing standardized concentrations of potent drugs. In anesthesia practice the drugs administered as infusions are usually potent cardiac, vasoactive, or narcotic drugs. The revised USP standard requires that drugs for infusion must be prepared under controlled conditions to ensure sterility and consistency of the diluent, volume, and final drug concentration. Drug infusions may only be prepared in the pharmacy or purchased as infusion ready products. This is far safer than when multiple individuals were making drug infusions in the OR while also attending to patient needs [14].

Complying with the standards has implications for anesthesia practices, particularly with OR workflow. Anesthesiologist directors need effective communication from hospital pharmacists to their clinical staff to ensure drug administration practice is accurate and compliant with the USP standards for the safest care of patients.

14.3.4 Drug Education in the OR

The education of anesthesiologists, CRNAs, Anesthesia Assistants and trainees includes considerable material regarding the pharmacology and administration of drugs. This is not the case with everyone who works in the OR and procedural areas where patients are receiving anesthesia. Most often the nurses helping take care of patients understand little about the practice of anesthesia or specific medications. Anesthesiologists have a tremendous OR and hospital leadership opportunity by holding regular educational sessions with the OR nurses. The topics for joint sessions with the OR staff are never ending but the OR nursing staff usually values educational programs that explaining basics of anesthesia, including the purpose and action of anesthetic drugs. By extension, the hospital nursing administration appreciates the attention and interest the anesthesia department takes in professional teambuilding in the OR.

Scheduling sessions with the OR nursing staff should occasionally include hospital pharmacists. Hospital pharmacy has many interactions with the OR but rarely is there an opportunity for all parties to openly share concerns and present issues. In addition to clinical practice and process issues, there is always a need to openly discuss the problem of substance abuse and drug diversion in the OR. Reviewing drug safety and compliance is important and is important for professional well-being of all who work in the OR and procedural areas.

14.3.5 Emergency Medication Management

Trauma patient care may be primarily surgical in nature and anesthesiologists are essential to deliver emergency surgical care. Emergency cases range from single individuals to mass casualty events with the potential to overwhelm an individual hospital. Anesthesia for trauma cases is challenging and places greater demands on anesthesia personnel due to its unpredictable and variable nature.

The American College of Surgeons (ACS) classifies hospital trauma centers according to the resources they make available for treating injured patients. The ACS defines the resource and compliance requirements for each level, Level I trauma centers providing the most comprehensive care of all types of injuries with most Level I centers based in university-affiliated academic medical centers. Level II centers provide care for a wide variety of injuries and have fewer educational, research, and community responsibilities of Level I centers. The Level III trauma centers manage mild to moderate injuries and are typically located in remote or rural areas [15].

Trauma program management and mass casualty event planning involves clinical and hospital administrative groups. The ACS trauma program specifies resource requirements by trauma level that must be available, and this includes the OR staffing and resources, emergency department and imaging resources, transfusion services, and ICU requirements for trauma care. The resources vary with the trauma level designation, but Level I and II designated centers have specific requirements for blood products and cardiopulmonary bypass availability. The ACS trauma requirements do not specify requirements for hospital pharmacy services, but as the intensity of trauma care rises to higher levels at medical centers, the pharmaceutical needs almost certainly increase. Collaboration on trauma planning with pharmacy services is another opportunity for anesthesiology groups to demonstrate greater value in hospitals.

14.3.6 Cost Management and Service to the Hospital Community

The Pharmacy and Therapeutics Committee (P&T committee) is responsible for determining the medications available for use in the hospital. Their primary function is maintaining and updating the hospital formulary. When evaluating requests for adding new drugs to the formulary, the P&T committee must consider both efficacy and cost for every new drug added. The P&T committee is usually a function of the institution's medical staff organization and reports regularly at medical staff meetings. Membership is often by appointment and includes physicians, pharmacists, nurses, quality managers, and hospital administrators. The Centers for Medicare and Medicaid Services require hospitals to have active P&T committees to receive payments from the Centers for Medicare and Medicaid Services and the Joint Commission requires them for certification.

P&T committee members vote to approve formulary decisions, and the decision to add a new drug or remove an old one from the hospital formulary involves more than just cost considerations. Reviewing changes to the formulary involves justifying the need and presenting pharmacological and clinical efficacy data. Hospital pharmacists present the information, but the process requires contributions from physicians. While the medical staff doctors share responsibility for formulary additions, unfortunately gaining physician involvement on the P&T Committee is often difficult. P&T committee chairs and hospital CMOs often find it difficult to involve hospital staff physicians.

Anesthesiologists have experience with all patient populations, knowledge and expertise with multiple drug classes, and firsthand familiarity with pharmacology, setting them apart from clinicians of other specialties. The anesthesiologists' management of controlled substances addresses one of the most important concerns of hospital pharmacists. However, anesthesiologists' reluctance to serve on a P&T committee may stem from limited exposure to antibiotics and anticancer drugs that are frequently brought before the P&T committee. This should not deter anesthesiologists from serving on this important committee as they frequently evaluate data and assess medication efficacy. Anesthesiologists are qualified to evaluate the clinical arguments for any new drug making P&T committee participation an opportunity for them to demonstrate their value to hospital leadership.

14.4 Summary

Hospitals in the USA are in a crisis with financial struggles and closures, especially in rural areas, exacerbated by the COVID-19 pandemic, rising costs and declining reimbursements. The hospital pharmacy is responsible for managing drug supplies and budgets, but it is often separated from anesthesia departments because of hospital organization structure and financial accounting systems. Anesthesiologists can develop productive relationships with hospital pharmacists that can help control drug cost control, improve patient safety, and demonstrate their value through collaboration.

References

1. Levinson M, Hulver S, Godwin J, Neuman T. Key facts about hospital. 2025. https://www.kff.org/key-facts-about-hospitals/?entry=overview-introduction. Accessed 23 Apr 2025.
2. Topchik M, Brown T, Pinette M, Balfour B, Wiesse A. Rural health state of the state. 2025. https://www.chartis.com/insights/2025-rural-health-state-state. Accessed 19 Apr 2025.
3. American Hospital Association. America's hospitals and health systems continue to face escalating operational costs and economic pressures as they care for patients and communities. 2024. https://www.aha.org/system/files/media/file/2024/05/Americas-Hospitals-and-Health-Systems-Continue-to-Face-Escalating-Operational-Costs-and-Economic-Pressures.pdf. Accessed 27 Mar 2025.
4. Speranzo A. Financial management of hospitals. Am J Hosp Pharm. 1984;41:935–41.
5. Definitive Healthcare. What is a hospital's biggest expense? https://www.definitivehc.com/resources/healthcare-insights/biggest-hospital-expenses#:~:text=The%20biggest%20

expense%20for%20hospitals,and%20third%20is%20employee%20benefits. Accessed 17 Mar 2025.

6. Tichy EM, Rim MH, Cuellar S, Tadrous M, Schumock GT, Johnson TJ, Newell MK, Hoffman JM. National trends in prescription drug expenditures and projections for 2025. Am J Hosp Pharm. 2025; https://doi.org/10.1093/ajhp/zxaf092.
7. Byrd JR, Singh L. No shortage of drug shortages: results of ASA survey. ASA Monit. 2011;75(7):56–7.
8. Ventola CL. The drug shortage crisis in the US: causes, impact, and management strategies. Pharm Ther. 2011;36(11):740–57.
9. Lampe JR. The controlled substances act (CSA): a legal overview for the 119th congress. Congressional Research Service; 2025. https://crsreports.congress.gov R45948. Accessed 19 Mar 2025
10. Wood D. Drug diversion. Aust Prescr. 2015;38(5):164–6.
11. Burnett G, Fry RA, Bryson EO. Emerging worldwide trends in substances diverted for person non-medical use by anesthetists. BJA Educ. 2020;20(4):114–9.
12. Fitzsimmons MG, de Sousa GS, Galstyan A, Quintao VC, Simoes CM. Prevention of drug diversion and substance use disorders among anesthesiologists: a narrative review. Braz J Anesthesiol. 2023;73(6):810–8.
13. Chui MA, Pohjanoksa-Mantyla M, Snyder ME. Improving medication safety in varied health systems. Res Social Adm Pharm. 2019;15(7):811–2.
14. US Pharmacopeia. USP compounding compendium. USP_HQS_797_FAQs_December2023_V6__002_pdf Accessed 19 Mar 2025.
15. American College of Surgeons. Resources for optimal care of the injured patient: 2022 standards. Chicago; 2023. p. 60611–3925.

Part IV

Postoperative Care and Recovery Management

The Post-anesthesia Care Unit: Clinical Stewardship, Systems Leadership, and the Expanding Role of the Anesthesiologist

15

Thomas Doss, Danny Jeong, Apoorva Amudhan, Bishoy Ezzat, and Daisy Munoz

15.1 Introduction: The Evolution and Purpose of the PACU

The Post-Anesthesia Care Unit (PACU) stands as one of the most critical nodes in the perioperative continuum—a space where physiology, vigilance, and systems management converge. As the patient emerges from the controlled environment of anesthesia and surgery, anesthesiologists assume a vital stewardship role that transcends airway and analgesia. They manage not only the physiologic recovery from anesthesia but also orchestrate workflow efficiency, interprofessional collaboration, and safety culture within a high-acuity, high-turnover environment. The PACU embodies anesthesiology's evolution from technical specialty to systems-oriented leadership discipline.

The PACU was born from necessity. In the early twentieth century, postoperative morbidity and mortality were largely attributed to respiratory depression, airway obstruction, and circulatory collapse. The pioneering work of Harold Griffith, who established one of the first recovery rooms in Canada, exemplified the transition from postoperative improvisation to structured observation. By the mid-twentieth century, anesthesiologists had assumed leadership in postoperative recovery, establishing monitoring standards, staffing protocols, and discharge criteria that remain the foundation of modern practice [1].

Today, the PACU functions not merely as a holding area but as an operational engine and safety checkpoint. It ensures physiological stability, expedites recovery, and serves as an early warning system for complications. For anesthesiologists, the PACU is where perioperative medicine culminates: patient safety, efficiency, quality assurance, and economic value converge. A well-run PACU safeguards patients, supports throughput, and generates institutional value.

T. Doss (✉) · D. Jeong · A. Amudhan · B. Ezzat · D. Munoz
Rutgers New Jersey Medical School, Newark, NJ, USA
e-mail: thomas.doss@rutgers.edu

G. Tewfik (ed.), *The Anesthesiologist as Perioperative Leader*,
https://doi.org/10.1007/978-3-032-18058-2_15

15.2 Clinical Stewardship and Patient Management

Anesthesiologists' clinical responsibilities in the PACU encompass airway management, hemodynamic stability, analgesia, and prevention of postoperative complications. These are not isolated tasks but interdependent functions demanding constant reassessment and anticipation.

15.2.1 Airway and Pulmonary Management

Respiratory complications remain among the leading causes of PACU morbidity. Residual neuromuscular blockade, opioid-induced hypoventilation, and airway obstruction dominate the list of preventable adverse events. Even at a train-of-four ratio greater than 0.8, partial paralysis can compromise ventilation and airway tone. The introduction of sugammadex revolutionized reversal by providing rapid, predictable restoration of neuromuscular function. Though more expensive per vial than neostigmine, sugammadex shortens PACU stay, reduces ICU transfers, and ultimately proves cost-effective by accelerating turnover and reducing adverse events.

Comprehensive postoperative airway management extends beyond reversal agents. Continuous capnography, early recognition of laryngospasm, and targeted interventions for hypoventilation underscore anesthesiologists' expertise in physiologic monitoring. The PACU is often the first line of defense against hypoxia-driven complications that might otherwise necessitate critical care transfer.

15.2.2 Hemodynamic Stability

Postoperative hemodynamic instability, whether hypotension from residual vasodilation or hypertension from pain and anxiety, directly influences PACU length of stay. Anesthesiologists apply nuanced understanding of autonomic physiology to differentiate between hypovolemia, medication effect, and occult hemorrhage. Early correction minimizes complications and accelerates discharge readiness. In doing so, anesthesiologists maintain continuity between intraoperative management and postoperative recovery—one of the defining characteristics of perioperative medicine.

15.2.3 Pain, Sedation, and Analgesic Stewardship

The PACU is a crucible for pain management strategy. Multimodal analgesia—incorporating acetaminophen, NSAIDs, dexmedetomidine, ketamine, and regional anesthesia—has become standard practice, reducing opioid consumption and adverse effects such as respiratory depression and postoperative nausea and vomiting (PONV). This strategy reflects a broader shift toward opioid stewardship in the wake of national crises.

Anesthesiologists are also responsible for titrating sedation. Over-sedation delays recovery, while under-sedation fosters agitation and pain-related hemodynamic surges. By individualizing analgesic regimens, anesthesiologists optimize patient comfort and PACU efficiency.

15.2.4 PONV and Recovery Optimization

PONV remains one of the most common PACU complications, impacting patient satisfaction and discharge readiness. Risk-stratified prophylaxis—combining serotonin antagonists, dexamethasone, and scopolamine when indicated—reduces incidence significantly. Through anticipatory management and standardized protocols, anesthesiologists reduce unplanned admissions and turnaround delays.

15.2.5 Neurocognitive Recovery and Delirium Prevention

Postoperative delirium, particularly among older adults, often first manifests in the PACU. Anesthesiologists' vigilance in assessing emergence behavior and cognitive status facilitates early intervention and communication with surgical and nursing teams, reducing downstream morbidity and length of stay.

15.3 Quality Assurance, Safety Culture, and Governance

Modern PACUs exemplify structured quality governance. The anesthesiologist's leadership ensures that standards for monitoring, discharge, and staff training are continuously met. The ASA's *Standards for Postanesthesia Care* mandate immediate evaluation of airway patency, ventilation, oxygenation, circulation, and level of consciousness upon arrival [1]. These standards form the bedrock of a safety culture where no patient leaves PACU without explicit sign-off by a qualified provider.

Anesthesiologists frequently chair PACU or perioperative governance committees, integrating clinical oversight with administrative strategy. These roles entail developing standardized discharge criteria such as the modified Aldrete or fast-track scores—quantitative tools that correlate physiologic readiness with safe disposition. Consistent use of such systems improves throughput and minimizes variability.

Quality assurance extends beyond metrics. Root-cause analysis of adverse events, near-miss reporting, and simulation-based team debriefings reinforce a learning culture. Anesthesiologists' systems-oriented mindset—derived from their intraoperative vigilance—translates seamlessly into structured improvement processes.

The PACU functions as a critical surveillance node where early recognition of physiologic deterioration prevents escalation of care. Timely identification and intervention for problems such as hypoventilation, airway obstruction, hemodynamic instability, and uncontrolled pain in PACU can reduce unplanned intensive-care admissions and shorten downstream resource use; dedicated PACU pathways and fast-track models have been associated with decreased ICU utilization and faster transfer to lower-acuity units compared with routine ICU admission [5, 7].

The PACU is where many potentially catastrophic postoperative events are intercepted before they become refractory. Respiratory complications (e.g., opioid-related hypoventilation, laryngospasm, aspiration, and evolving respiratory failure) and immediate cardiac events frequently manifest in the immediate postoperative period [4]. These events respond well to rapid bedside recognition and management in a staffed PACU environment; studies and reviews underscore that meticulous monitoring, structured assessment, and protocolized responses in PACU lower the incidence and severity of these adverse outcomes [6].

Standardized scoring systems and structured handoffs are foundational to safe PACU practice. The Aldrete Post-Anesthetic Recovery Score and its modified/"fast-track" adaptations provide an objective, reproducible framework for assessing physiologic recovery (consciousness, activity, respiration, circulation, and oxygen saturation) and for making disposition decisions [3, 8]. Comparative work shows that modified Aldrete and fast-track criteria reliably identify patients ready for phase-II recovery or discharge and facilitate safe, efficient throughput when used together with local protocols [2]. Equally important are ASA practice standards and formal OR to PACU handoff expectations, which require re-evaluation on arrival and a concise verbal transfer of critical information to the responsible PACU clinician—both measures that improve situational awareness and reduce missed problems.

15.4 Interdisciplinary Team Leadership and Education

PACU management demands constant collaboration. Nurses, respiratory therapists, surgeons, and anesthesiologists must function as a cohesive unit. As medical directors or supervising physicians, anesthesiologists serve as clinical mentors and operational leaders. Simulation-based education—covering airway rescue, malignant hyperthermia, and hemodynamic emergencies—has proven effective in improving response times and reducing error rates.

Moreover, anesthesiologists foster interdisciplinary communication frameworks modeled after aviation checklists and crew resource management principles. Structured handoffs between the OR and PACU ensure that critical data—airway status, medications, blood loss, and intraoperative events—are consistently conveyed. This communication mitigates information gaps that underlie preventable harm.

15.5 Economic and Operational Value of PACU Leadership

The PACU's function as both clinical and economic fulcrum cannot be overstated. Prolonged PACU stays increase labor costs, impede OR turnover, and generate opportunity loss when recovery beds are unavailable. Each hour of PACU hold time translates into delayed surgeries, overtime staffing, and decreased throughput. Conversely, efficient PACU management supports revenue generation through enhanced capacity utilization.

Pharmacologic and staffing decisions have measurable economic implications. For instance, judicious use of sugammadex, while more costly per unit, enables faster recovery and reduces the need for unplanned ICU admissions—yielding net institutional savings. Similarly, early mobilization and ERAS compliance reduce length of stay and readmission costs.

From a systems perspective, anesthesiologists bring financial literacy to PACU management. Their awareness of cost drivers—staffing ratios, drug utilization, and equipment maintenance—aligns patient safety goals with institutional sustainability. As members of perioperative services committees, they link clinical operations with hospital financial strategy, reinforcing anesthesiology's role as both a clinical and administrative discipline.

15.6 Integration with Hospital-Wide Initiatives

The PACU does not exist in isolation. It serves as a bridge between surgery and the broader hospital system. Through involvement in the Perioperative Surgical Home (PSH) model, anesthesiologists integrate PACU processes with preoperative optimization and post-discharge follow-up. The PSH's multidisciplinary framework has demonstrated reduced complications, improved pain control, and decreased hospital costs.

PACU alignment with Enhanced Recovery After Surgery (ERAS) protocols represents another key integration. Anesthesiologists champion ERAS principles—fluid management, opioid-sparing analgesia, and early mobilization—to promote continuity of care from OR to recovery. These initiatives exemplify how anesthesiology leadership drives institution-wide outcomes and financial value.

15.7 Technology and the Future of PACU Practice

Emerging technologies are redefining PACU operations. Predictive analytics now enable early detection of hypoventilation and hemodynamic instability, while artificial intelligence (AI) systems synthesize physiologic data to generate real-time alerts. Machine learning algorithms trained on EHR metadata can identify patients at risk for delayed recovery, prompting proactive interventions.

Anesthesiologists are uniquely equipped to interpret and operationalize these technologies. Their expertise in monitoring, data integration, and patient physiology makes them natural stewards of AI-driven PACU systems. Beyond in-hospital care, telemedicine platforms extend PACU follow-up into patients' homes, monitoring pain control, nausea, and vital signs remotely. These innovations enhance continuity, reduce readmissions, and align with value-based care imperatives.

15.8 The PACU as a Model for Systems Thinking

The PACU exemplifies anesthesiology's transition from task-based to systems-based practice. It is simultaneously a microcosm of patient safety science, workflow optimization, and economic stewardship. Within this environment, anesthesiologists function as clinician-leaders—balancing clinical acumen with data analytics, operational insight, and empathy.

Their leadership in the PACU demonstrates the specialty's broader trajectory: from the introduction of pulse oximetry to modern ERAS programs, anesthesiology has consistently pioneered safety and efficiency innovations that reshape perioperative care. As hospitals evolve toward integrated service-line models, anesthesiologists' ability to connect clinical outcomes to financial and strategic performance ensures their continued centrality.

15.9 Conclusion

The PACU is more than a recovery room; it is the crucible of perioperative medicine. Here, anesthesiologists blend physiology, leadership, and economics into a unified practice that safeguards patients and strengthens institutions. Through vigilance and systems design, they transform transient postoperative care into a sustainable, value-generating component of hospital operations. As healthcare systems embrace data-driven, value-based paradigms, anesthesiologists' leadership in the PACU embodies the essence of the essential perioperative physician.

References

1. American Society of Anesthesiologists. Standards for postanesthesia care. ASA Publications; 2024.
2. Dahake JS, Verma N. Comparative analysis of the modified aldrete score and fast-track criteria for post-general anaesthesia recovery: a narrative review. Cureus. 2024;16(7):e64439. https://doi.org/10.7759/cureus.64439. PMID: 39139348; PMCID: PMC11319724
3. Ding D, Ishag S. Aldrete scoring system [Updated 2023 Jul 8]. In: StatPearls [Internet]. Treasure Island: StatPearls Publishing; 2025. Available from: https://www.ncbi.nlm.nih.gov/books/NBK594237/.
4. Karcz M, Papadakos PJ. Respiratory complications in the postanesthesia care unit: a review of pathophysiological mechanisms. Can J Respir Ther. 2013;49(4):21–9. PMID: 26078599; PMCID: PMC4456822
5. Koning NJ, JLC L, Roovers L, Kallewaard JW, van Harten WH, Kalkman CJ, Preckel B. Introduction of a post-anaesthesia care unit in a teaching hospital is associated with a reduced

length of hospital stay in noncardiac surgery: a single-centre interrupted time series analysis. J Clin Med. 2024;13(2):534. https://doi.org/10.3390/jcm13020534. PMID: 38256668; PMCID: PMC10816897

6. Palermo J, Tingey S, Khanna AK, Segal S. Evaluation and prevention of perioperative respiratory failure. J Clin Med. 2024;13(17):5083. https://doi.org/10.3390/jcm13175083. PMID: 39274295; PMCID: PMC11396761
7. Probst S, Cech C, Haentschel D, Scholz M, Ender J. A specialized post anaesthetic care unit improves fast-track management in cardiac surgery: a prospective randomized trial. Crit Care. 2014;18(4):468. https://doi.org/10.1186/s13054-014-0468-2. PMID: 25123092; PMCID: PMC4243831
8. White PF, Song D. New criteria for fast-tracking after outpatient anesthesia: a comparison with the modified Aldrete's scoring system. Anesth Analg. 1999;88(5):1069–72. https://doi.org/10.1097/00000539-199905000-00018. PMID: 10320170

Adverse Event Analysis: The Role of the Perioperative Clinician

16

Karolina Brook

16.1 Introduction

Anesthetic care has become exceedingly safe, with a mortality rate estimated at 0.5 per 100,000 patients [1] in the 2000s compared to 64 per 100,000 in the 1940s and 1950s [2]. Despite this, adverse events (AEs) remain a relatively frequent perioperative occurrence [3]. Exact numbers of perioperative AEs are not known and vary depending on definitions of the AE and the method used to detect AEs [3, 4]. An older study from 1995 found an AE rate of about 19% perioperatively [4], while a more recent study found that 24% of surgical patients experience an intraoperative adverse event [5]. Numbers of adverse events directly attributable to the anesthesiology team are even less well characterized, for a variety of reasons discussed below. One type of anesthetic-related perioperative AE that has been frequently documented is medication errors: it is estimated that 1 in 20 perioperative medication administrations are associated with a medication error [6]. These AEs have potentially significant financial implications; the total additional cost of care due to perioperative medication errors is estimated to be $5.33 billion per year [7]. Considering that medication errors are just one type of AE, the prevention of AEs has significant financial implications not just for any individual anesthesia department, but also for healthcare systems across the United States and the globe.

This chapter will review definitions and classifications of adverse events, discuss *why* perioperative clinicians have a vital role in AE analysis, categorize financial implications of AEs, and provide an overview of the AE analysis process.

K. Brook (✉)
Boston University Chobanian & Avedisian School of Medicine, Boston, MA, USA

Boston Medical Center, Department of Anesthesiology, Boston, MA, USA

G. Tewfik (ed.), *The Anesthesiologist as Perioperative Leader*,
https://doi.org/10.1007/978-3-032-18058-2_16

16.2 Definitions and Classification of Adverse Events

The U.S. Department of Health and Human Services defines an adverse event (AE) as an event in which care resulted in an undesirable clinical outcome—an outcome not caused by underlying disease—that prolonged the patient stay, caused permanent patient harm, required life-saving intervention, or contributed to death [8]. The Institute for Healthcare Improvement (IHI) has a similar definition; the IHI Global Trigger Tool includes "any noxious or unintended event occurring in association with medical care" that results in harm, defined as "unintended physical injury resulting from or contributed to by medical care that requires additional monitoring, treatment or hospitalization, or that results in death" [9]. AEs are subdivided into preventable events, non-preventable events, and ameliorable events, where there could have been a reduction in the severity of the AE through alternative actions or procedures [10]. A sentinel event is a type of AE defined by the Joint Commission as a safety event that resulted in death, permanent harm, or severe temporary harm [11]. A near miss (NM), also known as a potential AE, as defined by the World Health Organization, is "an error that has the potential to cause an adverse event (patient harm) but fails to do so because of chance or because it is intercepted." [12] Similarly, the Institute of Medicine classifies a NM as "an act of commission or omission that could have harmed the patient but did not cause harm as a result of chance, prevention, or mitigation." [13]

Various organizations have attempted to standardize the taxonomy of AEs. The World Health Organization, for example, has developed a conceptual framework for an international classification for patient safety [14]. Their taxonomy includes two classes: "incident type" which groups incidents with shared features, and "patient outcomes" describing the impact attributable to the incident. Descriptive information is then further broken down to contributing factors, patient characteristics, incident characteristics, and organizational outcomes. This taxonomy is then used to inform actions taken to reduce future risk.

In the United States, the Joint Commission (a licensing body that regulates countless healthcare facilities) has terminology that is commonly used in healthcare institutions, with the goal of standardizing the process and allowing for systematic analyses across a variety of hospital systems [15]. Healthcare Performance Improvement, a consulting firm under Press Ganey which provides healthcare performance improvement solutions, has a different taxonomy [16]. Currently however, there is no one standardized classification system, limiting data exchange about similar issues and corresponding effective systems changes [17].

16.3 Why Analyze AEs? What Role Does the Perioperative Clinician Have in Adverse Events?

The goals for reporting and analyzing AEs and NMs are multifactorial and include:

- To assess whether there are any remediable actions on the part of the clinician(s) involved in the AE

David Marx, a mechanical systems engineer and lawyer, was one individual who popularized the concept of just culture, which is a human-centered system of accountability [18]. He argues that in situations where there was a negative outcome, it is essential to consider the original intention behind the behavior. Based on definitions from the moral penal code, he differentiates between behaviors where there is an intention to harm versus those where there was no intent to harm [19]. Based on where a clinician's actions fall, the corresponding action or "punishment" may be to sanction the clinician (such as in cases of deliberate harm or recklessness), to coach at risk behavior, or to focus on improving the system in which the clinician is operating (in the case of human error) [20].

- To identify modifiable contributing factors

One of the ultimate goals of AE analysis should be to identify factors that contributed to the adverse event that can be modified. Once these risk factors are reduced or nullified, overall risk should be reduced. The World Health Organization provides a helpful conceptual framework that illustrates this concept [14], specifically looking at contributing factors, patient and incident characteristics that can be analyzed with the purpose of taking action to reduce risk.

- To make systems changes that can prevent a similar event recurrence

When human error occurs, there is likely no conscious choice to take an unjustifiable risk [19]. The solution to prevent human error is to make the system in which fallible humans operate safer—thereby reducing risk and improving the safety of patient care.

- To promote a safety culture

Psychological safety, a concept popularized by Amy Edmondson, describes an environment where frontline workers not only feel comfortable speaking up, voicing concerns and identifying at-risk situations, but are also encouraged to do so. In environments where psychological safety is promoted, these individuals are not punished or humiliated, but are rather elevated as safety champions in their work environment [21]. Psychological safety is an important component of safety culture [20, 22]. Reporting and discussing adverse events is an important component of an anesthesia department that fosters psychological safety and promotes a safety culture [23].

- To encourage further reporting

Humans want to know that their work is valued. If clinicians report adverse events but never hear or see any results of these reports, they may be discouraged from further reporting. However, clinicians that are not punished for reporting AEs or NMs and who learn of systems changes that resulted from their reports may be encouraged to continue reporting [20].

- To decrease the financial impact of AEs

Estimating costs attributable to AEs is challenging; accurate estimates are hard to find. Costs associated with AEs may come from a variety of reasons, including the cost of the AE itself and downstream effects (for example, sepsis or wound infection associated with missing prophylactic antimicrobial medications), increased time in the operating room and the hospital or intensive care unit, and litigation costs associated with a potential malpractice suit or settlement.

We have already given an example of how medication errors, a type of AE, contribute to healthcare costs ranging in the billions of dollars per annum across the United States [7]. In another study, perioperative AEs in spinal surgery was associated with over $8million in incremental costs; higher-severity AEs were more costly while less severe AEs have a substantial aggregate cost as well due to their frequency [24].

It is also important to recognize that perioperative care is often fragmented and lacks standardization, which in itself increases AE risk and cost [25]. The Triple Aim is based on the premise that, by improving the health of populations, enhancing the patient experience of care, and reducing the per capita cost of healthcare, providers and institutions will enhance and optimize healthcare delivery [26]. Anesthesiologists, as perioperative clinicians, are uniquely positioned to achieve the Triple Aim [27]. At the same time, clinicians should recognize that focusing on the triple aim of health care can place undue emphasis on efficiency and productivity at the expense of patient safety. It is therefore essential to maintain a healthy balance between interventions that reduce costs through a focus on productivity versus those that make the system safer and decrease costs through a reduction in risk and AEs. Balancing these priorities is an essential function of effective perioperative leadership, often championed with great success by anesthesiologists.

16.4 The Process of Adverse Event Analysis: From Reporting to Feedback

The adverse event analysis process consists of multiple steps. Figure 16.1 illustrates the cycle of adverse event reporting, analysis, building safer systems through a focus on systems change, and feedback. At the core of this process is a well-established safety culture.

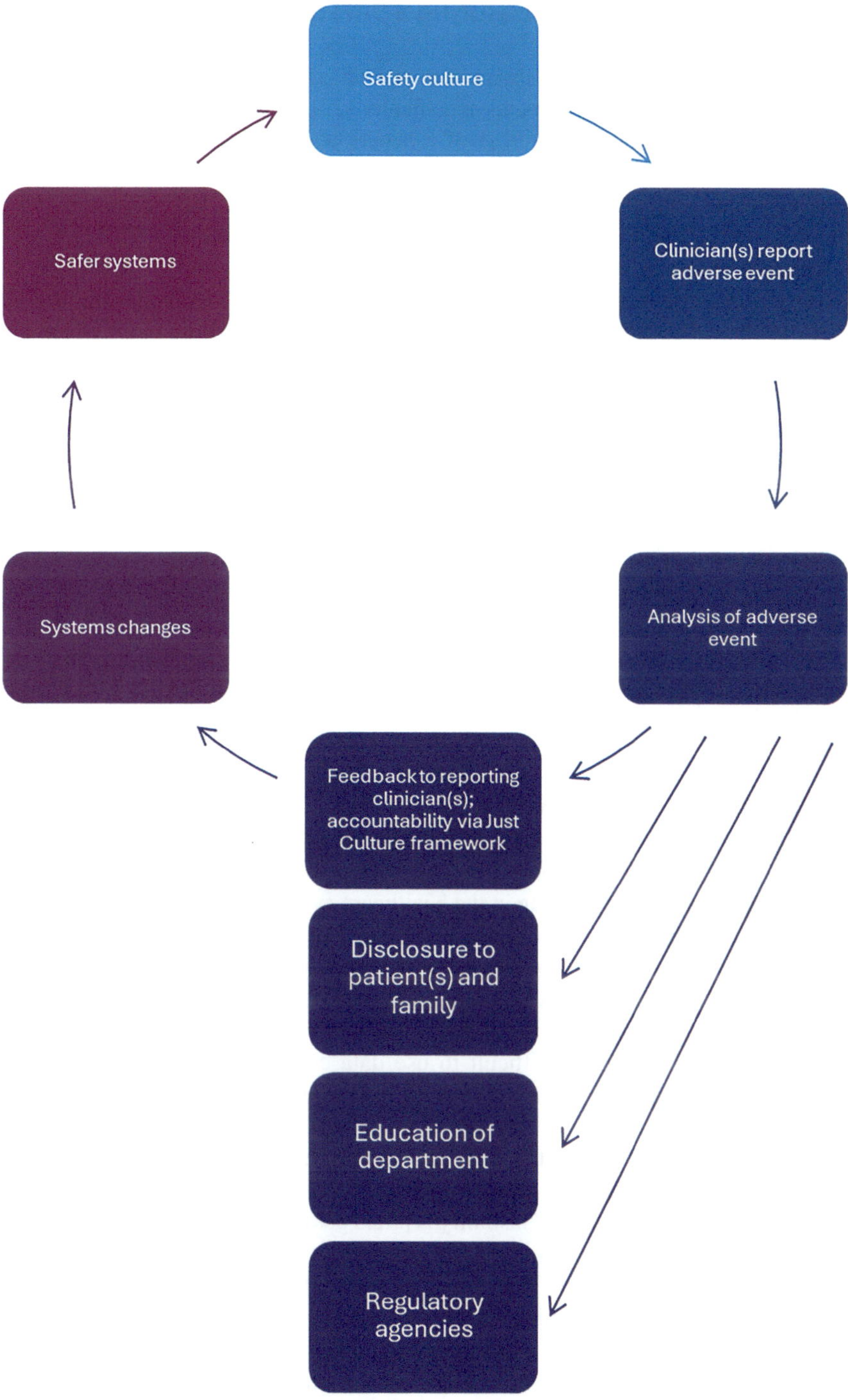

Fig. 16.1 Illustrating the cycle of adverse event reporting, analysis and feedback to clinician(s), education of the department and disclosure to patient(s) and family members, and a focus on systems changes (rather than individual fault) to make the system safer as a whole. Trust and understanding of the process and seeing change as a result of one's reports encourages further reporting. Safety culture and psychological safety are imperative components of this process

16.5 Establishing and Ensuring a Safety Culture

Much has been written about the importance of safety culture within hospitals in general and anesthesia departments specifically [22]. Clinicians need to feel safe to report AEs and NMs, without fear of retribution and with confidence that their reports will not only be taken seriously, but will lead to meaningful system change that will lead to a safer system. Developing and sustaining a safety culture requires consistent effort both departmentally and across an institution.

Tangible steps include educating both frontline clinicians and leaders about the principles of safety culture, demonstrating commitment to safety culture through both words and actions (for instance, by integrating safety culture into mission and vision statements, or by hiring leaders who similarly value safety culture), ensuring accountability (specifically in the manners in which AE reports are handled), and promoting open communication (both bottom-up, i.e., frontline clinicians reporting safety concerns and AEs to departmental and hospital leadership; and top-down, where hospital and department leaders are transparent about changes made as a result of AEs) [28]. These and other practical suggestions have been described in detail elsewhere [20].

A transparent process for AE analysis [28], the use of a reporting mechanism that provides clinicians ease of use, sharing findings of the AE analysis process with the clinicians and department as a whole, and continually focusing on systems changes (rather than individual blame) are some specific aspects to the AE analysis process that can contribute to fostering a safety culture.

16.6 Reporting of Adverse Events

Reporting AEs forms the foundation for the analysis process, because without knowledge of the AEs occurring in the healthcare system, identifying the contributing factors to fix the system and thereby prevent event recurrence is difficult. However, reporting of AE is challenging in many fields including anesthesiology [29]. Barriers to reporting AEs in anesthesiology include general apprehension about reporting, concern about how the collected data will be used, poor safety culture, fear of blame, and difficult to use data collection mechanisms [30–32]. Table 16.1 (adapted from source [33]) summarizes the different potential ways to collect data on AEs.

Each anesthesiology department must consider their various possible data reporting instruments and decide which avenue best facilitates the greatest number of accurate AE reports in a timely fashion [34]. It is possible that more than one system may be needed. Conceptually, these data collection mechanisms are divided into automated and self-reporting systems. There are several options within automated systems, including Anesthesia Information Management Systems (AIMS), national registries, billing coding data, and artificial intelligence. While data collection using an automated system removes the onus on clinicians to report events, using automated systems relies heavily on documentation in the patient's chart [33]. Although

Table 16.1 Automated versus self-reporting mechanisms to collect data on AEs

Automated	Self-reporting
Anesthesia Information Management Systems	Active surveillance
National Registries (MPOG, NACOR)	Complications/Outcomes tab in EHR
ICD-10 Coding	National incident reporting systems
Artificial Intelligence	Hospital-wide incident reporting systems
	Department-specific reporting systems

Abbreviations: *MPOG* Multicenter Perioperative Outcomes Group, *NACOR* National Anesthesia Clinical Outcomes Registry, *ICD*-10 International Classification of Diseases, Tenth Revision, *EHR* Electronic Health Record

an automated system can easily extract laboratory markers and vital signs, details about an event may rely on the clinician's documentation of an AE in the chart, which they may be hesitant to do for medico-legal reasons. For example, AIMS were initially considered to be the "solution" to AE data collection; however, it became clear that AIMS fell far short of an ideal AE data collection mechanism as it is estimated that only about 20% of AEs can be captured by AIMS [32, 35–38]. Similarly, data from billing/coding may capture less than one third of total AEs and is often delayed temporally from the actual AE [36].

In contrast, self-reporting mechanisms range from direct communication with department leadership (such as via in-person communication or e-mail), to an electronic health record (EHR)-embedded report (such as via a "Complications" or "Outcomes" tab), to national, hospital-wide or department-specific reporting interfaces that are separate from the patient's medical record [33]. Self-reporting places the onus of reporting on the clinician, which rests on the clinician being able to identify an AE or NM and recognizing the importance of reporting the AE. Clinical duties may decrease or delay reporting [33]. Each of these options has potential positives and drawbacks; for example, EHR-databases are easy to use but may be part of the patient record, which may deter clinicians [39]; national registries may be helpful to institutions nationally and provide data security, but may be limited in assisting in AE analysis within the hospital or department [33, 40–42].

Hospital incident-reporting systems is another self-reporting option which may be anonymous, tend to be separate from the patient record and have helpful features such as allowing non-anesthesia personnel to report AEs and may be able to generate reports for long-term analysis; however, these reporting systems are viewed by the hospital's risk management team and are somewhat less accessible to the anesthesia department [43, 44]. These reporting systems may be difficult to use and may put a large time burden on the clinician to file the report; however one recent study showed that customizing the hospital incident-reporting system and creating an anesthesia-specific section (or "software module") increased the number of AEs reports and the ability to analyze the categories of the report [45]. Finally, department-specific reporting systems may allow for the most customization, but may be costly and timely to build [33].

In deciding which type of AE reporting mechanism to adopt, the anesthesia department should consider several additional aspects, including:

- The ease of collecting AE data in a timely manner;
- The option for anonymous reporting;
- Whether they would like to utilize a voluntary or mandatory reporting mechanism, each with their own advantages and disadvantages [33, 39, 46]
- The option to report NM as well as AEs;
- The possibility of non-anesthesia personnel to report AEs and NMs.

One final important aspect of AE reporting is education of staff on the general value and importance of AE and NM reporting, the tools available to report, the categorization of AEs, and the importance of the timeliness of reporting. Departments can develop specific protocols for clinician referral and anesthesia departments should consider review of the AE reporting system an essential component of the onboarding process for new clinicians.

16.7 The Adverse Event Analysis Process

Establishing a standardized process for AE analysis is a crucial step toward patient safety for clinician leadership. Safety leaders need to have a firm understanding of the various conceptual frameworks, such as Safety-I, II and III, and the mechanisms to analyze AEs within these constructs [47]. Root cause analysis (RCA), introduced in the 1990s and associated with the Safety-I framework, continues to be a common analysis approach that incorporates a focus on systems factors that can be altered to make systems safer. The overarching concept is that it includes three core questions: "What happened?", "Why did it happen?", and "What action can we take to prevent it from happening again?" [48] While safety leaders should consider exploring Safety-II and Safety-III tools to analyze AEs, use of these alternate frameworks is not common practice in the medical field at this time [47]. Of note, collaborative case review (CCR) is emerging as another approach that tends to be multispecialty, allowing for the development of integrated systems changes throughout the hospital [49]. Table 16.2 summarizes the components of the AE analysis process.

The entire AE analysis process should be conducted confidentially, and involved clinicians should be aware of their organization's policies and any relevant state laws regarding the how to protect these discussions from legal purview. In the United States, peer review usually occurs for: 1) establishing privileges for new physicians or new privilege requests by existing physicians, 2) evaluating substandard clinical performance or questionable care, and 3) analyzing specific cases, possibly with poor outcomes, to review root causes [50–53].

Ideally, this should include various members of the anesthesia care team such as anesthesiologists, anesthesiologist assistants, certified registered nurse anesthetics and anesthesia residents. A clearly identified team lead will be responsible for reporting findings to department leadership and to risk managers within the institution as appropriate. This individual may also coordinate feedback and disclosure (discussed below). Clinicians involved in the event should not be part of the analysis team.

Table 16.2 A summary of the components of the AE analysis process

Components of adverse event analysis process
Ensure protected discussion (i.e. peer review protection, confidentiality)
Establish analysis team
Regular review of adverse event reports
Regular versus *ad hoc* meetings
Standardize analysis method
System of shared organizational & individual accountability
Focus on systems changes: create hierarchy of most impactful changes
Analyze trends over time
Follow up on actionable items

As part of the CCR, analysis could occur across multiple departments or specialties (e.g., nursing, surgery, or pharmacy). Although difficult to organize in a timely manner, a multi-department and/or multi-disciplinary analysis may be necessary to comprehensively assess the AE contributors and develop actionable systems changes.

In the same way that timeliness of reporting is essential, so is analysis of AE. Depending on the AE data collection mechanism, the reported AEs should be reviewed regularly (ideally, at least daily) to assess for the importance of immediate action. The AE analysis teams may choose to meet regularly or *ad hoc* in response to a serious AE.

Each event should be analyzed consistently within a standard framework. The World Health Organization's conceptual framework may be helpful in this regard and may be modified or adjusted to be made more anesthesia-specialty specific [14]; for example, one may start by defining the incident type and patient outcomes. An example would be Incident type "Medication/Wrong Drug," and patient outcome would involve a range of Degree of harm (ranging from none to death). Patient and incident characteristics need to be considered. Systemically and objectively evaluating all contributors, such as via a cause and effect diagram (also known as a fishbone or Ishikawa diagram) [54], is an important tool in the root cause analysis process to avoid any outcome biases.

Using a just culture framework of accountability, analysis teams should reflect on the *intent* of the behavior rather than solely on the outcome [19]. Situations where there is concern for reckless behavior, or deliberate harm, need to be addressed with the relevant clinician(s) immediately [18]. If a technical or educational deficiency is suspected, a broad plan for re-education of the entire department should be considered. While educating clinicians is important, it should not be the sole improvement strategy. Systems should ideally be designed to prevent human error and reflect the resilience of an organization [55, 56], namely, "'the degree to which a system continuously prevents, detects, mitigates or ameliorates hazards or incidents' so that an organization can 'bounce back' to its original ability to provide core functions" [14]. The focus should therefore be on broad systems fixes that should prevent a similar occurrence from occurring, remove unnecessary tasks and streamline workflows to reduce clinician burden. Frontline clinicians outside of the analysis teams could participate in developing systems solutions to avoid "top-down" enforcement. In a situation of many potential systems fixes, a prioritization matrix can help identify the solution that is most impactful with the least amount of effort and time to implement [49].

At the conclusion of the analysis, actionable items, responsible personnel and timelines should be made clear, with regular follow-up to ensure the completion of these tasks.

16.8 Disclosure, Feedback and Follow-Up

It is important to differentiate from the immediate versus longer-term actions surrounding an AE. For instance, the World Health Organization conceptual framework [14] describes mitigating factors that can "prevent or moderate the progression of an incident toward harming the patient", and ameliorating actions that attempt to compensate any harm after an incident (such as apologizing to the patient, staff debriefs, etc.) [14]. These short-term/immediate actions would, as their name suggests, occur within a short time frame after the AE. There are several sources to guide these disclosure discussions with affected patient(s) and family members using a structured approach [57, 58]. Over the longer-term, and after AE analysis, it may be important to return to the patient/family members with the proposed action plan to prevent recurrence of the AE [59].

While certain AEs may require specific remediation and education, when possible, it is important to move away from "blame and shame" mindsets and focus instead on systems changes and, when applicable, broaden education to the department as a whole. In other words, not only is it important to share lessons learned directly with the involved clinicians, but with the other related parties as well. This is an important component of top-down transparency [60]. As mentioned above, educating the clinicians about AEs that have occurred and being transparent about lessons learned and resultant systems changes is an important part of a strong culture of safety (Fig. 16.1) [22, 28, 61]. There are various ways to share this information with the department; examples include via regular morbidity and mortality conferences [62], or an AE safety dashboard [60].

Finally, the AE team analysis likely reports to a hospital risk management team, which makes decisions about reporting to outside regulatory agencies. Thus, it is important to keep notes on the AE analysis process, and to document planned and implemented systems changes for transparent disclosure to these regulatory agencies [28].

16.9 Conclusions

The perioperative clinician plays a vital role in the adverse event analysis process. Whether the process occurs within the confines of the anesthesiology department or is expanded to include other disciplines and specialties, the analysis process is integral to developing actionable systems changes that prevent event recurrence and increase the resilience of the organization. While challenging to ascertain exact costs of adverse events, they are known to increase healthcare costs through downstream effects, longer length of stays, and potential liability. Thus, in making the hospital safer and potentially preventing adverse events from recurring, anesthesiologists play a crucial role in reducing the burden of healthcare costs.

References

1. Pollard RJ, Hopkins T, Smith CT, May BV, Doyle J, Chambers CL, et al. Perianesthetic and anesthesia-related mortality in a Southeastern United States population: a longitudinal review of a prospectively collected quality assurance data base. Anesth Analg. 2018;127(3):730–5.
2. Beecher HK, Todd DP. A study of the deaths associated with anesthesia and surgery: based on a study of 599, 548 anesthesias in ten institutions 1948–1952, inclusive. Ann Surg. 1954;140(1):2–35.
3. Jung JJ, Elfassy J, Jüni P, Grantcharov T. Adverse events in the operating room: definitions, prevalence, and characteristics. A systematic review. World J Surg. 2019;43(10):2379–92.
4. Ouchterlony J, Arvidsson S, Sjöstedt L, Svärdsudd K. Peroperative and immediate postoperative adverse events in patients undergoing elective general and orthopaedic surgery. The Gothenburg study of perioperative risk (PROPER). Part II. Acta Anaesthesiol Scand. 1995;39(5):643–52.
5. Gawria L, Jaber A, Ten Broek RPG, Bernasconi G, Rosenthal R, Van Goor H, et al. Appraisal of Intraoperative adverse events to improve postoperative care. J Clin Med. 2023;12(7):2546.
6. Nanji KC, Patel A, Shaikh S, Seger DL, Bates DW. Evaluation of perioperative medication errors and adverse drug events. Anesthesiology. 2016;124(1):25–34.
7. Langlieb ME, Sharma P, Hocevar M, Nanji KC. The additional cost of perioperative medication errors. J Patient Saf. 2023;19(6):375–8.
8. U.S. Department of Health and Human Services. Adverse events. [cited 2023 Nov 16]. Adverse events | HHS-OIG. Available from: https://oig.hhs.gov/reports-and-publications/featured-topics/adverse-events/
9. Griffin F, Resar R. IHI global trigger tool for measuring adverse events, second edition. IHI innovation series white paper. [Internet]. Cambridge MA: Institute for Healthcare Improvement.. Available from: https://app.ihi.org/webex/gtt/ihiglobaltriggertoolwhitepaper2009.pdf
10. Forster AJ, Murff HJ, Peterson JF, Gandhi TK, Bates DW. The incidence and severity of adverse events affecting patients after discharge from the hospital. Ann Intern Med. 2003;138(3):161–7.
11. Joint Commission. Sentinel events: comprehensive accreditation manual for hospitals [Internet]. Available from: https://www.jointcommission.org/-/media/tjc/documents/resources/patient-safety-topics/sentinel-event/camh_24_se_all_current.pdf.
12. World Health Organization. WHO draft guidelines for adverse event reporting and learning systems: from information to action [Internet]. WHO Press; 2005. [cited 2024 Mar 11]. Available from: https://iris.who.int/bitstream/handle/10665/69797/WHO-EIP-SPO-QPS-05.3-eng.pdf?sequence=1
13. Institute of Medicine (US) Committee on Data Standards for Patient Safety. Patient safety: achieving a new standard for care [Internet]. In: Aspden P, Corrigan JM, Wolcott J, Erickson

SM, editors. . Washington (DC): National Academies Press; 2004. [cited 2024 Mar 11]. Available from: http://www.ncbi.nlm.nih.gov/books/NBK216086/.

14. World Health Organization. The conceptual framework for the international classification for patient safety. Version 1.1. Final Technical Report, January 2009. [Internet]. WHO Press; 2009 [cited 2024 Oct 4]. Available from: https://iris.who.int/bitstream/handle/10665/70882/WHO_IER_PSP_2010.2_eng.pdf.
15. Chang A, Schyve PM, Croteau RJ, O'Leary DS, Loeb JM. The JCAHO patient safety event taxonomy: a standardized terminology and classification schema for near misses and adverse events. Int J Qual Health Care. 2005;17(2):95–105.
16. Healthcare Performance Improvement. The HPI SEC & SSER patient safety measurement system for healthcare, Revision 2. [Internet]. Healthcare Performance Improvement, LLC; 2009.. Available from: https://dl.icdst.org/pdfs/files4/870b0f29a989bc0aadb758876423f054.pdf.
17. Tjia IM, Greene N. Chapter 8: learning from adverse events: classification systems. In: Katz CB, Rampersad SE, editors. Patient safety and quality improvement in anesthesiology and perioperative medicine [Internet]. Cambridge: Cambridge University Press; 2023. p. 64–76. [cited 2025 Mar 10]. Available from: https://www.cambridge.org/core/books/patient-safety-and-quality-improvement-in-anesthesiology-and-perioperative-medicine/learning-from-adverse-events-classification-systems/D246BD281A11B6415FF0F779EFB69779.
18. Marx D. Patient safety and the "Just Culture": a primer for health care executives. Prepared by David Marx, JD David Marx consulting in support of Columbia University. [Internet]. 2001 [cited 2022 Feb 23]. Available from: https://psnet.ahrq.gov/issue/patient-safety-and-just-culture-primer-health-care-executives.
19. Marx D. Patient safety and the just culture. Obstet Gynecol Clin North Am. 2019;46(2):239–45.
20. Brook K, Lin DM, Agarwala AV. Practical approaches to implementing a safety culture. Int Anesthesiol Clin. 2024;62(2):34–40.
21. Edmondson A. The fearless organization: creating psychological safety in the workplace for learning, innovation, and growth. Hoboken: Wiley; 2019.
22. American Society of Anesthesiologists. Statement on safety culture. 2022 [cited 2023 Jul 18]. Statement on safety culture.. Available from: https://www.asahq.org/standards-and-guidelines/statement-on-safety-culture.
23. Schein EH& WGB. Personal and organizational change through group methods: the laboratory approach. 1st ed. New York: Wiley; 1965.
24. Hellsten EK, Hanbidge MA, Manos AN, Lewis SJ, Massicotte EM, Fehlings MG, et al. An economic evaluation of perioperative adverse events associated with spinal surgery. Spine J. 2013;13(1):44–53.
25. Gonzalez RM, Norris M, Brook K, Azocar RJ. The practice of anesthesiology. In: Barash, cullen, and stoelting's clinical anesthesia Edited: Bruce F Cullen, M Christine Stock, Rafael Ortega, Sam R Sharar, Natalie F Holt, Christopher W Connor, Naveen Nathan. 9th ed.
26. Berwick DM, Nolan TW, Whittington J. The triple aim: care, health, and cost. Health Affairs. 2008;27(3):759–69.
27. Boudreaux AM, Vetter TR. A primer on population health management and its perioperative application. Anesth Analg. 2016;123(1):63–70.
28. Wilde M, Agarwala AV, Thomas BJ, Brook K. Sharing is caring: the importance of transparency in adverse events. Curr Opin Anaesthesiol. 2025;
29. Heard GC, Sanderson PM, Thomas RD. Barriers to adverse event and error reporting in anesthesia. Anesth Analg. 2012;114(3):604–14.
30. Wacker J, Steurer J, Manser T, Leisinger E, Stocker R, Mols G. Perceived barriers to computerised quality documentation during anaesthesia: a survey of anaesthesia staff. BMC Anesthesiol. 2015;15:13.
31. Williams GD, Muffly MK, Mendoza JM, Wixson N, Leong K, Claure RE. Reporting of perioperative adverse events by pediatric anesthesiologists at a tertiary children's hospital: targeted interventions to increase the rate of reporting. Anesth Analg. 2017;125(5):1515–23.

32. Arnal-Velasco D, Barach P. Anaesthesia and perioperative incident reporting systems: opportunities and challenges. Best Pract Res Clin Anaesthesiol. 2021;35(1):93–103.
33. Brook K, Wilde M, Vannucci A, Agarwala AV. Beyond adverse events in anesthesiology: "Unanticipated Events" and strategies for improved reporting. Curr Opin Anaesthesiol. 2024;37(6):727–35.
34. Gupta K, Rivadeneira NA, Lisker S, Chahal K, Gross N, Sarkar U. Multispecialty physician online survey reveals that burnout related to adverse event involvement may be mitigated by peer support. J Patient Saf. 2022;18(6):531–8.
35. Vinson AE, Randel G. Peer support in anesthesia: turning war stories into wellness. Curr Opin Anaesthesiol. 2018;31(3):382–7.
36. Tewfik G, Naftalovich R, Kaushal N, Zhang K. Adverse event and complication tracking in anaesthesiology: dependence on self-reporting despite implementation of electronic health records. Br J Anaesth. 2022;128(1):e28–32.
37. Ehrenfeld JM, Rehman MA. Anesthesia information management systems: a review of functionality and installation considerations. J Clin Monit Comput. 2011;25(1):71–9.
38. Benson M, Junger A, Fuchs C, Quinzio L, Böttger S, Jost A, et al. Using an anesthesia information management system to prove a deficit in voluntary reporting of adverse events in a quality assurance program. J Clin Monit Comput. 2000;16(3):211–7.
39. Wanderer JP, Gratch DM, Jacques PS, Rodriquez LI, Epstein RH. Trends in the prevalence of intraoperative adverse events at two academic hospitals after implementation of a mandatory reporting system. Anesth Analg. 2018;126(1):134–40.
40. Anesthesia Quality Institute. AQI - Anesthesia Incident Reporting System [Internet]. [cited 2024 Jan 18].. Available from: https://www.aqihq.org/airsIntro.aspx
41. Wacker J. Measuring and monitoring perioperative patient safety: a basic approach for clinicians. Curr Opin Anaesthesiol. 2020;33(6):815–22.
42. Wu HHL, Lewis SR, Čikkelová M, Wacker J, Smith AF. Patient safety and the role of the Helsinki declaration on patient safety in anaesthesiology: a European survey. Eur J Anaesthesiol. 2019;36(12):946–54.
43. Rubin DS, Pesyna C, Jakubczyk S, Liao C, Tung A. Introduction of a mobile adverse event reporting system is associated with participation in adverse event reporting. Am J Med Qual. 2019;34(1):30–5.
44. Ituk U, Mueller R. Implementation and evaluation of an event reporting system in an academic anaesthesia department. BMJ Open Qual. 2023;12(4):e002389.
45. Brook K, Song SY, Richards J, Harrington L, Okyere-Tawiah NK, Gonzalez RM. Anesthesia-specific software module for voluntary adverse event reporting. J Patient Saf. 2025;21(1):48–55.
46. Peterfreund RA, Driscoll WD, Walsh JL, Subramanian A, Anupama S, Weaver M, et al. Evaluation of a mandatory quality assurance data capture in anesthesia: a secure electronic system to capture quality assurance information linked to an automated anesthesia record. Anesth Analg. 2011;112(5):1218–25.
47. Samost-Williams A, Brook K. Using safety-I, II, and III to level up patient safety. Curr Opin Anaesthesiol. 2025;
48. Wu AW, Lipshutz AKM, Pronovost PJ. Effectiveness and efficiency of root cause analysis in medicine. JAMA. 2008;299(6):685–7.
49. Lacson R, Khorasani R, Fiumara K, Kapoor N, Curley P, Boland GW, et al. Collaborative case review: a systems-based approach to patient safety event investigation and analysis. J Patient Saf. 2022;18(2):e522–7.
50. Vyas D, Hozain AE. Clinical peer review in the United States: history, legal development and subsequent abuse. World J Gastroenterol. 2014;20(21):6357–63.
51. Moore I, Pichert J, Hickson G, Federspiel C, Blackford J. Rethinking peer review: detecting and addressing medical malpractice claims risk. Vanderbilt Law Rev. 2006;59(4):1175.
52. Edwards MT. Clinical peer review program self-evaluation for US hospitals. Am J Med Qual. 2010;25(6):474–80.
53. The Joint Commission. Comprehensive accreditation manual for hospitals: the patient safety systems. Chapter, Update 2. 2015 Jan;

54. American Society for Quality. What is a Fishbone diagram? Ishikawa cause & effect diagram | ASQ [Internet]. [cited 2025 Mar 10]. Available from: https://asq.org/quality-resources/fishbone
55. Hollnagel E, Wears RL, Braithwaite J. From safety-I to safety-II: a white paper. 2015 [cited 2023 Apr 25]; Available from: https://psnet.ahrq.gov/issue/safety-i-safety-ii-white-paper
56. Hollnagel E. Resilience engineering. [cited 2023 Nov 21].. Resilience Engineering. Available from: https://erikhollnagel.com/ideas/resilience-engineering.html.
57. Cornelissen C, Call RC. Enhancing a culture of safety through disclosure of adverse events. Anesthesia Patient Safety Foundation [Internet]. [cited 2025 Mar 4]; Available from: https://www.apsf.org/article/enhancing-a-culture-of-safety-through-disclosure-of-adverse-events/
58. American Society of Anesthesiologists. American Society of anesthesiologists physician series: manual on professional liability. [Internet]. [cited 2024 Nov 14].. Available from: https://www.asahq.org/standards-and-practice-parameters/~/media/9bd16ced606247a19d31aa15236f842f.ashx.
59. Committee on Medical Liability and Risk Management, Council on Quality Improvement and Patient Safety. Disclosure of adverse events in pediatrics. Pediatrics. 2016;138(6):e20163215.
60. Benitez AC, Brook K. Using a safety dashboard to share adverse events and systems changes. Br J Anaesth. 2024;133(4):893–5.
61. Reason J. Managing the risks of organizational accidents. London: Routledge; 2016. p. 272.
62. Brook K, Agarwala AV, Tewfik GL. Reframing the morbidity and mortality conference: the impact of a just culture. J Patient Saf. 2024;20(4):280–7.

Acute Pain Services: Clinical Impact, Cost Efficiency, and Hospital Value

17

Julia DeLorenzo, Patrick Discepola, and Jean D. Eloy

17.1 Introduction to the Acute Pain Service

Acute pain imposes a significant burden on patients, their families and clinicians. When patients experience acute pain, they require an increase in healthcare facility resources to manage it, including expensive pain medications and increased utilization of nursing staff to assess the pain and administer pain medications. Pain can also prolong the length of stay in the hospital, as patients who do not recover enough before discharge are at risk for readmission due to pain and inability to care for themselves. Increased demands on a healthcare system due to pain can thus decrease hospital efficiency and profitability, as well as patient satisfaction with their treatment. Acute pain services have been implemented in many hospitals to help remedy this burden and have become a tremendous asset to patients and hospitals alike, when implemented by a thoughtful and conscientious physician anesthesiologist-led team.

An acute pain service is a team of healthcare professionals dedicated to managing acute pain in a hospital, typically in the setting of surgery, trauma, or an acute exacerbation of chronic pain. The service is led by physician anesthesiologists specialized in acute pain management who assess patients, diagnose the cause of their pain, and provide them with the best mode of analgesia for their unique needs. Common methods of treatment in acute pain include multimodal medication therapy, peripheral nerve blocks, neuraxial anesthetics and patient-controlled analgesia (PCA) regimens. Nurses and other frontline clinicians are responsible for monitoring patients' pain levels and administering medications as needed. In teaching hospitals, resident anesthesiologists also work under the attending anesthesiologist to

J. DeLorenzo (✉)
Rutgers New Jersey Medical School, Newark, NJ, USA
e-mail: jd1439@njms.rutgers.edu

P. Discepola · J. D. Eloy
Department of Anesthesiology, Rutgers New Jersey Medical School, Newark, NJ, USA

G. Tewfik (ed.), *The Anesthesiologist as Perioperative Leader*,
https://doi.org/10.1007/978-3-032-18058-2_17

assess and treat acute pain. Pharmacists play a key role in expertly guiding medication choice and dosing, working in cooperation with anesthesiologists to ensure proper access to analgesics. Additionally, surgeons can help guide perioperative pain management by suggesting pain services for select patients. Together, these professionals can safely and effectively treat acute pain in the hospital. These services are frequently utilized in perioperative patient care when acute pain can be predicted, targeted, and managed, often mitigating potential effects before they reach a patient. This chapter will discuss the most significant benefits of an acute pain service with a focus on the advantages for perioperative patients, and the anesthesiologist's critical role.

17.2 Cost Reduction

In addition to their baseline expense, adverse events related to opioid use for pain management can be extremely costly. One study found that, compared to cases without opioid-related adverse events, admissions that were complicated by these types of events were associated with an increased cost of $4,700 [1]. Acute pain services can decrease the amount of opioids used by implementing multimodal treatment plans and regional pain techniques that significantly reduce the utilization of opioids [2, 3]. In a study by Corman et al. on the expense related to pain control for total knee replacements, it was found that single-injection peripheral nerve blocks cost $41.88 and periarticular infiltration using a multidrug cocktail costs $16.38, while opioid-utilizing methods such as IV PCA with morphine cost $178.94 [4]. Welch-Coltrane et al. suggest a potential savings of nearly $1.4M at one facility by utilizing acute pain services compared to traditional opioid pain management [3].

Beyond the materials and drugs used for pain relief, acute pain services can impact other areas of patient care that affect the overall costs of patient treatment. Pain is one of the most important factors that may hinder a patient's functional status perioperatively. By controlling pain, patients can gain earlier mobilization and thus may become ready for discharge sooner, leading to decreased length of stay (LOS). Implementation of acute pain services, such as regional anesthesia, has been shown to reduce hospital stay and postoperative pain, and increase early functionality in surgical patients. One study conducted on total knee replacement patients showed that usage of a clinical pathway involving regional anesthesia reduced LOS by 1.0 day (3.4 vs 4.4 days; $P < 0.001$), with patients citing decreased pain and increased ease of activity during physical therapy sessions [5]. Importantly, improved mobility can hasten recovery time and return to work, reducing disability costs for both the patient and the broader healthcare system [6]. The aforementioned study also measured the impact of implementing the clinical pathway on cost for the hospital and found a reduction in total direct hospital costs of $956 per patient compared to total knee replacement patients who were not treated using the clinical pathway with regional anesthesia [5]. Another study conducted on acute pain management in sickle cell disease patients found that personalized care plans reduced their patients' hospitalizations by 1.23 days, which directly produced a potential decrease in cost of over $1,500 per admission and an estimated $1.3M per year in a single institution [3]. Managing pain appropriately may also decrease the time a patient spends in the hospital by reducing readmissions. A study conducted using a large sample of 211,231 surgeries showed a dose-dependent increase in readmissions and emergency department visits in patients who experienced persistently elevated levels of pain in the hospital as opposed to those who had well-managed pain [7]. Limiting readmissions is also beneficial to the hospital systems because it reduces financial penalties enforced by the Hospital Readmissions Reduction Program (HRRP), which can cost hundreds of millions of dollars per hospital per year [8]. Acute pain services, therefore, can increase patient satisfaction through improved comfort and mobility, reduce time to discharge and total time in the hospital, and limit the cost of care per patient for the hospital system.

17.3 Reduction in Complication Rates

Postoperative complications are detrimental to patients and the healthcare system, increasing cost and rates of morbidity and mortality. Extensive amounts of effort and money are put into preventing complications after surgery because of the risk to the patient's health and the cost to facilities. Surgical site infections (SSIs) are one of the most common and dangerous postoperative complications, increasing the risk of mortality by up to onefold. They have been estimated to add an average of $29,414 to the cost of each affected admission, and up to $10B per year in the US alone [9]. While there is not yet a clear consensus on this topic, some research suggests that adequate pain control may help reduce the risk and incidence of SSIs. Several studies have found that regional anesthesia, such as epidurals, is associated with decreased odds of SSIs compared to patients receiving general anesthesia. Some of the proposed mechanisms to explain this difference include the reduced use of opioids, which can lead to immunosuppression, and adequate pain control causing vasodilation near the injury site, allowing for efficient wound healing and thus less opportunity for infection [10, 11].

Other important perioperative complications that may affect patient outcomes include cardiovascular and pulmonary sequelae. Adequate pain control of the thoracic cavity is known to decrease the risk of infection and other pulmonary complications by encouraging larger tidal volumes and decreasing atelectasis [12]. Recent research suggests epidurals, especially thoracic epidurals, may be associated with a decrease in the odds of postoperative pneumonia by half, as well as a reduction in risk of postoperative myocardial infarction of about 3.8% [13, 14]. Additionally, a systematic review and meta-analysis of randomized controlled trials from 2014 concluded that epidural analgesia significantly reduced overall mortality in surgical patients and found a decreased risk of arrhythmias and deep vein thrombosis compared to patients who only received general anesthesia without an epidural [15]. These complications not only increase the mortality and morbidity of the surgery for the patient but also increase the cost of care by tens of thousands of dollars [16].

It is, therefore, in the best interest of hospital systems to invest in resources, such as an acute pain service, that can reduce the risk and incidence of complications.

17.4 Enhanced Revenue

Adequate pain management is positively correlated with improved patient satisfaction with their treatment [17–19]. Patients' perspectives of their care have been shown to significantly influence their choice to return to a healthcare facility in the future or recommend it to others [20–23]. Hospitals and other healthcare facilities, therefore, are more likely to attract larger volumes of patients and generate more revenue when they can provide high-quality patient care that earns patient approval. A healthcare system's ability to control pain may therefore be a crucial factor in its financial success. Acute pain services have been found to control pain more effectively than the doctor-nurse model, which can have implications for the level of patient satisfaction and revenue generation [24]. Furthermore, when patients are satisfied with their treatment, they are more likely to score higher on their Hospital Care Quality Information from the Consumer Perspective (HCAHPS) surveys, which strongly influences Centers for Medicare & Medicaid Services (CMS) reimbursement and thus may further increase revenue [25]. Conversely, low patient satisfaction and low HCAHPS can lead to financial penalties for the hospital, reducing overall hospital reimbursement. While many factors play into a patient's experience with their care, optimizing pain management by having an acute pain service is one way to improve both their quality of care and the hospital's ability to succeed financially. Having a dedicated pain management team frees other hospital staff, such as nurses, from constantly addressing pain issues. This improves staff productivity and efficiency, ultimately enhancing revenue by supporting higher patient throughput

17.5 Cost Effectiveness

Launching a new service in healthcare can be costly; ensuring its profitability is important when making such an investment. While starting an acute pain service requires an initial investment to purchase supplies and hire appropriate staff, these services are often cost-effective and produce revenue for a healthcare facility. A study conducted on the implementation of acute pain management practices for patients with hip fractures produced a $1,500 cost reduction per inpatient stay compared to patients receiving standard pain management, which they noted more than offset the price of implementing the practice [26]. This chapter has previously outlined several of the many mechanisms behind the financial benefit of having an acute pain service, including increased revenue and reimbursements, improved patient satisfaction and volume, decreased readmissions and penalties, reduced length of stay and complication rates, lower cost of individual treatment plans, and enhanced hospital productivity and resource utilization.

17.6 Conclusion

The widespread success of acute pain services is not accidental; it is the direct result of anesthesiologists applying their expertise in perioperative physiology, regional anesthesia, and opioid stewardship to a collaborative, systems-level model of care. Anesthesiologists are uniquely trained to balance safety, efficiency, and patient experience using evidence-based strategies that reduce complications, shorten length of stay, and elevate the quality of postoperative recovery. Their leadership ensures regional techniques are performed safely, multimodal pathways are optimized, and frontline staff receive timely guidance and education.

Sustaining the value of an acute pain service requires continuous innovation, performance monitoring, and strategic alignment with hospital goals—areas in which anesthesiologists excel as stewards of perioperative improvement. Through their commitment to quality, cost-effective analgesia, and compassionate patient-centered care, physician anesthesiologists transform a pain service from a procedural offering into a durable institutional asset.

In this way, the acute pain service becomes not only a means of relieving suffering, but a cornerstone of modern perioperative medicine—strengthening hospital financial performance, supporting staff productivity, and ultimately enhancing the recovery and well-being of every surgical patient it touches. Anesthesiologists ensure these programs do not simply exist, but thrive, evolve, and continue to deliver measurable value to patients and healthcare systems alike.

References

1. Geller RJ, Espinoza TR, Horwitz D, Finkelstein Y, Kleinschmidt KC, Wax PM, Brent J. Opioid analgesic adverse drug events reported to a national poison data system. Ann Emerg Med. 2014;64(3):282–90. https://doi.org/10.1016/j.annemergmed.2014.01.018.
2. Said ET, Sztain JF, Abramson WB, Meineke MN, Furnish TJ, Schmidt UH, et al. A dedicated acute pain service is associated with reduced postoperative opioid requirements in patients undergoing cytoreductive surgery with hyperthermic intraperitoneal chemotherapy. Anesth Analg. 2018;127(4):1044–50. https://doi.org/10.1213/ANE.0000000000003342.
3. Welch-Coltrane JL, Wachnik AA, Adams MCB, Avants CR, Blumstein HA, Brooks AK, Farland AM, Johnson JB, Pariyadath M, Summers EC, Hurley RW. Implementation of individualized pain care plans decreases length of stay and hospital admission rates for high utilizing adults with sickle cell disease. Pain Med (Malden, Mass). 2021;22(8):1743–52. https://doi.org/10.1093/pm/pnab092.
4. Corman S, Shah N, Dagenais S. Medication, equipment, and supply costs for common interventions providing extended post-surgical analgesia following total knee arthroplasty in US hospitals. J Med Econ. 2018;21(1):11–8. https://doi.org/10.1080/13696998.2017.1371031.
5. Duncan CM, Moeschler SM, Horlocker TT, et al. A self-paired comparison of perioperative outcomes before and after implementation of a clinical pathway in patients undergoing total knee arthroplasty. Reg Anesth Pain Med. 2013;38:533–8.
6. Chowdhury AR, Graham PL, Schofield D, Costa DSJ, Nicholas M. Productivity outcomes from chronic pain management interventions in the working age population; a systematic review. Pain. 2024;165(6):1233–46. https://doi.org/10.1097/j.pain.0000000000003149.

7. Hernandez-Boussard T, Graham LA, Desai K, Wahl TS, Aucoin E, Richman JS, Morris MS, Itani KM, Telford GL, Hawn MT. The fifth vital sign: postoperative pain predicts 30-day readmissions and subsequent emergency department visits. Ann Surg. 2017;266(3):516–24. https://doi.org/10.1097/SLA.0000000000002372.
8. Alvarado M, Lahijanian B, Zhang Y, Lawley M. Penalty and incentive modeling for hospital readmission reduction. Oper Res Health Care. 2023;36:100376. https://doi.org/10.1016/j.orhc.2022.100376.
9. Shambhu S, Gordon AS, Liu Y, Pany M, Padula WV, Pronovost PJ, Hsu E. The burden of health care utilization, cost, and mortality associated with select surgical site infections. Jt Comm J Qual Patient Saf. 2024;50(12):857–66. https://doi.org/10.1016/j.jcjq.2024.08.005.
10. Chang C-C, Lin H-C, Lin H-W, Lin H-C. Anesthetic management and surgical site infections in total hip or knee replacement: a population-based study. Anesthesiology. 2010;113(2):279–84. https://doi.org/10.1097/ALN.0b013e3181e2c1c3.
11. Zorrilla-Vaca A, Grant MC, Mathur V, Li J, Wu CL. The impact of neuraxial versus general anesthesia on the incidence of postoperative surgical site infections following knee or hip arthroplasty: a meta-analysis. Reg Anesth Pain Med. 2016;41(5):555–63. https://doi.org/10.1097/AAP.0000000000000437.
12. Dogrul BN, Kiliccalan I, Asci ES, Peker SC. Blunt trauma related chest wall and pulmonary injuries: an overview. Chin J Traumatol = Zhonghua chuang shang za zhi. 2020;23(3):125–38. https://doi.org/10.1016/j.cjtee.2020.04.003.
13. Beattie WS, Badner NH, Choi P. Epidural analgesia reduces postoperative myocardial infarction: a meta-analysis. Anesth Analg. 2001;93(4):853–8. https://doi.org/10.1097/00000539-200110000-00010.
14. Pöpping DM, Elia N, Marret E, Remy C, Tramèr MR. Protective effects of epidural analgesia on pulmonary complications after abdominal and thoracic surgery: a meta-analysis. Arch Surg (Chicago, Ill: 1960). 2008;143(10):990–1000. https://doi.org/10.1001/archsurg.143.10.990.
15. Pöpping DM, Elia N, Van Aken HK, Marret E, Schug SA, Kranke P, Wenk M, Tramèr MR. Impact of epidural analgesia on mortality and morbidity after surgery: systematic review and meta-analysis of randomized controlled trials. Ann Surg. 2014;259(6):1056–67. https://doi.org/10.1097/SLA.0000000000000237.
16. Ludbrook GL. The hidden pandemic: the cost of postoperative complications. Curr Anesthesiol Rep. 2022;12(1):1–9. https://doi.org/10.1007/s40140-021-00493-y.
17. Bijur PE, Berard A, Esses D, Calderon Y, Gallagher EJ. Pain management: association with patient satisfaction among emergency department patients. Ann Emerg Med. 2014;64(5):537–43. https://doi.org/10.1016/j.annemergmed.2014.05.028.
18. Aubrun F, Mazoit JX, Riou B, Langeron O, Coriat P, Fletcher D. Determinants of patient satisfaction regarding pain care. Eur J Anaesthesiol. 2013;30(4):161–7. https://doi.org/10.1097/EJA.0b013e32835f7eb6.
19. Miner JR, Biros M, Trainor A, Hubbard J, Beltram M. Patient and physician perceptions as risk factors for satisfaction with pain management in the emergency department. Ann Emerg Med. 2010;56(6):785–93. https://doi.org/10.1016/j.annemergmed.2010.04.019.
20. Rahmqvist M, Bara A-C. Patient characteristics and quality dimensions related to patient satisfaction. Int J Health Care Qual Assur. 2010;23(2):188–202. https://doi.org/10.1108/09526861011017038.
21. Davis BA, Kiesel CK, McFarland JM, Collard AF, Maul D. Relationships among patient satisfaction, intent to return, and intent to recommend services provided by an academic nursing center. J Prof Nurs. 2003;19(1):11–7. https://doi.org/10.1053/jpnu.2003.6.
22. Otani K, Herrmann PA, Kurz RS. Improving patient satisfaction in hospital care settings. Health Serv Manag Res. 2010;23(4):163–9. https://doi.org/10.1258/hsmr.2010.010015.
23. Xie Z, Or C, Yan X, Li H, Zhang Z. Effect of inpatient experience on patient satisfaction and the willingness to recommend a hospital: the mediating role of patient satisfaction. Front Public Health. 2022;10:937441. https://doi.org/10.3389/fpubh.2022.937441.
24. Chen L, Zhang Y, Li X. Acute pain service for postoperative pain in adults: a network meta-analysis. Int J Surg. 2025;111(6):4009–19. https://doi.org/10.1097/JS9.0000000000002419.

25. Chen H-C, Cates T, Taylor M. The effect of patient quality measurements and HCAHPS patient satisfaction on hospital reimbursements. Hum Syst Manag. 2022;42(3):1–15. https://doi.org/10.3233/HSM-220042.
26. Brooks JM, Titler MG, Ardery G, Herr K. Effect of evidence-based acute pain management practices on inpatient costs. Health Serv Res. 2009;44(1):245–63. https://doi.org/10.1111/j.1475-6773.2008.00912.x. PMID: 19146567; PMCID: PMC2669631.

Part V

Systems of Safety: Technology, Oversight, and Critical Care Leadership in Modern Anesthesiology

18 Crisis Medicine: The Anesthesiologist's Role in Airway, Trauma, and Emergency Preparedness

Maeve Muldowney, David A. Leon, and Ireana C. Ng

18.1 Airway

Anesthesiologists are widely regarded as airway experts, skilled in advanced techniques to safely manage difficult airways. This expertise extends beyond the operating room (OR) to include intensive care units (ICUs), emergency departments (EDs), and other clinical environments.

18.1.1 The Role of Anesthesiologists in Difficulty Airway Management

The 2019 Anesthesia Closed Claims Project analysis by the American Society of Anesthesiologists (ASA) on difficult tracheal intubation management, along with findings from the Fourth National Audit Project (NAP4), highlights that difficult or failed airway management remains a major contributor to patient morbidity and mortality—as well as a significant source of liability for anesthesiologists [1, 2]. While tracheal intubation is generally a safe and straightforward procedure, complications can arise from an anatomically challenging airway or physiologically difficult airway, a newer concept that considers the patient's underlying critical physiological status (e.g., hypoxemia, hypotension, severe metabolic acidosis, or right heart failure). Both these scenarios may increase the risk of adverse events

M. Muldowney · I. C. Ng (✉)
Department of Anesthesiology and Pain Medicine, Harborview Medical Center, University of Washington, Seattle, WA, USA
e-mail: mmuldow@uw.edu; ireanang@uw.edu

D. A. Leon
Department of Anesthesiology and Pain Medicine and Department of Emergency Medicine, University of California Davis School of Medicine, Sacramento, CA, USA
e-mail: davleon@health.ucdavis.edu

G. Tewfik (ed.), *The Anesthesiologist as Perioperative Leader*,
https://doi.org/10.1007/978-3-032-18058-2_18

during airway management [3, 4]. When primary techniques fail, the situation can deteriorate rapidly, leading to poor outcomes.

Anesthesiologists have long led several professional societies to develop guidelines and algorithms for both anticipated and unanticipated difficult airway management. Notable examples include:

1. The 2015 Difficult Airway Society (DAS) guidelines on the management of unanticipated difficult intubation, produced by anesthesiologists and critical care specialists from various countries [5].
2. The 2022 ASA Practice Guidelines for the Management of the Difficult Airway, developed by an international task force representing multiple medical organizations [6].
3. The Anesthesia Patient Safety Foundation (APSF)—Patient Safety Priorities Advisory Group on airway management, who advocates for best practices in airway safety.

These national and international organizations serve as important platforms for education, evidence-based recommendations, and multidisciplinary collaboration to improve patient safety during challenging airway scenarios.

18.1.2 The Role of Anesthesiologists in Facility Airway Management

In most hospitals, the anesthesiology team responds to the emergency airway response call. These teams may be activated via overhead announcement, paging system, or designated emergency airway phone numbers. They often respond to Code Blue, trauma activations, emergent airway support outside OR, and surgical or difficult airway emergencies throughout hospital. The model of deployment depends on institutional resources and structure. This collaboration is particularly critical when anesthesiologists provide backup airway management for other specialties. For example, clear guidelines are needed for when the Emergency Department should request anesthesia management for anticipated difficult airway cases. Anesthesiologists work closely with other specialty departments to develop comprehensive guidelines to ensure minimal response time and effective airway management while minimizing risks to patient safety.

One example is the Difficult Airway Response Team (DART)—a quality improvement initiative led by anesthesiologists, otolaryngologists, trauma surgeons, and risk managers at Johns Hopkins Hospital. Implemented in 2005, the DART program focuses on operations, safety, and education related to airway emergencies. Its success underscores the value of structured airway response teams in improving outcomes and reducing adverse events [7].

With support from hospital leadership, anesthesiologists provide simulation training and regular drills to maintain team effectiveness. These team-based interventions emphasize role clarity, closed-loop communication, and interdisciplinary coordination. Recent efforts have also emphasized high-fidelity simulations, crisis resource management, and cognitive aids to support decision-making during perioperative arrests and airway emergencies [8].

In ICUs and EDs, airway management is often performed by appropriately trained clinicians, including intensivists, emergency physicians, and in some cases, advanced medical practitioners. Due to the critically ill nature of these patients, non-airway-related complications (e.g., hemodynamic instability, hypoxemia) are prevalent during intubations. As Mort reported, out-of-OR intubations carry a complication rate 40 times higher than intubations in the OR [9]. Jaber and colleagues found that 50% of ICU intubations were associated with complications, including severe complications in 28% of cases with no significant difference in outcomes between anesthesiologists and experienced intensivists performing the procedures [10].

Who can and should perform emergency intubation depends on state regulations and institutional policies. The anesthesiology team often assists with airway management in Code Blue situations in many hospitals. In many states, licensed respiratory therapists (RTs) are also authorized to perform intubation, while in some states, registered nurses who are appropriately trained and competent may perform intubation in accordance with local clinical practice standards. Additionally, emergency medicine technicians (EMTs) and paramedics are trained to perform intubations in the prehospital setting.

However, there is a clear distinction between certification and competency. Certification typically reflects completion of a training program, while competency involves demonstrated, sustained performance in clinical settings. Local credentialing bodies and professional associations are responsible for assessing and maintaining this competency. In many institutions, anesthesiologists have an important role in credentialing, privileging, and ongoing airway education for non-anesthesiologist providers, including emergency physicians, intensivists, EMTs, and paramedics.

Ensuring safe airway management requires not only well-trained and credentialed personnel, but also the appropriate infrastructure to support them. Competent providers are most effective when supported by reliable systems and standardized access to equipment. Thus, attention must extend beyond individual training to the institutional resources and technological tools that enable providers to deliver safe, timely, and effective airway care. Many institutions maintain portable "grab bags/boxes" with essential airway tools for emergencies outside the OR. Code/crash carts are equipped with basic airway supplies and direct laryngoscopy (DL) intubation equipment. The increasing use of video laryngoscopy (VL) has transformed traditional approaches to airway management. Compared to DL, VL is associated with higher first-pass success, fewer failed attempts, and reduced complications such as hypoxemia [11]. Many institutions have adopted VL as a rescue airway technique and integrated it into their airway response teams. However, VL adoption may be limited by factors such as cost, insufficient training, airway decontamination challenges, and concerns about skill degradation in use of DL. Some providers also perceive VL to be less effective in "bloody airways," although techniques exist to mitigate these limitations [12].

The availability of a difficult airway cart is another critical component of emergency airway preparedness. Typically organized by anesthesiologists and anesthesia technicians, these carts are stocked according to institutional protocols and difficult airway guidelines. They contain a range of advanced airway devices, including emergency invasive airway access kit, for example, cricothyroidotomy kit or percutaneous tracheostomy kit. They are strategically placed in ORs, ICUs, and EDs to enable rapid response to anticipated or unexpected airway challenges.

All airway providers must be familiar with the location, contents, and proper use of airway equipment. Regular training, orientation, and simulation exercises, often led by anesthesiologists, are essential for ensuring team readiness and patient safety.

18.1.3 Billing, Legal, and Liability Considerations in Shared Airway Management

According to the National Correct Coding Initiative (NCCI), elective endotracheal intubation performed as part of general anesthesia is considered integral to the procedure and not separately reimbursable. However, national and local Medicare rules allow emergency endotracheal intubation—performed by anesthesiologist in patients with rapidly deteriorating respiratory function requiring emergent airway protection or mechanical ventilation—to be billed separately [13, 14]. Additional anesthesia modifiers may apply based on the provider type and whether the anesthesia team is responsible for managing ventilation settings and initiating sedation prior to handing over patient care to the RT or ICU team [15–17].

Many institutions designate an Anesthesiologist-in-Charge (AIC) or an equivalent role to oversee daily operational efficiency and anesthesia team assignments in the OR. AICs may have minimal room assignments to ensure they are available to respond immediately to airway emergencies outside the OR, helping to minimize disruptions to scheduled surgical cases. In larger facilities, the AIC may be supported by CRNAs or residents assigned to non-operating room anesthesia (NORA) or airway rotations. In states where CRNAs practice independently, they may manage airway emergencies without anesthesiologist supervision, in accordance with state-specific regulations. Intensive care physicians or emergency physicians are also among those who can perform emergency intubations in the NORA setting, further helping to minimize frequency of OR disruptions.

A national survey by the Eastern Association for the Surgery of Trauma (EAST) and the Trauma Anesthesiology Society (TAS) revealed 81% of surveyed institutions reported that emergency medicine physicians were the primary providers for ED intubations. In 98.2% of the surveyed institutions where an anesthesiology team was not in the primary airway team, a member of the anesthesiology department was available on a 24-hour in-house basis to assist with difficult airways [18]. These data highlight the interdisciplinary nature of complex airway management and the necessity for effective communication between teams. While roles may not be explicitly defined, collaboration between the anesthesiology team and other departments is essential to ensure optimal patient outcomes.

Emergency airway management frequently involves shared responsibility between departments such as anesthesiology, emergency medicine, and intensive care. When anesthesiology is consulted for a rescue airway following a failed intubation—especially in NORA settings—the liability assessment, particularly in cases with airway complications, is highly dependent on institutional policies, the sequence of events and outcome, as well as the nature of the intervention.

A retrospective study of emergency intubations performed by anesthesiologists outside the OR reported that 10.3% (351 out of 3423 cases) were classified as difficult [19]. Difficult or failed intubation is a well-documented source of patient harm and professional liability for anesthesia providers [2]. The 2019 Anesthesia Closed Claims Analysis identified inadequate airway assessment or planning and errors in clinical judgment to be linked with undesired outcomes [2].

Legal claims related to airway complications may involve individual practitioners (anesthesiologists or other healthcare professionals) as well as the institutions where the care was provided. Liability is typically determined by evidence of a breach in the standard of care that results in morbidity or mortality.

Best practices for anesthesiologists in rescue airway situations include honest documentation on all attempts and interventions in a factual and neutral manner, as well as ensuring transparent communication about team roles and the sequence of events. Anesthesiologists also actively participate in institutional airway incident quality improvement reviews and root cause analyses to enhance patient safety. At the institutional level, they provide continuous education on recognition of difficult intubation predictors and establish escalation pathways and thresholds for involving anesthesia for emergency/difficult airway management by non-anesthesia providers. This includes determining the assignment of the first airway responder based on experience and knowing when to seek anesthesia assistance. The value of an experienced anesthesiologist in difficult airway scenarios is indisputable. Effective communication and collaboration between anesthesia and non-anesthesia airway providers are essential for managing the airway in challenging situations. The common goal should always be "primum non nocere"—first, do no harm to the patient.

18.2 Trauma Preparedness

18.2.1 The Role of the Trauma Anesthesiologist within the Trauma Team

The designation of trauma centers is the responsibility of the state or regional authorities. The verification of trauma center classification (Levels I to III) is carried out by the American College of Surgeons Committee on Trauma (ACS COT), assessed against the standards outlined in the *Resources for Optimal Care of the Injured Patient* [20]. This document specifies the criteria for levels of trauma team activation, the expected response time of the anesthesiologist, and the expected time for OR readiness. For example, at a level I and II trauma center, an anesthesia provider is expected to be available within 15 minutes of request and an OR ready within 15 minutes of decision to operate. Meeting these obligations has staffing and resource implications which must be addressed by anesthesiology leadership at an institutional level.

A further challenge is maintaining the availability of these resources outside of regular working hours. A study from one US level I trauma center examined the time of day patients required anesthesia care for emergency surgery [21]. The investigators found that patients with firearm injuries frequently underwent emergency surgery outside regular hours, with a peak between midnight and 4 am. This study represents a single center's experience but shows that traumatic injuries frequently occur outside of regular daytime hours, and these patients often require surgery soon after initial presentation. The onus is on individual institutions to examine their own data in this regard, but any center that cares for injured patients will have to ensure sufficient anesthesia staffing to meet their anticipated needs and trauma designation specifications. This will also require the availability of a suitable OR and trained OR staff to run it. Other critical services such as blood banking and laboratory staff will need to have the capabilities and staffing to rapidly mobilize blood products for transfusion and analyze blood samples. The need for operative anesthesia care is not confined to large level I trauma centers. In total 44% of patients with trauma managed in a level III–V designated trauma center required operative intervention [22]. Anesthesiologists are important stakeholders in OR readiness decision making. They serve on the institutional trauma council, where discussions focus on trauma outcomes, quality improvement initiatives, clinical research priorities, and strategies to optimize the delivery of trauma care.

In recent years, trauma anesthesiologists have been utilizing FAST (Focused Assessment with Sonography in Trauma). FAST is a Point of Care Ultrasound (POCUS) protocol used to detect hemoperitoneum and hemopericardium in trauma patients, and it has been expanded into Extended FAST (eFAST)—an evolution of the traditional FAST examination which incorporates thoracic window assessment to identify haemothorax and pneumothorax. Ultrasound is also used for intravascular central access as well as procedural guidance for peripheral nerve blocks. Trauma anesthesiologists actively contribute to education and clinical research in POCUS in trauma setting.

Not all trauma patients will be treated in the OR. Depending on injury patterns and hemodynamic conditions, some patients will require initial management in the Interventional Radiology (IR) suite. For example, patients with pelvic fractures and signs of hypovolemic shock may require NORA meaning the anesthesiologist must care for these patients in a potentially less familiar setting. The ASA issued practice standards for the provision of NORA, but there is no published guidance related specifically to trauma care [23]. IR staff may not have the same breadth of experience in caring for hemodynamically unstable injured patients and may need direction from the anesthesiology team. These locations tend to be more resource-limited with typically less space and anesthesia equipment compared to the OR. These sites are often remote from the main OR complex, which may result in challenges when additional personnel are needed. Access to the patient during the procedure will be limited, and the anesthesiology teams will have to carefully plan for this, as well as their own radiation safety.

The anesthesiology department should be involved in drafting and implementing guidance in managing trauma patients in the IR suite, ensuring the same level of care as would be provided in the OR. All anesthesiologists providing trauma care at a NORA location should be aware of the logistic considerations of this site. This includes such items as understanding how blood will be delivered, where the rapid infusion device is located, how the patient will be actively warmed in this setting, where all equipment will be positioned in relation to the IR table, and how the anesthesiology team will be able to access the patient during the procedure. This patient group has high needs, which must be anticipated in advance. The anesthesiology team contributes to the formulation of institutional guidelines governing the clinical management and safe transfer of these patients between clinical sites.

Anesthesiologists work closely with other specialties on the development of patient-centered protocols and policies for trauma patients. For example, the anesthesiology department may work with surgical teams and nutritionists to develop trauma-specific policies related to fasting times to minimize the interruption of nutrition on those requiring multiple operative interventions, especially for pediatric patients and those with major burns. Another example may be an agreement with neurosurgical teams on how external ventricular drains should be managed during patient transfer and in the OR.

ACS verification mandates the utilization of a trauma Performance Improvement and Patient Safety (PIPS) committee which runs in addition to any local Trauma Council [20]. This process allows the hospital to identify opportunities for improvement in trauma care. Trauma team stakeholders can benchmark performance and engage in cycles of audit and quality improvement. An anesthesiology representative is a critical member of such a committee.

18.2.2 The Role of the Trauma Anesthesiologist in Hemostatic Resuscitation

One of the key clinical roles of the trauma anesthesiologist is to guide the hemostatic resuscitation of severely injured patients. Anesthesiologists are responsible for the administration of blood products in balanced ratios, at least in the initial phases, and tailoring the transfusion strategy to meet specific deficits as individual patient information becomes available. Anesthesiologists will also decide on which hemostatic adjuncts are indicated. Away from this direct clinical role, anesthesiologists are an important voice in informing policies and procedures governing patient blood management.

On a local level, a member of the anesthesiology department sits on the local Transfusion Committee (TC). Membership of this committee also consists of physician representatives from transfusion medicine, surgery, emergency medicine and blood banking, and nursing staff. Here hospital-specific governance and policy issues are discussed. Applicable to trauma patients, anesthesiologists have a role in shaping the local Massive Transfusion Protocol (MTP), namely, what products and in what ratios will be delivered to the bedside and in what timeframe. Partnership with the blood bank and transfusion medicine is an opportunity to allow for a process of quality improvement such as identifying instances of noncompliance with crossmatching policies, blood wastage, and taking measures to improve performance on these fronts.

These TCs have also served as a platform for advancing resuscitation strategies in trauma care. For example, the TC at Harborview Medical Center, Seattle, WA, initiated a whole blood (WB) program in 2019 to make WB available for trauma resuscitation in the prehospital and hospital setting [24]. This partnership also opens the door for the institution to take part in multicenter randomized controlled trials. For example, retrospective data from military settings has suggested that WB may be a superior product for hemostatic resuscitation versus component therapy. The Trauma Resuscitation with Low Titre O WB or Products (TROOP) trial seeks to determine prospectively if this applies to civilian trauma [25]. Anesthesiologist representation on the TC allows for smooth communication with the anesthesia department who will be caring for patients enrolled in these trials. The results of such trials are an important component of improving resuscitation and patient outcomes.

During trauma resuscitation, anesthesiologists rely on rapid coagulation assessment to inform transfusion decisions and transition from empiric transfusion ratios to specific use of blood components to correct coagulation deficits. Local institutions decide on which rapid turnaround coagulation testing their laboratory is equipped to supply: conventional coagulation testing or viscoelastic testing. The anesthesiologist is responsible for interpreting the test results; in the case of viscoelastic testing, this will often require an educational component for those less familiar with this method. Through TC, anesthesiologists have an opportunity to partner with laboratory medicine on deciding what testing is most appropriate for their institution. Regardless of the method chosen, the laboratory team will have to prioritize the processing of samples from trauma patients undergoing active resuscitation.

On a national level, the ASA Committee on Patient Blood Management aims to advise on best practice for blood conservation strategies and the appropriate use of blood products. It also offers guidance on caring for special patient populations and issues blood status updates during times of resource constraint, such as during the COVID-19 pandemic [26]. Anesthesiologists with additional expertise and knowledge in patient blood management seek membership on this committee.

18.3 Emergency Preparedness

Disaster can strike at any time, and hospitals must be ready to adapt and respond at a moment's notice. Emergency preparedness encompasses activities designed to anticipate and effectively manage crisis situations, including mass casualty incidents (MCIs), natural disasters (e.g., earthquakes, hurricanes), terrorist attacks, chemical/biological warfare, pandemics (e.g., COVID-19), and hospital system failures (e.g., electrical grid collapse, cyberattacks) [27]. Emergency preparedness is a multidisciplinary effort aimed at ensuring rapid and effective responses to natural disasters, mass casualty events, pandemics, and other large-scale crises.

Anesthesiologists occupy a uniquely critical role due to their versatile skill set, acute clinical judgment, and experience managing critical care/crisis scenarios. Their contributions span the entire emergency preparedness cycle: planning, response, mitigation, and recovery. Anesthesiologists' knowledge and training provide them with the unique ability to respond during a disaster through their intrinsic roles in trauma and critical care, perioperative medicine, and pain management. In any public health emergency scenario, anesthesiologists are very likely to be directly involved in triaging, operative, and/or critical care of the victims. And while not every anesthesiologist will be directly involved in patient care during the mass disaster, most anesthesiologists will care for trauma patients at some point throughout the patient's acute resuscitation or chronic follow-up, be it in the ED, OR, ICU, or pain clinic, regardless if they work in a trauma center or not.

The ASA has remained engaged in improving public health and safety, including emergency preparedness. The best example of this is through the formation of the Committee on Trauma and Emergency Preparedness (COTEP), which was originally formed as a response to the 9/11 terrorist attacks more than 20 years ago [28]. Their mission statement reads: "ASA Committee on Trauma and Emergency Preparedness (COTEP) exists to improve the care of patients with traumatic injury and to educate anesthesiologists in disaster management" [29]. Through COTEP and other related groups within ASA, the greater community of anesthesiologists has been able to combine their expertise and knowledge regarding trauma, acute care, and emergency/disaster preparedness to the benefit of the medical community and the general public.

COTEP has led several large-scale initiatives since inception, including creation and distribution of the OR Mass Casualty checklist and a broader Emergency Preparedness.

Manual for Anesthesia Department Organizations and Management [30, 31]. Manuals and checklists such as these help guide OR staff with step-by-step instructions in situations of mass casualty and disaster events and is adaptable to individual facility's particular needs and capabilities. COTEP also leads significant efforts in the realm of public health and was integral during the COVID-19 pandemic, helping to provide resources and support for front-line clinicians, which included most anesthesiologists. COTEP has recently been the driving force behind the ReviveME campaign, is an advocacy initiative launched by the ASA to address the opioid epidemic. ReviveME campaign aims to provide information and tools to the public on how to recognize, react and revive a person experiencing an opioid emergency.

COTEP serves as a waypoint for information & resources regarding crisis management and disaster preparedness, for anesthesiologists at both an individual and a departmental level, including such topics as Active Shooter guides, OR power failure checklists and hurricane preparedness tools. COTEP additionally provides resources for personal and family preparedness, as well as hospital-level disaster management, in conjunction with such groups as Emergency Manuals

Implementation Collaborative (EMIC), Agency for Healthcare Research and Quality (AHRQ) and Centers for Disease Control (CDC).

COTEP (and by extension the ASA) wants to ensure that all anesthesiologists, their patients and their healthcare institutions, have access to accurate and timely information, practice guidelines and useful links for managing casualties from trauma, natural disasters, fires, industrial injuries, and weapons of mass destruction. Thus, COTEP has made collaborations with not only other groups charged with disaster and emergency preparedness, but also the other committees within ASA, such as the Committee on Patient Blood Management, and Committee on Critical Care Medicine, as well as other anesthesiology societies, such as TAS to ensure dissemination of information and resources to all anesthesiologists. In addition to anesthesia-specific organizations, COTEP also ensures active liaison with other specialty societies, both nationally and internationally, to establish unified consensus and work towards cooperative multi-disciplinary efforts in the immense task of system-wide preparation for mass casualty and disaster events. These groups include ACS COT, the World Association for Disaster and Emergency Medicine (WADEM), Committee on Accreditation of Educational Programs for the Emergency Medical Services Professions (CoAEMSP), the Pre-Hospital Blood Transfusion Coalition (PHBTIC), the Brain Trauma Foundation and Committee on Tactical Combat Casualty Care, amongst others. By maintaining these relationships, COTEP and ASA ensure anesthesiologists' concerns are heard and there is integration of anesthesiologists' perspective into trauma and disaster preparedness programs for multidisciplinary crisis protocols. The inclusion of the anesthesiologist in developing disaster management plans for hospitals is increasingly recognized as a vital component of perioperative readiness [32].

An additional critical component of emergency preparedness is education and research. To this end, COTEP and ASA have made substantial efforts in increasing familiarity with disaster management within not only the anesthesiology community but in collaboration with organizations of different disciplines. Numerous educational initiatives within anesthesiology include the development of a trauma curriculum for junior and senior anesthesiology residents, as well as collaboration with the American Board of Anesthesiology (ABA) to expand the number of topics in the ABA content outline and maintenance of certification in anesthesiology (MOCA) curriculum [33]. Additionally, there has been increasing numbers of scientific sessions in trauma and emergency preparedness at annual meetings as well as workshops in advanced trauma skills, emergency preparedness, and mass casualty events. In collaboration with various other organizations, anesthesiologists can help build multi-disciplinary best practice guidelines regarding disaster management, including prehospital, ED and OR team members. Anesthesiologists are also helping advance the science behind disaster management and emergency preparedness with active engagement in research in the field. By building educational standards and providing supporting research, anesthesiologists help foment their crucial role in maintaining emergency preparedness standards.

18.4 Conclusion

Anesthesiologists are more than perioperative physicians—they are crisis leaders, airway specialists, and critical care experts. Their ability to manage complex airway scenarios, lead resuscitative efforts, and provide life-sustaining care in trauma and intensive care settings underscores their indispensable role. Anesthesiologists play a central role in education, guiding best practices and provide patient-centered care. The role of the anesthesiologist remains indispensable—not just in the OR but also in the NORA setting. Their unique skill set, and adaptability make them vital contributors to any emergency preparedness and response system.

References

1. Cook TM, Woodall N, Frerk C, Fourth National Audit Project. Major complications of airway management in the UK: results of the fourth National Audit Project of the Royal College of Anaesthetists and the difficult airway society. Part 1: anaesthesia. Br J Anaesth. 2011;106(5):617–31. https://doi.org/10.1093/bja/aer058. Epub 2011 Mar 29. PMID: 21447488
2. Joffe AM, Aziz MF, Posner KL, Duggan LV, Mincer SL, Domino KB. Management of difficult tracheal intubation: a closed claims analysis. Anesthesiology. 2019;131(4):818–29. https://doi.org/10.1097/ALN.0000000000002815. PMID: 31584884; PMCID: PMC6779339
3. Fonseca D, Inês Graça M, Salgueirinho C, Pereira H. Physiologically difficult airway: how to approach the difficulty beyond anatomy. Trends Anaesth Crit Care. 2023;48:101212. ISSN 2210-8440. https://doi.org/10.1016/j.tacc.2023.101212.
4. Mosier JM, Joshi R, Hypes C, Pacheco G, Valenzuela T, Sakles JC. The physiologically difficult airway. West. J Emerg Med. 2015;16(7):1109–17. https://doi.org/10.5811/westjem.2015.8.27467. Epub 2015 Dec 8. PMID: 26759664; PMCID: PMC4703154
5. Frerk C, Mitchell VS, McNarry AF, Mendonca C, Bhagrath R, Patel A, O'Sullivan EP, Woodall NM, Ahmad I, Difficult Airway Society intubation guidelines working group. Difficult Airway Society 2015 guidelines for management of unanticipated difficult intubation in adults. Br J Anaesth. 2015;115(6):827–48. https://doi.org/10.1093/bja/aev371. Epub 2015 Nov 10. PMID: 26556848; PMCID: PMC4650961
6. Apfelbaum JL, Hagberg CA, Connis RT, Abdelmalak BB, Agarkar M, Dutton RP, Fiadjoe JE, Greif R, Klock PA, Mercier D, Myatra SN, O'Sullivan EP, Rosenblatt WH, Sorbello M, Tung A. 2022 American Society of anesthesiologists practice guidelines for management of the difficult airway. Anesthesiology. 2022;136(1):31–81. https://doi.org/10.1097/ALN.0000000000004002.
7. Mark LJ, Herzer KR, Cover R, Pandian V, Bhatti NI, Berkow LC, Haut ER, Hillel AT, Miller CR, Feller-Kopman DJ, Schiavi AJ, Xie YJ, Lim C, Holzmueller C, Ahmad M, Thomas P, Flint PW, Mirski MA. Difficult airway response team: a novel quality improvement program for managing hospital-wide airway emergencies. Anesth Analg. 2015;121(1):127–39. https://doi.org/10.1213/ANE.0000000000000691. PMID: 26086513; PMCID: PMC4473796
8. Weinger MB, Banerjee A, Burden AR, McIvor WR, Boulet J, Cooper JB, Steadman R, Shotwell MS, Slagle JM, DeMaria S Jr, Torsher L, Sinz E, Levine AI, Rask J, Davis F, Park C, Gaba DM. Simulation-based assessment of the management of critical events by board-certified anesthesiologists. Anesthesiology. 2017;127(3):475–89. https://doi.org/10.1097/ALN.0000000000001739. PMID: 28671903
9. Mort TC. The incidence and risk factors for cardiac arrest during emergency tracheal intubation: a justification for incorporating the ASA guidelines in the remote location. J Clin Anesth. 2004;16(7):508–16. https://doi.org/10.1016/j.jclinane.2004.01.007. PMID: 15590254

10. Jaber S, Amraoui J, Lefrant JY, Arich C, Cohendy R, Landreau L, Calvet Y, Capdevila X, Mahamat A, Eledjam JJ. Clinical practice and risk factors for immediate complications of endotracheal intubation in the intensive care unit: a prospective, multiple-center study. Crit Care Med. 2006;34(9):2355–61. https://doi.org/10.1097/01.CCM.0000233879.58720.87. PMID: 16850003
11. Hansel J, Rogers AM, Lewis SR, Cook TM, Smith AF. Videolaryngoscopy versus direct laryngoscopy for adults undergoing tracheal intubation: a Cochrane systematic review and meta-analysis update. Br J Anaesth. 2022;129(4):612–23. https://doi.org/10.1016/j.bja.2022.05.027. Epub 2022 Jul 9. PMID: 35820934; PMCID: PMC9575044
12. Saul SA, Ward PA, McNarry AF. Airway management: the current role of Videolaryngoscopy. J Pers Med. 2023;13(9):1327. https://doi.org/10.3390/jpm13091327. PMID: 37763095; PMCID: PMC10532647
13. Chapter 5, Centers for Medicare & Medicaid Services Medicaid National Correct Coding Initiative Policy Manual [Internet]. Place unknown: American Medical Association; 2023. [Revised Jan 2024, cited March 20, 2025]. Available from: https://www.cms.gov/files/document/medicaid-ncci-policy-manual-2024-chapter-5.pdf
14. Current Procedural Terminology Code [Internet]. Place unknown: MD Clarity; Unknown publication date [Cited March 20, 2025]. Available from: https://www.mdclarity.com/cpt-code/31500?10534572_page=64#what-is
15. Chapter 12, sections 50I and 140.3.3, Medicare claims processing manual [internet]. Place unknown: Centers for Medicare & Medicaid Services; December 19, 2024. [Cited 20 March 2025]. Available from: https://www.cms.gov/Regulations-and-Guidance/Guidance/Manuals/downloads/clm104C12.pdf
16. Anesthesia Payment Basics Series Codes and Modifiers [Internet]. Place unknown: American Society of Anesthesiologist. June 2019 [Updated June 12, 2024, cited March 24, 2025]. Available from: https://www.asahq.org/quality-and-practice-management/managing-your-practice/timely-topics-in-payment-and-practice-management/anesthesia-payment-basics-series-codes-and-modifiers
17. Medical Learning Network. Evaluation and Management Services Guide. MLN006764 [Internet]. Place unknown: Centers for Medicare & Medicaid Services; September 2024 [Cited 20 March 2025]. Available from: https://www.cms.gov/outreach-and-education/medicare-learning-network-mln/mlnproducts/downloads/eval-mgmt-serv-guide-icn006764.pdf
18. Chiaghana C, Giordano C, Cobb D, Vasilopoulos T, Tighe PJ, Sappenfield JW. Emergency department airway management responsibilities in the United States. Anesth Analg. 2019;128(2):296–301. https://doi.org/10.1213/ANE.0000000000003851.
19. Martin LD, Mhyre JM, Shanks AM, Tremper KK, Kheterpal S. 3,423 emergency tracheal intubations at a university hospital: airway outcomes and complications. Anesthesiology. 2011;114(1):42–8. https://doi.org/10.1097/ALN.0b013e318201c415. PMID: 21150574
20. American College of Surgeons. Resources for optimal care of the injured patient 2022 standards [Internet]. Chicago (US): American College of Surgeons; 2022. [Updated Dec 2023, cited Apr 18, 2025]. Available from: https://www.facs.org/quality-programs/trauma/quality/verification-review-and-consultation-program/standards/
21. Walters AM, Aichholz P, Muldowney M, Van Cleve W, Hess JR, Stansbury LG, Vavilala MS. Emergency anesthesiology encounters, care practices, and outcomes for patients with firearm injuries: a 9-year single-center US level 1 trauma experience. Anesth Analg. 2025;140(3):554–63. https://doi.org/10.1213/ANE.0000000000007152. Epub 2024 Aug 23. PMID: 39178169
22. Sunshine JE, Humbert AT, Booth B, Bowman SM, Bulger EM, Sharar SR. Frequency of operative anesthesia care after traumatic injury. Anesth Analg. 2019;129(1):141–6. https://doi.org/10.1213/ANE.0000000000003651. PMID: 30004933
23. American Society of Anesthesiologists. Statement on nonoperating room anesthesia services [Internet]. [Place unknown]: American Society of Anesthesiologists; 1994. [Updated 2023, cited Apr 18, 2025]. Available from: https://www.asahq.org/standards-and-practice-parameters/statement-on-nonoperating-room-anesthesia-services

24. Addams J, Arbabi S, Bulger EM, Stansbury LG, Tuott EE, Hess JR. How we built a hospital-based community whole blood program. Transfusion. 2022;62(9):1699–705. https://doi.org/10.1111/trf.17018. Epub 2022 Jul 11. PMID: 35815552
25. Jansen JO, University of Alabama at Birmingham. Trauma Resuscitation with Low-Titer Group O Whole Blood or Products (TROOP) [Internet]. Bethesda (US): National Library of Medicine ClinicalTrials.gov; [Updated Mar 4, 2025, cited Apr 18,2025]. Clinical trial number NCT05638581. Available from:. https://clinicaltrials.gov/study/NCT05638581
26. American Society of Anesthesiologists. National Blood Shortage – Optimization and Minimization Techniques for Patient Blood Management (PBM) [Internet]. [Place unknown]: American Society of Anesthesiologists Committee on Patient Blood Management; [Updated Apr 1,2025, cited Apr 18, 2025]. Available from: https://www.asahq.org/standards-and-practice-parameters/resources-from-asa-committees#bm
27. Chandler D, et al. Anesthesiologists' role in disaster management. In: The role of anesthesiology in global health: a comprehensive guide; 2015. p. 305–21.
28. Raiten J, Fleisher LA. Anesthesiologists in times of disaster: a rich history, a busy future. Anesthesiol Clin. 2021;39(2):xi–xii. https://doi.org/10.1016/j.anclin.2021.03.005. Epub 2021 Apr 28. PMID: 34024439; PMCID: PMC9760558
29. Steurer MP, Kaslow O, Varon AJ. Overview of COTEP/trauma/emergency preparedness. ASA Monit. 2022;86(3):27. https://doi.org/10.1097/01.ASM.0000823080.77926.d8.
30. McIssac, J; Section on Emergency Preparedness for Anesthesiologists, Manual for Anesthesia Department Organization and Management [Internet]. [Place unknown]: American Society of Anesthesiologists; Unknown [Updated September 16, 2022, cited Apr 18, 2025]. Available from: https://www.asahq.org/quality-and-practice-management/qmda-regulatory-toolkit/guide-to-anesthesia-department-administration
31. Mcisaac J. Operating room management during mass casualties: a new checklist. Prehosp Disaster Med. 2017;32(S1):S104. https://doi.org/10.1017/S1049023X17002667.
32. Kelley KM, Toscano N, Gestring ML, Capella J, Newton C, Bukur M, Shatz DV, Winfield RD, Fox A, Fallat ME, Kuhls DA, Glinik G, Doucet J, Gates J, Remick KN. Disaster planning for a surgical surge: when mass trauma threatens to overwhelm your operating rooms. Trauma Surg Acute Care Open. 2023;8(1):e001224. https://doi.org/10.1136/tsaco-2023-001224. PMID: 38020853; PMCID: PMC10649914
33. Dutton RP, Varon AJ. Five decades of trauma anesthesiology. Anesth Analg. 2023;136(5):949–56. https://doi.org/10.1213/ANE.0000000000006099. Epub 2023 Apr 14

19 Sedation Governance: The Anesthesiologist's Role in Oversight and Credentialing

Charlota Jurcik, Nikhil Kaushal, George Tewfik, and Andres Zuniga

19.1 Introduction

Sedation has become an integral component of modern medical practice, extending well beyond the traditional confines of the operating room. In endoscopy suites, interventional radiology, cardiology labs, emergency departments, dental offices, and ambulatory surgery centers, procedural sedation enables clinicians to perform diagnostic and therapeutic interventions safely and effectively. While anesthesiologists may not personally administer sedation in every setting, their oversight is essential to ensuring that these services are delivered within a framework of safety, quality, and regulatory compliance. This role—best described as *sedation supervision*—represents one of the key nonclinical contributions of anesthesiologists to the broader healthcare system.

Supervision of sedation encompasses more than immediate bedside care. It includes *developing and enforcing institutional policies*, establishing *credentialing and privileging standards* for non-anesthesiologist providers, ensuring *appropriate training and competency assessment*, and leading *quality assurance and adverse event review* processes. From a regulatory standpoint, accrediting bodies such as the *Joint Commission* and the *Centers for Medicare & Medicaid Services (CMS)* hold hospitals accountable for safe sedation practices, and these requirements are most effectively met through anesthesiologist leadership [1].

C. Jurcik (✉)
University of Arizona, Banner – University Medical Center, Tucson, AZ, USA
e-mail: cj397@njms.rutgers.edu

N. Kaushal
Rutgers New Jersey Medical School, Newark, NJ, USA

G. Tewfik
Department of Anesthesiology, Rutgers New Jersey Medical School, Newark, NJ, USA

A. Zuniga
Saint Peter's University, Jersey City, NJ, USA

G. Tewfik (ed.), *The Anesthesiologist as Perioperative Leader*,
https://doi.org/10.1007/978-3-032-18058-2_19

The economic and strategic importance of this oversight is significant. Adverse events related to sedation—airway compromise, hypoxemia, aspiration, hemodynamic collapse—can rapidly escalate into catastrophic outcomes, with downstream costs in terms of morbidity, liability, and resource utilization [2]. By contrast, anesthesiologist-driven sedation programs standardize safety practices, minimize variability, and improve throughput, thereby protecting patients while creating measurable value for institutions.

This chapter explores the multiple dimensions of sedation supervision: the *regulatory frameworks* that define the anesthesiologist's role, the *safety considerations* unique to sedation, the *models of oversight* that exist across healthcare systems, and the *economic value* that derives from well-structured sedation services. In doing so, it highlights how anesthesiologists, as essential perioperative physicians, extend their influence far beyond the operating room, shaping the safety and efficiency of patient care across the healthcare continuum.

In the sections that follow, we will first review the *regulatory and accreditation standards* that shape institutional policies on sedation, highlighting the requirements of CMS, the Joint Commission, and other accrediting bodies. Next, we will examine *professional guidelines*, including those from the ASA and multispecialty collaborations, which delineate safe practices and clarify the scope of non-anesthesiologist sedation. We will then explore the *safety concerns unique to sedation*, ranging from airway compromise to the medicolegal implications of inadequate monitoring. Building on this, we will outline the various *models of sedation oversight* employed across healthcare settings, focusing on how anesthesiologists contribute to credentialing, competency assessment, and ongoing quality assurance. Finally, we will consider the *economic value* that effective sedation supervision generates—through prevention of adverse events, improved throughput, and alignment with value-based care initiatives—before looking ahead to *future directions* such as AI-enabled monitoring and tele-sedation. Together, these elements illustrate how anesthesiologists' leadership in sedation supervision exemplifies the broader theme of this book: advancing patient safety while delivering measurable value to healthcare systems.

19.2 Regulatory and Accreditation Framework

The safe administration of procedural sedation is not only a clinical priority but also a regulatory requirement. Accrediting and oversight bodies hold healthcare institutions accountable for sedation practices, and anesthesiologists play a central role in ensuring compliance.

19.2.1 Centers for Medicare and Medicaid Services (CMS)

CMS Conditions of Participation mandate that hospitals establish policies governing anesthesia services, including *sedation and analgesia* [1]. These regulations require that institutions clearly delineate responsibilities for providers who administer moderate or deep sedation, specify credentialing requirements, and define monitoring standards. Importantly, CMS emphasizes that providers of sedation must be trained to rescue patients from one level deeper than the intended level of sedation. Anesthesiologists, by virtue of their training, are uniquely qualified to develop and oversee these institutional policies, ensuring that credentialing and competency standards align with federal requirements.

19.2.2 The Joint Commission (TJC)

The Joint Commission sets detailed standards for sedation and anesthesia care that apply to accredited hospitals and ambulatory surgery centers [3]. Key requirements include:

- Written policies for patient assessment, informed consent, monitoring, and discharge after sedation.
- Continuous monitoring of oxygenation, ventilation, circulation, and temperature, with escalation protocols if adverse events occur.
- Documentation of sedation depth, medications administered, and recovery scores.
- Institutional privileging processes for non-anesthesiologists who administer moderate sedation.

TJC surveys routinely include a review of sedation records and credentialing files. Hospitals that lack robust sedation oversight programs face citations that may jeopardize accreditation. Anesthesiologists often serve as chairs or members of *sedation committees*, ensuring compliance and reducing institutional risk.

19.2.3 Other Accrediting Bodies

Other organizations, including the *Accreditation Association for Ambulatory Health Care (AAAHC)* and *DNV GL Healthcare*, impose similar requirements for sedation services in ambulatory and office-based settings. Each emphasizes the need for ongoing monitoring, availability of resuscitation equipment, and regular review of adverse events. In these environments, anesthesiologists provide expertise in protocol development and emergency preparedness.

19.2.4 Institutional Policies and Bylaws

Beyond national regulations, hospitals develop bylaws that govern who may provide sedation and under what circumstances. These often reflect ASA guidelines and specify competency requirements for credentialed providers. Anesthesiologists frequently take the lead in drafting these policies, advising medical staff committees, and reviewing adverse events through quality assurance processes. By shaping institutional policies, anesthesiologists safeguard both patients and the organization.

19.2.5 Summary

Regulatory and accreditation requirements establish a clear expectation that sedation must be performed within a framework of safety and accountability. Anesthesiologists, through their leadership in policy development, credentialing, and quality oversight, ensure that institutions meet these standards. This supervisory role reinforces their position as essential perioperative physicians and underscores the value they add beyond direct patient care.

19.3 ASA and Professional Guidelines

In addition to federal regulations and accreditation requirements, professional society guidelines provide the clinical framework for safe and effective sedation. Among these, the American Society of Anesthesiologists (ASA) has been the most prominent authority, publishing statements, and practice guidelines that define the scope of sedation practice and the supervisory role of anesthesiologists.

19.3.1 ASA Practice Guidelines for Moderate Procedural Sedation and Analgesia (2018)

The most comprehensive multispecialty document on sedation is the 2018 *Practice Guidelines for Moderate Procedural Sedation and Analgesia*, jointly developed by the ASA, American Gastroenterological Association (AGA), American College of Radiology (ACR), American Society for Gastrointestinal Endoscopy (ASGE), Society of Cardiovascular Anesthesiologists (SCA), Society of Interventional Radiology (SIR), and Society for Academic Emergency Medicine (SAEM) [4]. These guidelines emphasize several critical points:

- *Continuum of sedation*: Sedation exists on a continuum from minimal sedation to general anesthesia, and unintended progression to deeper levels is common. Providers must be prepared to rescue patients who enter deeper sedation than intended.
- *Patient monitoring*: Continuous assessment of oxygenation, ventilation, circulation, and temperature is required, with capnography strongly recommended for moderate and deep sedation to detect hypoventilation early.
- *Provider training and competency*: Clinicians who are not anesthesia professionals may administer moderate sedation only if they have demonstrated competence in patient assessment, pharmacology of sedatives and analgesics, monitoring, and rescue techniques.
- *Institutional policies*: Hospitals and ambulatory facilities must have credentialing systems in place, often led or overseen by anesthesiologists, to ensure provider competency and adherence to monitoring standards.

19.3.2 ASA Statements on Sedation

Several ASA position statements further clarify the anesthesiologist's role:

- *Statement on Granting Privileges for Administration of Moderate Sedation to Practitioners Who Are Not Anesthesia Professionals*—affirms that hospitals may credential non-anesthesiologists but must ensure appropriate training, monitoring, and oversight [5].
- *Statement on Safe Use of Propofol*—highlights the risks of propofol when administered by non-anesthesia professionals, underscoring that only individuals trained in general anesthesia should administer drugs with narrow safety margins [6].
- *Statement on Monitored Anesthesia Care (MAC)*—differentiates MAC, an anesthesia service that requires readiness to manage all levels of sedation and anesthesia, from moderate sedation provided by non-anesthesiologists [7].

19.3.3 Multispecialty and International Guidelines

Other professional societies also publish sedation guidelines—such as the ASGE for endoscopy, the ACR for imaging, and the ACEP for emergency medicine [8]. While these documents provide specialty-specific recommendations, most endorse the principles of the ASA guidelines, particularly regarding the continuum of sedation and the need for rescue capability. International guidelines, such as those from the Royal College of Anaesthetists (UK) and the European Society of Anaesthesiology, echo similar themes and reinforce anesthesiologists' leadership role in oversight.

19.3.4 Summary

Taken together, ASA and multispecialty guidelines reinforce the principle that safe sedation requires not only technical skill in drug administration but also systems of supervision, credentialing, and rescue preparedness. Anesthesiologists, with their expertise in airway management and perioperative medicine, are best positioned to lead these systems.

19.4 Safety Concerns in Sedation

Sedation is generally safe when provided within structured systems of oversight; however, it carries inherent risks that can escalate quickly if unrecognized or mismanaged [9, 10]. Unlike in the operating room, where anesthesiologists have immediate access to advanced airway equipment and a controlled environment, sedation in procedural suites, emergency departments, and ambulatory settings often occurs in less-resourced environments [11]. This makes vigilance and appropriate supervision even more critical.

19.4.1 Airway Compromise

Airway obstruction, hypoventilation, and hypoxemia remain the most common and serious sedation-related complications [2]. Even with moderate sedation, patients may slip into deeper levels of sedation with the loss of airway reflexes. Capnography has been shown to improve early detection of hypoventilation, yet its use is inconsistent outside anesthesia-led environments. Anesthesiologists' training in airway rescue uniquely positions them to guide policy and training for all sedation providers.

19.4.2 Respiratory and Cardiovascular Events

Adverse events such as laryngospasm, bronchospasm, aspiration, and hypotension are well documented in sedation claims analyses. These complications are particularly concerning in high-risk populations such as pediatrics, patients with obstructive sleep apnea, the elderly, and those with ASA class III–IV status. Sedation-related cardiac arrest, while rare, is most often associated with inadequate monitoring and delayed recognition of airway compromise.

19.4.3 Closed Claims and Medicolegal Insights

The ASA Closed Claims Project highlights that a significant proportion of anesthesia malpractice cases involve sedation outside the operating room, particularly in GI endoscopy and interventional radiology [2]. The recurring themes include inadequate monitoring, lack of rescue capability, and use of propofol by non-anesthesiologists. These findings underscore the medicolegal vulnerability of institutions without structured sedation oversight and reinforce the economic and safety value of anesthesiologist supervision.

19.4.4 Population-Specific Risks

- *Pediatrics*: Increased risk of hypoxemia and airway obstruction, particularly with propofol or opioids. Data from the Pediatric Sedation Research Consortium show an adverse event rate of ~1 per 89 sedations, with rare but serious events requiring airway intervention [10].
- *Elderly*: Increased sensitivity to sedatives, greater risk of delirium, hypoxemia, and hemodynamic instability.
- *Patients with OSA*: Particularly vulnerable to airway collapse and postoperative hypoxemia.

- *High BMI patients*: More likely to require advanced airway maneuvers, prolonged recovery, and unplanned admission.

19.4.5 Summary

Sedation is not risk-free, and the line between moderate sedation and general anesthesia can blur quickly [12]. The presence of anesthesiologists in supervisory roles—through credentialing, protocol development, and real-time consultation—creates an essential safety net that protects patients, reduces institutional liability, and reinforces the anesthesiologist's role as the perioperative safety leader.

19.5 Models of Sedation Oversight

Supervision of sedation services within a healthcare facility can take many forms, reflecting local resources, case mix, and institutional culture. Regardless of the model employed, anesthesiologists play a pivotal role in ensuring that oversight aligns with regulatory requirements and maintains patient safety.

19.5.1 Anesthesiologist-Administered Sedation

In this model, an anesthesiologist or certified registered nurse anesthetist (CRNA) under anesthesiologist supervision provides sedation. This is the gold standard for high-risk patients, procedures requiring deep sedation, or when propofol is used. Advantages include:

- Full ability to manage any level of sedation up to general anesthesia.
- Immediate airway rescue capability.
- Enhanced safety in complex cases (e.g., pediatrics, ASA III–IV patients).

- Limitations include higher cost and limited availability, which may not be feasible for all low-acuity procedures.

19.5.2 Non-anesthesiologist Administered Sedation (with Anesthesiologist Oversight)

Common in gastroenterology, cardiology, and interventional radiology, this model involves trained non-anesthesia physicians (e.g., gastroenterologists) administering moderate sedation, typically with benzodiazepines and opioids. The anesthesiologist's role here is supervisory, often through:

- Developing institutional sedation policies.

- Credentialing and privileging providers.
- Training and periodic competency assessment.
- Reviewing adverse events and quality metrics.

- This model balances efficiency and safety but requires strong governance to prevent scope creep into deep sedation.

19.5.3 Nurse-Administered Procedural Sedation (NAPS)

In some institutions, nurses administer moderate sedation under the direct supervision of proceduralists [13]. While cost-efficient, this model poses risks if training, monitoring, and rescue capabilities are inadequate. Anesthesiologist involvement is critical in:

- Defining scope of practice and medication limitations.
- Establishing monitoring protocols, including capnography.
- Ensuring availability of resuscitation equipment and trained personnel.

- Evidence shows that structured nurse-administered sedation programs can be safe when embedded in strong oversight systems.

19.5.4 Propofol Administration by Non-anesthesiologists [14]

The use of propofol outside anesthesiology remains controversial. Some GI and interventional practices employ “anesthesia teams” or nurse-administered propofol sedation under non-anesthesiologist supervision [6]. However, numerous closed claims analyses link adverse outcomes to inadequate airway management in these settings. The ASA maintains that propofol should be administered only by providers trained in general anesthesia. Oversight by anesthesiologists reduces institutional liability and ensures rapid response to adverse events.

19.5.5 Office-Based Sedation Models

With the rise of office-based surgery, sedation supervision in this setting has become an area of concern. State medical boards and accrediting bodies vary widely in requirements. Anesthesiologists’ roles may include:

- Assisting in accreditation processes (AAAHC, Joint Commission).
- Reviewing office protocols and emergency preparedness.
- Providing consultation on patient selection and rescue capability.

- This model underscores the expanding reach of anesthesiologist leadership beyond hospitals into ambulatory and office practices.

19.5.6 Summary

Each sedation oversight model carries distinct trade-offs between safety, efficiency, and cost. Across all models, anesthesiologists' involvement—whether through direct patient care or supervisory oversight—ensures compliance, reduces adverse events, and builds trust with institutional leadership and patients alike.

19.6 Credentialing and Competency

19.6.1 Purpose and Guiding Principles

Credentialing and competency systems for sedation are the operational backbone of safe sedation programs [15]. Their goals are to (1) ensure individual providers possess the knowledge and technical skills to deliver the intended level of sedation and to rescue patients who progress to deeper levels, (2) delineate scope of practice and privileges consistently across sites and specialties, and (3) create measurable, auditable standards for initial privileging, ongoing maintenance, and remediation. These systems protect patients and institutions, and they formalize the anesthesiologist's supervisory role in sedation programs.

19.6.2 Core Components of a Sedation Credentialing Program

A comprehensive program typically includes the following administrative and clinical components:

1. *Delineation of privileges (scope of practice)*
   - Explicit privilege categories (examples):
     - *Moderate sedation (benzodiazepine/opioid) for adults.*
     - *Moderate sedation for pediatrics.*
     - *Deep sedation with propofol* (often requires anesthesia training or additional privileges).
     - *Sedation for specific locations* (ED, endoscopy, IR, dental/office-based).
   - Each privilege should specify permitted agents, patient selection limits (age, ASA class), and required supervision level.
2. *Initial privileging pathway*
   - *Application and documentation*: current CV, medical license, DEA, board certification/eligibility, BLS/ACLS/PALS certifications, letters of training/verification.
   - *Training verification*: documentation of relevant training (residency, fellowship, focused course). For non-anesthesiologists, evidence of institutional training courses and supervised sedation experience.

- *Proctoring/supervised cases*: institution-defined number of directly observed, proctored cases (commonly used ranges: 3–10 depending on institution and complexity). Proctor assessment should include direct observation of monitoring, airway management readiness, documentation, and communication with the team.
- *Knowledge assessment*: short written test or simulation-based assessment covering pharmacology, airway rescue, monitoring interpretation (including capnography), and local policies.

3. *Core competency domains (what to assess)*

- *Medical knowledge*: pharmacology of sedatives/analgesics, pharmacokinetic considerations, interactions, patient selection, and risk stratification.
- *Technical skills*: airway maneuvers (chin lift/jaw thrust), bag-mask ventilation, supraglottic airway placement, endotracheal intubation (if privileged), use of airway adjuncts, and management of ventilatory failure.
- *Monitoring skills*: continuous interpretation of pulse oximetry, noninvasive blood pressure, ECG, and capnography; recognition of early hypoventilation and hypoxemia.
- *Rescue skills*: ACLS/PALS algorithms, use of reversal agents (naloxone, flumazenil), management of aspiration, anaphylaxis, hemodynamic collapse.
- *Non-technical skills*: team communication, escalation and call-for-help behavior, documentation, informed consent, and situational awareness.

4. *Maintenance of competency (ongoing requirements)*

- *Periodic re-credentialing*—typically every 1–2 years depending on institutional policy. This should include: maintenance of certifications (BLS/ACLS/PALS), updated CME in sedation/airway courses, review of case logs, and participation in QA activities.
- *Minimum case volumes*—many institutions set a target or minimum number of sedations per year to maintain privileges (numbers vary; consider institution-specific thresholds or demonstrated equivalence via simulation if volumes are low).
- *Continuing education*—mandatory CME hours in sedation-related topics and attendance at departmental simulation refreshers or airway workshops.
- *Quality metrics*—providers must meet or not exceed departmental thresholds for predefined safety KPIs (see section on Metrics below).

5. *Assessment methods and tools*

- *Direct observation* using standardized checklists during proctoring and periodic peer observation.
- *Simulation-based assessment* for airway rescue and crisis management—can be used for both initial privileging and remediation. Simulation is particularly valuable for low-volume providers or for assessing rare but critical events (e.g., refractory airway obstruction).

- *Objective structured clinical examination (OSCE)* or case-based oral exams for knowledge and decision-making.
- *Chart review and case audits* focusing on documentation completeness, monitoring adherence (capnography use), and adverse events.
- *360° evaluations* from nursing, proceduralists, and supervising anesthesiologists to assess teamwork and communication.
- *Dashboard analytics*: automated EMR queries to flag events (e.g., naloxone/flumazenil administration, unplanned admissions, oxygen desaturation events) for provider-level review.

6. *Documentation and administrative systems*

- *Privileges form and privileging file* maintained by the Medical Staff Office with all supporting documentation.
- *Centralized tracking* (credentialing software or EMR flag) that shows active sedation privileges, expirations, proctoring status, and QA flags.
- *Sedation committee oversight*—an interdisciplinary committee (anesthesiology, nursing, procedural specialties, risk management) that reviews privileging criteria, adverse events, and appeals.

7. *Special situations*

- *Propofol/deep sedation*: many institutions require anesthesiologist-level qualifications or additional stringent proctoring and competency demonstration for non-anesthesiologist use of agents like propofol. The program should document explicit criteria for granting or denying such privileges.
- *Locums and temporary providers*: brief but rigorous onboarding is required—site-specific orientation, proctored first cases, restricted or time-limited privileges until competency is validated, and EMR flags indicating supervision requirements.
- *Nurse-administered sedation programs*: must include defined training curricula, standing orders, supervised practice, and explicit limitations on medications and patient selection.

19.6.3 Suggested Practical Templates and Checklists

Below are sample elements you can adapt into institutional forms.

19.6.3.1 Sample Initial Privileging Checklist (Sedation Privileges)

- Valid medical license, DEA, board status.
- Current BLS and ACLS (and PALS if pediatric cases).
- CV and training verification.
- Completion of institutional sedation orientation (policy review + simulation).
- Proctored cases: documentation of X directly observed cases with proctor sign-off (proctor checklist attached).
- Knowledge assessment completed (pass).

- Approved by sedation committee/medical staff office.

19.6.3.2 Sample Proctor Observation Checklist (Items to Score During Proctored Case)

- Pre-procedure assessment and risk stratification documented.
- Proper consenting for sedation documented.
- Correct setup: monitors, capnography, airway equipment, reversal drugs.
- Appropriate medication dosing and timing.
- Timely recognition and management of respiratory compromise.
- Clear communication with team and escalation when needed.
- Appropriate documentation and discharge decision-making.

19.6.4 Performance Metrics Tied to Credentialing

Tie privileging and maintenance to a small set of measurable KPIs (benchmarked quarterly/annually). Examples:

- *Adverse respiratory events per 1000 sedations* (e.g., episodes requiring airway intervention).
- *Unplanned escalation of care rate* (transfer to PACU longer than X hours / unplanned ICU transfer per 1000 cases).
- *Rate of naloxone/flumazenil administration per 1000 sedations.*
- *Incomplete monitoring documentation* (percentage of sedation cases missing capnography or SpO_2 charts).
- *Time to escalation* (time from event recognition to senior anesthesiologist notification).
- *Patient satisfaction/proceduralist satisfaction scores* related to sedation.

Providers who exceed safety thresholds should be engaged for targeted education; repeated exceedance should trigger remediation (see below).

19.6.5 Remediation, Restrictions, and Suspension Process

A transparent remediation pathway protects patients and provides a fair process for providers:

1. *First event/minor deficiency*: targeted feedback, focused education, and increased observation for next N cases.
2. *Repeated or serious event*: mandatory simulation-based retraining, proctored clinical cases, and focused CME. Temporary restriction of privileges (e.g., no unsupervised deep sedation) may be applied.

3. *Severe adverse event or failure to remediate*: temporary suspension of sedation privileges pending investigation; the sedation committee reviews and recommends actions, up to permanent revocation if indicated.
4. *Appeals*: allow providers to appeal findings through standard medical staff processes; remediation plans should be documented and time-bound.

19.6.6 Implementation Considerations and Operational Tips

- *Make privileging practical*: avoid excessively burdensome numeric thresholds that deter collaboration; prefer competency-based assessments supplemented by reasonable case volume expectations.
- *Standardize across sites*: in multi-hospital systems, harmonize privileging criteria so locums and staff move between sites without confusion.
- *Leverage simulation*: simulation is efficient for both initial assessment and rapid retraining. Use standardized scenarios (airway loss, aspiration, unanticipated apnea).
- *EMR integration*: create sedation procedure templates that capture required monitoring fields and auto-flag missing items. Use automated queries to populate dashboards.
- *Engage stakeholders*: include proceduralists, nurses, risk management, and administration in creating and approving privilege frameworks—this increases buy-in and compliance.
- *Transparency with providers*: publish privilege requirements and maintenance expectations. Clear expectations reduce surprise and defensiveness during QA.

19.6.7 Example Credentialing Timeline (Illustrative, Adapt Locally)

- *Day 0*: Application received; orientation assigned.
- *Days 1–7*: Complete online orientation modules and simulation module.
- *Week 2*: Proctored cases scheduled and completed (number per institutional policy).
- *Week 3*: Proctor signs off; privileges activated with EMR flag.
- *Ongoing*: Quarterly QA dashboard review; annual re-credentialing with case log and 360° review.

19.6.8 Conclusion

Credentialing and competency systems are not bureaucratic barriers—they are essential mechanisms that operationalize safe sedation practice. Effective systems are competency-based, pragmatic, and integrated with departmental QA. Anesthesiologists should lead design and governance: They bring the appropriate clinical expertise to set standards, evaluate competence, and ensure rescue capability—thereby protecting patients and enabling broader access to safe sedation across the health system.

19.7 Quality Assurance and Data Collection

Quality assurance (QA) and data collection form the backbone of safe and accountable sedation services. Because sedation is performed by a wide variety of clinicians in diverse settings, it is essential to establish structured systems for collecting outcomes, identifying trends, and implementing improvements. Anesthesiologists are uniquely positioned to design, oversee, and interpret these systems, ensuring that data translate into actionable improvements in both patient safety and operational efficiency.

19.7.1 Core Principles of QA in Sedation

- *Transparency*: QA programs must be standardized, consistently applied across providers and sites, and transparent in expectations.
- *Continuous learning*: Data collection should not only identify failures but also highlight successes and enable dissemination of best practices.
- *System-level focus*: QA should prioritize system improvement over individual blame, except in cases of repeated unsafe practice.
- *Benchmarking*: Institutions benefit from comparing local sedation performance to internal standards and external registries when available.

19.7.2 Key Metrics to Track

Effective QA programs monitor both *process* and *outcome* metrics (Table 19.1):

Table 19.1 Sample of both process and outcomes metrics that may be used to track efficacy of a sedation supervision program

Process metrics	Outcome metrics
Compliance with required monitoring (SpO_2, NIBP, capnography use)	Rates of hypoxemia, hypotension, and bradycardia
Completion of pre-procedure risk assessment and consent	Incidence of airway intervention (jaw thrust, bag-mask ventilation, intubation)
Adherence to NPO guidelines	Rescue medication use (naloxone, flumazenil, vasopressors)
Documentation completeness (drug dosing, recovery scores, discharge criteria)	Unplanned admission, escalation of care, or procedure cancellation
	Patient satisfaction scores
	Proceduralist and nursing satisfaction regarding sedation safety/efficiency

19.7.2.1 Process Metrics

- Compliance with required monitoring (e.g., continuous SpO_2, NIBP, capnography use).
- Completion rates of pre-procedure risk assessments and consent documentation.
- Adherence to NPO guidelines.
- Documentation completeness (drug dosing, recovery scores, discharge criteria).

19.7.2.2 Outcome Metrics

- Rates of hypoxemia, hypotension, and bradycardia.
- Incidence of airway intervention (jaw thrust, bag-mask ventilation, LMA/intubation).
- Rescue medication use (naloxone, flumazenil, vasopressors).
- Unplanned admission, escalation of care, or procedure cancellation.
- Patient satisfaction scores.
- Proceduralist and nursing team satisfaction regarding sedation safety and efficiency.

19.7.3 Data Collection Systems

- *Electronic Medical Records (EMR)*: Sedation modules should include structured fields for monitoring, events, and interventions, enabling automated queries. Drop-down menus and hard stops can reduce missing data.
- *Automated Dashboards*: Periodic dashboards displaying trends in adverse events, compliance, and outcomes provide visibility to clinical leaders.
- *Event Reporting Systems*: Critical incidents and near misses should be captured in institutional reporting systems, reviewed by the sedation committee and categorized by contributing factors.
- *Prospective Registries*: When available, participation in multicenter registries (e.g., Pediatric Sedation Research Consortium) allows for benchmarking against national data.

19.7.4 Review Processes

- *Sedation Committee Oversight*: A multidisciplinary committee (anesthesiology, nursing, proceduralists, risk management) should meet regularly to review data, adverse events, and opportunities for improvement.
- *Root Cause Analysis*: Sentinel or serious events warrant structured analysis using standardized tools to identify system vulnerabilities.
- *Feedback Loops*: Providers should receive individual feedback on performance metrics, with confidentiality maintained but patterns of repeated deficiencies addressed transparently.

- *Policy Revision*: QA findings should feed directly into updates of sedation policies, credentialing requirements, and education curricula.

19.7.5 Challenges in Locums and Multi-site Environments

Collecting and reviewing sedation data for *locum tenens providers* or clinicians rotating across multiple sites presents additional challenges. Institutions must:

- Ensure locum providers are entered into the same EMR workflows to capture complete data.
- Flag locum cases in QA systems for pattern recognition.
- Incorporate locum event data into the same review pathways to ensure consistency and accountability.

19.7.6 Summary

Robust QA and data collection systems protect patients, improve institutional reliability, and reduce medicolegal risk. By leading these processes, anesthesiologists demonstrate their unique value as perioperative safety leaders—moving beyond direct patient care to systemic improvements that safeguard every patient undergoing sedation.

19.8 Economic and Strategic Value

While sedation services are often viewed as routine and low-acuity, their management has important implications for hospital economics, institutional liability, and strategic positioning. Anesthesiologists, through supervision and oversight, add measurable value by reducing costs associated with adverse events, optimizing efficiency, and aligning sedation programs with system-wide strategic goals.

19.8.1 Cost Avoidance Through Safety

Sedation-related complications, though infrequent, can be catastrophic and costly. Unplanned ICU admissions, litigation, and regulatory penalties carry significant financial burdens.

- *Closed claims analyses* show that sedation-related malpractice cases often involve inadequate monitoring and lack of airway rescue capability [2]. Each case not only incurs direct legal costs but also damages institutional reputation.
- Preventing a single sentinel event may offset the annual cost of maintaining a robust sedation oversight infrastructure.

- By ensuring credentialing, competency, and adherence to monitoring standards, anesthesiologists reduce institutional exposure to both direct and downstream costs.

19.8.2 Operational Efficiency

Efficient sedation services directly impact hospital throughput and revenue:

- *Procedure completion rates*: Avoidance of cancellations and premature terminations translates to more predictable case volumes and fewer wasted resources.
- *Patient flow optimization*: Timely recovery and discharge from sedation-dependent units (e.g., endoscopy suites, interventional radiology) prevent bottlenecks that delay subsequent cases.
- *Length of stay reduction*: Effective sedation management decreases unplanned admissions and facilitates same-day discharge, aligning with ambulatory surgery trends and value-based care initiatives.

19.8.3 Strategic Value in Competitive Markets

Sedation services can differentiate an institution in increasingly competitive outpatient markets:

- *Patient satisfaction*: Safe and comfortable sedation contributes to higher HCAHPS scores and greater patient loyalty.
- *Proceduralist satisfaction*: Reliable sedation oversight improves collaboration, builds trust, and attracts proceduralists seeking efficient practice environments.
- *Market expansion*: Robust sedation programs allow hospitals and ASCs to expand into higher-complexity cases (e.g., advanced endoscopy, complex interventional radiology), broadening service lines and revenue streams.

19.8.4 Alignment with Value-Based Care

As healthcare shifts toward bundled payments and value-based purchasing, sedation oversight contributes to system-level cost savings:

- Reduced adverse events → fewer penalties and readmissions.
- Optimized workflows → higher case throughput with the same resources.
- Standardized practices → measurable improvements in quality metrics that align with payer incentives.

19.8.5 The Anesthesiologist's Value Proposition

Anesthesiologist-led sedation supervision demonstrates how perioperative physicians extend their impact beyond the operating room. By ensuring safety, preventing costly complications, and improving efficiency, anesthesiologists directly influence both the *financial bottom line* and the *strategic reputation* of healthcare organizations. Their leadership in this domain is a prime example of how specialized expertise translates into institutional economic value.

19.9 Future Directions

As healthcare delivery continues to evolve, the landscape of sedation practice is likely to undergo significant transformation. Advances in technology, changes in workforce dynamics, and shifts in patient expectations will all shape how sedation is supervised in the coming years.

19.9.1 Technology Integration and Automation

Artificial intelligence (AI)-driven monitoring systems and closed-loop drug delivery platforms are emerging tools that may reduce variability in sedation practice. Automated systems capable of titrating sedatives to physiologic targets have already shown promise in pilot studies. In the future, anesthesiologists may oversee teams using such platforms, ensuring safety while optimizing efficiency.

19.9.2 Expanded Use of Tele-Sedation

Telemedicine platforms are increasingly being applied to procedural sedation, especially in geographically underserved or resource-limited settings. Remote anesthesiologist supervision through video-enabled monitoring and integrated physiologic data streams could allow broader access to safe sedation without requiring an on-site specialist at every location.

19.9.3 Workforce and Scope-of-Practice Evolution

The ongoing shortage of anesthesiologists in many regions underscores the need for optimized models of supervision. Clear delineation of roles among anesthesiologists, nurse anesthetists, and proceduralists will remain a central theme. Collaborative team-based models—potentially supported by national guidelines and credentialing bodies—will likely expand.

19.9.4 Data-Driven Quality Improvement

As health systems emphasize value-based care, sedation practices will increasingly be assessed through quality metrics, patient satisfaction scores, and cost-effectiveness analyses. Large-scale data collection from electronic health records and registries will inform best practices and refine supervision models.

19.9.5 Patient-Centered Care

Future models of sedation supervision will need to incorporate patient-centered outcomes, including recovery profiles, cognitive function, and long-term safety. Personalized sedation strategies—guided by genetic markers, comorbidities, and predictive analytics—may become standard of care.

19.10 Conclusion

Sedation supervision represents a critical intersection of patient safety, clinical judgment, and systems-based practice. The anesthesiologist's role is not confined to medication administration but extends to ensuring competency among providers, establishing standards of monitoring, and aligning practices with institutional and regulatory requirements. The balance between efficiency, patient-centered care, and safety continues to evolve as new technologies, data-driven approaches, and workforce models emerge.

Looking forward, the future of sedation supervision will depend on the integration of innovation with thoughtful oversight. Automated drug delivery systems, telemedicine platforms, and predictive analytics hold promise, but they must be guided by anesthesiologists who can interpret data, anticipate complications, and intervene when necessary. Ultimately, maintaining high standards in sedation practice ensures that patient outcomes remain at the forefront while also delivering measurable economic and strategic value to health care institutions.

Key Takeaways: Sedation Supervision

- *Anesthesiologists play a central role* in maintaining safety, competency, and oversight in sedation practice.
- *Supervision extends beyond drug administration*, encompassing credentialing, monitoring standards, and quality assurance.
- *Economic and strategic benefits* arise from optimized sedation supervision, including efficiency, cost savings, and institutional value.
- *Future directions* include automation, tele-sedation, workforce evolution, and data-driven quality improvement.
- *Patient-centered care* and individualized sedation strategies will define the next era of sedation supervision.

References

1. Centers for M, Medicaid S. Conditions of participation for hospitals (42 CFR part 482). U.S. Department of Health and Human Services; 2020.
2. Robbertze R, Posner KL, Domino KB. Closed claims review of anesthesia for procedures outside the operating room. Curr Opin Anaesthesiol. 2006;19(4):436–42. (In eng). https://doi.org/10.1097/01.aco.0000236146.46346.fe.
3. The Joint C. Comprehensive accreditation manual for hospitals. The Joint Commission; 2022.
4. Anesthesiologists ASo. Practice guidelines for moderate procedural sedation and analgesia 2018: a report by the American Society of Anesthesiologists Task Force on Moderate Procedural Sedation and Analgesia, the American Association of Oral and Maxillofacial Surgeons, American College of Radiology, American Dental Association, American Society of Dentist Anesthesiologists, and Society of Interventional Radiology. Anesthesiology. 2018;128(3):437–79. (In eng). https://doi.org/10.1097/aln.0000000000002043.
5. Anesthesiologists ASo. Statement on granting privileges for Administration of Moderate Sedation to practitioners who are not anesthesia professionals. 2021.
6. Anesthesiologists ASo. Statement on Safe Use of Propofol. 2024.
7. Anesthesiologists ASo. Statement on distinguishing monitored anesthesia care ("MAC") from moderate sedation/analgesia (conscious sedation). 2023.
8. Early DS, Lightdale JR, Vargo JJ 2nd, et al. Guidelines for sedation and anesthesia in GI endoscopy. Gastrointest Endosc. 2018;87(2):327–37. (In eng). https://doi.org/10.1016/j.gie.2017.07.018.
9. Cote CJ, Wilson S. Guidelines for monitoring and management of pediatric patients before, during, and after sedation for diagnostic and therapeutic procedures. Pediatrics. 2016;138(1):e20161212. https://doi.org/10.1542/peds.2016-1212.
10. Cravero JP, Beach ML, Blike GT, Gallagher SM, Hertzog JH. The incidence and nature of adverse events during pediatric sedation/anesthesia with propofol for procedures outside the operating room: a report from the Pediatric Sedation Research Consortium. Anesth Analg. 2009;108(3):795–804. (In eng). https://doi.org/10.1213/ane.0b013e31818fc334.
11. Godwin SA, Burton JH, Gerardo CJ, et al. Clinical policy: procedural sedation and analgesia in the emergency department. Ann Emerg Med. 2014;63(2):247–58.e18. (In eng). https://doi.org/10.1016/j.annemergmed.2013.10.015.
12. Hinkelbein J, Schmitz J, Lamperti M, Fuchs-Buder T. Procedural sedation outside the operating room. Curr Opin Anaesthesiol. 2020;33(4):533–8. (In eng). https://doi.org/10.1097/aco.0000000000000885.
13. Lightdale JR, Mahoney LB, Fredette ME, Starkey E, Nagle D. Nurse-administered propofol sedation: feasibility and safety in the pediatric population. Gastrointest Endosc. 2005;62(5):692–7. https://doi.org/10.1016/j.gie.2005.07.020.
14. Gross JB, Benumof JL, Caplan RA, Connis RT, Nickinovich DG, Praetel CR. Practice guidelines for sedation and analgesia by non-anesthesiologists. Anesthesiology. 2002;96(4):1004–17. https://doi.org/10.1097/00000542-200204000-00031.
15. O'Connor RE, Sama A, Burton JH, et al. Procedural sedation and analgesia in the emergency department: recommendations for physician credentialing, privileging, and practice. Ann Emerg Med. 2011;58(4):365–70. (In eng). https://doi.org/10.1016/j.annemergmed.2011.06.020.

Non-operating Room Anesthesia Oversight and Management

20

Aaron N. Primm, Dane Saksa, and Patricia Fogarty Mack

20.1 Introduction

Non-operating room anesthesia (NORA) is a general term for the practice of anesthesia that is outside of the traditional operating rooms (ORs) or obstetric suites. Sites such as gastrointestinal (GI) endoscopy, bronchoscopy, and diagnostic or interventional radiology (IR) suites are prime examples (Table 20.1). In the past, NORA was also referred to as "offsite anesthesia" or "out-of-OR anesthesia" and was not a central focus of physician education and training. The evolution in naming and recognition is emblematic of its growing importance in perioperative care. Though ambulatory surgery centers and office-based procedures fall under the umbrella of NORA, this chapter will primarily discuss hospital-based NORA oversight and management.

Case volumes in NORA have grown immensely and will almost certainly exceed 50% of all cases requiring anesthesia care in the next decade [1]. NORA has become an increasingly significant part of anesthesia practice due to multiple factors, including technological advancements, economic pressures, and patient and clinician convenience. Continual refinements in procedural techniques and the introduction of new technology enable less invasive procedures to be performed and enable the care of patients who would have been deemed "too sick" for routine operative care. These refinements expand the range of patients and procedures that can be safely performed at NORA sites. Additionally, hospital systems are interested in following payer incentives for ambulatory surgery, with subsequent shorter length of stay, to

A. N. Primm (✉)
Department of Anesthesiology, Perioperative Care, and Pain Medicine, NYU Grossman School of Medicine, New York, NY, USA

D. Saksa
UCLA Health, Los Angeles, CA, USA

P. F. Mack
Weill Cornell Medicine, New York Presbyterian Hospital, New York, NY, USA

G. Tewfik (ed.), *The Anesthesiologist as Perioperative Leader*,
https://doi.org/10.1007/978-3-032-18058-2_20

Table 20.1 Non-operating room anesthesia (NORA) locations and common procedures

NORA location	Common procedures
Gastrointestinal endoscopy	Esophagoduodenoscopy (EGD) Colonoscopy Endoscopic ultrasound Endoscopic retrograde cholangiopancreatography (ERCP)
Interventional pulmonology	Bronchoscopy Endobronchial ultrasound Electromagnetic navigational bronchoscopy Endobronchial stent
Interventional radiology	Angioplasty and stenting Transjugular intrahepatic portosystemic shunt (TIPS) Nephrostomy and ureteric stent
Interventional neuroradiology	Angiography and embolization Aneurysm coiling Thrombectomy Kyphoplasty
Radiologic imaging	Magnetic resonance imaging (MRI) Computed tomography (CT) Positron emission tomography
Electrophysiology laboratory	Electrophysiology studies and radiofrequency ablation Implantation of cardioverter defibrillators Transesophageal echocardiogram
Cardiac catheterization/structural heart	Transcatheter aortic valve replacement Balloon valvuloplasty Percutaneous coronary interventions
Radiotherapy	External beam radiation therapy Brachytherapy
Other	In vitro fertilization Electroconvulsive therapy Dental procedures

decrease costs and increase value. Adding to these factors, concerns about a workforce shortage for anesthesiologists and hospital systems further emphasize the need to manage NORA case volumes effectively. In many hospital systems, anesthesiologists are tasked with leading the optimization of preoperative evaluation, scheduling, and staffing, thereby enhancing procedural throughput and streamlining communication while providing training and guidelines [2].

This chapter aims to address the oversight and management of NORA locations and processes. After reviewing known safety and communication concerns in NORA, the discussion will turn to navigating the complex regulatory system and optimizing preoperative evaluation, scheduling, and staffing. Finally, we will discuss the value that strong anesthesiologist leadership can bring to the field through directing the NORA workflow.

20.2 Oversight and Management in the NORA Environment

20.2.1 General Safety and Communication Concerns

It is well-recognized among anesthesia clinicians that NORA locations present a unique set of challenges related to patient safety, team-based communication, and care coordination. Closed claims analyses have consistently shown that patients undergoing NORA procedures have a higher incidence of morbidity and mortality [3, 4]. Several factors contribute to the increased safety concerns. First, the procedural suites where NORA care takes place were typically not built or designed to accommodate the increase in anesthesia cases being performed [5]. At the same time, procedural sites may be located on separate floors or at a considerable distance from the ORs, creating an environment where obtaining backup anesthesia or technical support is more difficult. Factors related to the procedure itself can also present challenges to the safe administration of anesthesia care: Radiographic equipment can hinder access to the patient and their airway; endoscopic procedures routinely involve a shared airway; magnetic resonance imaging (MRI) safety concerns can require an entire wall between clinician and patient; and evolving technologies and procedures can leave the anesthesiologist guessing about procedural needs and case duration.

Beyond these ergonomic and procedural challenges, patient-specific factors are well-documented drivers of patient safety concerns in NORA. NORA patients tend to be older and of higher ASA status classification than OR patients, presumably because a sicker patient may be a better candidate for a less-invasive procedure than a more-invasive surgery [1]. The proceduralist often receives the patient as a referral, rather than one they evaluated in the clinic, implying that the intimate pre-op workup the anesthesiologist is accustomed to in the operating room may be absent.

Fostering effective teamwork and communication in NORA procedural settings is perhaps the most influential way an anesthesiologist can improve patient safety. In the NORA environment, patient-specific preoperative considerations are often not discussed, and critical procedural steps or concerns are frequently assumed. The proceduralist and nursing teams may not be as comfortable working with anesthesia teams, especially if a significant portion of their workload is performed without anesthesia and they are constantly switching between anesthesia and non-anesthesia cases. This feeling of being a "visitor to the team" or a "stranger in a strange land" can present an impediment to team-based communication and contribute to safety issues [6]. Quite often, the anesthesiologist must initiate these discussions and establish the standard for effective communication before the induction of anesthesia. A 2019 article in the APSF newsletter highlighted the importance of pre-procedural time-out checklists for NORA cases, specifically focused on "the issues proceduralists, anesthesia professionals, nurses, technicians, and patients have determined to be important" [7]. This time-out can also be an opportunity to define roles, emergency response protocols, and specific needs of the anesthesiologist, such as nursing support during induction, requirements for muscle relaxation, and the need to place additional vascular access lines before the patient is prepped and positioned (Fig. 20.1).

20.2.2 Navigating Regulation

In addition to the call for anesthesia engagement in the realms of patient safety and team-based communication in NORA, there is also a significant role for anesthesiologists to support their health systems in adhering to the growing body of regulatory standards regarding patient care in NORA locations. The Joint Commission (TJC), and other accrediting agencies, suggests that the same quality and safety standards prescribed to the OR should be upheld in NORA locations. This includes an appropriate pre-procedural evaluation, the same monitoring standards and

PRE-PROCEDURE VERIFICATION	SAFETY SIGN-IN	FINAL TIME-OUT
Location: PTU or Outside IR Suite (for inpatients) Who: • Procedure Nurse • PTU Nurse (or Bedside Nurse for inpatients)	Location: In the IR suite Who: • Initiated by RN • Anesthesia Attending, CRNA, or Resident Physically Present • IR Fellow/Resident Physically Present • IR Attending Present or On Speaker Phone or Immediately Available by Pager (***if not physically present, all items below will have been explicitly discussed with Fellow/Resident night before***) When: prior to induction of anesthesia or start of sedation.	Location: In the IR suite Who: • Initiated by Procedural MD • RN • Anesthesia Attending, CRNA, or Resident • IR Fellow/Resident or Attending Physically Present When: immediately before vascular access or skin incision **All other activities/conversation should be suspended during Final Time-Out except in case of emergency*
Checklist: o Patient Identifier x 2 o Planned Procedure o Procedure site, if relevant o Review consents/plan to obtain o Review Important exam findings, labs, imaging, and medications due o Review patient allergies o Ensure special equipment, devices, and/or device reps are present prior to patient in room.	Checklist: o Patient Identifier x 2 o Introduction of all team members by name o Planned Procedure o Procedure Site (if relevant) o Plan for Vascular Access o Patient Allergies o Antibiotic Prophylaxis o Blood Status (RN to call Blood Bank in advance) o Anticipated Blood Loss o Specific BP Goals (most relevant in Neuro IR cases) o Need for arterial line for tight BP control, who will obtain? o Heparinization required? Plan? Timing? Hourly Checks? Who will administer? o Need for muscle relaxation, breath holds? o **Specific to lung ablations: bronchial blocker available in room?* o Anesthesia-specific concerns, major patient comorbidities o High-Risk Procedural Steps or Concerns o Need for ICU bed	Checklist: o Patient Identifier x 2 o Procedure (as listed on consent displayed on a computer) o Procedure Site (if relevant) o Plan for Vascular Access o Patient Allergies o Antibiotic Prophylaxis Given? o Review any outstanding questions about specific procedural or anesthetic needs o "**If anyone has any concerns now or at any point during the surgery/procedure, please voice them immediately.**" • *Joint Commission Guidelines advise that, if the attending was not present for Safety Sign-In or Final Time-Out, there be another brief time-out to confirm patient and procedure.*

Fig. 20.1 Comprehensive pre-procedural checklist (interventional radiology)

vigilance, consistent documentation, and similar post-procedure recovery and discharge standards. In accordance with Center for Medicare and Medicaid Services (CMS) Conditions of participation, which require that all anesthesia and sedation services in a hospital or ASC be "organized under the direction of a qualified doctor of medicine or osteopathy," TJC surveys require that sedation practices throughout the hospital be "monitored and evaluated by the Department of Anesthesia" to ensure that any type of sedation practice, whether provided by an anesthesia clinician, sedation nurse, or other licensed professional, adheres to a minimum basic standard of monitoring, safety, and quality [8, 9]. This mandate positions the anesthesiologist as the primary voice in setting safety and quality standards across all NORA sites.

At the same time, national anesthesiology organizations have been paying attention to the growth of NORA and the need for effective local oversight and governance to ensure safety, quality, and operational efficiency. A recently updated set of guidelines from the ASA was published in 2023 and leads with the theme that has permeated the above discussion: "Perianesthesia services, including perioperative care as it related to NORA locations, requires similar leadership, management, and oversight structures as those in the operating rooms" [10]. The 2023 ASA statement moves beyond simple patient safety and monitoring recommendations to also highlight the potential role of the anesthesiologist in perioperative leadership and management in NORA locations [11]. Similarly, the Anesthesia Patient Safety Foundation (APSF) released Consensus Recommendations for the Safe Conduct of Nonoperating Room Anesthesia in 2023 that range from facility and equipment concerns to specific standards for pre-, intra-, and post-procedural care [12]. These two expert consensus statements serve as excellent guides to the safe development and expansion of NORA services and should be consulted by every hospital with a significant NORA practice.

20.2.3 Preoperative Evaluation, Scheduling, and Staffing

20.2.3.1 Preoperative Evaluation

As anesthesiologists step into leadership roles within NORA services, their role in optimizing patient safety, communication, and adherence with regulatory expectations begins in the pre-procedural phase. As discussed above, TJC and the ASA all explicitly state that NORA patients must undergo the same preoperative evaluation as any patient going to the OR. This oversight is a critical role of the anesthesiologist. NORA locations bring an added layer of complexity because the patients are often critically ill, and the proposed NORA procedure may be a "last resort" for a patient who is not deemed a good surgical candidate [1]. The onus is often on the anesthesia clinician to possess the most thorough knowledge about the comorbidities and medications of these complex patients, as proceduralists are typically consultants. The complexity of NORA patients and the disparate and uncoordinated nature of the procedural subgroups included under the NORA umbrella present a critical void that anesthesiologists can uniquely address, given their breadth of knowledge and experience.

Unfortunately, most anesthesia pre-operative clinics lack the bandwidth to screen every NORA patient to assess for procedural optimization, venue appropriateness, and the most suitable sedation plan and personnel. Therefore, the most successful health systems will have a triage system in place that allows non-physician staff to be trained and educated on protocols and guidelines directing certain patients toward procedural sedation and others toward an anesthesia consultation. Moving forward, there will likely be a role for artificial intelligence systems to support clinicians in this triaging process. Guidelines and triaging protocols should also clearly define, which patients are best suited to inpatient versus outpatient facilities. For example, Peterson describes a "grid model" at her large children's hospital in which patients and procedures can be evaluated based on risk, with the understanding that a low-risk patient for a low-risk procedure can likely be performed under procedural sedation, and a high-risk patient for a high-risk procedure will most likely require anesthesia support and an inpatient venue [13]. Patients in the intermediate grids may need a closer review by an anesthesiologist. Any direction the anesthesiologist can provide in triaging both sedation/anesthesia requirement type and venue of care will add significant value to the health system and for hospital leadership. Pre-operative involvement by the anesthesiologist has been shown to lead to cost savings and improved performance by optimizing patients to allow for same-day admissions, avoid same-day cancellations, and improve patient outcomes and satisfaction [14, 15].

20.2.3.2 Scheduling and Staffing

The goal of scheduling and staffing anesthetics outside of the OR is to cover growing case needs and maximize revenue. A successful NORA service will enable hospitals to expand their physician practices, increase market share, and meet the community's needs [16]. Likewise, NORA scheduling should prioritize patient safety, patient and healthcare team satisfaction, scheduling efficiency and cost effectiveness [17]. The OR management literature is heavily leaned on to provide logistical and tactical direction. However, there are still gaps in knowledge on how to schedule NORA optimally. For example, scheduling one anesthesiologist to work a 10-h shift covering GI, MRI, and electrophysiology at different sites across a hospital with low volumes or large gaps between cases is grossly inefficient. This will lead to underutilized time and low productivity. In fact, the increasing number of NORA locations to be staffed has resulted in a decrease of more than 11% in net medical revenues per full-time equivalent physician [18]. Along with decreasing reimbursements and staff shortages, it is unsurprising that 85–95% of all hospitals have needed to subsidize their anesthesia services.

Anesthesiology departments must contend with staffing restrictions due to remote locations, variations in daily workloads, and specialized knowledge required for individual sites (Table 20.2). As hospitals and health systems differ in their service lines and culture, the best approach is to discuss general strategies that have

Table 20.2 Common challenges in NORA scheduling

Challenges
Sites may be located at great distances from each other, making it challenging to cover multiple sites with multiple anesthesia staff or impossible with a single anesthesiologist
Procedures not requiring anesthesia services interrupt case flow
Sites may be highly specialized (e.g., MRI safety), limiting the staff that can be assigned
Turnover time can be longer: difficult to access area of the hospital (patient or equipment transportation), preanesthesia evaluation must sometimes be done immediately prior to the procedure, and postanesthesia recovery is far from the site
Case times may be difficult to estimate (new procedures, sicker patients), resulting in inefficiency in anesthetic duration or technique
Scheduling system software and data analytics may be unavailable
Daily case volumes, as well as proceduralist availability, may vary substantially

been proven successful. Site-specific issues must always be addressed individually, as specific equipment and staff are needed.

The scheduling and staffing of NORA can take many different forms, but a critical branching point is managing services with higher versus lower case volumes. An approach by Dexter and Wachtel [19] advocates for allowing proceduralists in remote locations to schedule in blocks of time reserved specifically for them, assuming the case volumes are higher. As anesthesiology departments typically plan for around 8- to 10-h workdays, they argue that these offsites can be allocated 10 h of cases no longer than once every 2 weeks. Any "add-on" cases that do not fit in this block would then go into an "overflow" anesthesia time block. The schedule should aim to reduce over-utilized time with sequential case scheduling. If multiple services cannot fill a whole block, they can be combined to avoid underutilization. Under this system, it is proposed that the anesthesiology department will realize financial gain from increased productivity. Borrowing from the OR literature, a sensible goal is to have open anesthesia time available within 2 weeks of any request, as surveys have deemed this the most acceptable amount of time for patients to wait for an elective procedure [20]. This flexibility promotes patient and team satisfaction overall.

GI endoscopy is the most common NORA site and has been the background for much of the scheduling research in the literature. Tsai et al. [21] introduced a new block time system, where weekly allocated blocks were determined by gastroenterologists' historical utilization rates, procedural volumes, and scheduling limitations. Additionally, unused time was released to other services (radiology). They reported improved block time utilization and productivity, which benefited the hospital financially. Navidi and Kiai [22] reported increases in efficiency in their GI endoscopy suites by standardizing block times and adopting a 4:1 certified registered nurse anesthetist (CRNA) to anesthesiologist model, which transitioned from conscious sedation to solely propofol sedation. In their review, the costs associated with the anesthesia care team are more than offset by increased revenue and patient satisfaction, resulting in a 16% increase in case productivity over two years.

An alternative and more traditional model for scheduling low volumes of cases involves a central anesthesia scheduler who fills in cases to a block of anesthesia time for any requesting service [23]. Instead of being assigned to a single area, anesthesiologists can potentially visit multiple areas in a single day. Though the model utilizes the anesthesiologists' time well, it may cause inefficiencies at the different NORA sites, particularly when the site has a larger-than-normal or growing volume of cases. If, for example, the bronchoscopy suite has an endobronchial ultrasound case at the end of the workday, but the anesthesiologist is significantly delayed from 9 colonoscopies at another site, there will be frustration. A study that calculated site utilization, physician efficiency (minutes utilized divided by minutes staffed), and scheduling efficiency (staff anesthesiologists divided by staffed sites) found that scheduling and physician efficiency do not correspond with each other in NORA as they do in the ORs [24]. These metrics are better aligned when travel between NORA sites is limited. Ultimately, the feasibility of any system will be site-specific. Many anesthesiology departments operate in a hybrid system with daily blocks for high-volume services and more ad hoc scheduling for very low-volume services [23].

The ASA Statement on Non-Operating Room Anesthesia Services also provides baseline expectations for optimizing scheduling and staffing [10]. In addition to the methods discussed above, the statement emphasizes practical and actionable items. The expectations highlight the need to triage patients who may not require anesthesia services. Importantly, these procedural sedation cases should not interrupt the anesthesia schedule. Hospitals should utilize the same organizational and data analytics (scheduling software) to drive perioperative efficiency. This may include real-time scheduling and the ability to adjust preoperative fasting times. Finally, the statement promotes scheduling complex patients and procedures during times of optimal staffing and availability of ancillary services when possible. Data from the Anesthesia Quality Institute's National Anesthesia Clinical Outcomes Registry (NACOR) has shown that patients with a higher ASA physical status classification were more likely to have procedures during after-hours shifts [25].

Staffing models vary according to local needs and regulations, but they follow the same principles as those of the ORs. As nursing and support staff at NORA sites may be unfamiliar with the anesthesiologist's expertise, adequate training and support must be provided to ensure their understanding. According to the APSF, a NORA team should include at least two individuals with appropriate certification (ACLS, BLS, PALS, PeRLS) and defined roles in case of emergency [12].

The proper selection of anesthesia personnel to work at these sites is essential to a successful NORA program. Many anesthesiologists view the production pressure at NORA sites as more labor-intensive and stressful, preferring the conventions of the traditional OR. For example, working in a combined MRI-OR room reduces perceptions of safety while increasing stress and anxiety [26]. Avoiding burnout, staff turnover, and the costs associated with replacing physicians requires careful staff selection and effective support. This may include assigning dedicated NORA anesthesiologists with proper staffing ratios, assisting with turnovers, and providing adequate breaks. The concept of a "NORA specialist" who could lead a particular NORA site has been proposed to enhance communication, safety, and efficiency [27].

20.2.4 Anesthesiology Leadership in NORA

Given the growing volume and the associated safety and efficiency concerns that arise across disparate clinical areas throughout the hospitals, there is a significant opportunity for anesthesiologists to step into their role as perioperative leaders. While an interventional cardiologist, gastroenterologist, and interventional radiologist may rarely find themselves around the same table, a designated anesthesia leader within NORA is uniquely poised to engage stakeholders across disciplines and bridge the gaps to support more coordinated clinical efforts. As stated in a 2024 call to action for NORA leadership, it is critical that the anesthesiologist not be "swept away by the tide" but rather "take up the challenge to organize, manage, and improve NORA workflow" [27]. An anesthesiologist in this role, which many refer to as "NORA Director," can work with hospital leadership, proceduralists, anesthesiology department chairpersons, and schedulers to build a unified schedule and workflow that optimizes clinician productivity and patient throughput. Any operational efficiency achieved will be viewed as a significant value-added benefit by health system leadership. Expediting patient throughput for inpatients awaiting NORA procedures and increasing the ability to schedule profitable outpatient procedures have been, and will continue to be, top priorities for hospitals. An anesthesiologist NORA Director will have a meaningful and positive impact in both regards. As service lines expand and new physical spaces are constructed, the NORA Director will be intimately involved in the planning and design to ensure that minimum standards for the provision of anesthesia care are met and to advocate for an ergonomic workspace that facilitates safe patient care and enhances clinician well-being [10].

In addition to the urgent need for operational and organizational coordination within NORA, the NORA Director will also play a crucial role in ensuring consistent quality and safety across all NORA locations [11]. By adopting the same quality metrics tracked in the OR, such as first-case on-time starts, turnover time, and incidence of unplanned admissions or upgrades of care, the NORA Director is positioned to reverse the trend of increased adverse events in NORA. Additionally, the most successful programs will undertake the same detailed systems-based quality review after adverse events in NORA. The current critical period of increasing NORA volume and anesthesia workforce constraints should serve as a call to action for anesthesiologists at hospitals of all sizes to embrace this role and take ownership of leadership within this space [5].

20.3 Conclusions

The practice of anesthesia in NORA environments demands a nuanced and proactive approach to ensure patient safety, procedural efficiency, and regulatory compliance. Unlike the traditional operating room, NORA settings often present physical, procedural, and communication challenges that require anesthesiologists to function not only clinically but also as leaders in care coordination and safety standardization. The evolving complexity of both patients and procedures necessitates meticulous preoperative evaluation, thoughtful communication strategies, and strong interprofessional collaboration. By taking the initiative in pre-procedure discussions, establishing clear protocols, and utilizing tools such as time-out checklists and post procedure debriefings, anesthesiologists can mitigate risks and foster safer, more cohesive procedural environments.

Anesthesiologists play a critical role in supporting the broader health system through effective scheduling, staffing, and triage models tailored to the unique demands of NORA services. From preoperative triage to real-time scheduling systems and specialized staffing approaches, anesthesiologists are uniquely positioned to lead in developing high-performing NORA programs. When empowered with leadership opportunities and supported by institutional investment, anesthesiologists can transform NORA from a fragmented collection of procedural sites into a unified extension of high-quality perioperative care.

References

1. Nagrebetsky A, Gabriel RA, Dutton RP, Urman RD. Growth of nonoperating room anesthesia care in the United States: a contemporary trends analysis. Anesth Analg. 2017;124:1261–7.
2. Harter RL. Be the solution: anesthesiologists lead the way in ensuring safe and efficient growth of NORA. ASA Monitor. 2025;89:11.
3. Metzner J, Posner KL, Domino KB. The risk and safety of anesthesia at remote locations: the US closed claims analysis. Curr Opin Anaesthesiol. 2009;22:502–8.
4. Walls JD, Weiss MS. Safety in non-operating room anesthesia. APSF Newsl. 2019;34(3-4):21.
5. Abdelmalak B, Burkle C, Marco A, Mathews D. Non-operating room anesthesia: patient safety, scheduling, efficiency and effective leadership. SAMBA. 2019:1–18.
6. Schroeck H, Taenzer AH, Schifferdecker KE. Team factors influence emotions and stress in a non-operating room anaesthetising location. Br J Anaesth. 2021;127:e95–8.
7. Chang C, Dudley R. Time-out checklists promote safety in nonoperating room anesthesia (NORA). APSF Newsl. 2021;36(120):122.
8. 42 CFR 482.52 Condition of Participation: Anesthesia Services. 1986.
9. Kelly JS. Sedation by non-anesthesia personnel provokes safety concerns; anesthesiologists must balance JCAHO standards, politics, & safety. APSF Newsl. 2001;16:2.
10. American Society of Anesthesiologists Committee on Standards and Practice Parameters. Statement on nonoperating room anesthesia services. 2023.
11. Primm A, Anca D. Updates in non-operating room anesthesia. Curr Opin Anaesthesiol. 2025;38:297–302.
12. Beard J, Methangkool E, Angus S, Urman RD, Cole DJ. Consensus recommendations for the safe conduct of nonoperating room anesthesia: a meeting report from the 2022 stoelting conference of the anesthesia patient safety foundation. Anesth Analg. 2023;
13. Enabling growth in nonoperating room anesthesia procedures amid workforce shortages. American Hospital Association. 2024.
14. Pollard JB. Economic aspects of an anesthesia preoperative evaluation clinic. Curr Opin Anaesthesiol. 2002;15:257–61.
15. Talbot M. Launching a preanesthesia clinic at the University of Wisconsin. ASA Monit. 2024;88:32.
16. Urman RD. Anesthesia outside the operating room. 2nd ed. Oxford: Oxford University Press USA – OSO; 2018.

17. Warner ME, Martin DP. Scheduling the nonoperating room anesthesia suite. Curr Opin Anaesthesiol. 2018;31:492–7.
18. Galati MF. Financial aspects of providing anesthesia in nonoperating room locations. Int Anesthesiol Clin. 2009;47:93–103.
19. Dexter F, Wachtel RE. Scheduling for anesthesia at geographic locations remote from the operating room. Curr Opin Anaesthesiol. 2014;27:426–30.
20. Dexter F, Macario A, Traub RD, Hopwood M, Lubarsky DA. An operating room scheduling strategy to maximize the use of operating room block time: computer simulation of patient scheduling and survey of patients' preferences for surgical waiting time. Anesth Analg. 1999;89:7–20.
21. Tsai MH, Hall MA, Cardinal MS, Breidenstein MW, Abajian MJ, Zubarik RS. Changing anesthesia block allocations improves endoscopy suite efficiency. J Med Syst. 2020;44:1.
22. Navidi B, Kiai K. Efficiency and scheduling in the nonoperating room anesthesia suite: implications from patient satisfaction to increased revenue operating room a common (Dollars and Sense) approach. Curr Opin Anaesthesiol. 2019;32:498–503.
23. Trummel JM, Gentz BA, Furman WR. Non-operating room locations. In: Kaye AD, Urman RD, Fox ICJ, editors. Operating room leadership and perioperative practice management. 2nd ed. Cambridge University Press; 2018. p. 147–55.
24. Tsai MH, Huynh TT, Breidenstein MW, O'Donnell SE, Ehrenfeld JM, Urman RD. A systemwide approach to physician efficiency and utilization rates for non-operating room anesthesia sites. J Med Syst. 2017;41:112.
25. Gabriel RA, Burton BN, Tsai MH, Ehrenfeld JM, Dutton RP, Urman RD. After-hour versus daytime shifts in non-operating room anesthesia environments: national distribution of case volume, patient characteristics, and procedures. J Med Syst. 2017;41:140.
26. Schroeck H, Whitty MA, Martinez-Camblor P, Voicu S, Burian BK, Taenzer AH. Anaesthesia clinicians' perception of safety, workload, anxiety, and stress in a remote hybrid suite compared with the operating room. Br J Anaesth. 2023;131:598–606.
27. Primm AN, Schroeck H, Methangkool E, Anca D. Out of sight, out of mind? A call to action for leadership in nonoperating room anesthesia. Anesth Analg. 2024;139:857–62.

Electronic Health Records/Anesthesia Information Management Services

21

Franklin Chiao

Almost every medical and hospital system has some electronic health or medical record system (EHR/EMR) in place (Fig. 21.1). Anesthesia practices may utilize anesthesia information management systems (AIMS), often as a component of an institution's EHR to record and store procedural anesthesia records. The anesthesiology leadership team and individual providers have a major role in selecting, integrating, and maintaining the AIMS [10, 12, 19]. The anesthesia team, working in concert with the EHR/AIMS team, contributes via work with the EHR to increase patient safety, ensure compliance with regulatory requirements, and promote efficient management of staff and resources. Effective use of EHR by anesthesiologists improves scheduling, billing, quality control, quality improvement, research data, evidence-based medicine integration, and strategic interdisciplinary care.

Ensuring comprehensive documentation is essential for capturing patients' medical problems, enabling proper decision-making based on accurate information, and to optimize billing. Anesthesiologists must collect and enter the data for their patient notes in the preoperative, intraoperative, and postoperative phases. Their efforts are important to provide accurate and comprehensive documentation to help meet regulatory, legal, and compliance requirements as well as to reduce workloads for billing staff. These requirements overlap with financial and billing requirements for documentation such as American Society of Anesthesiologists (ASA) physical status, and medications administered. With surgeries providing a relatively large source of hospital revenue, it becomes paramount to have the anesthesia team include both required and supplemental items for billing to improve net income per surgical case and charge capture [22]. The "low hanging fruit" can add a significant amount of revenue in a hospital system.

Coordinating the activities of the operating room often requires a system to organize case schedules, estimate appropriate staffing numbers, and assist in determining coverage for emergency surgeries. The anesthesia department often has a clinical

F. Chiao (✉)
Westchester Medical Center Health Network, Valhalla, NY, USA

G. Tewfik (ed.), *The Anesthesiologist as Perioperative Leader*,
https://doi.org/10.1007/978-3-032-18058-2_21

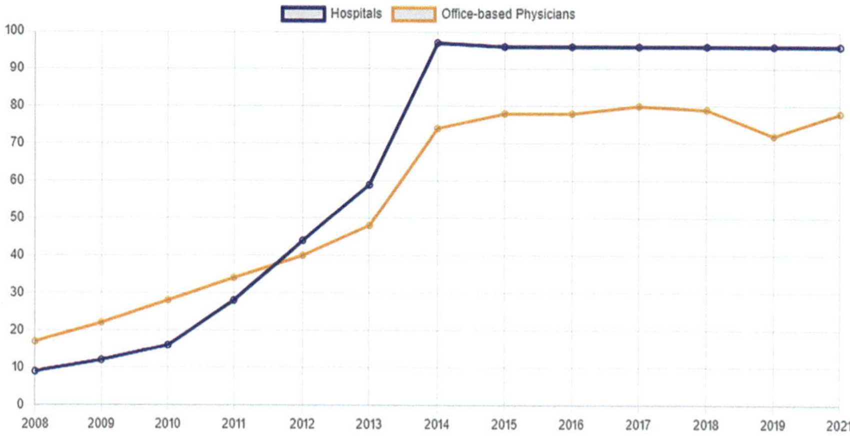

Fig. 21.1 Trends in Hospital & Physician EHR Adoption (American Hospital Association (AHA) Annual Survey Information Technology Supplement, 2008–present. National Center for Health Statistics (NCHS) National Ambulatory Care Survey (2008–2011) and National Electronic Health Record Survey (2012–present)

leader each day to provide these services, and they may use the AIMS to better visually understand the schedule [8, 11]. An effective AIMS may even enable departmental leaders to look ahead and forecast resource needs, while enabling staffing to be proactively adjusted up or down. However, this requires anesthesia involvement to ensure estimates about case times are accurate and appropriate staff members are made available for specialized cases [17]. A potential reduction in operating room staff on slower days enables the hospital to clearly reduce costs and redundancies which enables adaptive staffing models where anesthesia team members can be assigned to different locations or hospitals in a flexible manner when one site is busier than another site. Effective use of AIMS for schedule management can provide increased efficiency and utilization of resources.

Cost containment and increased revenue may also result from effective data analysis through use of AIMS and EHR. Analysis of drug utilization by anesthesiologists is important for cost analysis, and inefficiencies may be addressed to yield cost containment. More sophisticated systems can account for supplies used during the surgery, improving systemic supply chains. Improved documentation using EHR and AIMS also improves revenue; for example, anesthesiologist-designed pager alerts improved charting from 98.7% to 99.96% while increasing revenue by an estimated $400,000 per year in one hospital system [6, 22]. Recommendations for other cost savings measures derived from EHR and AIMS use may be made based on anesthesiologist input.

The anesthesia team further increases patient safety with their ability to customize, design, and improve EHR/AIMS. EHR/AIMS are not static systems and rely on user feedback. This dynamic and malleable nature allows physicians and other users to provide ongoing feedback. For example, clinical decision support systems are often initiated by users who are familiar with the latest evidence-based guidelines and protocols [5, 16]. These alerts can be displayed in real time on the user interface and can warn users about dosing, or serve as reminders for medications such as postoperative nausea vomiting prophlyaxis [18, 22]. In more advanced systems, artificial intelligence and machine learning can provide additional safety alerts or warn anesthesiologists to avoid concurrency [1, 16]. Predictions using artificial intelligence regarding the risk of postoperative nausea and vomiting and other adverse events are critically helpful [2]. Operationally, end of the surgery prediction times can also be predicted with artificial intelligence [14]. The basis of these warnings or reminders are often guided by anesthesiologists [20]. Ultimately, this has led to reduction in errors, and improved patient outcomes [22]. Anesthesiologists may also integrate customized macros into AIMS for starting cases and handoff checklists when transitioning between providers. This ensures accurate and efficient documentation and that a comprehensive handoff is performed.

AIMS and EHR provide vast depositories of data that may be utilized by the anesthesia team to make major decisions related to quality improvement/assurance and clinical research. Hospital and perioperative quality improvement projects are frequently original ideas from the anesthesia department and rely on data from patient care [7]. For example, efforts to improve turnover time, first case on-time starts, and antibiotic compliance may be championed by anesthesiologists [2]. Antibiotic compliance increased from 82 to 89%, and missing allergy information decreased from 30% to 8% in one study [18]. Moreover, arterial line documentation compliance improved from 75 to 88 to 99% in an additional paper [16]. Quality assurance documentation compliance increased from 55 to 78% with anesthesiologist education and workflow integrations [22]. Rare events are also captured with large data collection [17]. Even the terminology and standardization of anesthesia data elements are dependent on anesthesiologists' input. If data is not consistent, the collection is too varied and hard to analyze. Communication is also enhanced with the standardization of clinical terminology.

At a management or health system executive level, anesthesiologists participate in clinical informatics where they help choose vendors, assist in implementation and process improvement. The process can be managed with an AIMS steering committee, often 1 to 2 years in advance of deployment. Decision about best of breed versus best fit may have to be made [13]. There are about 10–15 vendors that have some market share so the choices are not always straightforward [9]. For large hospitals, 2–3 vendors are often competing for selection, and anesthesiologists provide valuable industry insight for the selection process [13]. Smooth transitions from legacy systems to more advanced EHR/AIMS are essential to ensure all revenue is captured and compliance goals are met [4]. It is a large undertaking to transition electronic systems, and anesthesiologists often become superusers who educate and assist other users in their transitions [21].

On a performance level, anesthesiologist operations leaders create personalized feedback reports for their staff. This often involves extracting data from the EHR/AIMS. For example, in one quality improvement effort to reduce gas flow levels, e-mail reports were sent to anesthesia providers outlining quantities they had used and how much could have been saved by using less [3]. Moreover, MPOG also provides individual and department wide analytics reports. For example, linking data from the AIMS can demonstrate how many paralytic cases checked train of four (an effective, but often overlooked metric) before reversal of muscle paralysis. The content of the reports are emailed to providers and ultimately allow for better practices, cost savings, and coaching of providers. In other national programs, similar data access helps in the National Surgical Quality Improvement Program, Wake Up Safe, and most recently the Anesthesia Community Registry with its link to EPIC EHR (Faulkner, J. 1999, EPIC (Electronic Health Record) Epic Systems Corporation). Anesthesiologists contribute to the setup of data transfer automation in these data registries [2].

There are other service lines also dependent on AIMS anesthesiology assistance. Anesthesiologists in this role serve as gatekeepers and collaborators. For example, transfusion medicine may access the operating room schedule, review CPT codes and diagnoses, and use this information to predict how many units of blood will be needed for cases. In more advanced systems, there would be no need to order blood products as they would automatically be ready based on the AIMS data [15]. Furthermore, pharmacies utilize the AIMS to surveil drug diversion risk factors.

From a professional liability perspective, anesthesiologists have a major role in optimizing the EHR/AIMS to reduce risk. Ensuring documentation of the appropriate elements of a case, reviewing adverse events, and documenting relevant findings allow more transparency. The ASA closed claims reviews from anesthesiologists shed insight into adverse events that occur. The customizable pop-up reminders, alerts, and soft and hard stops rely on anesthesiologists input and reduce medical errors.

EHR and AIMS are an integral and vital part of medical ecosytems. Anesthesiologists play a critical role in the selection, implementation, maintenance, and utilization of these systems.

References

1. Amici LD, van Pelt M, Mylott L, Langlieb M, Nanji KC. Clinical decision support as a prevention tool for medication errors in the operating room: a retrospective cross-sectional study. Anesth Analg. 2024; https://doi.org/10.1213/ane.0000000000007058.
2. Dutton RP, DuKatz A. Quality improvement using automated data sources: the anesthesia quality institute. Anesthesiol Clin. 2011;29(3):439–54. https://doi.org/10.1016/j.anclin.2011.05.002.
3. Epstein RH, Dexter F, Patel N. Influencing anesthesia provider behavior using anesthesia information management system data for near real-time alerts and post hoc reports. Anesth Analg. 2015;121(3):678–92). Lippincott Williams and Wilkins. https://doi.org/10.1213/ANE.0000000000000677.
4. Epstein RH, Dexter F, Schwenk ES. Provider access to legacy electronic anesthesia records following implementation of an electronic health record system. J Med Syst. 2019;43(5) https://doi.org/10.1007/s10916-019-1232-6.
5. Harutyunyan R, Jeffries SD, Ramírez-Garcíaluna JL, Hemmerling TM. Clinical performance of decision support systems in anesthesia, intensive care, and emergency medicine: a systematic review and meta-analysis. Anesth Analg. 2023;136(6):1084–95. https://doi.org/10.1213/ANE.0000000000006500.

6. Jang J, Yu SH, Kim CB, Moon Y, Kim S. The effects of an electronic medical record on the completeness of documentation in the anesthesia record. Int J Med Informatics. 2013;82(8):702–7. https://doi.org/10.1016/j.ijmedinf.2013.04.004.
7. Kadry B, Feaster WW, MacArio A, Ehrenfeld JM. Anesthesia information management systems: past, present, and future of anesthesia records. Mount Sinai J Med. 2012;79(1):154–65. https://doi.org/10.1002/msj.21281.
8. Kahn RA, Gal JS, Hofer IS, Wax DB, Villar JI, Levin MA. Visual analytics to leverage anesthesia electronic health record. Anesth Analg. 2022;135(5):1057–63. https://doi.org/10.1213/ANE.0000000000006175.
9. Kazemi P, Lau F, Matava C, Simpao AF. An environmental scan of anesthesia information management systems in the American and Canadian marketplace. J Med Syst. 2021;45(12) https://doi.org/10.1007/s10916-021-01781-0.
10. Kheterpal S, Tremper KK. Information technology comes to anesthesiology. Anesthesiol Clin. 2011;29(3) https://doi.org/10.1016/j.anclin.2011.05.011.
11. Kruger GH, Tremper KK. Advanced integrated real-time clinical displays. Anesthesiol Clin. 2011;29(3):487–504. https://doi.org/10.1016/j.anclin.2011.05.004.
12. Lai M, Kheterpal S. Creating a real return-on-investment for information system implementation: life after HITECH. Anesthesiol Clin. 2011;29(3):413–38. https://doi.org/10.1016/j.anclin.2011.05.005.
13. Muravchick S, Caldwell JE, Epstein RH, Galati M, Levy WJ, O'Reilly M, Plagenhoef JS, Rehman M, Reich DL, Vigoda MM. Anesthesia information management system implementation: a practical guide. Anesth Analg. 2008;107(5):1598–608. https://doi.org/10.1213/ane.0b013e318187bc8f.
14. Olsen RM, Aasvang EK, Meyhoff CS, Dissing Sorensen HB. Towards an automated multimodal clinical decision support system at the post anesthesia care unit. Comput Biol Med. 2018;101:15–21. https://doi.org/10.1016/j.compbiomed.2018.07.018.
15. Rinehart JB, Lee TC, Kaneshiro K, Tran MH, Sun C, Kain ZN. Perioperative blood ordering optimization process using information from an anesthesia information management system. Transfusion. 2016;56(4):938–45. https://doi.org/10.1111/trf.13492.
16. Shah NJ, Tremper KK, Kheterpal S. Anatomy of an anesthesia information management system. Anesthesiol Clin. 2011;29(3):355–65. https://doi.org/10.1016/j.anclin.2011.05.013.
17. Simpao AF, Rehman MA. Anesthesia informatics in 2018. In: Advances in anesthesia, vol. 37. Academic; 2019. p. 145–62. https://doi.org/10.1016/j.aan.2019.08.006.
18. Simpao AF, Tan JM, Lingappan AM, Gálvez JA, Morgan SE, Krall MA. A systematic review of near real-time and point-of-care clinical decision support in anesthesia information management systems. J Clin Monit Comput. 2017;31(5):885–94). Springer. https://doi.org/10.1007/s10877-016-9921-x.
19. Springman SR. Integration of the enterprise electronic health record and anesthesia information management systems. Anesthesiol Clin. 2011;29(3):455–83. https://doi.org/10.1016/j.anclin.2011.05.007.
20. St. Jacques P, Rothman B. Enhancing point of care vigilance using computers. Anesthesiol Clin. 2011;29(3):505–19. https://doi.org/10.1016/j.anclin.2011.05.008.
21. Vigoda MM, Rothman B, Green JA. Shortcomings and challenges of information system adoption. Anesthesiol Clin. 2011;29(3):397–412. https://doi.org/10.1016/j.anclin.2011.05.010.
22. Wanderer JP, Sandberg WS, Ehrenfeld JM. Real-time alerts and reminders using information systems. Anesthesiol Clin. 2011;29(3):389–96. https://doi.org/10.1016/j.anclin.2011.05.003.

22 Quality Management and the Anesthesiologist's Role in Advancing Perioperative Excellence

Vilma Joseph and Terry Chambers

22.1 Introduction

Quality management in anesthesiology is not merely a set of compliance activities—it is the systematic pursuit of safer, more efficient, and patient-centered perioperative care. Anesthesiologists, uniquely positioned at the crossroads of surgery, critical care, and hospital operations, are natural leaders in translating clinical excellence into measurable outcomes. Our practice spans the operating room, post-anesthesia care unit (PACU), intensive care unit (ICU), labor and delivery, interventional suites, and procedural areas such as cardiology, endoscopy and radiology. Across these environments, anesthesiologists drive patient safety initiatives, develop quality indicators, and integrate data analytics that shape the delivery of modern healthcare.

The imperative for anesthesiologists to engage in quality management stems from both internal motivations—professional stewardship and ethical duty—and external forces such as regulatory programs, reimbursement models, and accreditation requirements. This chapter explores the multifaceted role of anesthesiologists in leading quality improvement (QI), from evidence-based measure development to systems-based innovation.

V. Joseph (✉) ·
Department of Anesthesiology, Montefiore Medical Center, Weiler Hospital, New York, NY, USA
Department of Anesthesiology, Albert Einstein College of Medicine/Montefiore Medical Center/Moses Campus, New York, USA

T. Chambers
Department of Anesthesiology, Albert Einstein College of Medicine/Montefiore Medical Center/Moses Campus, New York, USA

G. Tewfik (ed.), *The Anesthesiologist as Perioperative Leader*,
https://doi.org/10.1007/978-3-032-18058-2_22

22.2 The Foundation of Quality Management in Anesthesiology

Quality in healthcare encompasses six domains defined by the Institute of Medicine: safety, effectiveness, patient-centeredness, timeliness, efficiency, and equity [1]. Within anesthesiology, these dimensions intersect daily practice—from medication administration to multidisciplinary collaboration.

22.2.1 Historical Context

The specialty's longstanding commitment to patient safety dates to the formation of the Anesthesia Patient Safety Foundation (APSF) in 1985—the first medical foundation dedicated exclusively to safety improvement. The APSF's ethos, "that no patient shall be harmed by anesthesia," catalyzed a global transformation in medical quality, leading to widespread adoption of monitoring standards such as pulse oximetry and capnography.

22.2.2 The Anesthesiologist as Systems Leader

Anesthesiologists are uniquely trained in real-time risk management and crisis response. These skills position them as "systems thinkers," capable of bridging operational silos. Their influence extends into hospital quality committees, surgical services governance, and performance improvement programs that tie directly into reimbursement and public reporting.

22.3 Core Domains of Quality in Anesthesiology

22.3.1 Clinical Effectiveness and Evidence-Based Practice

Quality management begins with adherence to evidence-based clinical guidelines. Anesthesiologists enhance outcomes by implementing protocols for the following:

- Maintenance of perioperative normothermia
- Prophylaxis for postoperative nausea and vomiting (PONV)
- Preoperative antibiotic timing and redosing
- Smoking cessation counseling
- Prevention of venous thromboembolism (VTE)

Each of these measures not only reduces morbidity but also qualifies under the Centers for Medicare & Medicaid Services (CMS) Quality Payment Program.

22.3.2 Patient Safety and Event Prevention

Safety culture in anesthesiology relies on continuous monitoring, root-cause analysis, and proactive risk identification. Near-miss tracking systems—integrated through the Anesthesia Quality Institute's (AQI) *Anesthesia Incident Reporting System (AIRS)*—allow benchmarking of events such as airway difficulties, medication errors, or equipment failures. These data feed directly into national safety alerts and best-practice updates.

22.3.3 Operational Efficiency

Anesthesiologists' expertise in workflow optimization extends beyond the OR. By analyzing start-time accuracy, turnover time, and PACU throughput, anesthesiologists help hospitals identify inefficiencies that impact case volume and cost. Integration of OR dashboards and predictive scheduling analytics further illustrates how quality and efficiency intersect to create institutional value.

22.4 National Quality Frameworks and Programs

22.4.1 CMS Quality Payment Program

The CMS Quality Payment Program (QPP) links physician reimbursement to performance on selected quality measures. Anesthesiologists participate via the following:

1. **Merit-Based Incentive Payment System (MIPS)**—assesses clinicians across Quality, Improvement Activities, Cost, and Promoting Interoperability categories.
2. **MIPS Value Pathways (MVPs)**—streamline reporting by aligning specialty-specific measures.
3. **Alternative Payment Models (APMs)**—reward groups assuming financial risk for patient outcomes.

Anesthesia-specific MIPS measures include normothermia maintenance, prophylaxis for PONV, pediatric vomiting prevention, and perioperative smoking abstinence counseling. Consistent participation enhances both payment and institutional standing in public reporting databases.

22.4.2 Hospital Value-Based Purchasing (HVBP)

Under HVBP, hospitals receive financial incentives tied to performance on clinical outcomes, patient experience, and efficiency. Anesthesiologists influence several domains—particularly those affecting surgical complications, readmissions, and patient satisfaction. Their leadership in optimizing perioperative workflows directly supports HVBP metrics.

22.4.3 The Role of Accreditation and Certification

Accrediting bodies such as *The Joint Commission* increasingly evaluate anesthesia-related safety protocols as part of hospital certification. Demonstrating adherence to national guidelines on PONV prophylaxis, infection prevention, and Enhanced Recovery After Surgery implementation strengthens institutional readiness for certification audits.

22.5 Quality Infrastructure: ASA, AQI, and CPOM

The American Society of Anesthesiologists (ASA) plays a pivotal role in advancing the specialty's quality infrastructure. Its *Committee on Performance and Outcomes Measurement (CPOM)* and the *Anesthesia Quality Institute (AQI)* anchor national efforts to define, collect, and analyze performance data.

22.5.1 ASA CPOM

CPOM helps to develop anesthesia-relevant quality metrics that are scientifically valid, clinically meaningful, and aligned with CMS requirements. Each metric undergoes rigorous validation, literature review, and stakeholder input. Examples include the following:

- Postoperative hypothermia avoidance
- Timely antibiotic administration
- Multimodal pain management adherence

CPOM's collaboration with CMS ensures anesthesia's voice is represented in national policymaking. Members also participate in the *Partnership for Quality Measurement*, which reviews and approves CMS-endorsed metrics.

22.5.2 ASA Anesthesia Quality Institute (AQI)

Founded in 2008, the AQI collects data from thousands of practice sites through the *National Anesthesia Clinical Outcomes Registry (NACOR)*. NACOR serves as the most comprehensive repository of anesthesia data worldwide, encompassing over 60 million cases. It provides the following:

- Benchmarking reports comparing institutional performance
- Data for CMS QPP submissions

- Insights for academic research and guideline development

Anesthesiologists can use AQI dashboards to identify performance gaps and design targeted interventions. In partnership with electronic health record vendors like EPIC, the AQI is expanding its analytic capability, integrating structured data fields for real-time performance feedback.

22.6 Measure Development and Data-Driven Improvement

The process of developing new anesthesia quality measures follows a rigorous pathway:

1. **Concept Identification**: Emerging clinical concerns or research findings are reviewed to identify performance gaps.
2. **Measure Specification**: Each measure defines the numerator (compliant cases), denominator (eligible patients), and exclusion criteria.
3. **Testing and Validation**: Measures undergo pilot testing for reliability, validity and feasibility.
4. **Implementation and Maintenance**: Finalized measures are updated annually with new evidence.

Anesthesiologists are encouraged to participate in measure development workgroups, ensuring relevance and feasibility for real-world practice.

22.7 Quality in Practice: From Metrics to Meaning

Collecting data is only the first step; translating insights into practice change is the true hallmark of quality management.

22.7.1 Clinical Dashboards

Real-time dashboards integrate OR data, physiologic monitoring, and EHR metrics to provide continuous feedback. Institutions using anesthesia-led dashboards have reported measurable improvements in case start times, antibiotic compliance, and PACU throughput.

22.7.2 Peer Review and Morbidity/Mortality Conferences

Structured peer review is central to maintaining safety culture. Modern Morbidity & Mortality conferences emphasize system analysis over individual blame, identifying latent factors such as communication breakdowns or workflow flaws. Anesthesiologists, due to their cross-disciplinary role, often lead these reviews.

22.7.3 Continuous Professional Development

The Maintenance of Certification in Anesthesiology (MOCA 2.0) program includes QI projects as core components. These initiatives encourage anesthesiologists to document performance improvement within their own practice, promoting lifelong learning.

22.8 The Economics of Quality: Aligning Safety and Sustainability

Quality improvement is not only ethically imperative but economically strategic. Hospitals face increasing financial risk from readmissions, complications, and inefficiencies. Anesthesia-led QI projects—such as reducing PONV-related admissions or optimizing PACU throughput—demonstrate measurable return on investment.

Anesthesiologists who link QI metrics to operational savings strengthen the specialty's position in institutional negotiations. As hospital systems transition toward value-based purchasing, quality metrics become currency for advocacy, leadership, and resource allocation.

22.9 Leveraging Informatics and Artificial Intelligence

The next frontier of quality management lies in informatics. Advanced analytics enable identification of patterns invisible to human review—such as subtle correlations between intraoperative hypotension and postoperative kidney injury. AI-driven surveillance systems can generate predictive alerts, guiding anesthesiologists toward proactive interventions.

The integration of EPIC Community with AQI represents a major step toward automated quality reporting. This real-time data linkage will allow for continuous risk stratification and outcome prediction, fundamentally transforming how anesthesiologists engage with quality improvement.

22.10 Education, Leadership, and the Human Factor

Effective quality management requires cultivating leadership skills. Anesthesiologists should actively participate in hospital quality councils, perioperative governance boards, and institutional accreditation teams. Serving on such committees not only advances the specialty's visibility but ensures that anesthesia-relevant quality domains—airway safety, hemodynamic control, and postoperative pain management—receive institutional attention.

Educational initiatives in residency and fellowship programs now include QI methodology, Lean and Six Sigma principles, and data literacy. Trainees who master these frameworks become future leaders capable of transforming systems, not just delivering care.

22.11 Challenges and Future Directions

Despite robust infrastructure, the following challenges remain:

- **Data Overload**: Clinicians often face "metric fatigue." Future systems must prioritize actionable data rather than sheer volume.
- **Equity and Access**: Quality must also address disparities in care delivery across patient demographics and institutions.
- **Integration Across Care Continuum**: Linking preoperative optimization, intraoperative management, and postoperative outcomes remains a work in progress.

Emerging innovations—AI-enabled monitoring, precision medicine, and predictive analytics—offer opportunities to refine these systems and further enhance safety.

22.12 Conclusion

Anesthesiologists stand at the nexus of clinical performance and organizational strategy. Through rigorous quality management, they translate data into decisions that safeguard patients, improve efficiency, and strengthen institutional value. From national quality programs to bedside initiatives, anesthesiology exemplifies how medicine can lead in continuous improvement. As healthcare evolves toward transparency, accountability, and value-based care, anesthesiologists will remain indispensable architects of safer, smarter, and more sustainable perioperative systems.

Reference

1. Institute of Medicine (IOM). Crossing the quality chasm: a new health system for the 21st century. Washington, DC: National Academy Press; 2001.

At the Crossroads of Safety: The Anesthesiologist's Leadership in Preventing Harm

23

Emily Methangkool

23.1 Introduction

Patient safety is "the absence of preventable harm to a patient and reduction of risk of unnecessary harm associated with health care to an acceptable minimum" [1]. Although often conflated with one another, patient safety and quality are distinct but related concepts. The Agency for Healthcare Research and Quality (AHRQ) defines six domains of high-quality care: safety, effectiveness, patient-centered care, timeliness, efficiency, and equity [2]. While safety is an essential component of high-quality care, it is primarily focused on preventing and mitigating harm to patients.

Anesthesiology has long been lauded as an exemplar in patient safety [3]. However, critical issues in anesthesia patient safety continue to persist, ranging from technical complications such as unplanned reintubation, aspiration, and medication error to nontechnical issues such as communication, teamwork, and production pressure. As such, it is critical that the perioperative physician understand the history of anesthesia patient safety, concepts in safety science, as well as how to effectively implement a patient safety program.

23.2 History of Anesthesia Patient Safety

Anesthesia is an area in which very impressive improvements in safety have been made.— Institute of Medicine report, "To Err is Human" [3]

The potentially fatal consequences of anesthesia began to be recognized not long after its first demonstration in Boston in 1846. The epidemiologist John Snow

E. Methangkool (✉)
Department of Anesthesiology and Perioperative Medicine, University of California, Los Angeles, Los Angeles, CA, USA
e-mail: emethangkool@mednet.ucla.edu

G. Tewfik (ed.), *The Anesthesiologist as Perioperative Leader*,
https://doi.org/10.1007/978-3-032-18058-2_23

documented several cases of the fatal administration of chloroform, beginning with Hannah Greener in 1848. Greener was a 14-year-old undergoing an ingrown toenail removal; within half a minute of chloroform administration, she became unarousable, and within 2 minutes from the start of the procedure she was dead [4]. Another case occurred in 1848 due to airway obstruction from application of the ether cloth. These are some of the first documented cases of a medication error in anesthesiology, likely attributable to lack of education and training on anesthetic dosing.

Despite the well-recognized risks of anesthesia, there was little progress in patient safety until a commission convened in 1945 found that 67% of anesthetic deaths were preventable. They stated that "The probable foremost benefit [of the finding] is the direction of the attention of the medical profession to fatalities occurring from improper anesthesia and its mismanagement which otherwise would be considered attributable to other causes." [5] In 1954, Beecher and Todd published their study on anesthetic mortality using a data set of 599,548 cases from 10 institutions from 1948 to 1952, finding that 1 in 1560 deaths were directly attributable to anesthetic care [6]. Subsequently, there was much blame placed on individual practitioners for errors; Keats wrote in 1979 about the "error-seeking bias" of these early investigations, which focused primarily on individual errors rather than the potential toxicity of anesthetic medications [7].

The turning point in anesthesia patient safety came in the 1980s, when several things happened simultaneously. In 1982, the television news program 20/20 brought the issue of anesthesia safety to the forefront of public consciousness; the program began, "If you are going to go into anesthesia, you are going on a long trip and you should not do it, if you can avoid it in any way. General anesthesia is safe most of the time, but there are dangers from human error, carelessness, and a critical shortage of anesthesiologists. This year, 6000 patients will die or suffer brain damage." [8] Given the public outcry, the American Society of Anesthesiologists (ASA) established a new committee, the Committee on Patient Safety and Risk Management. Around the same time, the chiefs of anesthesia at the Harvard hospitals embarked on an effort to reduce risks associated with anesthesia, as well as to decrease malpractice costs [9]. Their work eventually led to standards for basic anesthetic monitoring that were subsequently adopted by the ASA in 1986 and disseminated nationally [10]. The Anesthesia Patient Safety Foundation was founded in 1985, focused on funding research and education in patient safety through a multidisciplinary approach involving anesthesiologists, nurse anesthetists, and industry representatives. Separately, maturation of technologies such as pulse oximetry and capnography allowed improved intraoperative monitoring of patients. Taken together, these events brought about improved mortality statistics and decreased anesthetic morbidity. The tremendous improvements in anesthesia patient safety led Lucian Leape to write that anesthesiology is "the only system in health care that begins to approach the vaunted 'six-sigma' level of perfection" [11].

23.3 Foundations of Safety in Anesthesia Practice

> *The single greatest impediment to error prevention in the medical industry is that we punish people for making mistakes.—Lucian Leape* [12]

23.3.1 Safety Culture, Just Culture, and Psychological Safety

A detailed understanding of safety culture, Just Culture, and psychological safety are fundamental to understanding patient safety. Just Culture and psychological safety are essential elements of safety culture, which is typically defined as the set of attitudes, values, and patterns of behavior shared by providers within an organization that are related to the pursuit of patient safety [13, 14]. A positive safety culture is characterized by the following key elements:

- Acknowledgment that the practice of medicine is high risk.
- Dedication to patient safety in spite of that risk.
- Engagement from everyone in finding solutions to problems.
- Commitment from leadership to providing resources to improve patient safety.
- Ability to report adverse events and near-misses without fear of blame or punishment [15]

A culture of blame, cited as early as the 1970s by Arthur Keats, is detrimental to the pursuit of patient safety because it makes individuals much less likely to report errors [7, 16]. Without reports of errors, it is impossible to identify interventions to improve safety.

A Just Culture is one in which individuals involved in adverse events are not blamed for errors related to poor system design or failures, but are held accountable when reckless action is the underlying root cause [17]. Psychological safety is an environment in which individuals are able—even obligated—to speak up about concerns and one where colleagues build trust, respect one another, and have the freedom to be candid [18, 19]. A robust culture of safety, along with Just Culture and psychological safety, provides the foundation to pursue patient safety.

23.3.2 Errors at the Blunt End

The British psychologist James Reason is well known for his work on human error, which has been applied across diverse fields such as aviation, healthcare, and manufacturing. His "Swiss cheese" model is often cited as a model for envisioning how adverse events occur [20]. Reason describes two approaches to error: the person approach, which focuses on individual mistakes, and the systems approach, which acknowledges that systemic failures are often at the root of many errors. The person approach posits that errors are due to the actions of those at the "sharp end" (e.g., closest to the patient), and are usually the result of forgetfulness, inattention, carelessness, negligence, or recklessness. These are also known as *active* errors. In contrast, the systems approach acknowledges that humans are fallible, and errors are inevitable. These errors occur at the "blunt end" and are often the result of underlying issues or design failures that may take time to manifest—also known as *latent* errors. In the Swiss cheese model, there are multiple layers of defense between an error and a patient—process, protocol, procedure, vigilance, alarms, etc.; however, each layer of defense may have a weakness (the "hole") (Fig. 23.1). In usual circumstances, harm may not come to a patient; however, when the holes align, an adverse outcome may occur [21].

23.3.3 Threats to Patient Safety: Cognitive Errors, Cognitive Overload, and Production Pressure

Decision-making is most commonly thought to occur via two mechanisms: fast (System 1) and slow (System 2) thinking [22]. System 1 thinking is often unconscious and effortless and based on pattern recognition or experience; however, it may also be susceptible to cognitive bias. Such bias may result in the exclusion of certain perspectives or alternative choices. System 2 thinking, on the other hand, requires more conscious effort and involves logical thinking, deduction, and processing. Common cognitive biases include premature closure, confirmation bias, omission bias, anchoring, overconfidence bias, framing effect, availability bias, and fixation error (Table 23.1) [23]. An unfortunate example of fixation error contributing to grave patient harm is that of Elaine Bromiley, an otherwise healthy mother of 2 who presented for routine otolaryngologic surgery [24]. After induction of

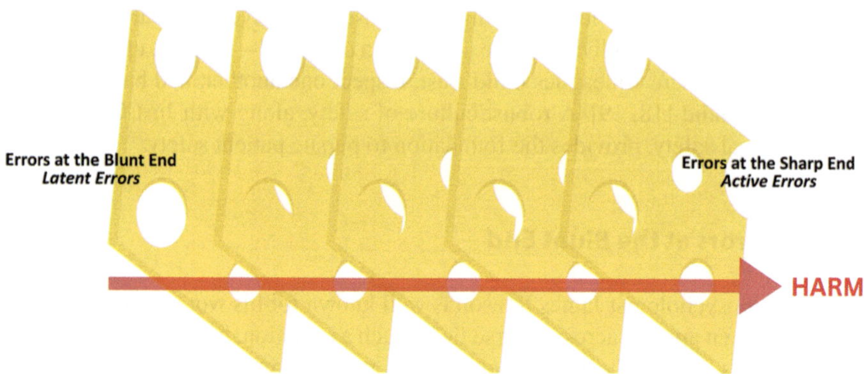

Fig. 23.1 Swiss cheese model of error. In the Swiss cheese model of error, multiple layers, such as process, procedure, equipment, or design, help prevent patient harm. However, each of these layers may also have a weakness (the "hole"). When the holes align, or when circumstances expose the weaknesses of each layer all at once, harm may come to a patient

Table 23.1 Common cognitive biases

Cognitive bias	Description
Premature closure	Accepting a diagnosis before alternatives have been considered and before verification of all the facts; "jumping to conclusions"
Confirmation bias	Seeking information to support a preconceived diagnosis or idea
Omission bias	Judging harm from action more negatively than harm from inaction
Anchoring bias	Fixating on the initial diagnosis despite new information
Overconfidence bias	Overestimating knowledge, judgment or management ability
Framing effect	Making different decisions based on how options are presented
Availability bias	Relying on information, diagnoses, or options that most easily come to mind
Fixation error	Focusing on a single aspect of a case, diagnosis or solution, to the exclusion of other diagnoses or options

anesthesia, she was unable to be ventilated or intubated, leading to 23 minutes of hypoxia. She developed anoxic brain injury and expired 7 days later. While there were several issues during the case that contributed to her injury, including strict hierarchical gradients and lack of psychological safety, the medical team's fixation on securing her airway, neglecting to proceed down the difficult airway algorithm, played a key role.

The high-pressure, time-sensitive, and elevated stakes nature of the operating room can exacerbate the patient safety impact of cognitive biases. Strategies to reduce potential cognitive biases include cognitive forcing strategies, clinical decision support, and cognitive aids [25, 26]. Cognitive forcing strategies encourage slower thinking by engaging in exercises to reason, test hypotheses, entertain alternative possibilities, and reflect [27]. Examples include the rule of three (three alternative explanations for a diagnosis should be considered) and prospective hindsight (imagine a situation where the decision is wrong, and ask "What did I miss?") [23, 28]. Both cognitive aids and clinical decision support may help aid in exploring alternative possibilities. Ultimately, the design of a safe working environment must keep in mind the human propensity for these cognitive biases.

Another psychological phenomenon called cognitive overload may also significantly impact patient safety. Cognitive overload occurs when a plethora of sensory input threatens to overwhelm an individual's ability to process information and make decisions [29]. In the operating room environment, there can many competing factors for an anesthesiologist's attention: hemodynamics, ranging from routine vital signs such as blood pressure and heart rate to measurements of cardiac index, systemic vascular resistance, and cerebral oximetry; requests from the surgeon for table height or position; information passed from the circulator nurse about critical lab values; background music; conversation among the surgical team; the presence of medical students or other trainees; the transesophageal echocardiogram or noninvasive cardiac output monitor; and all the various alarms associated with operating room devices. Managing all these inputs requires continuous multitasking; however, only 13% of clinicians report that they are able to multitask without performance decrement [30]. In particular, cognitive overload may impact medication safety; 23.1% of medication errors are attributed to distraction and cognitive overload, and each interruption of a medication-related task increases risk of error by 25% [31–34]. Task interruptions, in particular, are frequent and have a negative impact on patient safety [35–38]. Poor ergonomics may also increase cognitive overload; having to manage medication preparation in cardiac catheterization laboratories with poor lighting, for example, increases cognitive processing requirements and is a prime environment for medication errors.

Technological improvements designed to improve clinical care may also contribute to cognitive overload. Documentation in the electronic medical record has been known to distract from patient care [39, 40]. Over the course of a standard shift, a clinician may be exposed to over 1000 alarms, 80–90% of which are nonactionable [41, 42]; as a result, alarm fatigue ensues and increases response times to patient changes [43, 44]. Each sensory input may require the clinician to switch tasks cognitively; however, this readjustment often slows response and increases risk for error [45]. After each task interruption, it can take several seconds to reorient to another complex task [46–48].

Production pressures may also contribute to errors and may occur when overt or covert pressures place incentives on personnel to prioritize efficiency, throughput, or productivity over safety. Contributors to production pressure include financial considerations, excessive surgical backlogs, and inadequate staffing, which can, in turn, engender a poor safety culture and clinician burnout and attrition. Eric Hollnagel describes the Efficiency and Thoroughness Tradeoff (ETTO) Spectrum: one can have a high degree of thoroughness but low efficiency, or a low degree of thoroughness and high efficiency (Fig. 23.2) [49]. At the far left of the spectrum, safety may be maintained, but patients will not receive efficient or timely care; at the far right of the spectrum, productivity is maximized, but safety may be sacrificed. The middle of the spectrum, therefore, should be the goal to maintain patient safety while providing high-quality care.

Production pressure is a daily occurrence in the operating room; in a study of California anesthesiologists, 49% had observed an anesthesiologist pressured to conduct anesthesia in an unsafe fashion given the level of urgency, and 63% had made errors due to the workload within a case [50]. Other studies have confirmed pressures on clinicians to perform tasks in as little time as possible and to yield to surgeon demands to proceed with cases even if not in the patient's best interest [51]. However, these pressures are not isolated to anesthesiology; in a survey study, many

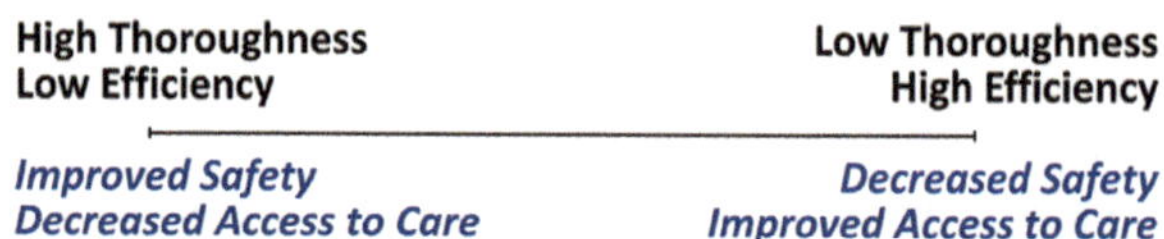

Fig. 23.2 Efficiency and thoroughness tradeoff spectrum. When there is high thoroughness, there may be improved safety but decreased efficiency and access to care; when there is low thoroughness, there may be decreased safety but improved efficiency and access to care

gastroenterologists admitted to altering normal practices to speed the start of procedures or to get through the patient list for the day [52].

23.3.4 Safety-1, -2, -3 and Resilience

Approaches to safety are often thought of in a spectrum from Safety-1, to Safety-2, to Safety-3 (Fig. 23.3). Most organizations have now moved beyond Safety 0, where individuals were thought to be the primary point of failure. Safety-1 is the approach most commonly used in modern adverse event analysis, and looks into *how things went wrong*. It provides a reactive and retrospective perspective, looking at the chain of events and taking into account both individual and systems failures. Safety-2 is an approach that looks into *how things went right*. It is a prospective look into processes that work well, and investigates how individuals adapt and modify to changing clinical environments to improve safety [53]. Safety-2, however, may be more challenging to implement practically than Safety-1 [54]. Safety-3 has not yet been adopted into healthcare; it is primarily focused on preemptive control and design to promote safety, with elements of both Safety-1 and Safety-2. Both Safety-1 and Safety-2 are needed in a patient safety program; when events occur, there must be mechanisms to identify systematic and/or individual contributors; however, workflows must also be analyzed prospectively to prevent errors before they occur.

Resilience is an essential concept in Safety-2, and it relates to the ability to adapt to dynamic clinical situations in order to maintain or improve safety [55]. It requires proactive anticipation of issues, adaptation to new scenarios, and learning from these changes. Safety-2 also recognizes that there may be a gap between

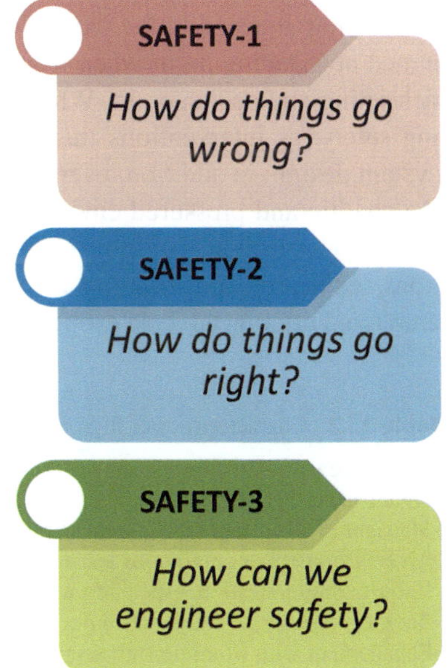

Fig. 23.3 Approaches to safety. Safety-1 primarily focuses on analyzing adverse events and attempting to minimize individual or system failures. Safety-2 seeks to understand how clinicians adapt to dynamic clinical situations, and how safe situations result the majority of the time. Safety-3 includes both Safety-1 and Safety-2 and incorporates proactive system design to prevent errors

"work-as-imagined" and "work-as-done"; that is, the processes and workflows envisioned by leaders within an organization may differ significantly from what is done at the frontline [56, 57]. As a result, standardization should not necessarily always be the goal, as variability and adaptability can lend some measure of safety. What may, in fact, be needed are flexible protocols that allow adaptation while minimizing omission of critical safety steps.

This model of safety has formed the basis for principles behind high-reliability organizations (HROs), which often have nearly error-free performance in the setting of challenging and dynamic high-risk environments [58, 59]. Characteristics of HROs are presented in Table 23.2. HROs are often preoccupied with failure and error, and in so doing are able to anticipate and prepare for those failures. However, this strategy necessitates a proactive orientation toward error and safety, which is not yet consistently implemented within healthcare.

Human factors engineering (HFE) takes into account the propensity for human fallibility, as well as usual human behavior and ability, when designing devices, workflows, protocols, or processes for healthcare. The basic principle behind HFE is to "make it easy to do the right thing" and "impossible to do the wrong thing." [60] HFE relies on four basic principles, ranging from most effective in terms of promoting patient safety to least effective: design, barriers, mitigation, and education and training (Fig. 23.4) [61]. Work environments designed with safety in mind are most likely to be the most effective in promoting patient safety. One potential area where design can make a significant improvement is with "lookalike vials," which pose a significant threat to medication safety; concerted effort can be made among drug manufacturers to adhere to a uniform design per class of medication, rather than having small vials of different medications with similar colored tops and labels. Physical or administrative barriers can prevent harm from coming to a patient, for example, the pin index safety system that prevents a nitrous oxide tank from being attached to the oxygen port of the anesthesia machine. Mitigations are aimed at reducing harm when it occurs. Examples of mitigation strategies include debriefing and peer support. While education and training are critical for maintaining safety, as interventions they are not able to overcome challenges from poor system design; in addition, overreliance on staff to "remember" to do something in the chaotic and pressured environment of the operating room may lead to critical failures more often than not. Unfortunately, for many departments and organizations, education and training are often the first and most frequent intervention employed after an adverse event.

Table 23.2 Characteristics of high-reliability organizations

Characteristics of high-reliability organizations
Deference to experts for decision-making in urgent situations, regardless of position in the organization
Manager involvement in decision-making only when absolutely required
An environment of continuous learning
Robust communication, especially when related to safety
Back-up systems available when needed
Engagement with frontline staff on perspectives about safety

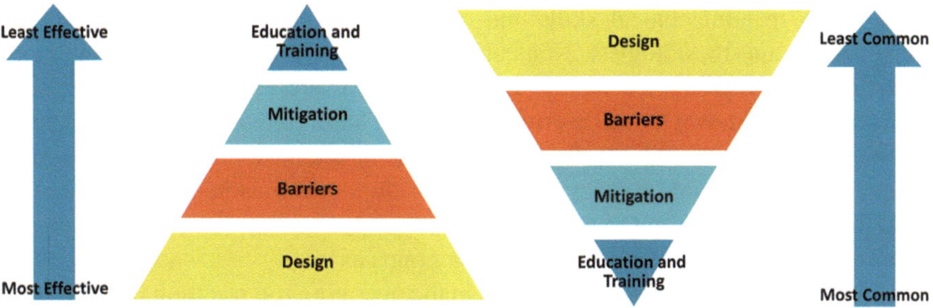

Fig. 23.4 Human factors principles to improve patient safety. Deliberate systems design is the most effective intervention to improve safety, but is often the one least utilized; in contrast, education and training are the least effective interventions to improve safety, but often the easiest to implement and most frequently used

Table 23.3 Elements of a patient safety program

Incident reporting
Adverse event analysis
Training and education
Tracking of key performance indicators
Safety culture assessment
Dedicated leadership

23.4 Creation of a Patient Safety Program

> *The same situation keeps producing the same errors ... even though different people are involved. That surely indicates we are dealing with error prone circumstances rather than error prone people.—James Reason* [20]

A dedicated patient safety program is critical for departments and institutions to maintain patient safety. Elements of a patient safety program are listed in Table 23.3. As incident reporting and adverse event analysis are covered elsewhere in this book, this section will focus primarily on training, metrics, leadership, and assessment.

23.4.1 Education and Training in Patient Safety

While quality improvement and patient safety is an essential topic for certification by the American Board of Anesthesiology, education in patient safety varies from training program to training program. In addition, faculty who completed residency prior to the addition of quality improvement and patient safety to the certification outline may not have the background necessary to guide trainees. As a result, departments should make concerted efforts to implement robust patient safety education for both faculty and trainees. Participation in adverse event analysis and process improvement can help provide hands-on practical experience [62].

Training in nontechnical skills and crew resource management is absolutely essential for anesthesiologists. Nontechnical skills include communication, teamwork, decision-making, leadership, and situational awareness. Deficiencies in such skills have been known to lead to errors and patient harm [63–67]. The Anaesthetists' Non-Technical Skills (ANTS) framework is one of the most commonly used tools and can provide a guide for elements to assess during a simulated or real operative case [68, 69]. Crew resource management is the application of nontechnical skills, and can be incorporated into simulation programs as well.

Communication failures are common in the operating room setting [63, 70]; barriers to communication include perceived hierarchy, incivility, unfamiliarity among team members, and distractions [71]. Simulation, especially when involving other disciplines such as nursing and surgery, can help break down these barriers to communication. In addition, simulation may be particularly helpful to teach "speaking up" behaviors and debriefing. "Speaking up" behaviors occur in the presence of a perceived patient safety incident and facilitate communication about safety concerns, especially when there may be barriers to communication such as an authority gradient between resident and attending (Fig. 23.5). Debriefing after a critical incident can help identify opportunities for improvement while allowing team members to reflect, discuss, and support one another [72].

23.4.2 Key Performance Indicators in Anesthesia Patient Safety

A departmental patient safety program should track anesthesia-specific metrics to identify opportunities for improvement. Many national societies have published indicators, which can provide a starting point. The Anesthesia Quality Institute, for example, utilizes published measures such as preoperative older adult cognitive assessment; neuromuscular blockade and quantitative train-of-four; patient-reported experience with anesthesia; and avoidance of cerebral hyperthermia during

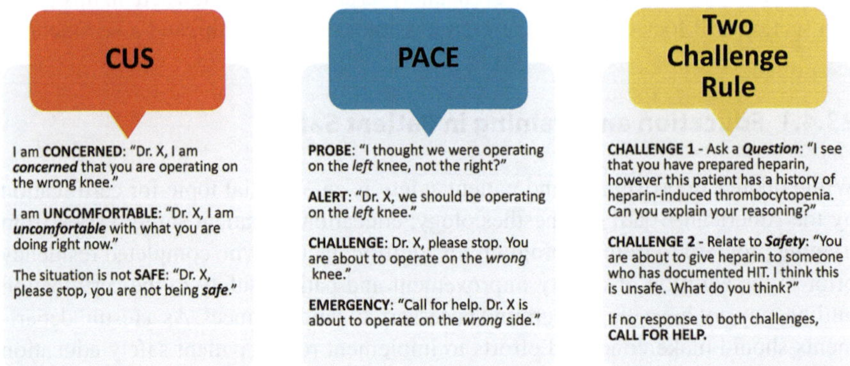

Fig. 23.5 "Speaking up" algorithms. Examples of "speaking up" algorithms—CUS, PACE, and the two-challenge rule. These algorithms can help facilitate communication when a patient safety event occurs, especially when there may be barriers such as unfamiliarity or hierarchical gradients

cardiopulmonary bypass [73]. Other metrics for tracking and intervention are listed in Table 23.4. Metrics should be shared on a regular basis with departmental and institutional leadership as well as among departmental staff members, ideally on a widely available and easily accessible electronic dashboard.

23.4.3 Leadership

A successful departmental patient safety program relies on having personnel with dedicated resources with time to manage adverse event analysis, education, tracking of metrics, and interventions. A Patient Safety Officer should be designated, and should work in close collaboration with the departmental Vice Chair of Quality and Safety [74]. The Patient Safety Officer ideally would have training in safety science, and may pursue designations such as the Certified Professional in Patient Safety (CPPS) offered by the Institute for Healthcare Improvement (IHI) [75]. Importantly, the work of the Patient Safety Officer can only be successful if fully supported by departmental leadership, who should emphasize psychological safety, inclusive leadership behaviors, transparency, honesty, and approachability.

23.4.4 Safety Culture Assessments

Measurement of pre-existing safety culture can help guide work of the departmental patient safety program. Such assessments can help identify strengths and weaknesses in communication, leadership, teamwork, and error reporting and provide avenues for intervention. Several tools exist, including the Survey on Patient Safety Culture from the Agency for Healthcare Research and Quality, the Safety Attitudes Questionnaire, and the Manchester Patient Safety Framework [76, 77]. These tools allow comparisons between departments and national benchmarks and provide a

Table 23.4 Selected patient safety indicators

Patient safety indicators for departmental tracking
Perioperative cardiac arrest
Administration of prophylactic antibiotics
Perioperative mortality
Postdural puncture headache after epidural anesthesia
Unplanned escalation of care
Postanesthesia recovery unit re-intubation
Postoperative renal failure after cardiac surgery
Corneal injury
Central line-associated infections

starting point for intervention. In addition, the implementation of such assessments can promote positive attitudes toward, and engagement in, local safety interventions.

23.5 Conclusion

Patient safety is not a fad. It is not a preoccupation of the past. It is not an objective that has been fulfilled or a reflection of a problem that has been solved. Patient safety is an ongoing necessity. It must be sustained by research, training, and daily application in the workplace.—Ellison C. "Jeep" Pierce, founding president of the Anesthesia Patient Safety Foundation [78]

Patient safety is at the heart of the work of every anesthesiologist. In the operating room, patients are subjected to profound insults, from loss of consciousness to surgical trauma, and it is through the continued and persistent vigilance of dedicated anesthesiologists that, in the overwhelming majority of cases, patients come through their surgery safe and unharmed. While as a specialty anesthesiology no longer faces the hazards of lack of adequate monitoring or technology, errors continue to occur due to contributors such as communication failures, lack of situational awareness, and suboptimal teamwork. In order to mitigate these challenges, perioperative physicians should be educated in safety science and encourage the dedication of resources to safety programs and interventions.

References

1. World Health Organization. Patient Safety. 2023. Available at: https://www.who.int/newsroom/fact-sheets/detail/patient-safety. Accessed 1 May 2025.
2. Agency for Healthcare Quality and Research. Six Domains of Quality. 2025. Available at: https://www.ahrq.gov/talkingquality/measures/six-domains.html. Accessed 1 May 2025.
3. Institute of Medicine (US) Committee on Quality of Health Care in America. In: Kohn LT, Corrigan JM, Donaldson MS, editors. To err is human: building a safer health system. Washington, DC: National Academies Press (US); 2000.
4. Snow J. On the fatal cases of inhalation of chloroform. Edinb Med Surg J. 1849;72:75–87.
5. Ruth HS, Haugen FP, Grove DD. Anesthesia study commission: findings of eleven years' activity. JAMA J Am Med Assoc. 1947;135:881–4.
6. Beecher HK, Todd DP. A study of the deaths associated with anesthesia and surgery. Ann Surg. 1954;140:2–33.
7. Keats AS. What do we know about anesthetic mortality? Anesthesiology. 1979;50:387–92.
8. Pierce EC. Looking back: doctor pierce reflects. APSF Newsl. 2007;22:2.
9. Pandya AN, Majid SZ, Desai MS. The origins, evolution, and spread of anesthesia monitoring standards: from Boston to across the world. Anesthesia Analg. 2020;132:890–8.
10. American Society of Anesthesiologists. Standards for Basic Anesthetic Monitoring. 2020. Available at: https://www.asahq.org/standards-and-practice-parameters/standards-for-basic-anesthetic-monitoring. Accessed 30 Apr 2025.
11. Leape LL, Berwick DM, Bates DW. What practices will most improve safety? Evidence-based medicine meets patient safety. JAMA. 2002;288:501–7.

12. Agency for Healthcare Research and Quality. Individual Clinician Performance. 2025. Available at: https://psnet.ahrq.gov/primer/individual-clinician-performance-issues. Accessed 17 May 2025.
13. Reason J, Hobbs A. Managing maintenance error: a practical guide. Aldershot, Hampshire, England: Ashgate; 2003.
14. Joint Commission. Patient Safety systems. 2025. Available at: https://www.jointcommission.org/-/media/tjc/documents/standards/ps-chapters/2025/number-2-camhospital_ps_jan_2025.pdf. Accessed 1 May 2025.
15. Agency for Healthcare Research and Quality. Culture of Safety. 2024. Available at: https://psnet.ahrq.gov/primer/culture-safety. Accessed 8 May 2025.
16. Heard GC, Sanderson PM, Thomas RD. Barriers to adverse event and error reporting in anesthesia. Anesth Analg. 2012;114:604–14.
17. Marx D. Patient Safety and the "just culture": a primer for health care executives. New York: Trustees of Columbia University, 2001.
18. Edmondson A. Psychological safety and learning behavior in work teams. Adm Sci Q. 1999;44:350–83.
19. Edmondson A. The fearless organization. New York: Wiley & Sons; 2018.
20. Reason J. Managing the risks of organizational accidents. London: Ashgate; 1997.
21. Reason J. Human error: models and management. BMJ. 2000;320:768.
22. Kahneman D. Thinking, fast and slow. New York: Farrar, Straus, and Giroux; 2011.
23. Stiegler MP, Neelankavil JP, Canales C, Dhillon A. Cognitive errors detected in anaesthesiology: a literature review and pilot study. Br J Anaesth. 2012;108:229–35.
24. Mcintosh E. The implications of diffusion of responsibility on patient safety during anaesthesia, 'so that others may learn and even more may live'—Martin Bromiley. J Perioper Pr. 2019;29:341–5.
25. Stiegler MP, Tung A. Cognitive processes in anesthesiology decision making. Anesthesiology. 2014;120:204–17.
26. Yan L, Karamchandani K, Gaiser RR, Carr ZJ. Identifying, understanding, and minimizing unconscious cognitive biases in perioperative crisis management: a narrative review. Anesth Analg. 2024;139:68–77.
27. Mamede S, Schmidt HG. The structure of reflective practice in medicine. Med Educ. 2004;38:1302–8.
28. Singh H, Graber M. Reducing diagnostic error through medical home-based primary care reform. JAMA. 2010;304:463–4.
29. Sewell JL, Santhosh L, O'Sullivan PS. How do attending physicians describe cognitive overload among their workplace learners? Med Educ. 2020;54:1129–36.
30. Van Pelt M, Weinger MB. Distractions in the anesthesia work environment. Anesth Analg. 2017;125:347–50.
31. Wahr JA, Abernathy JH, Lazarra EH, Keebler JR, Wall MH, Lynch I, Wolfe R, Cooper RL. Medication safety in the operating room: literature and expert-based recommendations. Br J Anaesth. 2017;118:32–43.
32. Webster CS, Merry AF, Larsson L, McGrath KA, Weller J. The frequency and nature of drug administration error during Anaesthesia. Anaesth Intensive Care. 2001;29:494–500.
33. Cooper L, DiGiovanni N, Schultz L, Taylor AM, Nossaman B. Influences observed on incidence and reporting of medication errors in anesthesia. Can J Anesthesia. 2012;59:562–70.
34. Westbrook JI, Coiera E, Dunsmuir WTM, Brown BM, Kelk N, Paoloni R, Tran C. The impact of interruptions on clinical task completion. Qual Saf Heal Care. 2010;19:284.
35. Campbell G, Arfanis K, Smith AF. Distraction and interruption in anaesthetic practice. Br J Anaesth. 2012;109:707–15.
36. Jothiraj H, Howland-Harris J, Evley R, Moppett IK. Distractions and the anaesthetist: a qualitative study of context and direction of distraction. Br J Anaesth. 2013;111:477–82.
37. Compère V, Croizat G, Popoff B, Allard E, Durey B, Dureuil B, Besnier E, Clavier T, Selim J. Clinical impact of task interruptions on the anaesthetic team and patient safety in the operating theatre. Br J Anaesth. 2023;131:e55–7.

38. Compère V, Besnier E, Clavier T, Byhet N, Lefranc F, Jegou F, Sturzenegger N, Hardy JB, Dureuil B, Elie T. Evaluation of the time spent by anesthetist on clinical tasks in the operating room. Front Med. 2022;8:768919.
39. Arndt BG, Beasley JW, Watkinson MD, Temte JL, Tuan W-J, Sinsky CA, Gilchrist VJ. Tethered to the EHR: primary care physician workload assessment using EHR event log data and time-motion observations. Ann Fam Med. 2017;15:419–26.
40. Sittig DF, Wright A, Ash J, Singh H. New unintended adverse consequences of electronic health records. Yearb Med Inform. 2016;25:7–12.
41. Borowski M, Görges M, Fried R, Such O, Wrede C, Imhoff M. Medical device alarms. Biomed Tech Biomed Eng. 2011;56:73–83.
42. Drew BJ, Harris P, Zègre-Hemsey JK, Mammone T, Schindler D, Salas-Boni R, Bai Y, Tinoco A, Ding Q, Hu X. Insights into the problem of alarm fatigue with physiologic monitor devices: a comprehensive observational study of consecutive intensive care unit patients. PLoS One. 2014;9:e110274.
43. Bailey JM. The implications of probability matching for clinician response to vital sign alarms: a theoretical study of alarm fatigue. Ergonomics. 2015;58:1487–95.
44. Bonafide CP, Lin R, Zander M, Graham CS, Paine CW, Rock W, Rich A, Roberts KE, Fortino M, Nadkarni VM, Localio AR, Keren R. Association between exposure to nonactionable physiologic monitor alarms and response time in a children's hospital. J Hosp Med. 2015;10:345–51.
45. Monsell S. Task switching. Trends Cogn Sci. 2003;7:134–40.
46. Foroughi CK, Werner NE, McKendrick R, Cades DM, Boehm-Davis DA. Individual differences in working-memory capacity and task resumption following interruptions. J Exp Psychol Learn Mem Cogn. 2016;42:1480–8.
47. Monk CA, Trafton JG, Boehm-Davis DA. The effect of interruption duration and demand on resuming suspended goals. J Exp Psychol Appl. 2008;14:299–313.
48. Altmann EM, Trafton JG. Timecourse of recovery from task interruption: data and a model. Psychon Bull Rev. 2007;14:1079–84.
49. Hollnagel E. The ETTO principle: efficiency-thoroughness trade-off: why things that go right sometimes go wrong. London: Ashgate; 2009.
50. Gaba DM, Howard SK, Jump B. Production pressure in the work environment. Anesthesiology. 1994;81:488–500.
51. Chai J, Chong S. Production pressures among anaesthesiologists in Singapore. Singapore Med J. 2018;59:271–8.
52. Whitson MJ, Bodian CA, Aisenberg J, Cohen LB. Is production pressure jeopardizing the quality of colonoscopy? A survey of U.S. endoscopists' practices and perceptions. Gastrointest Endosc. 2012;75:641–648.e8.
53. Kanjia MK, Kurth CD, Hyman D, Williams E, Varughese A. Perspectives on anesthesia and perioperative patient safety: past, present, and future. Anesthesiology. 2024;141:835–48.
54. Leveson N. Safety III: a systems approach to Safety and resilience. 2020. Available at: http://sunnyday.mit.edu/safety-3.pdf. Accessed 8 May 2025.
55. Staender S. Safety-II and resilience. Curr Opin Anaesthesiol. 2015;28:735–9.
56. Arnal-Velasco D, Heras-Hernando V. Learning from errors and resilience. Curr Opin Anaesthesiol. 2023;36:376–81.
57. Smith AF, Plunkett E. People, systems and safety: resilience and excellence in healthcare practice. Anaesthesia. 2019;74:508–17.
58. Serou N, Sahota LM, Husband AK, Forrest SP, Slight RD, Slight SP. Learning from safety incidents in high-reliability organizations: a systematic review of learning tools that could be adapted and used in healthcare. Int J Qual Heal Care. 2021;33:mzab046.
59. Bagnara S, Parlangeli O, Tartaglia R. Are hospitals becoming high reliability organizations? Appl Ergon. 2010;41:713–8.
60. Shorrock S, Williams C. Human factors and ergonomics in practice: improving system performance and human wellbeing in the real world. New York: CRC Press; 2017.

61. Kelly FE, Frerk C, Bailey CR, Cook TM, Ferguson K, Flin R, Fong K, Groom P, John C, Lang AR, Meek T, Miller KL, Richmond L, Sevdalis N, Stacey MR. Human factors in anaesthesia: a narrative review. Anaesthesia. 2023;78:479–90.
62. Harbell MW, Methangkool E. Patient safety education in anesthesia: current state and future directions. Curr Opin Anaesthesiol. 2021;34:720–5.
63. Hu Y-Y, Arriaga AF, Peyre SE, Corso KA, Roth EM, Greenberg CC. Deconstructing intraoperative communication failures. J Surg Res. 2012;177:37–42.
64. Anderson O, Davis R, Hanna GB, Vincent CA. Surgical adverse events: a systematic review. Am J Surg. 2013;206:253–62.
65. Mazzocco K, Petitti DB, Fong KT, Bonacum D, Brookey J, Graham S, Lasky RE, Sexton JB, Thomas EJ. Surgical team behaviors and patient outcomes. Am J Surg. 2009;197:678–85.
66. Catchpole K, Mishra A, Handa A, McCulloch P. Teamwork and error in the operating room. Ann Surg. 2008;247:699–706.
67. Weller J, Boyd M, Cumin D. Teams, tribes and patient safety: overcoming barriers to effective teamwork in healthcare. Postgrad Med J. 2014;90:149–54.
68. Boet S, Larrigan S, Martin L, Liu H, Sullivan KJ, Etherington N. Measuring non-technical skills of anaesthesiologists in the operating room: a systematic review of assessment tools and their measurement properties. Br J Anaesth. 2018;121:1218–26.
69. University of Aberdeen. Framework for Observing and Rating Anaesthetists' Non-Technical Skills. 2012. Available at: https://www.jeehp.org/upload/media/jeehp-13-44-supple1.pdf. Accessed 7 May 2025.
70. Lingard L, Espin S, Whyte S, Regehr G, Baker GR, Reznick R, Bohnen J, Orser B, Doran D, Grober E. Communication failures in the operating room: an observational classification of recurrent types and effects. Qual Saf Heal Care. 2004;13:330.
71. Shi R, Marin-Nevarez P, Hasty B, Roman-Micek T, Hirx S, Anderson T, Schmiederer I, Fanning R, Goldhaber-Fiebert S, Austin N, Lau JN. Operating room in situ interprofessional simulation for improving communication and teamwork. J Surg Res. 2021;260:237–44.
72. Sullivan L, Park R, Staffa SJ, Cravero J, Vinson AE. Rapid debriefings following critical incidents in pediatric anesthesiology. Pediatr Anesthesia. 2023;33:319–20.
73. Anesthesia Quality Institute. Measures & Metrics. 2025. Available at: https://www.asahq.org/aqi/quality/measures. Accessed 8 May 2025.
74. Cohen JB, Patel SY. The successful anesthesia patient Safety officer. Anesth Analg. 2021;133:816–20.
75. Institute for Healthcare Improvement. Certified Professional in Patient Safety (CPPS). Available at: https://www.ihi.org/education/certified-professional-patient-safety-cpps. Accessed 6 June 2025.
76. Agency for Healthcare Quality and Research. Manchester Patient Safety Framework (MaPSaF). 2008. Available at: https://psnet.ahrq.gov/issue/manchester-patient-safety-framework-mapsaf. Accessed 9 May 2025.
77. Agency for Healthcare Improvement and Quality. Surveys on Patient Safety Culture. Available at: https://www.ahrq.gov/sops/index.html. Accessed 1 May 2025.
78. Eichhorn J, Cooper J. A tribute to Ellison C. (Jeep) Pierce, Jr., MD, the beloved founding leader of the APSF. APSF Newsl. 2011;26:23–5.

The Anesthesiologist as Intensivist: Integrating Perioperative and Critical Care Medicine

24

Shivani Patel and Sofia Gilels

Critical care anesthesiologists undergo additional specialized training in critical care medicine upon completion of the training to become an anesthesiologist. This is a board certifying fellowship that highlights the unique skill set that is required to take care of critically ill patients in the intensive care unit in the hospital.

As anesthesiologists, we are trained to monitor and treat consciousness, hemodynamics, respiratory status, metabolic derangements, and perioperative complications in the setting of multiple comorbid conditions. Naturally, this extends well into the intensive care unit (ICU). Many times the primary reason for admission is an overlap with the above: shock requiring vasopressors, respiratory failure necessitating intubation and ventilator management, titration of sedation and pain control, and postoperative bleeding or complications. These are conditions we have been diagnosing and treating in the operating room as anesthesiologists. For surgical patients, this also allows a unique opportunity for continuity of care as their intensivist. Every patient is unique in their physiology and response to certain therapies; caring for them in the operating room allows us to understand what works for them and carry it forward to postoperative care. Procedurally, we perform transesophageal echocardiograms, bronchoscopies, fiber-optic intubations, and percutaneous tracheostomies (among countless other procedures) in either setting.

Our understanding of pharmacodynamics and pharmacokinetics gives us an advantage as we regularly administer many of the sedatives and analgesic medications first-hand. Our experience with advanced physiology and monitoring lends us well to care for these patients. For example, pulmonary artery catheters were ubiquitously present to guide fluid resuscitation in the past. Their use in recent years has declined in favor of more noninvasive approaches [2, 12]. Numerous studies have shown a lack of mortality benefit and increased risk of complications for many of

S. Patel
Anesthesia Specialists of Bethlehem, Bethlehem, PA, USA

S. Gilels (✉)
Montefiore Medical Center, Bronx, NY, USA

G. Tewfik (ed.), *The Anesthesiologist as Perioperative Leader*,
https://doi.org/10.1007/978-3-032-18058-2_24

the previous indications such as severe chronic heart failure and acute respiratory distress syndrome [9–11]. Nevertheless, there are still circumstances during which data from a pulmonary artery catheter may be helpful. Anesthesiologists and cardiologists have the most familiarity with placement and interpretation given their ongoing use in procedural settings. Similarly, our exposure to transesophageal echocardiography and mechanical support devices (i.e., ventricular assist devices, intra-aortic balloon pumps, extracorporeal membrane oxygenation) in the operating room allow for an ease of transition to the cardiothoracic ICU. Intracranial pressure monitoring devices provide analogous movement to the neurocritical care unit. And while not most important, certainly not inconsequential, is a trusting relationship with the respective surgeons.

Critical care anesthesiologists are uniquely positioned given the skill set and training required to take care of the sickest patients in the hospital. Specifically before, during, and after surgery, the specialty training allows for coordinated care between the operating room, recovery room, and the intensive care unit. As such, this creates pathways to streamline patient care. Efficiency improvements exist in determining the appropriate level of care for patients to minimize hospital cost, optimize recovery, and overall provide improvement in the care for patients [18]. When there are unanticipated complications intraoperatively, the anesthesiologist responsible for the recovery room can facilitate the care of the patient. However, a critical care anesthesiologist can facilitate the admission of such a patient directly to the critical care unit to minimize turnover of the patient care team and shorten the time for necessary interventions for the patient.

Anesthesiologists are airway experts, translating that specific skill to intubated patients in the ICU. This advanced training may fast-track extubation in critically ill patients at times. This allows patients progress through recovery without delay and promotes improved outcomes. In the intensive care unit, it is also invaluable to be able to deal with difficult airways, and both anticipate and prevent negative outcomes in airway manipulation. This makes a critical care anesthesiologist a crucial component to the successful intervention in a patient with respiratory distress or failure in any part of the hospital. In more recent years, the skills have continued to evolve and the goal is always to streamline and facilitate patient care. Performing percutaneous tracheostomies bedside has become another skill and opportunity available to a critical care anesthesiologist. The ability to perform the procedure can decrease intubation days, decrease need for OR availability, surgeon availability, and the need to move the patient between locations in the hospital [18]. Early tracheostomies are crucial in a patient's ICU trajectory. Having a team able to plan and schedule the procedure without requiring a consult to an otolaryngology or trauma surgical service team expedites the timing of the performance of the tracheostomy [19].

Within the specialized field of critical care medicine, anesthesiologists function as intensivists that work within a collaborative team inclusive of surgeons, nurse practitioners (NPs), physician assistants (PAs), residents, and pharmacists to cultivate clinical care plans for patients. As a team, each member contributes in their own capacity to create a more thorough and comprehensive approach to patient care. Systemic and protocolized rounding, vent weaning, and infection prevention protocols are developed within surgical, medical, cardiothoracic, and neurological intensive care units to optimize patient care. To that end, critical care anesthesiologists serve a crucial role in improvement of the quality of the patient care received. By creating protocols and standardizing each sphere of patient recovery, more opportunity exists to better the care of patients in the ICU [20]. Different institutions have various types of intensive care units. Some smaller community hospitals have mixed ICUs in which both patients that have and have not undergone surgery would be in the same unit if they have critical care needs. In larger academic institutions, there are intensive care units that are dedicated to specific needs that patients could have following specific types of surgery, such as neurological or cardiothoracic.

Specialized units allow the benefit of highly trained nurses, technicians, advanced practice practitioners to optimize their experience and skills to cater to one patient group. For example, a Neurosurgical Intensive Care Unit (NSICU) would take care only of patients following neurosurgical intervention, or a unit only for patient populations that have undergone a stroke. This allows more protocolization of specific patient needs following these specific cases. Ultimately, this can improve patient outcomes [21].

Rounds are conducted throughout the unit on a regular basis with the team to systematically optimize and progress the care of a patient during their stay in the intensive care unit. The goal is to minimize ICU stay and implement patient care pathways as early as possible, to ultimately facilitate a patient's safe discharge from the hospital. The surgical patients specifically benefit as a function of the relationship between anesthesiologists and surgeons that facilitates care plans and open clear communication among the entire team to optimize patient care. In specifically oriented intensive care units such as cardiac, transplant, or surgical general ICUs, the surgeons play a critical role in dictating care specifically related to the surgical procedure. As dual-trained anesthesiologists, the intensivists are able to seamlessly understand the intraoperative course and inform their clinical decision-making more cogently.

The natural overlap makes anesthesiologists the primary base for intensivists outside of the United States. Alternatively, intensivists within this country are largely pulmonary critical care physicians or surgical critical care physicians [17]. Multiple factors have been suggested to influence this—reimbursement, lifestyle for anesthesiologists, and preference for private practice versus academia [1]. For example, while compensation may favor practicing anesthesiology full time, critical care may allow for more time off. With the rarity of the anesthesiologist presence in the ICU, the majority of career options remain in academic institutions. In academic institutions, the increased availability in resources can open the door for more staff intensivists and required on site physicians. The structure of the split of time varies greatly for critical care anesthesiologists. Some choose to practice primarily in their capacity as a critical care physician, while others prefer to work in the operating room. Most will have a varied schedule allowing them to work in both the operating room and in the intensive care unit. In recent years, the takeover of many anesthesiology practices by private equity firms, insurance companies, or healthcare systems often prevents restructuring to involve time away from the operating room, limiting options for those critical care anesthesiologists hoping to practice in a split capacity. Still, there are many opportunities for the critical care anesthesiologist to integrate easily into many units. Specifically, the recovery units, and intensive care units, are the mainstay of the critical care anesthesiologists' area coverage. Additionally, innovative care models, including tele-critical care, are allowing critical care anesthesiologists to broaden their opportunities to care for patients across the country in low-access facilities - specifically those which may be more isolated and lack the necessary skilled physicians to best care for patients.

As anesthesiologists, critical care physicians can implement medication protocols even preoperatively to help facilitate the postoperative care of patients. Specific use of ketamine in chronic pain patients can help minimize postoperative pain [6]. Protocols that incorporate regional anesthesia and multimodal analgesia to optimize patients' postoperative courses are instrumental in fast-tracking recovery. These tools translate to the intensive care unit where minimization of sedation and better control of patients' pain can result in short days on the ventilator and faster discharges from both the ICU and the hospital. As intensivists, the experience of dealing with multiorgan systemic pathologies in the intensive care unit helps prepare and inform the management of critically ill patients undergoing surgery in a more comprehensive manner.

Various hospitals and institutions have assessed care models that differ with respect to in house versus home call for intensivists. In one study, it was found that having specialized and dedicated 24/7 intensivist coverage was associated with decreased ventilator time, and decreased hospital stay [3]. The important difference is whether the trained critical care attending is "in house" or on "home call." This speaks specifically to the response time and availability of the physician to take care of and coordinate care for patients outside of "business hours." The intensive care unit does not adhere to standard hours as critically ill patients require admission and care at all hours of the day. Given the importance of maintaining the continuity of care throughout the stay, irrespective of the time of day, it reasonably stands that the physician coverage should remain the same as well.

The Leapfrog Group that has worked to initiate improvements in hospital safety, quality, and cost-effective changes has advocated for 24/7 intensivist hospital coverage. However, there remains a significant lag in the implementation in many US hospitals. A significant concern is cost; however, there have been recent investigations suggesting a favorable cost-benefit analysis given the improvement in quality metrics that outweigh the necessary salary costs associated with hiring the required number of physicians to provide the coverage [4].

As anesthesiologists can cross cover the intensive care unit, the recovery unit, and work in the operating room, there is both increased flexibility and options for coverage in the field.

Within the scope of critical care, the care of patients who do not improve medically is a challenging but necessary component. As such, palliative care is a significant aspect of critical care medicine. Admission to an ICU is stressful to both patients and families. Early introduction to palliative care, regardless of severity of condition, provides an outlet for stress and mitigation of suffering. Managing symptoms of anxiety and pain are commonplace for an anesthesiologist—both elective and emergent surgeries are nerve-racking conditions, and we are given a short time to establish connection and provide relief. As critical care anesthesiologists, this translates well to quickly manifest trust and provide the basis for ongoing goals of care conversations. This specific skill is honed both in the operating room in which case the anesthesiologist meets a patient the morning of their surgery and must immediately establish rapport prior to the patient undergoing anesthesia, and in the ICU. In the critical care unit, at times, patients can be significantly incapacitated and unable to participate in their own medical care decisions; in these cases, an intensivist must establish rapport with the families immediately in order to make the best choices for the care of the patient.

24.1 Palliative Care

Critically ill patients require intensive immediate interventions in order to improve their disease states and resolve or improve pathological processes. At times, the severity of the disease or organ dysfunction can progress beyond what can be reasonably able to improve. The priority of the care of the patient at that time becomes to coordinate the wishes of the patient and to coordinate with the family to ensure the best options for the patient are offered. It is difficult to navigate the challenging discussions and decisions that families must make for their loved ones, and it is at this juncture that a critical care anesthesiologist is able to best facilitate the conversation.

Palliative care is in and of itself a specialized field that requires additional training and board certification. The field produces specialists that offer patients and families throughout their medical care journeys the support needed to navigate end-of-life decision-making. Given the necessity and emergency of such needs that arise specifically in the ICU, it is often that the overnight or weekend services can be limited and not available necessarily at the time of a patient's decompensation. This is why critical care physicians strive to excel in their own skill set to be able to help patients at any time.

Critical care anesthesiologists are uniquely trained and qualified to facilitate difficult and necessary conversations regarding end-of-life care in the ICU. At times, the most important and appropriate management plan is one that requires the cessation of invasive interventions in line with the goals and wishes of the patient/family. These decisions and action plans are made in a multidisciplinary fashion involving the surgical teams, social workers, family members, and any other pertinent team members with respect to the care of the specific patient. Spiritual support members such as priests or rabbis also play a critical role in the care of the patient and the appropriate transition of care from full intervention to end of life.

The initiation of comfort measures with the goal of transfer to specific hospital units geared toward the specialty end-of-life care is also within the scope of the field. Ultimately, there are patients that are too critically ill to be moved and necessitate the end-of-life care to be carried out in the critical care unit. As such, both the clinical acumen and social sensitivity for the patient and family must exist in the abilities of the critical care anesthesiologist. Many end-of-life symptoms are related to pain, anxiety/delirium, and dyspnea. In addition to psychosocial support, our familiarity with medications can help make the transition for patients as comfortable as possible.

Once decisions are made by the patient or the family members to shift the focus of care from invasive interventions to providing comfort and pain relief, the critical care anesthesiologist would work with the intensive care team to facilitate that transition. In some institutions, there are designated palliative care units which specifically specialize in end-of-life care. In other institutions, the intensive care unit directly provides palliative services. Many times, patients are too unstable to move and ultimately do require the care of the staff of the intensive care unit even with the modification in the care plan to opt out of any continued medical interventions. Ultimately, the goal is to provide the best care that is most appropriate for each patient.

24.2 Sleep Medicine

Another aspect of critical care anesthesiology may include sleep medicine. It is important to consider that the maintenance of physiologic sleep is an important modifiable risk factor for delirium prevention. Sleep medicine (especially with respect to obstructive sleep apnea [OSA]) has overlap with the management skills of a critical care anesthesiologist. Many patients with OSA undergo surgery, both emergently, and electively, and at times require admission to the ICU. Obstructive sleep apnea, among other sleep disorders, is important to treat and manage appropriately to prevent or treat respiratory failure or distress in patients. An anesthesiologist has the opportunity to further specialize in sleep medicine for additional board certification to master the necessary skills to specifically treat patients affected by pathological disease states of the wake-sleep cycle.

Delirium in the ICU is a multifaceted and complicated disease process that can prolong hospital stay, worsen outcomes, and be frightening for the patients and their families [13]. Better sleep hygiene, sleep protocols, and initiatives that prioritize the prevention of delirium have been shown to have better outcomes for patients [5]. In the ICU, the beeping machines, continuous testing, monitoring, and overall interruptions in sleep significantly affect the sleep-wake cycle of patients. The effects are deleterious and can delay recovery. Delirium may be addressed in the ICU; nonetheless, it has been shown that long-term sequelae can result in neurocognitive impact on patients long after they are discharged home [14, 15].

Given this, the importance of the implementation of protocols that minimize the evolution of delirium in patients is paramount. As critical care anesthesiologists within the intensive care unit, the goal is to spread awareness, knowledge, and formulate team-based approaches to optimize the care provided. In order to decrease delirium, adherence to sleep-promoting habits has been shown to improve outcomes [16]. Specially, it is critical to have patients adhere to a day/night regime even in the intensive care unit as best as possible. Sleep order sets or "delirium precautions" help to standardize the interventions and to minimize disturbances in the sleep of patients.

Anesthesiologists have, in recent years, moved to become more comprehensive in their care of patients. While sleep medicine is typically an outpatient centered practice, the knowledge overlaps to the inpatient care that anesthesiologists provide. The physiology of sleep, specific sleep-related disorders, and the effects of anesthetics on patients postoperatively all combine to become significant for the ultimate care of the patient—specifically in the intensive care units and is an area that critical care anesthesiologists can excel in [7]. Patients who have OSA, narcolepsy, or central sleep apnea can have increased risks in the perioperative period and can be more significantly impacted afterwards [8].

There is significant variability within the care that is standardized for patients postoperatively and subsequently in the ICU. Optimization and standardization within the ICUs nationally can improve patient outcomes by educating clinicians regarding the optimal approaches for patients with sleep disorders. This may include the use of machinery such as Bipap, CPAP, or other respiratory interventions that can facilitate the care of patients with sleep disorders in the intensive care unit postoperatively. Many of the covered topics within the separate subspecialty of sleep medicine are relevant for anesthesiologists and critical care physicians. For example, the pathophysiology of upper airway collapse, influence of opioids on respiratory center modulation, as well as implications of sleep disturbances to patient health are of increased importance to clinicians of varying specialties. In the ICU, where there is regular disturbance of sleep, it is vital to learn the subsequent detriments that could arise as a result.

The critical care anesthesiologist plays a vital role both in and out of the operating room. Our familiarity with many aspects of medical and surgical specialties provides flexibility in coverage options and streamlining patient care throughout the hospital. Patients can rest assured that our unique compilation of skills will keep them and their families as safe as possible during what may be their most trying times.

References

1. Flynn BC. Anesthesiology critical care: current state and future directions. J Cardiothorac Vasc Anesth. 2023;37(8):1478–84.
2. Chatterjee K. The Swan-Ganz catheters: past, present, and future: a viewpoint. Circulation. 2009;119(1):147–52. https://doi.org/10.1161/CIRCULATIONAHA.108.811141.
3. Pronovost PJ, Needham DM, Waters H, Birkmeyer CM, Calinawan JR, Birkmeyer JD, Dorman T. Intensive care unit physician staffing: financial modeling of the Leapfrog standard. Crit Care Med. 2004;32:1247–53.
4. Kamdar BB, Martin JL, Needham DM, Ong MK. Promoting sleep to improve delirium in the ICU. Crit Care Med. 2016;44(12):2290–1. https://doi.org/10.1097/CCM.0000000000001982. PMID: 27858818; PMCID: PMC5599108.

5. Radvansky BM, Shah K, Parikh A, Sifonios AN, Le V, Eloy JD. Role of ketamine in acute postoperative pain management: a narrative review. Biomed Res Int. 2015;2015:749837. https://doi.org/10.1155/2015/749837. Epub 2015 Oct 1. PMID: 26495312; PMCID: PMC4606413.
6. Bhattacharya PK, Nair SG, Kumar N, Natarajan P, Chhanwal H. Critical care as a career for anaesthesiologists. Indian J Anaesth. 2021;65(1):48–53. https://doi.org/10.4103/ija.IJA_1490_20. Epub 2021 Jan 20. PMID: 33767503; PMCID: PMC7980238.
7. Singh M, Gali B, Levine M, Strohl K, Auckley D. Integrating sleep knowledge into the anesthesiology curriculum. Anesth Analg. 2021;132(5):1296–305. https://doi.org/10.1213/ANE.0000000000005490. PMID: 33857971.
8. Binanay C, Califf RM, Hasselblad V, et al. Evaluation study of congestive heart failure and pulmonary artery catheterization effectiveness: the ESCAPE trial. JAMA. 2005;294:1625–33.
9. Harvey S, Harrison DA, Singer M, et al. Assessment of the clinical effectiveness of pulmonary artery catheters in management of patients in intensive care (PAC-Man): a randomised controlled trial. Lancet. 2005;366:472–7.
10. Rajaram SS, Desai NK, Kalra A, et al. Pulmonary artery catheters for adult patients in intensive care. Cochrane Database Syst Rev. 2013;2013:CD003408.
11. Coverdale G, Patteril M. Do pulmonary artery catheters have a role in the 21st century intensive care unit? Br J Anaesth. 2022;129(1):3–7.
12. Ely EW, Gautam S, Margolin R, et al. The impact of delirium in the intensive care unit on hospital length of stay. Intensive Care Med. 2001;27(12):1892–900. https://doi.org/10.1007/s00134-001-1132-2.
13. Brummel NE, Jackson JC, Pandharipande PP, et al. Delirium in the ICU and subsequent long-term disability among survivors of mechanical ventilation. Crit Care Med. 2014;42(2):369–77. https://doi.org/10.1097/CCM.0b013e3182a645bd.
14. Jackson JC, et al. Depression, post-traumatic stress disorder, and functional disability in survivors of critical illness in the BRAIN-ICU study: a longitudinal cohort study. Lancet Respir Med. 2014;2(5):369–79.
15. Watson PL, Ceriana P, Fanfulla F. Delirium: is sleep important? Best Pract Res Clin Anaesthesiol. 2012;26(3):355–66. https://doi.org/10.1016/j.bpa.2012.08.005. PMID: 23040286; PMCID: PMC3808245.
16. Flynn BC, et al. Sustainability of the subspecialty of anesthesiology critical care: an expert consensus and review of the literature. J Cardiothorac Vasc Anesth. 2024;38(8):1753–9.
17. Bennett S, Grawe E, Jones C, Josephs SA, Mechlin M, Hurford WE. Role of the anesthesiologist-intensivist outside the ICU: opportunity to add value for the hospital or an unnecessary distraction? Curr Opin Anaesthesiol. 2018;31(2):165–71. https://doi.org/10.1097/ACO.0000000000000560. PMID: 29341963.
18. Khammas AH, Dawood MR. Timing of tracheostomy in intensive care unit patients. Int Arch Otorhinolaryngol. 2018;22(4):437–42. https://doi.org/10.1055/s-0038-1654710. Epub 2018 Aug 9. PMID: 30357027; PMCID: PMC6197980.
19. Mehta C, Mehta Y. Percutaneous tracheostomy. Ann Card Anaesth. 2017;20(Supplement):S19–25. https://doi.org/10.4103/0971-9784.197793. PMID: 28074819; PMCID: PMC5299824.
20. Chang B, Lorenzo J, Macario A. Examining health care costs: opportunities to provide value in the intensive care unit. Anesthesiol Clin. 2015;33(4):753–70. https://doi.org/10.1016/j.anclin.2015.07.012. PMID: 26610628.
21. Mirski MA, Chang CW, Cowan R. Impact of a neuroscience intensive care unit on neurosurgical patient outcomes and cost of care: evidence-based support for an intensivist-directed specialty ICU model of care. J Neurosurg Anesthesiol. 2001;13(2):83–92. https://doi.org/10.1097/00008506-200104000-00004. PMID: 11294463.

Peripartum Excellence: The Anesthesiologist's Role in Quality, Safety, and Equity of Maternal Care

25

Sangeeta Kumaraswami, Christine Chen, and Mark Zakowski

25.1 Introduction

The specialty of obstetric anesthesiology has contributed significantly to improving maternal and neonatal health and well-being, beyond the intraoperative and peripartum time periods. In addition to providing neuraxial analgesia or anesthesia, these specialists improve maternal and neonatal outcomes and reduce complications, readmissions, and costs. Obstetric anesthesiologists provide high-risk consultation, coordinate multidisciplinary care, and participate in quality improvement initiatives. They contribute to reducing disparities, shortening length of hospital stay, and ensuring better quality of recovery via Enhanced Recovery After Cesarean (ERAC) protocols [1–4]. Indeed, a study from Scotland showed that receiving epidural analgesia reduced by 54% the incidence of severe maternal morbidity (SMM) and critical care admission [5]. This improvement in maternal outcomes stems from both the physiologic benefits of labor analgesia and the obstetric anesthesiologist's cognitive

S. Kumaraswami
Westchester Medical Center/New York Medical College, Valhalla, NY, USA

ASA Committee on Quality Management and Departmental Administration, ASA Representative to the DNV Healthcare Advisory Board, Schaumburg, IL, USA

C. Chen
Cedars-Sinai Medical Center, Los Angeles, CA, USA

M. Zakowski (✉)
Department of Anesthesiology, Cedars-Sinai Medical Center, Los Angeles, CA, USA

ASA Committee on Obstetric Anesthesia, Past ASA Liaison to ACOG CC-OB, ASA Committee on Quality Management and Departmental Administration, ASA Educational Track Subcommittee on Obstetric Anesthesia, Schaumburg, IL, USA

Society for Obstetric Anesthesia and Perinatology, Lexington, KY, USA

California Society of Anesthesiologists, Sacramento, CA, USA

CSA Foundation for Education, Sacramento, CA, USA

G. Tewfik (ed.), *The Anesthesiologist as Perioperative Leader*,
https://doi.org/10.1007/978-3-032-18058-2_25

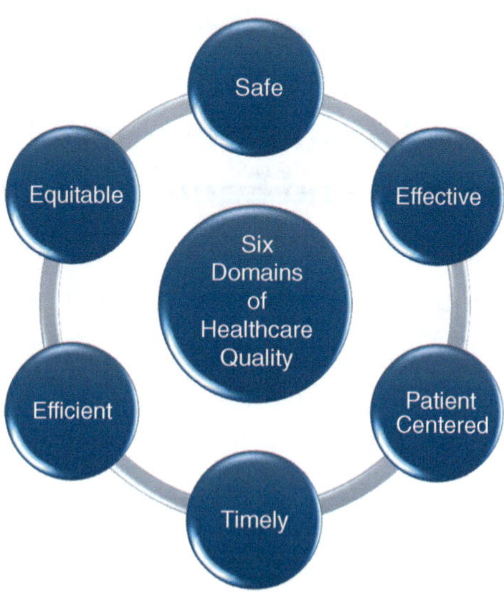

Fig. 25.1 Institute of Medicine's six domains of healthcare quality

involvement. Previous studies have also found that anesthesiologists' involvement decreased SMM and postpartum hemorrhage [6, 7]. Obstetric anesthesiologists' involvement also helps to provide consultations, risk-appropriate care, and collaborative relationships, all aligned with the American College of Obstetrics and Gynecology (ACOG)'s Levels of Maternal Care (LoMC) [8]. Associated benefits may even extend to the almost half million babies born in counties in the United States that are maternity care deserts or have limited maternity care. In these areas, consultation and coordination of care occurs with tertiary referral centers where obstetric anesthesiologists add their expertise [9]. Anesthesiologists may even provide remote patients with telehealth services for antenatal anesthesia consults [10]. Indeed, these benefits can, and should, translate into high-value payment models for hospitals, with measures, performance targets, and value-based payments [11].

The Institute of Medicine defines the six domains of healthcare quality as safe, effective, patient-centered, timely, efficient, and equitable (Fig. 25.1) [12]. Anesthesiologists play a major role in providing quality driven evidence-based peripartum care.

25.2 Safe Care

One mother dies every 2 min from childbirth worldwide. Alarmingly, the maternal mortality rate in the United States is higher than other high-income counties and continues to increase [13, 14]. In 2014, the National Partnership for Maternal Safety (NPMS) was formed to focus on improving maternal care with multidisciplinary collaboration between organizations including the American Society of Anesthesiologists (ASA) and Society for Obstetric Anesthesia and Perinatology (SOAP) [15, 16]. NPMS produced several evidence-based consensus bundles that resulted in improved care [17]. Anesthesiologists have been an integral part of the NPMS multidisciplinary groups, creating bundles for obstetric hemorrhage, severe hypertension, venous thromboembolism, reduction of peripartum racial and ethnic disparities, and opioid use disorder [18–23]. Anesthesiologists provide necessary critical care to improve perioperative and long-term outcomes in preeclamptic patients undergoing cesarean deliveries [24].

Delays in diagnosis, treatment, and even misdiagnosis continue to contribute to maternal mortality. Obstetric early warning systems (EWS) facilitate timely recognition, diagnosis, and treatment of critical illnesses in the peripartum period by using changes in vital signs and level of consciousness to assist with timely assessment, intervention, and transfer to a higher level of care [25–27]. EWS includes protocols for observation in the peripartum period, detection of an abnormality, and the triggering of a response [28]. SOAP was one of eight women's healthcare organizations that formed the NPMS Subcommittee on Vital Sign Triggers creating Maternal EWS [25], along with differential diagnoses and methods for local implementation [16–22, 25].

ACOG LoMC classification (Table 25.1) helps provide safe, risk-appropriate care to patients. Births occur in accredited birth centers or hospitals providing basic care (Level I), specialty care (Level II), subspecialty care (Level III), or at regional perinatal centers (Level IV) [8]. The LoMC program helps facilitate safe birth depending upon the risk of pregnancy while also providing support when higher level of resources and skill are needed [8]. It is recommended that pregnant patients at risk for severe morbidities (e.g., heart failure, massive hemorrhage) give birth at ACOG LoMC III or IV hospitals [29], which have the appropriate personnel and resources. Anesthesiologists with obstetric anesthesia fellowship training or [significant] experience in obstetric anesthesia are part of the LoMC III or IV requirements [8, 29]. Involvement of obstetric anesthesia fellowship-trained

Table 25.1 ACOG levels of maternal care

ACOG LoMC	Definition	Implications for anesthesia professionals
Level I (basic care)	Low to moderate risk pregnancies	Anesthesia provider readily available at all times.
Level II (specialty care)	Moderate to high risk antepartum, intrapartum, or postpartum conditions	Anesthesiologist readily available at all times.
Level III (subspecialty care)	Complex maternal medication conditions, obstetric complications, fetal conditions	Board-certified anesthesiologist physically present at all times. Director of obstetric anesthesia services is board-certified with obstetric anesthesia fellowship training or experience in obstetric anesthesia.
Level IV (regional perinatal health center)	On-site medical and surgical care of the most complex conditions and critical ill pregnant women and fetuses	Board-certified anesthesiologist with obstetric anesthesia fellowship training or experience physically present at all times. Director of obstetric anesthesia services is board-certified with obstetric anesthesia fellowship training or experience in obstetric anesthesia.

Adapted from Obstetrics & Gynecology [8]

anesthesiologists was associated with decreased rates of general anesthesia for cesarean deliveries [30, 31]. Thus, sub-specialty training improves outcomes [32]. Patients with placenta accreta spectrum disorders, a leading contributor of maternal hemorrhage, have better outcomes when delivered in ACOG LoMC III or IV hospitals [33]. For these patients, obstetric anesthesiologists contribute to successful outcomes through preparation, use of guidelines and protocols, and management of postpartum pain and improving postoperative disposition [34, 35]. Since the majority of hospital births in the United States occur at lower volume hospitals, anesthesiologists use their understanding of perioperative medicine to guide risk stratification so that patients can be appropriately referred to a higher level of care.

The majority of women undergoing cesarean delivery in the United States receive neuraxial morphine for postoperative analgesia [36]. Neuraxial morphine is considered the most effective form of analgesia for cesarean deliveries but might be associated with a risk for respiratory depression [36]. As part of SOAP's mission to improve outcomes in pregnancy, a consensus statement was published in 2019 on recommendations for the prevention and detection of respiratory depression after administration of neuraxial morphine [36]. The statement recommends decreased respiratory monitoring in healthy mothers while simultaneously focusing on those with a high risk for respiratory depression.

In 2019, SOAP started awarding "Center of Excellence"(COE) designation to institutions that provide high-quality obstetric anesthesia care [37]. The process guides institutions to achieve higher quality metrics, with numerous criteria covering domains such as personnel and staffing, policies and equipment, simulation and team training, management of obstetrical emergencies, and care of patients undergoing vaginal deliveries and cesarean deliveries, along with quality processes and systems for follow-up (Table 25.2) [37]. The SOAP COE designation helps benchmark the quality of obstetric anesthesia care nationally and internationally.

25.3 Effective Care

Obstetric anesthesiologists lead in providing effective, evidence-based care throughout the peridelivery period. This section is divided into subsections as we highlight examples of effective care. Obstetric anesthesiologists are directly involved in all six domains of healthcare quality (Table 25.3).

25.3.1 Predelivery Optimization

Predelivery assessment of high-risk patients is essential [38], as it reduces delays and cancellations and improves patient satisfaction while diminishing costs [39, 40]. Obstetric preanesthesia clinics help identify and manage the high-risk parturient. The UK Confidential Enquiry into Maternal and Child Health report emphasizes early identification and management, highlighting examples of maternal deaths from poor recognition of life-threatening illnesses by inexperienced

Table 25.2 Key recommendations for SOAP centers of excellence

Personnel and staffing	Equipment, protocols, policies	Cesarean delivery management	Labor analgesia	Guidelines implementation	Quality assurance and patient follow-up
Obstetric anesthesiologist leadership In-house 24/7 dedicated coverage of obstetric patients Ability to mobilize additional anesthesia personnel in case of emergencies and high volume	Massive transfusion protocol with rapid-infuser device available Difficult airway cart on unit Multidisciplinary team-based approach with emergency simulation drills and daily rounds or huddles Obstetric emergency response team Additional operating room with personal available at all times	Standardized clinical care pathway Routine utilization of pencil-point needle, 25 gauge or less for spinal anesthesia Multimodal analgesia protocols Strategies to prevent maternal and fetal intraoperative hypothermia Appropriate antibiotic prophylaxis Spinal hypotension, nausea, vomiting, prophylaxis, and treatment	Use of low-concentration local anesthetic solutions with neuraxial opioids Combined-spinal epidural techniques available. Patient-controlled epidural analgesia utilized Routine utilization of flexible epidural catheters Regular assessment of labor analgesia effectiveness	Implementation of the practice guidelines for obstetric anesthesia by the ASA task force on obstetric anesthesia and SOAP	An anesthesiologist serves on a team that develops and implements multidisciplinary clinical policy Follow-up with all patients who received anesthesia services A system to evaluate and treat a postdural puncture headache in a timely fashion

Adapted from Carvalho and Mhyre [37]

Table 25.3 Six domains of healthcare quality and examples demonstrating involvement of obstetric anesthesiologists

Domains of healthcare quality	Involvement of obstetric anesthesiologists
Safe care	Consensus bundles Maternal early warning systems SOAP statement: monitoring recommendations for prevention & detection of respiratory depression from neuraxial morphine administration in cesarean delivery Anesthesiologists part of criteria for ACOG levels of maternal care SOAP Centers of Excellence institutions providing high-quality care
Effective care	Preanesthesia Clinics for optimizing high-risk patients Statements/guidelines: Enhanced recovery after cesarean, PDPH, quality metrics Patient safety bundles and toolkits Medications and drugs (statements on sugammadex, opioid use disorder, cannabis and cannabinoids use) Point-of-care ultrasound
Patient-centered care	Trauma-informed care Unique considerations for certain patient populations (e.g., Jehovah's witness) SOAP statements: patients with thrombocytopenia, thromboprophylaxis ASA statements: pain during cesarean delivery, psychological support in obstetrics
Timely care	Patient educational materials on professional anesthesia society websites Multidisciplinary huddles in the labor and delivery unit Simulation training of emergencies and adverse events
Efficient care	Decrease adverse environmental consequences from volatile inhaled anesthetic agents Resources on ASA website to guide use of nitrous oxide for labor analgesia Considerations on care during major events such as COVID-19, shortage of intravenous fluids and medications (local anesthetics, oxytocin)
Equitable care	Reducing racial and ethnic disparities in obstetric care

SOAP Society for Obstetric Anesthesia and Perinatology, *ACOG* American College of Obstetricians and Gynecologists, *PDPH* postdural puncture headache, *ASA* American Society of Anesthesiologists

clinicians, and lack of timely input from other specialties [41]. Evaluation of high-risk pregnant patients should be done by an anesthesiologist. A preanesthesia clinic provides an opportunity for optimizing high-risk patients and for allowing collaboration between various specialties [42]. The ACOG Practice Bulletin on Obstetric Analgesia and Anesthesia contains a broad list of medical conditions that warrant anesthesiology consultation for improving outcomes [43], including cardiovascular conditions such as valvular abnormalities, aortopathies, arrhythmias, and cardiomyopathies [44–46]. For some cardiac conditions, collaboration between an obstetric and cardiothoracic anesthesiologist may be helpful for optimal outcomes [47]. Additional comorbidities that may need preanesthesia evaluation include pulmonary conditions such as obstructive sleep apnea and cystic fibrosis [48, 49], as well as preexisting neuromuscular and skeletal disorders [50–52]. Patients with implanted hardware after surgical repair of scoliosis are often unnecessarily denied neuraxial anesthesia [53]. Interdisciplinary discussions that include obstetricians and orthopedists or neurosurgeons guide both providers and patients to be better informed about anesthetic options for delivery. Optimizing coagulation status in pregnant patients with disorders like von Willebrand disease and factor XI deficiency is also an example [54, 55]. In these patients, consultation with hematologists can be valuable in formulating a plan and assessing the safety of neuraxial anesthesia. These discussions will foster confidence in pregnant patients and improve patient satisfaction.

25.3.2 ERAC and Quality Metrics

SOAP has developed an ERAC statement in order to standardize clinical care pathways for cesarean deliveries [56]. Components include preoperative patient education, limited fasting, preoperative oral fluid and carbohydrate loading, intraoperative vasopressor infusions, and prophylactic antiemetics. ERAC protocols reduce length of stay and improve maternal and neonatal outcomes [2, 57]. Additionally, guidelines for intraoperative care in cesarean delivery as part of the Enhanced Recovery After Surgery recommendations were published in April 2025 [58]. Representatives from several societies including obstetric anesthesiologists from ASA and SOAP were involved in drafting these guidelines.

Another clinically useful document is the Statement on Quality Metrics approved by the ASA Committee on Obstetric Anesthesia in 2022 with input from a broad group of obstetric anesthesiologists [59]. This statement outlines six areas of quality improvement to measure obstetric anesthesia care and recommends best practices that cover six areas including mode of anesthesia for cesarean delivery, neuraxial-induced hypotension, post-cesarean opioid consumption, responsiveness to the request for labor analgesia, postdural puncture headache (PDPH) rates and accountability, and labor epidural replacements [59].

The issue of PDPH has also been addressed by evidence-based clinical practice multisociety guidelines that were published in 2023. Experts from different national and international societies including anesthesiologists from SOAP and the American Society of Regional Anesthesia and Pain Medicine were involved in formulating these guidelines [60, 61].

25.3.3 Medications and Drugs

Adequate reversal of neuromuscular blockade is essential for patients receiving non-depolarizing muscle relaxants in order to prevent residual neuromuscular blockade, a common cause of postoperative complications. Sugammadex is associated with faster reversal of neuromuscular blockade than neostigmine, with improved recovery of postoperative respiratory muscle strength, shorter operating room time, and shorter length of stay in the post-anesthesia care unit [62, 63]. SOAP published a statement regarding considerations for the use of sugammadex during pregnancy and the postpartum period, which serves as a valuable resource for anesthesiologists that care for this patient population [64].

The opioid crisis has been declared a public health emergency in the United States. About 1 in 300 opioid naïve women become persistent opioid prescription users after cesarean delivery [65]. ERAC reduces postpartum opioid consumption and decreases opioid prescriptions given to patients during discharge [56]. Care of pregnant patients with opioid use disorder presents unique anesthetic considerations. In 2022, SOAP, the Society for Maternal-Fetal Medicine, and the American Society of Regional Anesthesia and Pain Medicine (ASRA) published a consensus statement on the management of pregnant patients with opioid use disorder [66]. Antenatal consultation is essential to reassure patients that their pain management needs will be addressed along with developing a plan for the intrapartum and postpartum period that involves multimodal analgesia [67].

With increasing societal use of cannabis and cannabinoids, ASRA recently published much needed guidelines on anesthetic considerations for this patient population which included considerations for parturients with chronic cannabis use presenting for labor or cesarean delivery [68]. While there is currently no evidence to suggest changes in neuraxial anesthesia, its use during pregnancy and the peripartum period should be discouraged, and women counseled about maternal, fetal, and neonatal effects [68].

25.3.4 Patient Safety Bundles

In 2014, ACOG implemented a quality improvement initiative that became the Alliance for Innovation on Maternal Health (AIM) [69]. AIM released several patient safety bundles with specific actionable steps and resources to assess metrics including the recent sepsis in obstetric care which was spearheaded by a critical care-obstetric anesthesiologist [70]. Anesthesiologists have been involved in the California Maternal Quality Care Collaborative (CMQCC), an organization founded in 2006 that develops quality improvement toolkits and other initiatives to reduce maternal morbidity and mortality. Toolkits exist for maternal cardiovascular disease, substance use disorder, hemorrhage, hypertensive disorders of pregnancy, sepsis, support of vaginal births and reduction of cesarean, and thromboembolism. Since the inception of CMQCC, the maternal mortality rate between 2006 and 2016 declined by 65% in California, while the national maternal mortality rate continued to rise [71].

25.3.5 Point-of-Care Ultrasound (POCUS)

Anesthesiologists are at the forefront in using POCUS in the management of high-risk obstetrics [72]. Uses include the measurement of optic nerve sheath diameter in preeclampsia, and its evaluation in predicting postdural puncture headache (PDPH) [73, 74]. Applications also include airway, lung, cardiac, vascular, abdomen, and neuraxial ultrasound [75]. Lung ultrasound plays a potential role in the management of preeclampsia complicated by pulmonary edema [72, 76]. Cardiac ultrasound is used in the management of pulmonary hypertension, peripartum cardiomyopathy, and in assessment of fluid status during hemorrhage, a common cause of maternal morbidity and mortality [77]. Use of ultrasound for neuraxial procedures has also been found to increase efficacy without a clinically significant prolongation of the total time required for the procedure [78].

25.4 Patient-Centered Care

Patient-centered care involves incorporating patients' values and sharing decision-making responsibilities. Patients may request labor analgesia with varying goals for partial or complete pain relief based on their desire to stay in touch with the birthing process. Using principles of trauma-informed care within anesthesia care can improve psychological outcomes [79]. The Substance Abuse and Mental Health Services Administration or SAMHSA defines trauma-informed care using the 4 Rs: *realize* the pervasive and widespread nature of trauma in our society; *recognize* what unresolved trauma looks like in adult survivors; *respond* by incorporating knowledge into practices, protocols, and principles; and *resist* retraumatization [80, 81]. The role of the obstetric anesthesiologist in recognizing and responding to acute stress responses and safeguarding the emotional well-being of the pregnant patient is crucial [81].

Another example of patient-centered care is the unique considerations for patients who refuse blood products. For example, Jehovah's Witnesses' refusal of blood transfusion is a constitutionally protected right [82]. These individuals should be able to decide on acceptability of plasma derivatives or cellular blood components and autologous blood management. Education regarding personal choice items including albumin, cryoprecipitate, factor concentrates, and intraoperative cell salvage should be part of shared decision-making [82, 83]. Anesthesiologists should ensure that patients' desires are communicated, respected, and documented in the medical record [82, 83].

National and international quality metrics also emphasize patient-centered care and help to achieve excellence in obstetric anesthesia care. Examples include the ASA's Statement on Quality Metrics [in Obstetric Anesthesia] [59], Obstetric Anaesthetists Association's (OAA) national quality indicators in the United Kingdom [84], and SOAP Center of Excellence designation [37]. Data from these metrics should help to drive meaningful improvements in the quality of maternal care [85].

Anesthesiologists have also led quality initiatives by attaching cognitive aids to anesthesia carts or embedding reminders into electronic health records (EHR) such as timing of local anesthetic administration (e.g., repeat administration of 3% 2-chloroprocaine during cesarean delivery). EHR can also provide clinical decision support by generating patient-specific assessments and recommendations, thereby improving care. Several obstetric anesthesia groups have integrated the collection, tracking, and reporting of these metrics into their EHR [86, 87].

Many parturients have been denied neuraxial anesthesia because of low platelet counts due to medical concerns for safety. SOAP published a consensus statement on the feasibility of neuraxial procedures in obstetric patients with thrombocytopenia to guide discussions on the risks and benefits of neuraxial anesthesia [88]. Another common clinical conundrum occurs when parturients are on anticoagulants. The pharmacology, safety, and timing of neuraxial procedures relative to thromboprophylaxis have been addressed by SOAP [89]. These statements help clinicians provide safe care and guide treatment.

Recent literature has stressed the importance of recognition and treatment of pain during cesarean delivery [90–92]. The ASA COBA published a statement on intraoperative pain during cesarean delivery thus joining other international organizations in addressing this important issue [93–95]. The ASA statement contains information on the use of adjuvant medications and management of intraoperative pain during cesarean delivery to help disseminate information [93]. The ASA also published a statement on providing psychological support to obstetric patients given that about 6% of patients can have a childbirth-related posttraumatic stress disorder (CR-PTSD) [96]. Anesthesiologists can help address psychological needs of patients with preexisting mental health conditions or past traumatic experiences, thereby decreasing the odds of CR-PTSD [96, 97].

25.5 Timely Care

Care for obstetric patients should be timely. Ideal staffing of obstetric anesthesia services involves prioritization of multiple time-varying demands based on labor epidural utilization, cesarean delivery rate and duration, delivery volume, and availability of support services [98–100]. Preoperative optimization of pregnant patients can help avoid delays and cancellations, reduce costs, and streamline care. Explaining the benefits and risks of neuraxial anesthesia and analgesia during predelivery visits decreases the time needed for education prior to delivery in the hospital. Professional society-based patient educational materials for labor analgesia are often shown to be significantly more readable and understandable than other websites [101]. The SOAP, OAA, and ASA websites have free, easy-to-read, high-quality patient education information provided by obstetric anesthesiologists. Education by anesthesiologists can also help allay anxiety [102], and improve the patient experience. Anesthesiologists may discuss side effects and complications when a patient is undergoing painful labor [84]. Some women may want to know about every complication [103]. Giving detailed information during labor could delay delivery of neuraxial labor analgesia. Availability of high-quality patient education materials that patients can access beforehand may reduce the time spent by anesthesiologists in navigating the informed consent process and may improve retention of information and maternal satisfaction [103].

Another example of timely care is multidisciplinary huddles that allow for effective communication and safety in the workplace when clinical care could rapidly change [104], such as prior to urgent cesarean deliveries [105].

Anesthesiology societies often collaborate with other societies to release statements in response to issues that cause concern in pregnant patients or the general public. For example, in 2020, the ASA, SOAP, ACOG, Society for Maternal-Fetal Medicine, and Society for Pediatric Anesthesia released a joint statement in response to an article concerning labor epidurals and autism [106]. During the COVID-19 pandemic, obstetric anesthesiology experts published a review on anesthesia considerations in caring for patients with COVID-19 [73, 107]. SOAP also established a registry and published timely information on obstetric and neonatal outcomes in patients with COVID-19 [108].

Anesthesiologists have led simulation training of emergencies and adverse events, a valuable tool for training and assessing multidisciplinary care teams [109], including implementation of a mobile simulation program for improving obstetric emergency skills in rural hospitals in Iowa [100]. Augmented reality, virtual reality, and mixed reality help provide remote [110], and asynchronous, simulation-based training [111]. Simulation has been crucial in addressing high rates of maternal mortality in low-resource settings and in improving global peripartum and perinatal outcomes [112].

25.6 Efficient Care

Efficient care avoids wastage of equipment, supplies, time, and energy. Anesthesiologists lead in reducing operating room delays related to scheduling, improving revenues and decreasing waste. Indeed, the Royal College of Anaesthetists and the ASA statements on deactivating central piped nitrous oxide describe pipeline connection leaks as a 70–95% waste of N_2O, with a recommendation to transition to portal systems, if needed, to decrease adverse environmental consequences and save money [113, 114]. In support of patients' requests, the ASA COBA published a document on nitrous oxide use for obstetric patients which is a valuable resource for institutions considering introduction of nitrous oxide on their obstetric units as a modality for labor analgesia [115]. The ASA Committee on Environmental Health also offers a sustainability checklist for greening the OR [116].

As of 2025, the United States continues to experience medication shortages in the perioperative environment. The ASA statement on neuraxial medications shortages and alternatives provides possible solutions for anesthesiologists [117]. SOAP also released a similar statement during a shortage of hyperbaric bupivacaine used in spinal anesthesia and offered alternative anesthetic options for cesarean deliveries [118], as well as guidance pertaining to a shortage of oxytocin [119]. These statements are a valuable resource for practicing anesthesiologists and suggest continuing involvement of national anesthesia societies in optimizing obstetric anesthesia care.

The 2024 shortage of intravenous fluids following Hurricane Helene required conservation and prioritization of intravenous fluids to minimize cancelling needed surgeries and procedures. ASA suggested conservation, alternatives, and guidance without compromising patient safety or quality of care [120]. SOAP also encouraged oral hydration during labor and discouraged the routine use of preloading of intravenous fluids and reducing infusion rates during labor [121]. SOAP has also addressed epidural kit shortages and alternative strategies [122].

25.7 Equitable Care

Pregnancy-related maternal mortality rates have been increasing in the United States [123], with significantly higher rates in Native Hawaiian, Black, and American Indian or Alaska Native women [123–125]. Disparities exist in several aspects of obstetric anesthesia care, including neuraxial administration for labor pain, rates of general anesthesia for cesarean delivery, post-neuraxial anesthesia complications, postpartum pain management, and PDPH treatment practices [126, 127].

Hispanic and non-Hispanic Black patients are more likely to receive general anesthesia for a cesarean delivery, receive fewer postpartum pain assessments than White patients, and are less likely to receive postpartum opioid analgesia or opioid prescriptions at the time of discharge [124]. However, note that for laboring patients with epidural catheters in situ that underwent cesarean delivery, no disparity by race or ethnicity existed [128].

Racial and ethnic disparities were found to exist in the management of PDPH and use of epidural blood patches (EBP) for obstetric patients in the state of New York, with lower rates and delayed timing [129]. In another analysis of patients with PDPH from 2016 to 2020, racial and ethnic disparities were identified in the utilization of epidural blood patches with minority patients being less likely to receive an epidural blood patch [130]. Black race, Hispanic ethnicity, and delivering at Black-serving delivery-units increased the odds of severe maternal morbidity, thus emphasizing the need for multi-level public policies to address disparities in maternal healthcare [131]. Proposed solutions require multifaceted efforts to restructure how obstetrical care is provided at the societal, hospital, and patient levels [132]. The ASA published a statement on reducing maternal peripartum racial and ethnic disparities in anesthesia care [133]. Recommendations include use of preanesthesia clinics to work with obstetricians to identify high-risk patients, multidisciplinary efforts to optimize peripartum anesthetic management, and implementation of ERAC recommendations, as enhanced recovery protocols in non-obstetric settings have been shown to minimize variations in care and reduce disparities [134]. Tools are necessary to reduce peripartum racial and ethnic disparities on both patient and structural levels, including quality improvement efforts, education, implicit bias training, and creation of new models of antenatal care [21, 134]. Anesthesiologists are often at the forefront of these efforts, and their expertise is essential in charting a path forward to minimize disparities in access to healthcare.

25.8 Conclusion

Obstetric anesthesiologists play a major role in driving safe, effective, patient-centered, timely, efficient, and equitable peripartum care with improved outcomes and cost savings. Delays in the incorporation of society guidelines to common clinical practice may be common; therefore, quality improvement initiatives can expedite evidence-based care. These initiatives reduce maternal morbidity and mortality rates, mitigate long-term health issues, and contribute to reducing disparities. There is a profound economic cost associated with safe and effective peripartum care. The medical and nonmedical costs from outcomes associated with maternal morbidity was estimated to total $32.3 billion over a 5-year postpartum period when looking at births in 2019 in the United States alone [134]. Thus, anesthesiologists play a crucial role in improving outcomes and quality, contributing to the patient experience, decreasing costs, and reducing maternal morbidity and mortality.

References

1. Shinnick JK, Ruhotina M, Has P, Kelly BJ, Brousseau EC, O'Brien J, et al. Enhanced recovery after surgery for cesarean delivery decreases length of hospital stay and opioid consumption: a quality improvement initiative. Am J Perinatol. 2020. https://doi.org/10.1055/s-0040-1709456.
2. Pinho B, Costa A. Impact of enhanced recovery after surgery (ERAS) guidelines implementation in cesarean delivery: a systematic review and meta-analysis. Eur J Obstet Gynecol Reprod Biol. 2024;292:201–9. https://doi.org/10.1016/j.ejogrb.2023.11.028.
3. Kleiman AM, Chisholm CA, Dixon AJ, Sariosek BM, Thiele RH, Hedrick TL, et al. Evaluation of the impact of enhanced recovery after surgery protocol implementation on maternal outcomes following elective cesarean delivery. Int J Obstet Anesth. 2020;43:39–46. https://doi.org/10.1016/j.ijoa.2019.08.004.
4. Tepper JL, Harris OM, Triebwasser JE, Ewing SH, Mehta AD, Delaney EJ, et al. Implementation of an enhanced recovery after surgery pathway to reduce inpatient opioid consumption after cesarean delivery. Am J Perinatol. 2023;40(9):945–52. https://doi.org/10.1055/s-0041-1732450.
5. Kearns RJ, Kyzayeva A, Halliday LOE, Lawlor DA, Shaw M, Nelson SM. Epidural analgesia during labour and severe maternal morbidity: population based study. BMJ. 2024;385:e077190. https://doi.org/10.1136/bmj-2023-077190.
6. Guglielminotti J, Landau R, Daw J, Friedman AM, Chihuri S, Li G. Use of labor Neuraxial analgesia for vaginal delivery and severe maternal morbidity. JAMA Netw Open. 2022;5(2):e220137. https://doi.org/10.1001/jamanetworkopen.2022.0137.
7. Driessen M, Bouvier-Colle MH, Dupont C, Khoshnood B, Rudigoz RC, Deneux-Tharaux C, et al. Postpartum hemorrhage resulting from uterine atony after vaginal delivery: factors associated with severity. Obstet Gynecol. 2011;117(1):21–31. https://doi.org/10.1097/AOG.0b013e318202c845.
8. Levels of maternal care: obstetric care consensus no, 9. Obstet Gynecol. 2019;134(2):e41–55. https://doi.org/10.1097/AOG.0000000000003383.
9. Brigance C, Lucas R, Jones E, Davis A, O'Inuma MKM, et al. Nowhere to go: maternity care deserts across the U.S. (Report no. 3). https://www.marchofdimes.org/research/maternity-care-deserts-report.aspx. March of Dimes; 2022.
10. Scharf K, Toledo P. The integration of telehealth in antenatal anesthesia consults. Curr Opin Anaesthesiol. 2025. https://doi.org/10.1097/ACO.0000000000001460.

11. Birth Settings in America: outcomes, quality, access, and choice. Washington: National Academies of Sciences, Engineering, and Medicine; 2020.
12. Six Domains of Healthcare Quality. https://www.ahrq.gov/talkingquality/measures/six-domains.html (2022). Accessed 2 Jan 2025.
13. Nathan N. Maternal mortality: here and abroad. Anesth Analg. 2024;139(6):1132. https://doi.org/10.1213/ANE.0000000000007310.
14. Sultan P. The 2023 Gerard W. Ostheimer lecture. A contemporary narrative review of maternal mortality and morbidity: opportunities to improve peripartum outcomes. Anesth Analg. 2024;139(6):1133–42. https://doi.org/10.1213/ANE.0000000000006885.
15. D'Alton ME, Main EK, Menard MK, Levy BS. The national partnership for maternal safety. Obstet Gynecol. 2014;123(5):973–7. https://doi.org/10.1097/AOG.0000000000000219.
16. Kacmar RM. Safety interventions on the labor and delivery unit. Curr Opin Anaesthesiol. 2017;30(3):287–93. https://doi.org/10.1097/ACO.0000000000000469.
17. Arora KS, Shields LE, Grobman WA, D'Alton ME, Lappen JR, Mercer BM. Triggers, bundles, protocols, and checklists–what every maternal care provider needs to know. Am J Obstet Gynecol. 2016;214(4):444–51. https://doi.org/10.1016/j.ajog.2015.10.011.
18. Main EK, Goffman D, Scavone BM, Low LK, Bingham D, Fontaine PL, et al. National Partnership for maternal safety: consensus bundle on obstetric hemorrhage. Anesth Analg. 2015;121(1):142–8. https://doi.org/10.1097/AOG.0000000000000869.
19. Bernstein PS, Martin JN Jr, Barton JR, Shields LE, Druzin ML, Scavone BM, et al. National partnership for maternal safety: consensus bundle on severe hypertension during pregnancy and the postpartum period. Anesth Analg. 2017;125(2):540–7. https://doi.org/10.1213/ANE.0000000000002304.
20. D'Alton ME, Friedman AM, Smiley RM, Montgomery DM, Paidas MJ, D'Oria R, et al. National partnership for maternal safety: consensus bundle on venous thromboembolism. Obstet Gynecol. 2016;128(4):688–98. https://doi.org/10.1097/AOG.0000000000001579.
21. Howell EA, Brown H, Brumley J, Bryant AS, Caughey AB, Cornell AM, et al. Reduction of peripartum racial and ethnic disparities: a conceptual framework and maternal safety consensus bundle. Obstet Gynecol. 2018;131(5):770–82. https://doi.org/10.1097/AOG.0000000000002475.
22. Krans EE, Campopiano M, Cleveland LM, Goodman D, Kilday D, Kendig S, et al. National partnership for maternal safety: consensus bundle on obstetric care for women with opioid use disorder. Obstet Gynecol. 2019;134(2):365–75. https://doi.org/10.1097/AOG.0000000000003381.
23. Garneau AW, Daly JL, Blair K, Minehart RD. Racism and inequities in maternal health. Anesthesiol Clin. 2025;43(1):47–66. https://doi.org/10.1016/j.anclin.2024.09.003.
24. Dennis AT, Xin A, Farber MK. Perioperative management of patients with preeclampsia: a comprehensive review. Anesthesiology. 2025;142(2):378–402. https://doi.org/10.1097/ALN.0000000000005296.
25. Mhyre JM, D'Oria R, Hameed AB, Lappen JR, Holley SL, Hunter SK, et al. The maternal early warning criteria: a proposal from the national partnership for maternal safety. Obstet Gynecol. 2014;124(4):782–6. https://doi.org/10.1097/AOG.0000000000000480.
26. Singh S, McGlennan A, England A, Simons R. A validation study of the CEMACH recommended modified early obstetric warning system (MEOWS). Anaesthesia. 2012;67(1):12–8. https://doi.org/10.1111/j.1365-2044.2011.06896.x.
27. Shields LE, Wiesner S, Klein C, Pelletreau B, Hedriana HL. Use of maternal early warning trigger tool reduces maternal morbidity. Am J Obstet Gynecol. 2016;214(4):527 e1–6. https://doi.org/10.1016/j.ajog.2016.01.154.
28. Zuckerwise LC, Lipkind HS. Maternal early warning systems-towards reducing preventable maternal mortality and severe maternal morbidity through improved clinical surveillance and responsiveness. Semin Perinatol. 2017;41(3):161–5. https://doi.org/10.1053/j.semperi.2017.03.005.

29. Silver RM, Fox KA, Barton JR, Abuhamad AZ, Simhan H, Huls CK, et al. Center of excellence for placenta accreta. Am J Obstet Gynecol. 2015;212(5):561–8. https://doi.org/10.1016/j.ajog.2014.11.018.
30. Cobb BT, Lane-Fall MB, Month RC, Onuoha OC, Srinivas SK, Neuman MD. Anesthesiologist specialization and use of general anesthesia for cesarean delivery. Anesthesiology. 2019;130(2):237–46. https://doi.org/10.1097/ALN.0000000000002534.
31. Wagner JL, White RS, Mauer EA, Pryor KO, Kjaer K. Impact of anesthesiologist's fellowship status on the risk of general anesthesia for unplanned cesarean delivery. Acta Anaesthesiol Scand. 2019;63(6):769–74. https://doi.org/10.1111/aas.13350.
32. Gelber K, Kahwajian H, Geller AW, Zakowski MI. Obstetric anesthesiology in the United States: current and future demand for fellowship-trained subspecialists. Anesth Analg. 2018;127(6):1445–7. https://doi.org/10.1213/ane.0000000000003809.
33. DeSisto CL, Ewing AC, Diop H, Easter SR, Harvey E, Kane DJ, et al. Maternal risk conditions and outcomes by levels of maternal care. J Womens Health (Larchmt). 2024. https://doi.org/10.1089/jwh.2024.0547.
34. Hess PE, Li Y. Anesthetic considerations and blood utilization for placenta accreta spectrum. Clin Obstet Gynecol. 2024. https://doi.org/10.1097/GRF.0000000000000921.
35. Warrick CM, Sutton CD, Farber MM, Hess PE, Butwick A, Markley JC. Anesthesia considerations for placenta accreta spectrum. Am J Perinatol. 2023;40(9):980–7. https://doi.org/10.1055/s-0043-1761637.
36. Bauchat JR, Weiniger CF, Sultan P, Habib AS, Ando K, Kowalczyk JJ, et al. Society for obstetric anesthesia and perinatology consensus statement: monitoring recommendations for prevention and detection of respiratory depression associated with administration of neuraxial morphine for cesarean delivery analgesia. Anesth Analg. 2019;129(2):458–74. https://doi.org/10.1213/ANE.0000000000004195.
37. Carvalho B, Mhyre JM. Centers of excellence for anesthesia care of obstetric patients. Anesth Analg. 2019;128(5):844–6. https://doi.org/10.1213/ANE.0000000000004027.
38. van Klei WA, Moons KG, Rutten CL, Schuurhuis A, Knape JT, Kalkman CJ, et al. The effect of outpatient preoperative evaluation of hospital inpatients on cancellation of surgery and length of hospital stay. Anesth Analg. 2002;94(3):644–9. Table of contents. https://doi.org/10.1097/00000539-200203000-00030.
39. Ferschl MB, Tung A, Sweitzer B, Huo D, Glick DB. Preoperative clinic visits reduce operating room cancellations and delays. Anesthesiology. 2005;103(4):855–9. https://doi.org/10.1097/00000542-200510000-00025.
40. Umeno Y, Ishikawa S, Kudoh O, Hayashida M. Effects of the multidisciplinary preoperative clinic on the incidence of elective surgery cancellation. J Med Syst. 2022;46(12):95. https://doi.org/10.1007/s10916-022-01883-3.
41. Knight M, Bunch K, Patel R, Shakespeare J, Kotnis R, Kenyon S, on behalf of MBRRACE-UK, et al. Saving lives, improving mothers' care core report - lessons learned to inform maternity care from the UK and Ireland confidential enquiries into maternal deaths and morbidity 2018–20. Oxford: National Perinatal Epidemiology Unit: University of Oxford; 2022.
42. Metzger L, Teitelbaum M, Weber G, Kumaraswami S. Complex pathology and management in the obstetric patient: a narrative review for the anesthesiologist. Cureus. 2021;13(8):e17196. https://doi.org/10.7759/cureus.17196.
43. American College of O, Gynecologists' Committee on Practice B-O. ACOG Practice Bulletin No. 209: obstetric analgesia and anesthesia. Obstet Gynecol. 2019;133(3):e208–e25. https://doi.org/10.1097/AOG.0000000000003132.
44. Sachs A, Aaronson J, Smiley R. The role of the anesthesiologist in the care of the parturient with cardiac disease. Semin Perinatol. 2014;38(5):252–9. https://doi.org/10.1053/j.semperi.2014.04.014.
45. Kostyk P, Kumaraswami S, Rajendran GP, Goldberg J. Management of a parturient with the ACTA2 gene mutation. Int J Obstet Anesth. 2021;47:103173. https://doi.org/10.1016/j.ijoa.2021.103173.

46. Bian W, Liu S, Zhou P, Yan K, Zhang J, Bian W, et al. Extracorporeal membrane oxygenation in obstetrical patients: a meta-analysis. J Artif Organs. 2024. https://doi.org/10.1007/s10047-024-01480-w.
47. Meng ML, Smiley R. The cardio-obstetrics patient and the cardiothoracic anesthesiologist. J Cardiothorac Vasc Anesth. 2022;36(2):546–8. https://doi.org/10.1053/j.jvca.2021.11.009.
48. Dominguez JE, Habib AS. Obstructive sleep apnea in pregnant women. Int Anesthesiol Clin. 2022;60(2):59–65. https://doi.org/10.1097/AIA.0000000000000360.
49. Deighan M, Ash S, McMorrow R. Anaesthesia for parturients with severe cystic fibrosis: a case series. Int J Obstet Anesth. 2014;23(1):75–9. https://doi.org/10.1016/j.ijoa.2013.10.006.
50. Garvey GP, Wasade VS, Murphy KE, Balki M. Anesthetic and obstetric management of syringomyelia during labor and delivery: a case series and systematic review. Anesth Analg. 2017;125(3):913–24. https://doi.org/10.1213/ANE.0000000000001987.
51. Waters JFR, O'Neal MA, Pilato M, Waters S, Larkin JC, Waters JH. Management of anesthesia and delivery in women with Chiari I malformations. Obstet Gynecol. 2018;132(5):1180–4. https://doi.org/10.1097/AOG.0000000000002943.
52. Camann W. Obstetric neuraxial anesthesia contraindicated? Really? Time to rethink old dogma. Anesth Analg. 2015;121(4):846–8. https://doi.org/10.1213/ANE.0000000000000925.
53. Landrum M, Nocka HR, Ashebo L, Hilmara D, MacAlpine E, Flynn JM, et al. Pregnancy and childbirth after spinal fusion for adolescent idiopathic scoliosis. J Pediatr Orthop. 2023;43(10):620–5. https://doi.org/10.1097/BPO.0000000000002499.
54. Reale SC, Farber MK, Lumbreras-Marquez MI, Connors JM, Carabuena JM. Anesthetic management of Von Willebrand Disease in pregnancy: a retrospective analysis of a large case series. Anesth Analg. 2021;133(5):1244–50. https://doi.org/10.1213/ANE.0000000000005502.
55. Handa S, Sterpi M, Sacchi De Camargo Correia G, Frankel DS, Beilin Y, Cytryn L, et al. Obstetric and perioperative management of patients with factor XI deficiency: a retrospective observational study. Blood Adv. 2023;7(10):1967–75. https://doi.org/10.1182/bloodadvances.2022008648.
56. Bollag L, Lim G, Sultan P, Habib AS, Landau R, Zakowski M, et al. Society for Obstetric Anesthesia and Perinatology: consensus statement and recommendations for enhanced recovery after cesarean. Anesth Analg. 2021;132(5):1362–77. https://doi.org/10.1213/ane.0000000000005257.
57. Patel K, Zakowski M. Enhanced recovery after cesarean: current and emerging trends. Curr Anesthesiol Rep. 2021;11(2):136–44. https://doi.org/10.1007/s40140-021-00442-9.
58. Caughey AB, Sultan P, Monks DT, Sharawi N, Bamber J, Panelli DM, et al. Guidelines for intraoperative care in cesarean delivery: enhanced recovery after surgery society recommendations (part 2)-2025 update. Am J Obstet Gynecol. 2025:S0002-9378(25)00121-8. https://doi.org/10.1016/j.ajog.2025.02.040. Epub ahead of print.
59. American Society of Anesthesiologists. Statement on quality metrics. In: Committee on Obstetric Anesthesia, editor. https://www.asahq.org/standards-and-guidelines/statement-on-quality-metrics. American Society of Anesthesiologists; 2022.
60. Uppal V, Russell R, Sondekoppam R, Ansari J, Baber Z, Chen Y, et al. Consensus practice guidelines on postdural puncture headache from a multisociety, international working group: a summary report. JAMA Netw Open. 2023;6(8):e2325387. https://doi.org/10.1001/jamanetworkopen.2023.25387.
61. Uppal V, Russell R, Sondekoppam RV, Ansari J, Baber Z, Chen Y, et al. Evidence-based clinical practice guidelines on postdural puncture headache: a consensus report from a multisociety international working group. Reg Anesth Pain Med. 2024;49(7):471–501. https://doi.org/10.1136/rapm-2023-104817.
62. Huang C, Wang X, Gao S, Luo W, Zhao X, Zhou Q, et al. Sugammadex versus neostigmine for recovery of respiratory muscle strength measured by ultrasonography in the postextubation period: a randomized controlled trial. Anesth Analg. 2023;136(3):559–68. https://doi.org/10.1213/ANE.0000000000006219.

63. Moss AP, Powell MF, Morgan CJ, Tubinis MD. Sugammadex versus neostigmine for routine reversal of neuromuscular blockade and the effect on perioperative efficiency. Proc (Bayl Univ Med Cent). 2022;35(5):599–603. https://doi.org/10.1080/08998280.2022.2079921.
64. Society for Obstetric Anesthesia and Perinatology. Statement on sugammadex during pregnancy and lactation. https://www.soap.org/assets/docs/SOAP_Statement_Sugammadex_During_Pregnancy_Lactation_APPROVED.pdf. Society for Obstetric Anesthesia and Perinatology; 2019.
65. Bateman BT, Franklin JM, Bykov K, Avorn J, Shrank WH, Brennan TA, et al. Persistent opioid use following cesarean delivery: patterns and predictors among opioid-naive women. Am J Obstet Gynecol. 2016;215(3):353 e1–e18. https://doi.org/10.1016/j.ajog.2016.03.016.
66. Lim G, Carvalho B, George RB, Bateman BT, Brummett CM, Ip VHY, et al. Consensus statement on pain Management for pregnant patients with opioid-use disorder from the Society for Obstetric Anesthesia and Perinatology, Society for Maternal-Fetal Medicine, and American Society of Regional Anesthesia and Pain Medicine. Anesth Analg. 2024. https://doi.org/10.1213/ANE.0000000000007237.
67. Landau R. Post-cesarean delivery pain. Management of the opioid-dependent patient before, during and after cesarean delivery. Int J Obstet Anesth. 2019;39:105–16. https://doi.org/10.1016/j.ijoa.2019.01.011.
68. Shah S, Schwenk ES, Sondekoppam RV, Clarke H, Zakowski M, Rzasa-Lynn RS, et al. ASRA pain medicine consensus guidelines on the management of the perioperative patient on cannabis and cannabinoids. Reg Anesth Pain Med. 2023 Mar;48(3):97–117.
69. Alliance for Innovation on Maternal Health. https://saferbirth.org (2024). Accessed 2 Jan 2025.
70. Bauer ME, Albright C, Prabhu M, Heine RP, Lennox C, Allen C, et al. Alliance for innovation on maternal health: consensus bundle on sepsis in obstetric care. Obstet Gynecol. 2023;142(3):481–92. https://doi.org/10.1097/AOG.0000000000005304.
71. Lagrew D, McNulty J, Sakowski C, Cape V, McCormick E, Morton C. Improving health care response to obstetric hemorrhage, a California maternal quality care collaborative toolkit. California Maternal Quality Care Collaborative; 2022.
72. Martins JG, Waller J, Horgan R, Kawakita T, Kanaan C, Abuhamad A, et al. Point-of-care ultrasound in critical care obstetrics: a scoping review of the current evidence. J Ultrasound Med. 2024;43(5):951–65. https://doi.org/10.1002/jum.16425.
73. Assu SM, Bhatia N, Jain K, Gainder S, Sikka P, Aditya AS. Sonographic optic nerve sheath diameter following seizure prophylaxis in pre-eclamptic parturients with severe features: a prospective, observational study. J Ultrasound Med. 2021;40(11):2451–7. https://doi.org/10.1002/jum.15632.
74. Osorio Cajes G, Belot-de Saint Leger F, Lefevre C, Clement D. Reevaluating optic nerve sheath diameter in predicting postdural puncture headache: exploring clinical implications beyond threshold values. J Clin Monit Comput. 2024;38(2):557–8. https://doi.org/10.1007/s10877-023-01086-2.
75. Van de Putte P, Vernieuwe L, Bouchez S. Point-of-care ultrasound in pregnancy: gastric, airway, neuraxial, cardiorespiratory. Curr Opin Anaesthesiol. 2020;33(3):277–83. https://doi.org/10.1097/ACO.0000000000000846.
76. Siddiqui MM, Banayan JM, Hofer JE. Pre-eclampsia through the eyes of the obstetrician and anesthesiologist. Int J Obstet Anesth. 2019;40:140–8. https://doi.org/10.1016/j.ijoa.2019.04.002. Epub 2019 Apr 13.
77. Padilla CR, Shamshirsaz AA, Easter SR, Hess P, Smith C, El Sharawi N, et al. Critical care in placenta accreta spectrum disorders-a call to action. Am J Perinatol. 2023;40(9):988–95. https://doi.org/10.1055/s-0043-1761638.
78. Young B, Onwochei D, Desai N. Conventional landmark palpation vs. preprocedural ultrasound for neuraxial analgesia and anaesthesia in obstetrics - a systematic review and meta-analysis with trial sequential analyses. Anaesthesia. 2021;76(6):818–31. https://doi.org/10.1111/anae.15255.

79. Mergler BD, Duffy CC, Mergler RJ. Patient-centered strategies in obstetric anaesthesia. BJA Educ. 2025;25(2):80–6. https://doi.org/10.1016/j.bjae.2024.09.007.
80. Substance Abuse and Mental Health Services Administration. Trauma -informed approaches and programs. https://www.samhsa.gov/mental-health/trauma-violence/trauma-informed-approaches-programs. Updated Dec 2024, Accessed Aug 2025.
81. Vogel TM, Coffin E. Trauma-informed care on labor and delivery. Anesthesiol Clin. 2021;39(4):779–91. https://doi.org/10.1016/j.anclin.2021.08.007.
82. Mason CL, Tran CK. Caring for the Jehovah's witness parturient. Anesth Analg. 2015;121(6):1564–9. https://doi.org/10.1213/ANE.0000000000000933.
83. Sween LK, West JM. Ethical issues in the care of patients whose personal, religious, or cultural beliefs impact clinical management strategies. Anesthesiol Clin. 2024;42(3):515–28. https://doi.org/10.1016/j.anclin.2023.12.002.
84. Bamber JH, Lucas DN, Plaat F, Allin B, Knight M, Collaborators for the Obstetric Anaesthetists' Association Q, et al. The identification of key indicators to drive quality improvement in obstetric anaesthesia: results of the Obstetric Anaesthetists' Association/National Perinatal Epidemiology Unit collaborative Delphi project. Anaesthesia. 2020;75(5):617–25. https://doi.org/10.1111/anae.14861.
85. Fedoruk KA, Sultan P. Obstetric anesthesia quality metrics: performance, pitfalls, and potential. Anesth Analg. 2024;139(6):1223–8. https://doi.org/10.1213/ANE.0000000000007054.
86. Pandya ST, Chakravarthy K, Vemareddy A. Obstetric anaesthesia practice: dashboard as a dynamic audit tool. Indian J Anaesth. 2018;62(11):838–43. https://doi.org/10.4103/ija.IJA_346_18.
87. Fedoruk K, Xie J, Wang E, Fowler C, Riley E, Carvalho B. Effect of an electronic medical record nudge to improve quality improvement program tracking of neuraxial catheter replacements in obstetric patients. BMJ Open Qual. 2023;12(4). https://doi.org/10.1136/bmjoq-2022-002240.
88. Bauer ME, Arendt K, Beilin Y, Gernsheimer T, Perez Botero J, James AH, et al. The Society for Obstetric Anesthesia and Perinatology interdisciplinary consensus statement on neuraxial procedures in obstetric patients with thrombocytopenia. Anesth Analg. 2021;132(6):1531–44. https://doi.org/10.1213/ANE.0000000000005355.
89. Leffert L, Butwick A, Carvalho B, Arendt K, Bates SM, Friedman A, et al. The Society for Obstetric Anesthesia and Perinatology consensus statement on the anesthetic management of pregnant and postpartum women receiving thromboprophylaxis or higher dose anticoagulants. Anesth Analg. 2018;126(3):928–44. https://doi.org/10.1213/ANE.0000000000002530.
90. Park YL, Clifton B, Ashraf R, Barlow R, Anderson A, Altamirano V, et al. Patient and provider perspectives on pain and other dimensions of anesthesia experience for cesarean delivery: a qualitative study. Res Sq. 2024. https://doi.org/10.21203/rs.3.rs-4814545/v1.
91. Orbach-Zinger S, Olliges E, Garren A, Azem K, Fein S, Heesen P, et al. Patient/anesthesiologist intersubjective experiences and intravenous supplementation during elective cesarean delivery: a prospective patient-reported outcome study. J Clin Anesth. 2025;100:111689. https://doi.org/10.1016/j.jclinane.2024.111689.
92. Charles EA, Carter H, Stanford S, Blake L, Eley V, Carvalho B, et al. Intraoperative pain during cesarean delivery under neuraxial anesthesia: a systematic review and meta-analysis. Anesthesiology. 2025;143(1):156–67. https://doi.org/10.1097/ALN.0000000000005486. Epub 2025 Apr 4.
93. American Society of Anesthesiologists. Statement on the use of adjuvant medications and management of intraoperative pain during cesarean delivery. In: Committee on Obstetric Anesthesia, editor. https://www.asahq.org/standards-and-practice-parameters. American Society of Anesthesiologists; 2024.
94. Keita H, Deruelle P, Bouvet L, Bonnin M, Chassard D, Bouthors AS, et al. French Practice Bulletin Taskforce: "Préconisations - insuffisance d'analgésie au cours de la césarienne sous anesthésie périmédullaire: prévention - prise en charge immédiate et différée". Raising awareness to prevent, recognise and manage acute pain during caesarean delivery: The French Practice Bulletin. Anaesth Crit Care Pain Med. 2021;40(5):100934. https://doi.

org/10.1016/j.accpm.2021.100934. Epub 2021 Aug 13. Erratum in: Anaesth Crit Care Pain Med. 2021;40(6):100954. https://doi.org/10.1016/j.accpm.2021.100954.

95. Plaat F, Stanford SER, Lucas DN, Andrade J, Careless J, Russell R, et al. Prevention and management of intra-operative pain during caesarean section under neuraxial anaesthesia: a technical and interpersonal approach. Anaesthesia. 2022;77(5):588–97. https://doi.org/10.1111/anae.15717. Epub 2022 Mar 24.
96. American Society of Anesthesiologists. Statement on providing psychological support for obstetric patients. In: Committee on Obstetric Anesthesia, editor. https://www.asahq.org/standards-and-practice-parameters/statement-on-providing-psychological-support-for-obstetric-patients. American Society of Anesthesiologists; 2024.
97. Kountanis JA, Vogel TM. Unveiling the anesthesiologist's impact on childbirth-related posttraumatic stress disorder. Anesth Analg. 2024;139(6):1156–8. https://doi.org/10.1213/ANE.0000000000006991.
98. Im M, Riley ET, Hoang D, Lim G, Zakowski M, Carvalho B. Obstetric anesthesia procedure-based workload and facility utilization of Society of Obstetric Anesthesia and Perinatology Centers of excellence designated institutions. Anesth Analg. 2022;135(6):1142–50. https://doi.org/10.1213/ane.0000000000006112.
99. Ginosar Y, Wimpfheimer A, Weissman C. Using mean anesthesia workload to plan anesthesia workforce allocations: the "flaw of averages". Anesth Analg. 2022;135(6):1138–41. https://doi.org/10.1213/ANE.0000000000006220.
100. Lim G, Lim AJ, Quinn B, Carvalho B, Zakowski M, Lynde GC. Obstetric operating room staffing and operating efficiency using queueing theory. BMC Health Serv Res. 2023;23(1):1147. https://doi.org/10.1186/s12913-023-10143-0.
101. Murphy J, Vaughn J, Gelber K, Geller A, Zakowski M. Readability, content, quality and accuracy assessment of internet-based patient education materials relating to labor analgesia. Int J Obstet Anesth. 2019;39:82–7. https://doi.org/10.1016/j.ijoa.2019.01.003.
102. Che YJ, Gao YL, Jing J, Kuang Y, Zhang M. Effects of an informational video about anesthesia on pre- and post-elective cesarean section anxiety and recovery: a randomized controlled trial. Med Sci Monit. 2020;26:e920428. https://doi.org/10.12659/MSM.920428.
103. Broaddus BM, Chandrasekhar S. Informed consent in obstetric anesthesia. Anesth Analg. 2011;112(4):912–5. https://doi.org/10.1213/ANE.0b013e31820e777a.
104. McQuaid-Hanson E, Pian-Smith MC. Huddles and debriefings: improving communication on labor and delivery. Anesthesiol Clin. 2017;35(1):59–67. https://doi.org/10.1016/j.anclin.2016.09.006.
105. Girnius A, Snyder C, Czarny H, Minges T, Stacey M, Supinski T, et al. Preoperative multidisciplinary team huddle improves communication and safety for unscheduled cesarean deliveries: a system redesign using improvement science. Anesth Analg. 2024;139(6):1199–209. https://doi.org/10.1213/ANE.0000000000006905.
106. Society for Obstetric Anesthesia and Perinatology, American Society of Anesthesiologists, Society for Pediatric Anesthesia, American College of Obstetricians Gynecologists, Society for Maternal-Fetal Medicine. Labor epidurals do not cause autism; safe for mothers and infants, say anesthesiology, obstetrics, and pediatric medical societies. https://soap.memberclicks.net/assets/docs/JAMAPeds_Epidurals_SOAP_ASA_SPA_ACOG_SMFM_Media_Response_101220%20%281%29.pdf. Society for Obstetric Anesthesia and Perinatology; 2020.
107. Bauer ME, Bernstein K, Dinges E, Delgado C, El-Sharawi N, Sultan P, et al. Obstetric anesthesia during the COVID-19 pandemic. Anesth Analg. 2020;131(1):7–15. https://doi.org/10.1213/ANE.0000000000004856.
108. Katz D, Bateman BT, Kjaer K, Turner DP, Spence NZ, Habib AS, et al. The Society for Obstetric Anesthesia and Perinatology coronavirus disease 2019 registry: an analysis of outcomes among pregnant women delivering during the initial severe acute respiratory syndrome Coronavirus-2 outbreak in the United States. Anesth Analg. 2021;133(2):462–73. https://doi.org/10.1213/ANE.0000000000005592.

109. Abrams J, Mahoney B. The importance of simulation-based multi professional training in obstetric anesthesia: an update. Curr Opin Anaesthesiol. 2024;37(3):239–44. https://doi.org/10.1097/ACO.0000000000001352.
110. Thenuwara K, Santillan D, Henkle J, Forman J, Dunbar A, Faro E, et al. A statewide mobile simulation program for improving obstetric skills in rural hospitals. Anesth Analg. 2024;139(5):931–9. https://doi.org/10.1213/ANE.0000000000006883.
111. Chan J, Chan C, Chia P, Goy R, Sng BL. Novice learners' perspectives on obstetric airway crisis decision-making training using virtual reality simulation. Int J Obstet Anesth. 2024;57:103926. https://doi.org/10.1016/j.ijoa.2023.103926.
112. Duffy CC, Kearsley R. Simulation-based training in obstetric anaesthesia. BJA Educ. 2024;24(12):468–75. https://doi.org/10.1016/j.bjae.2024.08.002.
113. American Society of Anesthesiologists. Statement on deactivating central piped nitrous oxide to mitigate avoidable health care pollution. https://www.asahq.org/standards-and-practice-parameters/statement-on-deactivating-central-piped-nitrous-oxide-to-mitigate-avoidable-health-care-pollution. American Society of Anesthesiologists; 2024.
114. Royal College of Anaesthetists. Consensus statement on the removal of pipeline nitrous oxide in the United Kingdom and Republic of Ireland. https://rcoa.ac.uk/sites/default/files/documents/2024-07/Consensus%20statement%20on%20removal%20of%20pipeline%20nitrous%20oxide.pdf. Royal College of Anaesthetists; 2024.
115. Rollins MD, Arendt K, Carvalho B, Vallejo MC, Zakowski M. Nitrous oxide. In: Anesthesia ACoO, editor. https://www.asahq.org/about-asa/governance-and-committees/asa-committees/committee-on-obstetric-anesthesia/nitrous-oxide. American Society of Anesthesiologists; 2018.
116. ASA Committee on Environmental Health. Anesthesiology sustainability checklist. https://www.asahq.org/about-asa/governance-and-committees/asa-committees/environmental-sustainability/greening-the-operating-room/checklists#/. American Society of Anesthesiologists; 2024.
117. American Society of Anesthesiologists. Statement on neuraxial medication shortage and alternatives. In: Anesthesia ACoO, editor. https://www.asahq.org/standards-and-practice-parameters/statement-on-neuraxial-medication-shortage-and-alternatives. American Society of Anesthesiologists; 2023.
118. Society for Obstetric Anesthesia and Perinatology. Advisory in response to shortages of local anesthetics in North America. https://soap.memberclicks.net/assets/docs/2018-bupivacaine-shortage-statement-1.pdf. Society for Obstetric Anesthesia and Perinatology; 2018.
119. Society for Obstetric Anesthesia and Perinatology. Statement on oxytocin shortage. In: Committee SE, editor. https://www.soap.org/soap-statement-on-oxytocin-shortage. Society for Obstetric Anesthesia and Perinatology; 2022.
120. American Society of Anesthesiologists. ASA suggested actions on conservation of IV solutions during ongoing shortage. https://www.asahq.org/advocating-for-you/hurricane-helene-baxter-shortages/asa-guidance-shortages#/. American Society of Anesthesiologists; 2024.
121. Society for Obstetric Anesthesia and Perinatology. SOAP recommendations for IV fluid conservation. https://soap.memberclicks.net/assets/docs/SOAP%20RECOMMENDATIONS%20FOR%20IV%20FLUID%20CONSERVATION.pdf. Society for Obstetric Anesthesia and Perinatology; 2024.
122. Society for Obstetric Anesthesia and Perinatology. It's a 'Kit'astrophe! TIps on Epidural Kit Shortage. In: Subcommittee SPS, editor. https://www.soap.org/assets/docs/Its_a_Kitastrophe_Epidural_Kit%20Shortage_final.pdf. Society for Obstetric Anesthesia and Perinatology; 2022.
123. Chen Y, Shiels MS, Uribe-Leitz T, Molina RL, Lawrence WR, Freedman ND, Abnet CC. Pregnancy-related deaths in the US, 2018–2022. JAMA Netw Open. 2025;8(4):e254325. https://doi.org/10.1001/jamanetworkopen.2025.4325.
124. Lee W, Martins MS, George RB, Fernandez A. Racial and ethnic disparities in obstetric anesthesia: a scoping review. Can J Anaesth. 2023;70(6):1035–46. https://doi.org/10.1007/s12630-023-02460-z.

125. Centers for disease control and prevention: pregnancy mortality surveillance system (PMSS). https://www.cdc.gov/reproductivehealth/maternal-mortality/pregnancy-mortality-surveillance-system.htm (2023). Accessed 2 Jan 2025.
126. Khusid E, Lui B, Ibarra A, Villegas K, White RS. Review of racial/ethnic disparities in obstetrics-related anesthesia administration and pain management. Pain Manag. 2023;13(7):415–22. https://doi.org/10.2217/pmt-2023-0034.
127. Toledo P, Sun J, Grobman WA, Wong CA, Feinglass J, Hasnain-Wynia R. Racial and ethnic disparities in neuraxial labor analgesia. Anesth Analg. 2012;114(1):172–8. https://doi.org/10.1213/ANE.0b013e318239dc7c.
128. Thomas CL, Lange EMS, Banayan JM, Zhu Y, Liao C, Peralta FM, et al. Racial and ethnic disparities in receipt of general anesthesia for cesarean delivery. JAMA Netw Open. 2024;7(1):e2350825. https://doi.org/10.1001/jamanetworkopen.2023.50825.
129. Lee A, Guglielminotti J, Janvier AS, Li G, Landau R. Racial and ethnic disparities in the management of postdural puncture headache with epidural blood patch for obstetric patients in New York state. JAMA Netw Open. 2022;5(4):e228520. https://doi.org/10.1001/jamanetworkopen.2022.8520.
130. Potnuru PP, Jonna S, Orlando B, Nwokolo OO. Racial and ethnic disparities in epidural blood patch utilization among obstetric patients in the United States: a Nationwide analysis, 2016–2020. Anesth Analg. 2024;139(6):1190–8. https://doi.org/10.1213/ANE.0000000000006754.
131. Sastow DL, Jiang SY, Tangel VE, Matthews KC, Abramovitz SE, Oxford-Horrey CM, et al. Patient race and racial composition of delivery unit associated with disparities in severe maternal morbidity: a multistate analysis 2007–2014. Int J Obstet Anesth. 2021;47:103160. https://doi.org/10.1016/j.ijoa.2021.103160.
132. White RS, Tangel VE, Lui B, Jiang SY, Pryor KO, Abramovitz SE. Racial and ethnic disparities in delivery in-hospital mortality or maternal end-organ injury: a multistate analysis, 2007–2020. J Womens Health (Larchmt). 2023;32(12):1292–307. https://doi.org/10.1089/jwh.2023.0245.
133. American Society of Anesthesiologists. Statement on reducing maternal peripartum racial and ethnic disparities in anesthesia care. In: Committee on Obstetric Anesthesia, editor. https://www.asahq.org/standards-and-practice-parameters/statement-on-reducing-maternal-peripartum-racial-and-ethnic-disparities-in-anesthesia-care. American Society of Anesthesiologists; 2021.
134. O'Neil SS, Platt I, Vohra D, Pendl-Robinson E, Dehus E, Zephyrin L, et al. Societal cost of nine selected maternal morbidities in the United States. PLoS One. 2022;17(10):e0275656. https://doi.org/10.1371/journal.pone.0275656.

Part VI

Advancing the Profession of Anesthesiology: Risk, Revenue, Workforce, Policy, and the Future of Perioperative Care

Risk Management, Medicolegal Considerations, and the Role of the Anesthesiologist

26

Ashley Eltorai

26.1 Risk Management in Anesthesiology

Anesthesiologists are masters, by trade, at quickly assimilating numerous complex data points into one cohesive clinical picture and decisively selecting courses of action for their patients. Who better, then, to review adverse events and recognize the best strategies and processes for quality improvement and risk management moving forward? Managing risk and weighing a patient's different interests against one another is a daily task of every anesthesiologist, and no small one when the level of risk often rises to life-threatening. For instance, the patient may have recently taken a GLP-1 inhibitor, increasing the risk of aspiration during anesthetic induction, but the decision to wait longer for surgery while holding that medication must be weighed against the risk of not addressing the surgical problem as quickly. Logistical and facility constraints, as well as socioeconomic factors such as access to care, may interplay with medical factors to add many layers of complexity to the question of what is best for a patient.

26.2 The Process of Quality Review

I. **What Is the Problem**? In order for anesthesiologists to propose solutions to manage risk and improve quality of patient care, they need to know which problems actually exist and the details of incidents that have occurred. Tracking adverse events in anesthesiology is challenging, due to the need to precisely define quality metrics and effectively categorize data, the inability of an electronic medical record to fully capture a complete clinical picture, and under-reporting by clinicians of adverse events encountered. Roadblocks to accurate

A. Eltorai (✉)
University of Connecticut School of Medicine, Hartford, CT, USA
e-mail: ashleyszabo@alumni.nd.edu

G. Tewfik (ed.), *The Anesthesiologist as Perioperative Leader*,
https://doi.org/10.1007/978-3-032-18058-2_26

and complete reporting include lack of a centralized, easily accessible reporting database; under-recognition of the importance of completing such reporting, perhaps representing an opportunity for clinical leadership to better communicate its utility in quality improvement; concerns about repercussions for "admitting mistakes"; and not detecting safety events in the first place. In what context could an involved anesthesiologist not even recognize that a safety event occurred? Near misses, a type of safety event where the chain of events is stopped before actually reaching and causing harm to the patient, are especially difficult to track or later investigate. The anesthesiologist may not know a near miss ever occurred if the chain of events was stopped not consciously by him or her, but by chance, or because the adverse occurrence was mitigated by a second one and its effects became unrecognizable. For example, if a phenylephrine infusion is programmed incorrectly and delivers a much lower dose than intended, but a sudden noxious surgical stimulus also occurs without adequate opioid on board to blunt its sympathetic effects, then the blood pressure may increase by an amount that makes sense for the amount of phenylephrine the anesthesiologist thought was programmed, so he or she never realizes it was programmed incorrectly. Because near misses are harder to identify and appear less dramatic than other adverse event types, they may capture less attention from anesthesiologists and hospital administrators, leading to less effort devoted to the implementation of quality measures meant to deter and mitigate the issues. The situation is analogous to the amount of press and recognition received for rescuing a person from a burning building versus recognizing and remedying a design flaw in an electrical device that would have almost certainly resulted in electrical fires for dozens of end users.

II. **The Anesthesia Record**. When adverse events occur, anesthesiologists begin from the first chapter of the story—the pre-anesthetic evaluation and data available about the patient at that time—and move through each chapter via the anesthesia record. Anesthesia records involve a large quantity of information from a variety of categories, including vital signs and medications administered; however, anesthesiologists during record review, just as in during clinical practice, are able to synthesize it all and distill it down to answer specific questions. Were vital signs just before induction a harbinger of problems to come, or was the onset of the problem more sudden? Does the timing of a drug's administration point to an allergic reaction as the cause of the patient's deterioration? During record review, it is vital to avoid hindsight bias, instead considering the data points and decision tree available to the anesthesiologist in real time, despite knowing what outcome eventually transpired.

III. **Evaluating Human Factors**. Human factors is the study of human behavior, abilities, and limitations and the design of systems, processes, and products to be as user-friendly as possible to maximize the quality of the work those people perform. Human factors represents a significant category of root causes of adverse events in anesthesiology, and anesthesiologists, even without formal psychology training, become informal experts in the area. Because anesthesiologists often perform cognitively demanding tasks under stress, they are aware of the vulnerabilities that exist within systems or processes that create increased likelihood of error. An anesthesiologist may significantly contribute to risk management by recognizing specific, nuanced, and detailed systems shortcomings—such as when the concentration of drug contained in a bag prepared by the pharmacy suddenly doubles, without an announcement made to anesthesiologists letting them know to expect something different. Equally, anesthesiologists are also positioned to recognize more global shortcomings, such as whether operating room production pressure, including on-time case starts, negatively impacts performance by discouraging thoroughness in favor of "cutting corners." Anesthesiologists interact extensively with all members of the perioperative care team and, as individuals present for the duration of surgery, are able to observe exactly how workplace culture and behaviors unfold and what outcomes are generated from them.

26.3 Medicolegal Considerations

I. **Understanding Malpractice Claims Against Anesthesiologists**. When adverse events occur in anesthesia, the involved patient and/or family may choose to bring legal action under the tort of medical malpractice. The requirements for a successful medical malpractice case are known as the four D's: duty, deviation, damages, and direct cause. A duty of care must have been owed to the patient by the defendant in the lawsuit; the care provided must have deviated from what the standard of care requires; and the patient must have suffered damages as a direct result of the standard-of-care deviation. Anesthesiologists do important work any time they develop and communicate standards of care for their profession, uniting their colleagues in the awareness of what is best practice and expected from each other so they may all work toward optimization of anesthesia practice and avoidance of substandard care. Examples include writing anesthesia society guidelines, drafting hospital bylaws, publishing peer-reviewed research on best practices, and participating in internal quality review meetings.

II. **The Role of Professional Societies and Guidelines in Medical Malpractice Defense**. Since bringing a successful medical malpractice case requires establishment that the medical provider deviated from the standard of care, the plaintiff's legal counsel may cite professional societal guidelines as evidence that reasonable providers follow a course of action that is different from the one chosen by the defendant. Conversely, the defendant medical provider may cite guidelines as support for his or her chosen course of action. If guidelines are being used against the defendant, then the defendant's legal counsel can establish why the specific clinical situation was one to which those guidelines could not reasonably apply, or an expert witness can testify that the defendant's choice of action, while different from the guidelines, was a reasonable one that still falls within the usual and customary contemporary practice of anesthesia.

III. **Informed Consent**. The key elements of informed consent in medicine are disclosure, competency, and voluntariness. With respect to anesthesia, the anesthesiologist discloses information to the patient regarding the proposed anesthetic plan and procedures, developed after considering the patient's medical conditions, and the risks and benefits involved. Competency involves ensuring that the patient can adequately comprehend the information that is given in order to make a decision about his or her anesthetic care. If a patient is incompetent to consent for anesthesia, then consent must come from a legally authorized representative. If no such representative is available and surgery is needed emergently to prevent death or serious harm, then the physicians can proceed with surgery and anesthesia under the legal doctrine of implied consent. This involves the assumption that were the patient able to consent, he or she would have, as proceeding is clearly in his or her best interest.

IV. **Documentation**. Documentation plays a key role in both quality review and medical malpractice case proceedings. Anesthesiologists are impactful when they work to develop and tailor their facilities' electronic medical record systems to provide accurate, and appropriately thorough, accounts of patient care. Documentation in real time is important, where the anesthesiologist clearly describes the aspects of the patient's condition (laboratory values, physical examination findings, vital signs, review of systems, and so on) that led him or her to a certain choice of anesthetic plan before that plan is actually executed; in that way, sound medical reasoning behind the decision is apparent, regardless of whether an adverse event later occurs. For instance, for an anesthesiologist choosing general anesthesia with a laryngeal mask airway (LMA) instead of an endotracheal tube, the preoperative evaluation can confirm no active gastroesophageal reflux disease symptoms, appropriate NPO status, and no nausea or emesis prior to the LMA being placed. However, the time between performing a preoperative evaluation and anesthetic induction is quite busy for many anesthesiologists, as the pursuit of operating room efficiency and minimal turnover time, coupled with the potential simultaneous supervision of multiple anesthetizing locations, can leave the anesthesiologist with little time to sit in front of a computer to draft the preoperative evaluation. For this reason, the development of user-friendly, efficient, appropriate EMR templates can mean the difference between an anesthesiologist documenting his or her preoperative evaluation and medical decision-making prior to the time of case start, versus after an adverse event has already occurred. Emergence from anesthesia at the end of the case is another busy time for the anesthesiologist, so when the EMR facilitates quick documentation of important clinical parameters like full neuromuscular blockade reversal with a simple click of a button, the likelihood that the anesthesiologist will complete this documentation prior to a potential failed extubation—not after the fact—increases significantly. Real-time documentation is the most accurate and reliable, where an anesthesiologist is reporting in the moment rather than relying upon recall later, and anesthesiologists make a large-scale difference by optimizing EMR systems and underscoring to colleagues the availability and importance of real-time documentation.

V. **Preoperative Clearance**. When a perioperative adverse event occurs, a major point of scrutiny is whether the patient should have been cleared to undergo that surgery and anesthetic in the first place. Risk reduction is accomplished via thorough preoperative evaluation, in which anesthesiologists play a substantial role. Anesthesiologists, with their broad medical knowledge base in physiology and pharmacology, are well-positioned to analyze a patient's comorbid medical conditions and their potential impact upon perioperative outcomes. They are experts in perioperative medical optimization, including holding or continuing medications the patient was already taking, repleting electrolytes that impact cardiac rhythm, or referring the patient to a new specialist. Anesthesiologists add tremendous value by using their expertise and medical knowledge to weigh in and avoid either over- or under-referral to specialists for additional preoperative optimization and clearance.

VI. **Legal Implications of New Models of Care**

A. **Perioperative Surgical Home (PSH) and Enhanced Recovery After Surgery (ERAS) Programs**

The Perioperative Surgical Home (PSH) is a team-based, multispecialty, coordinated care model (anesthesiology, surgery, nursing) that coordinates a patient's clinical experience before (beginning with the decision to operate), during, and after surgery, optimizing resource use to generate the best possible clinical outcomes [1]. Goals include "prehabilitating" the patient before surgery, delivering ideal care intraoperatively, performing adequate follow-up evaluations, and smoothly transitioning to either home or a post-acute care facility [1]. The emphasis is upon value-based rather than volume-based care [1]. Sample aspects of a PSH include limiting preoperative testing, such as labs, to only what is essential for optimizing care during surgery, and utilizing morbidity and mortality risk models for surgical procedures such as the Veterans Affairs Surgical Quality Improvement Program (VASQIP) calculator [1]. Preoperative patient education is another important component of a PSH, found independently to improve surgical outcomes [1]. Patient satisfaction also improves when PSH is utilized [1].

A subset of PSH includes enhanced recovery after surgery (ERAS) programs, multimodal programs whose goals are to make recovery faster, hospital stay shorter, and complication rates lower [1]. Clinical practices associated with ERAS include optimizing preoperative hydration by avoiding bowel preparations, instead conducting carbohydrate loading and continuing a clear liquid diet until 2 h preoperatively; performing thoughtful intraoperative fluid resuscitation by following metrics such as non-invasive volume responsiveness monitoring and urine output; and avoiding hypothermia or poor tissue oxygen perfusion [1].

The multidisciplinary, team-based structure of PSH creates shared liability for adverse perioperative outcomes. For instance, if a patient suffers an interoperative myocardial infarction, then medical malpractice litigators would examine what preoperative cardiac evaluation was performed and by whom, what tests were ordered, whether the patient was referred to a cardiologist, and what preoperative medication instructions were given and by whom. This would occur in addition to analysis of the surgery itself and of factors controlled intraoperatively by the anesthesia team such as drug administration and hemodynamic monitoring and management. Closed-loop communication is critical when multiple care providers and disciplines are involved in medical management and decision-making: both the pre-anesthesia testing clinic and surgeon's office may assume, for instance, that the other conveyed specific preoperative instructions to the patient, when in reality neither did, the surgeon may have assumed that the anesthesiologist seeing the patient in preoperative anesthesia testing clinic would have placed a cardiologist referral, whereas the anesthesiologist thought the surgeon was going to make that referral decision at his or her own preoperative clinic visit the following day.

B. **Artificial Intelligence in Perioperative Medicine**

As artificial intelligence (AI) becomes increasingly sophisticated and utilized in a variety of contexts, it may find places within anesthesiology. Ideas include decision-support tools that integrate vital sign monitor data into recommendations for clinical interventions, risk predictors for intraoperative and postoperative complications, and interfaces to optimize anesthetic drug dosing for individual patients [2].

When AI operates autonomously, the legal question becomes whether the technology is still considered an agent of some other person or entity, or if liability issues need to be decided on a basis different from agency because that AI technology engages in "thinking" that renders it an agent of no one [3]. Products liability law can be applied whenever an AI-caused adverse event appears to be the result of human error—in the design or production of the AI, or in the failure to properly instruct humans about its use [3]. Even if an adverse event does not appear to be the result of human error in any of the above respects, courts have precedent for using the doctrine of res ipsa loquitur (Latin for "the thing speaks for itself") to assert that the adverse event itself is proof there was a defect or shortcoming [3].

References

1. Kash BA, Zhang Y, Cline KM, Menser T, Miller TR. The perioperative surgical home (PSH): a comprehensive review of US and non-US studies shows predominantly positive quality and cost outcomes. Milbank Q. 2014;92(4):796–821.
2. Kambale M, Jadhay S. Applications of artificial intelligence in anesthesia: a systematic review. Saudi J Anaesth. 2024;18(2):249–56.
3. Vladeck DC. Machines without principals: liability rules and artificial intelligence. Wash Law Rev. 2014;89:117.

Foundation of Revenue Cycle Management Excellence for Today's Anesthesia Practices

27

Dean Polce and Frank Burns

27.1 Revenue Cycle Management System Investment

The anesthesia specialty brings unique challenges to the RCM workflow that may be difficult for billing systems to capture appropriately. Most services are billed through a combination of base and time units as well as modifiers that vary based upon care team structure and medical direction ratios, as well as the clinical complexity and length of the surgery. Additionally, the codes that get billed to payors explaining what services were performed are ASA codes instead of CPT® [1] Codes, as used in other specialties. Therefore, operating dictionaries within the RCM billing system must be updated regularly and audited to ensure the right codes are being billed. Adding to the uniqueness of the specialty, many cases may incorporate an "anesthesia care team" that includes an anesthesiologist and a resident physician, certified registered nurse anesthetist (CRNA), or a certified anesthesiology assistant (CAA). The care team cases require an RCM system with robust functionality to manage physician and care team concurrency while also incorporating appropriate modifiers to maximize revenue for services delivered.

Compliance is a major part of any revenue cycle system, and anesthesia is as challenging as any specialty to make sure invoices are billed correctly. The RCM system must be able to run a daily physician concurrency calculation for all cases that are billed to ensure the right modifiers are included with every claim. It is critical that anesthesia care team modifiers [2] are accurate as payor reimbursement levels vary depending on medical direction care team staffing ratios [3].

D. Polce
US Anesthesia Partners, Las Vegas, NV, USA
e-mail: dean.polce@usap.com

F. Burns (✉)
US Anesthesia Partners, Dallas, TX, USA
e-mail: Frank.burns@usap.com

G. Tewfik (ed.), *The Anesthesiologist as Perioperative Leader*,
https://doi.org/10.1007/978-3-032-18058-2_27

Modifier	Description
AA	Anesthesia services personally performed by an anesthesiologist
AD	Medical supervision by an anesthesiologist of more than four concurrent anesthesia services
QK	Medical direction of two, three, or four concurrent anesthesia procedures involving qualified individuals
QY	Medical direction of one qualified non-physician anesthetist by an anesthesiologist
QX	Qualified non-physician anesthetist service, with medical direction by a physician
QZ	CRNA service, without medical direction by a physician

The unique billing policies required by government and commercial payors need to be defined and monitored (audited) to ensure compliance with payor reimbursement contracts. Not monitoring or complying with these policies appropriately could result in financial penalties and/or fines from payors. It is also important to note that payment and reimbursement for services, as well as allowable modifiers, will vary greatly from payor to payor.

Another important aspect of a best-in-class revenue cycle operating system is the ability to develop custom edits that are necessary to ensure "clean claims" are being sent to payors. There are different definitions of clean billing claims in the industry, but for this discussion, we will define a "clean claim" as a new bill that can be correctly invoiced and accepted by the payor on the initial billing attempt with no manual manipulation. For the anesthesia practices that we manage today, we have built over 1500 custom edits to make sure new claims meet the unique criteria and policies for each payor nationally. The end result of these edits (which are actively managed and updated) is greater than 99.8% claim acceptance rate from the payor. Operational teams that do not have a clean billing process will waste thousands of extra hours annually correcting and reprocessing claims that do not have the required information needed from a payor the first time [4]. Ultimately, these denials cost the practice with delayed or possibly lost revenue if not worked timely and accurately by the operational team.

Arguably just as important is the ability for the billing system to appropriately interface with multiple third-party anesthesia records such as Epic or Cerner, but also multiple third-party vendor applications. This topic will be further addressed in the interoperability section, but it is worth noting the importance of a flexible system that has the right technology available to interface with all of these medical record systems simultaneously.

27.2 Robust Allowable Monitoring

There is an increased focus on physician and hospital Contracting Teams negotiating agreements with payors today as they work to navigate an ever-changing contracting environment between anesthesia practices and commercial payors. Today, it is not uncommon for payor policies to be updated in the middle of the current contract term that could materially impact negotiated reimbursement rates. Over the past year, major commercial payors have introduced national policies that have reduced payment by 15% from contracted fee schedule rates for non-medically directed (QZ billed) CRNA cases. Other examples include eliminating payment for physical status modifiers and qualifying circumstance codes. Combined, these policy changes will have a materially negative impact on your commercial revenue that you now need to understand as you renegotiate or renew your contracts.

Commercial payors have operational systems setup to process all specialties, each with different rates and custom terms across multiple product lines. The complexity of anesthesia time and unit-based billing as well as the care team and unique risk modifiers often make it challenging for commercial and government payors to correctly adjudicate claims at contracted rates.

When asked if they are getting paid at the correct rates, a practice administrator may respond by saying "yes, we audit a sample of cases each year to make sure we get paid the correct rate." While this process is better than not auditing any cases, experience may demonstrate that between 1% and 3% of all anesthesia cases are not paid correctly by a payor annually. While this may seem like a small number, it may put thousands or tens of thousands of dollars in underpaid claims at risk for a practice. Anesthesiologists who provide services should not suffer revenue leakage due to underpaid claims. Simple auditing of cases will not find all the underpaid claims. The RCM system or vendor that is supporting one's practice must ensure that 100% of all cases are paid at the contracted rate. This means having an RCM system that can verify that contracted rates for your cases match the allowable that is paid by the payor. The allowable monitoring system must be robust and sophisticated enough to manage contract rates that vary by payor and be able to differentiate between categories such as level of clinician, practice location, surgery risk factors, and modifiers as an example.

27.3 Interoperability

Healthcare is historically behind other business sectors in the adoption of new technology that will drive efficiency, cost savings, and overall program scalability. There are many reasons for this, including the complexity required to accommodate communication and data exchange between different care providers and vendors. Challenges often exist within a single health system because of competing priorities and lack of a cohesive and integrated strategic plan. Organizations historically have little tolerance for failure in these areas due to the high risk of increased cost and potential decrease in patient quality of care. Leaders must constantly evaluate the need to continue to invest in new technology while evaluating these risks. Also complicating this framework is the fact that anesthesia practices are often not the primary decision maker when it comes to purchasing EHR systems and can therefore be at the mercy of decisions made by other administrators. It is important for your anesthesia practice to have a seat at the table when your health system is considering purchases of capital software that will impact your practice and are unlikely to change for long time horizons.

A successful anesthesia practice today will need an interoperability platform that will allow you to interface with a number of external platforms and technology systems. These can often seem daunting in nature but at a minimum include:

1. Interaction with different electronic anesthesia record systems from multiple health systems
2. Data exchange with different vendors that will work to optimize your RCM claim processing systems
3. Interfacing with health system practice management system(s) to capture accurate scheduling and patient demographics
4. Interfacing with your data warehouse and reporting software systems

New technology, including artificial intelligence, is rapidly expanding within the area of interoperability. While there are many options available for you to evaluate, you need to select the interoperability technology that will interact with your other applications and workflows efficiently and at scale.

27.4 Strong Coding and RCM Compliance System

One of the most critical drivers to ensure appropriate anesthesia reimbursement is accurate procedure coding. Developing a complete procedure coding program starts well before submitting an ASA code to the payors. A complete anesthesia coding program includes the following areas:

A. **Review of Anesthesia Record Templates**

   The correct anesthesia record templates will make documentation for anesthesiologists, resident trainees, CRNA's, and CAA's more efficient while simultaneously providing a clearer picture of what happened during a case for the Procedure Coding Team to review and assign the appropriate ASA code. Automated coding has been in the industry for many specialties for decades, but anesthesia billing has lagged behind due to the complexity of the specialty including care team billing as well as required payor policies and unique billing requirements. Due to improvements in technology including AI, automated coding for anesthesia cases is being tested with increased success, and this will make standardized format of anesthesia record templates more important than ever as this technology and capability expands. All anesthesia records should be jointly reviewed at least annually to ensure that they meet the current requirements for all teams.

B. **Anesthesia Record Documentation Education**

   Anesthesiologists and nonphysician anesthesia clinicians have a great deal to manage in the operating room monitoring the patient through a successful surgery; asking them to also be experts in procedure coding is not practical. There are hundreds of surgery codes that could be billed by a practice during the course of a year and correctly selecting the appropriate procedure code and modifiers that will accurately report the right information for a case to the payor for correct reimbursement is critical. A successful RCM program must have a Coding Education Team that is available to meet with the anesthesia care team clinicians to share the documentation requirements and best practices. An important goal of the Coding Education Team is to create a partnership with clinicians to simultaneously help ensure both compliant anesthesia records while also supporting clear documentation of the anesthetic in such a way that will allow the procedure coding team to capture the information necessary to accurately procedure code the case, or for an automated system to ensure proper procedure coding selection and outputs.

C. **Coding Education for Anesthesia Procedure Coders**

Similar to an education program for anesthesia clinicians, a robust revenue cycle program will include routine education for anesthesia procedure coders within your RCM Department. With payor policies and national coding guidelines changing regularly, an anesthesia coder must receive and understand the new commercial and government policy information and implement new policies to keep up with the required industry changes.

D. **Coding Audit Program**

All RCM production coding staff should have a regular audit that is performed on the quality of the coding that is performed. This point is important to verify and complete regardless of a practice using an external vendor or internal employees to perform the procedure coding. An effective coding compliance plan should have an independent internal team to review a sample set of cases that are completed for each coder. The result of that audit should be shared with the coder being audited and he/she should have a chance to review and understand the results. If the coder is meeting targeted coding quality results vs. goal, they remain in the regular production coding team. If they are under goal, there should be follow-up remediation and education as well as re-auditing of current coding production until he/she is meeting targeted goals. The coding audits should also have a minimum threshold with removal of the coder from the production environment if the scores are below that threshold. As automated coding becomes more common within the anesthesia specialty with improved technology and AI, it will be important to audit these workflows and results with the same standards to ensure compliant coding and billing. This is true for any automated technology within the RCM workflows (AI Bots, large language models, etc.).

Coding audits should be a welcome part of an overall coding compliance plan. There should be regular education and training for the production coders so they remain current on all anesthesia coding guidelines and payor polices. Creating a culture of high-quality coding and on-going education in a collaborative and professional environment will result in meeting your desired outcomes and developing a more compliant revenue cycle management program.

E. **Anesthesia Clinician and Procedure Coder Communication**

Collaboration and clear communication between physicians, the anesthesia care team, and the production coders is an important part of an effective coding program. As highlighted earlier, although there is baseline anesthesia record documentation training completed by each physician, there will often be documentation questions on a case that need to be clarified to ensure all charges are captured accurately and completely. There should be a clear process in place regarding communication of questions or clarifications between clinicians, coders, and compliance personnel. This communication should be via a consistent and clear mechanism that is provided via HIPAA secure technology.

27.5 Hire the Right RCM Operations Team

A great anesthesia revenue cycle management program will have industry leading technology systems, automation, vendor support, as well as the most current and robust data and analytics. All of those components are foundational to a successful program, but the department and practice will not function optimally if proper leadership is not in place to operationalize the workflow. Personnel is a large part of your overall operational budget, often averaging 60%–65% of your departmental costs [5]. An experienced leadership team will establish clear operational pathways with robust training and audit programs for all department personnel. Daily, these operational leaders need to address areas such as appropriate hiring, staffing productivity, processing quality, payor compliance, and operational communication with key stakeholders.

The right leadership team will establish a positive culture that your organization exhibits every day. A department that has a clear vision and supportive culture with established goals that everyone manages to will have higher retention rates, increased quality, and ultimately higher overall program effectiveness.

27.6 Culture of Communication

Revenue cycle management is often considered the operational heartbeat of an independent physician practice. When not operating correctly, the RCM Department can negatively impact and threaten the financial stability of the entire physician group. Whether the decision is made to manage your revenue cycle processing internally or via an external vendor, your team must be open and transparent regarding communication with the critical departments that interact with revenue cycle daily. Several examples of these departments include Payor Contracting, Legal, Finance, Compliance, Information Technology, Human Resources, and Clinical Practice Operations. Revenue Cycle Management is difficult to manage because of the ever-changing payor policies, government regulations, and new payor agreements; it requires active and continuous engagement by leadership within anesthesia practices. These changes may lead to underpaid or delayed claim processing. New contracts and payor reimbursement levels mean new accrual rates that finance needs to update. Internal and external audits mean collaboration and alignment with the

Compliance and Legal Teams. Clear communication with all appropriate stakeholders is required to maximize practice overall performance.

27.7 Practice Reporting and Data Analytics

Reporting and analytics continue to grow in importance for the entire healthcare sector, and anesthesia practice management is no different. Specifically, within a successful anesthesia RCM practice, the operational team will be managing Key Performance Indicators (KPIs) that determine the operational health of your practice. Examples of these should include but not be limited to important areas such as:

1. Net collection rates
2. Initial and final payor denial rates
3. Vendor performance vs. established targets
4. Accounts receivable aging
5. Credit balances
6. Charge lag
7. Employee satisfaction and turnover ratios

Most of these functions must be monitored at a payor, and clinical location level to make sure any material changes in metrics vs. goal can be identified and addressed as soon as possible. Deviations in these measurements may impact cashflow and overall program effectiveness. The RCM leadership team should share these metrics with practice leadership on a regular (minimum monthly) basis and include explanations and action plans for any metric variances vs. published goals. It is important to periodically share practice goals for metrics with all stakeholders in the RCM value chain, to guarantee proper alignment among all relevant participants.

An effective analytics engine is receiving data daily to provide customers with the most complete and up to date information necessary to manage business needs. Successful leaders know that just supplying data is not as impactful as providing meaningful information that is actionable to the business and clinical leaders that are relying on it every day to run their business.

27.8 Automation and Artificial Intelligence Investments

It seems like every industry is implementing and testing how AI can help their business be more cost efficient and scalable in a very competitive environment. Revenue cycle management workflows and processes have an incredible opportunity to invest in AI technology to drive improved processing efficiency, accuracy, and overall program scalability.

Our current Information Technology and RCM Teams have partnered together for the past 5 years to develop and implement several automation workflows, which have resulted in millions of dollars of annualized cost savings. Basic workflows across multiple business unit departments such as payment posting, accounts receivable claim denials, eligibility, and many others have incorporated automation and AI workflows to improve overall productivity while simultaneously increasing quality. We have learned many lessons during this investment and have developed clear business plans on how we evaluate and assess workflow opportunities to automate before deciding to implement them. Once approved, we formalize business requirements and get formal sign-off from all impacted business unit leaders to ensure alignment and business unit accountability. There is also a significant investment in program monitoring and auditing to ensure processes are functioning as designed with approved outcomes.

AI programs continue to expand using additional technology such as machine learning. For example, the use of large language models (LLM) available in the RCM space can significantly improve patient satisfaction in the collections process. Another area of opportunity includes identifying high risk claim denial trends based upon historical payor claims data. Identifying these trends up front will allow practice administrators to address claim opportunities upstream before they are denied and improve overall practice cashflow.

The wait to realize the benefit of AI is over for RCM Leaders. There are many examples within the RCM industry of how investing in the right technology and department personnel will allow physician anesthesiology leaders to create significant improvements in the quality, efficiency, and overall program scalability of one's RCM Team.

27.9 Information Technology Strategic Partnership

The importance of a strategic partnership between the Information Technology (IT) and RCM Teams within your organization is critical to managing business challenges and future innovation within your organization. Alignment between these departments will ensure you have a defined set of mutual goals that all leaders are incentivized to drive towards and achieve. The business risks within your IT Team are significant. Areas such as cybersecurity, data loss prevention, and disaster recovery planning are more important than ever. Having a strategic partnership with the IT Leadership Team will allow you to meet current business demands, while you continue to invest in new technologies (AI) that will drive innovation, efficiency, and scalability.

27.10 Conclusion

There is not a single technological solution or personnel addition that an anesthesia physician practice may use to ensure an RCM Team is functioning at peak levels. As discussed throughout this chapter, a best-in-class RCM Department needs to utilize the correct technology as well as operational workflows, business controls, cross-departmental communication and collaboration, data analytics, and department leadership to maximize overall performance. It is also critical to balance AI innovation and cost savings with appropriate quality control metrics. Long-term investment in RCM operations is essential for optimal returns as shortcuts will often lead to lost revenue, increased cost, and higher compliance risks.

This is an exciting time to be working in the RCM space as new technology is available and being deployed that is changing the industry and driving a considerable amount of efficiency and improved performance. Focusing across your entire business, including the areas listed in this chapter will help ensure you maximize your net collection rate returns today while also positioning your anesthesia practice for the future.

References

1. AMA. CPT and ASA codes are a registered trademark of the American Medical Association. www.ama-assn.org/practice-management/cpt.
2. CMS. Anesthesia billing modifiers are a registered trademark of the American Medical Association. CMS IOM Pub. 100-04, Medicare claims processing manual, Chapter 12, section 50. www.cms.gov/Regulations-and-Guidance/Guidance/Manuals/downloads/clm104c12.pdf.
3. Novitas Solutions Anesthesia Modifiers. 12 Aug 2025. www.novitas-solutions.com/webcenter/portal/MedicareJL/pagebyid?contentId=00144514.
4. National Planning Cycles. By the National Planning Cycles Team. 11 Oct 2025. https://nationalplanningcycles.org/healthcare-claim-denial-statistics-state-of-claims-report-2025.
5. Healthcare Financial Management Association. The strategic role of revenue cycle management in battling rising healthcare costs. 3 Dec 2024. https://www.hfma.org/revenue-cycle/the-strategic-role-of-revenue-cycle-management-in-battling-rising-healthcare-costs.

Training the Next Generation: Education, Workforce Development, and the Future of Anesthesiology

28

Yohannes B. Getachew

28.1 An Overview

Anesthesiologists, or perioperative physicians, go through years of rigorous training to be consultants in the perioperative care of patients. Their expertise has a critical impact on the quality of patient outcomes, patient safety, and the efficiency of care provided. The greatest emphasis on the training of anesthesiologists is on patient care, but trainees also learn how to manage an operating room (OR), work with Physicians of various specialties, and interact with nurses and hospital administrative staff to provide optimal care and ensure efficient utilization of resources in healthcare institutions.

The terms 'anesthesiologists' and 'perioperative physicians' are used interchangeably, and the terms describe different aspects of the same specialty. Anesthesiology is the study of the science of anesthetic care of a patient (*'anesthesia' is an ancient Greek word meaning 'without pain'. In the present day it represents a medically induced 'insensitivity to pain'*). Perioperative physician describes the area of expertise of the physician for the period before, during, and after an operation or a procedure like colonoscopy, radiation therapy, interventional procedure, etc. Anesthesiologists also care for patients in procedure rooms that are not operating rooms (Radiology, GI suites, Labor, and Delivery) as well as patients in Critical Care settings (ICU). They also treat patients with chronic pain in-hospital and outpatient settings with procedures or medical management.

Y. B. Getachew (✉)
Perelman School of Medicine, University of Pennsylvania, Children's Hospital of Philadelphia, Philadelphia, PA, USA

General Anesthesiology, Children's Hospital of Philadelphia, Philadelphia, USA
e-mail: getachewy@chop.edu

G. Tewfik (ed.), *The Anesthesiologist as Perioperative Leader*,
https://doi.org/10.1007/978-3-032-18058-2_28

After high school, a future anesthesiologist has to complete a 4-year undergraduate degree before entering medical school. Four years of medical school is followed by a 4-year residency in anesthesiology and critical Care to become an attending (or consultant) anesthesiologist. Nearly 60% of residents pursue a fellowship afterwards, which is subspecialty training in a specific area of anesthesiology (e.g. pediatric or cardiac anesthesiology) [6]. The remaining 40% join the workforce immediately as practicing anesthesiologists.

The cost of undergraduate degree and medical school education is paid by the student and may be partially or fully supplemented by scholarships, financial aid, etc. Residency and fellowship training are salaried positions. Resident and fellowship salary, in addition to the majority of the cost of operating a residency program, is mostly covered by the federal government.

Although the primary reason to operate anesthesiology residency program is to produce high quality perioperative physicians, there are multiple financial and other benefits these programs provide to a healthcare institution in which they train.

Upon completion of training, and beginning the practice of anesthesiology, a perioperative physician also begins the career-long process of continuous learning, refinement of various skill sets and of exploring new ideas, processes, and innovation. Changes in models of learning and technology bring an ever-evolving opportunity for an anesthesiologists to provide safer and higher quality care more efficiently.

The breadth of knowledge that can be acquired in an anesthesiologist's career goes beyond clinical care. The complexity of the US healthcare finance system and its administration requires the anesthesiologist to educate themselves on a continuous basis while in practice. Understanding the impact of technology and other new developments that directly or indirectly influence the healthcare business environment should ideally start in medical school, continue through training and extend into one's career. Leadership is another area in which anesthesiologists can broaden their skill set. Anesthesiologists often participate in committees such as those in safety and quality in their institution and may go on to assume positions of various levels of leadership ranging from committee chair, directorship, department chair, chief medical officer to being part of the C-suite.

The American Society of Anesthesiologists (ASA) has various publications, courses, seminars, certificate programs that members can use to enhance their knowledge and skills in clinical and non-clinical fields. Some anesthesiologists supplement their educational needs from sources outside of the ones offered by the ASA. And others choose to obtain an advanced degree in various fields like business administration, education, public health, etc. A well-rounded anesthesiologist that is well-informed in these varied topics is best suited to provide excellent care with efficiency and successfully navigate the complex healthcare system that we practice within.

28.2 The Education of an Anesthesiologist

28.2.1 Medical School Education

In the USA, students are accepted to medical schools after completing a 4-year undergraduate degree [1]. Many proceed directly to medical school after getting their bachelor's degree. Some enter the work force before joining medical school, while others pursue further studies in a Masters, PhD or other programs. Some may choose to participate in research prior to enrolling. There are exceptions where a pre-medical education is integrated into medical school and students join this track right after high school [11, 14–16].

US medical students complete 4 years of medical school education that includes scientific study, clinical instruction, and hands-on training [1]. The greatest emphasis is on high-quality clinical care. They also learn teamwork and collaboration, ethics, etc. The learning process starts with basic medical concepts, the human body's structure and function under normal and abnormal situations, and the study of the various diseases and treatment options. In the later years, students get exposed to patients in clinical settings and learn diagnosis and treatment concepts, physician-patient interaction including taking medical histories, performing physical examinations and professional conduct [1]. Such education will prepare them for a residency training where they specialize in a certain field of medicine. The education style has evolved significantly in the last decades and, as a result, the teaching process has become more patient-oriented at an early stage of a medical student's education [5, 13].

Obtaining an undergraduate degree prior to joining medical school is an important feature of American medical education. An undergraduate degree often provides a unique perspective, culled from the arts, STEM, social studies, business, law or other fields, that has contributed to innovation and the advancement of the field of medicine. It also later makes anesthesiologists a resourceful partner in solving healthcare-related issues [5]. It is important to note that in many parts of the world, unlike the US system, students enter medical school right after graduating from high school.

In the United States, attending both college and medical school is expensive. On average, a medical school graduate carries debt of more than $200,000 [7–10, 12]. The prospect of such high debt discourages some students from considering applying to medical school. This is particularly prohibitive for students from lower income families. Paying the loan over years also means less money saved for the future, reducing a physician's net worth by a significant amount.

28.2.2 Residency in Anesthesiology and Perioperative Medicine

An anesthesiology residency program consists of 4 years of training to master the field of Perioperative Medicine. During the first year, referred to as an internship, residents work in basic clinical care (usually in internal medicine or surgery) under the supervision of an attending physician and different levels of senior residents. An intern spends the year rotating through different departments, and often a gradual entry into perioperative medicine often takes place in the last few months.

In the following 3 years, residents continue to learn and assume greater responsibilities towards becoming independent anesthesiologists.

The majority of the cost of operating an anesthesiology residency program is covered by the federal government through Medicare, Medicaid, and/or the Military [2]. Medicare divides the cost into 'direct' and 'indirect' costs. A direct cost is the trainee stipend, the teaching physician's time dedicated to preparation for and actual training of residents and administrative costs, etc [3]. Indirect costs provide compensation to reflect the higher cost of care that teaching hospitals incur compared to non-teaching hospitals. This includes potential inefficiencies in patient care, longer time to interpret results and increased resource utilization [2].

There are some expenses that may be covered by the institution that is sponsoring the training [4]. According to research done mostly in the 1990s, there is more financial benefit for the system, which often incentivizes this financial investment. Training future perioperative physicians has several benefits to the hospital system in addition to training future practitioners. Anesthesiology residents bring money to the hospital because their training is paid by different government entities. According to some studies performed in the late 1990s and early 2000s, the financial benefit from the revenue generated by a resident outweighs the cost of the training, as they cover clinical tasks that would otherwise be performed by other high-earning workers.

Another important advantage of having a residency program is the educational environment that is cultivated improves the overall standard of care provided, helping to achieve better quality and safety. Newly graduated anesthesiologists may find it appealing to work in a place where there is education and training for the next generation of clinicians; thus, a residency program is also an effective recruiting tool.

28.3 Entering the Workforce and Board Certification

New graduates enter a variety of practice settings, and board certification within a certain time, usually 5 years after joining the workforce, is often mandated in order to continue performing clinical care. An anesthesiologist has to pass a written exam first, then pass an oral exam to be board certified. Board certification has to be renewed (also called recertification) every 5–10 years via a process administered by the governing board for their profession. In the case of Anesthesiologists, it is the American Board of Anesthesiology (ABA). Part of the process is participating in

Continuing Medical Education (CME), a system for healthcare professionals to maintain and update their medical knowledge, skills, and professional performance to stay current in their field. The ABA guidelines specify what type of CME credits will be appropriate to fulfill the requirement for board re-certification. In addition to CME, anesthesiologists have to participate in performance and quality improvement projects that show their continued effort to maintain and improve their knowledge and skills.

28.4 The National Shortage of Anesthesiologists

There is a significant shortage of anesthesiologists in the USA. As of 2025, the gap between the demand and supply of anesthesiologists is large and growing [18]. This is due to several factors that worsened in the 1990s. There is a supply and demand mismatch that exacerbates the shortage.

One significant factor affecting the supply of anesthesiologists is the national push for a change in healthcare in the early 1990s. The proposal put more emphasis on primary care and would have reduced payment for specialty care. The federal government proposed a high percentage of medical school graduates enter primary care fields, and medical schools emphasized this goal and de-emphasized specialty care and training. The proposal was a hot topic and its impact on specialty physicians was national news that made medical students shy away from applying to specialty residencies, especially anesthesiology. For the next several years, anesthesiology residency programs barely filled their allotted positions [17–20].

Today, the slow pace with which new residency programs are opening, and the difficulty of increasing the number of trainees in a program, makes it difficult to graduate enough anesthesiologists to meet the demand.

Further, the retirement of a significant number of anesthesiologists due to COVID-19 exacerbated shortages. Procedures were postponed during the early days of the pandemic, creating a backlog of cases for clinicians when elective procedures resumed. As COVID restrictions ended, there were a large number of patients that needed procedures. Such a reduced number of anesthesiologists, coupled with significantly increased demand, put a strain on healthcare systems and the remaining clinicians. The ensuing physician burnout contributed to more retirements or reductions in work hours.

On the demand side, America's population is rapidly aging, increasing the need for more procedures. There has been rapid growth in minimally invasive procedures, procedures done in Non-Operating Room Anesthesia (NORA) locations and outpatient surgery centers creating logistical challenges and the need for more anesthesiologists.

The American Society of Anesthesiologists is leading a concerted effort to increase residency programs and the number of anesthesiologists graduating from training programs. The proposed strategy to address the shortage includes taking steps to enhance staff retention, expanding anesthesia coverage capacity through practice innovations and using artificial intelligence and emerging technologies to aid decision-making and deliver care more efficiently. It also requires easing financial constraints, including Medicare payment reform for anesthesiologist services, as well as steps to remove barriers to anesthesiologist provided and led care in rural communities and other inequities in patient care [18].

28.5 Conclusion

Anesthesiologists or perioperative physicians go through a rigorous dozen or more years of training after completing high school before start their career. Because of the duties of a perioperative physician and the type of unique training involved, anesthesiologists are well positioned to efficiently manage the complex perioperative environment, an environment that often generates half or more of a hospital system's revenue.

Departments with anesthesiology residency programs benefit from the educational environment that sets a high educational standard and encourages continuous learning, while the cost of administering such a program will bring federal money to an institution. It also creates an attractive environment for practicing anesthesiologists potentially increasing staff retention.

Anesthesiologists' participation in the administration of the perioperative environment also involves working with medical and administrative staff as a team, often assuming various leadership roles towards the goal of higher quality and safety, and improving efficiency. Their clinical and non-clinical work exposes them to a wide-ranging practice setting and requires them to routinely interact with a variety of physician specialties and non-physician personnel. The complex work environment also encourages them to seek further training in the form of advanced degree or a certificate program to improve their performance.

References

1. Aamc article on medical education. https://students-residents.aamc.org/choosing-medical-career/what-expect-medical-school.
2. Cost can be around 65–75K with a hidden cost of about $4,500. https://pmc.ncbi.nlm.nih.gov/articles/PMC4054764/#:~:text=We%20determined%20that%20direct%20costs,%2471%2C492%2C%20and%20%2475%2C636%2C%20respectively.
3. https://students-residents.aamc.org/financial-aid-resources/cost-applying-medical-residency.
4. The hidden cost of graduate medical education. https://pmc.ncbi.nlm.nih.gov/articles/PMC3399629/#:~:text=The%20average%20annual%20cost%20per,and%20Recruitment%20%24525%20(11.8%25).
5. The future of medical education. https://www.ama-assn.org/education/changemeded-initiative/precision-education-and-future-medical-education.
6. Percentage of residents going into fellowship and reasons for choosing fellowship. https://pmc.ncbi.nlm.nih.gov/articles/PMC10725004/.
7. College debt. https://www.usnews.com/education/best-colleges/paying-for-college/articles/see-how-student-loan-borrowing-has-changed.

8. Med school debt by state. https://students-residents.aamc.org/system/files/2024-09/MSAR014%20-%20MSAR%20Debt%20%20Information.pdf.
9. NIH rising med school debt—2012 article. https://pmc.ncbi.nlm.nih.gov/articles/PMC6179784/.
10. Student loan's effect on the economy. https://www.pgpf.org/article/how-does-student-debt-affect-the-economy/.
11. Laon should not deter from Med school—AMA. https://www.ama-assn.org/medical-students/preparing-medical-school/3-reasons-student-loan-debt-should-not-deter-you-med.
12. Borrow or serve? https://pmc.ncbi.nlm.nih.gov/articles/PMC5483978/.
13. GME financing. https://www.ncbi.nlm.nih.gov/books/NBK248024/.
14. Medical education in USA. https://en.wikipedia.org/wiki/Medical_education_in_the_United_States.
15. AMA residency acceptance rate. https://www.aamc.org/media/6091/download.
16. History and evolution of anesthesia education in the United States. https://www.longdom.org/open-access-pdfs/history-and-evolution-of-anesthesia-education-in-united-states-2155-6148-1000734.pdf.
17. Balanced Budget Act of 1997. https://jamanetwork.com/journals/jama/fullarticle/182532, https://pmc.ncbi.nlm.nih.gov/articles/PMC2690212/.
18. National shortage, causes and solutions. https://ascnews.com/2024/08/national-anesthesiologist-shortage-causes-solutions-and-strategies-for-asc-operators/.
19. ASA article on staff shortage—Aboulish. https://www.asahq.org/about-asa/newsroom/news-releases/2024/06/anesthesia-workforce-shortage-poses-threat-to-health-care.
20. Hx of healthcare in the 90s, U Michigan. https://medschool.umich.edu/sites/default/files/2023-08/anesthesiology-history.pdf.

29 Accountable Care Organizations: Integrating Anesthesiology into Value-Based Care

Diana C. Mosquera and Matthew J. Dellaquila

29.1 Definition of an ACO and Prevalence of ACOs

An Accountable Care Organization (ACO) is a collective of healthcare providers (e.g., physicians, hospitals, and other healthcare entities) that collaborate and align efforts to provide coordinated, high-quality care to a defined patient population. The primary aim of ACOs is to ensure that patients receive the right care, in the right place, and at the right time while avoiding unnecessary duplication of services and preventing medical errors. These organizations operate under financial models that incentivize providers to meet established quality benchmarks while reducing the growth of healthcare expenditures.

As of 2025, there are over 500 active ACOs in the United States, serving millions of beneficiaries [1]. Medicare and commercial insurers have implemented various ACO models that differ widely in scope and structure. The Medicare Shared Savings Program (MSSP) is a Medicare ACO model that has experienced exponential growth since its introduction in 2012, becoming a cornerstone of value-based care in the US healthcare system. Commercial payer ACOs and state-led Medicaid ACOs have contributed to the expanding footprint of this payment model.

29.1.1 Importance of ACOs in the Healthcare Ecosystem

The introduction of ACOs represented a critical shift in the healthcare paradigm from volume-based to value-based care. They paved the way for the management of

D. C. Mosquera
Northwell, New Hyde Park, NY, USA

M. J. Dellaquila (✉)
Henry Ford Jackson Hospital, Jackson, MI, USA

G. Tewfik (ed.), *The Anesthesiologist as Perioperative Leader*,
https://doi.org/10.1007/978-3-032-18058-2_29

defined populations by emphasizing preventive care, care coordination, patient satisfaction, quality improvement, and data transparency. ACOs aim to address long-standing inefficiencies created by siloed approaches to healthcare delivery. Their collaborative structure encourages multidisciplinary approaches to care, fostering improved communication among providers and enabling a more comprehensive understanding of patient needs.

29.2 History of ACOs

The concept of an ACO was introduced in 2006 as part of the broader conversation on health care reform that preceded the passage of the Affordable Care Act (ACA) in 2010 [2]. The three tenets of an ACO were defined as: shifting financial and health outcome accountability to healthcare providers, decoupling provider salaries from care intensity and utilization, and transparent and meaningful quality and cost measures [3]. Following a recommendation from the Medicare Payment Advisory Commission (MedPAC), policymakers included ACOs in the ACA for voluntary participation and instructed the Secretary for Health and Human Services to create the Medicare Shared Savings Program (MSSP) [4].

The Medicare Shared Savings Program (MSSP), the first ACO program, was launched in 2012 and is a statutory program under Medicare (Table 29.1). MSSP launched the first ACOs as part of the Pioneer ACO model and has evolved overtime with iterative demonstrations. The original ACO model had five tracks delineating the percent of shared savings and shared losses (risk) an ACO participant could choose. In the first year of the program, participants were allowed to select a track with no risk exposure to shared losses [5].The Pioneer ACO demonstration selected healthcare organizations that had experience managing risk, consisted of 32 ACOs at its peak, and ended in 2016. In addition, the Advanced ACO model was introduced in parallel to the Pioneer ACO model to allow smaller physician-based and rural first-time ACO participants to make the necessary investments to successfully participate in MSSP [6].

The Next Generation ACO model followed the Pioneer ACO demonstration, beginning in 2016 and ending in 2022. The model further shifted shared losses risk to participants, built on insights from the Pioneer ACOs and introduced new care

Table 29.1 Milestones in ACO development [4–10]

2012	MSSP launches with over 220 participants. Advanced ACO Model launched to support small ACOs with limited risk experience
2016	Introduction of the Next Generation ACO Model, allowing greater flexibility and higher levels of risk. ACO Investment model provides financial capital to ACOs serving underserved and rural areas
2019	Pathways to Success initiative introduces tiered risk structures and mandatory participation timelines
2021	CMS Innovation Center Strategy Refresh set a goal to have 100% of Medicare FFS beneficiaries in an ACO-type relationship by 2030 [10]
2023 and beyond	Expansion of direct contracting models, specialty care VBP models, and integration of digital health technologies to support ACO objectives

delivery transformations [7]. Additionally, the ACO Investment Model followed the Advanced ACO model and focused on ACOs serving underserved and rural areas. The ACO Investment Model provided the financial support required to create the infrastructure needed to improve the care of Medicare beneficiaries for 24 months and lasted through 2017 [8]. Currently, there are 480 Medicare ACO models serving about 10 million beneficiaries.

Since the first ACO models were introduced, CMS has continued to improve upon subsequent iterations with the goal of fostering greater financial accountability, integrating risk-adjustment advancements and responding to policy reforms [9]. For example, the Pathways to Success initiative, launched by the Centers for Medicare & Medicaid Services (CMS) in 2019, refined ACO participation rules to emphasize performance accountability and accelerate the transition to two-sided risk models. These changes reflect broader trends in healthcare policy aimed at promoting efficiency, enhancing quality, and reducing costs. In 2021, the CMS Innovation Center released their Strategy Refresh in which it announced the aim to have 100% of Medicare fee-for-service beneficiaries in an ACO relationship by 2030 [10].

29.2.1 Benefits of Membership in an ACO

Participation in an ACO offers numerous advantages for providers, patients, and the healthcare system (Fig. 29.1).

Shared Savings Opportunities: Providers can benefit financially by achieving cost and quality benchmarks, sharing in savings generated from improved efficiencies [3]

Improved Patient Outcomes: Coordinated care can facilitate better management of chronic diseases, reduce avoidable hospital readmissions, and enhance preventive care delivery.

Enhanced Data Analytics: ACOs can leverage advanced data analytic systems to track performance metrics, identify care delivery gaps, and implement evidence-based interventions.

Patient-Centered Care: The focus on value fosters a holistic approach to care, addressing social determinants of health and prioritizing patient satisfaction.

Diversified Revenue Stream: Shifting focus towards alternative payment models allows providers to tap into sources of revenue other than traditional fee-for-service (i.e. per member per month, prospective payments, capitation and global budgets.)

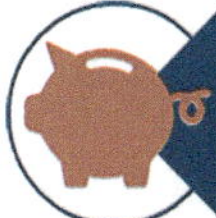

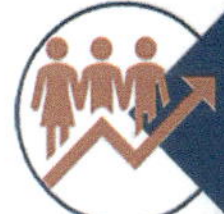

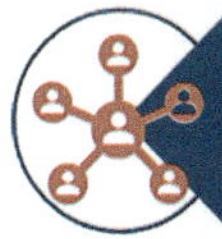

Fig. 29.1 Advantages of ACO membership [3]

29.3 Difference Between an ACO and a CIN

While Accountable Care Organizations (ACOs) and Clinically Integrated Networks (CINs) share similar goals of enhancing care quality and reducing costs, their structures and scopes differ:

- **ACO**: A legal entity that allows a group of providers to work together to manage the health and cost of care for a specific population. ACOs are often associated with the Medicare program but can exist to serve Medicaid and commercially insured populations [11]. ACOs can enter formal agreements for shared savings or losses, emphasizing accountability for a defined patient population.
- **CIN**: A broader network of healthcare providers aligned to meet quality and cost objectives across various payors, often focusing on commercial insurance markets. CINs typically emphasize clinical integration and data sharing rather than direct financial accountability [12]. An ACO can often serve as the platform on which a CIN operates.

29.4 ACOs and the Broader Payor Landscape

ACOs are integral to the transition from fee-for-service to value-based care models. They exist alongside other initiatives, such as bundled payment arrangements and alternative payment models (APMs). Together, these frameworks represent a unified effort to control healthcare costs while enhancing outcomes. ACOs began specifically targeting Medicare and Medicaid populations, though in present practice commercial insurers have adopted similar models to expand value-based care principles.

29.4.1 ACO Interaction with Other Value-Based Models

ACOs complement other payment models, such as bundled payments, and address longitudinal outcomes for patient populations at the performance year level rather than specific episodes of care. This holistic approach enables them to influence both acute and chronic care delivery, making them a critical component of the value-based care ecosystem. One area of integration that is still under development for ACOs involves alignment of programs to allow, in the case of Medicare, beneficiaries attributed to an ACO to also enroll in a bundled payment program. For example, a Medicare beneficiary may be enrolled in a Medicare ACO and requires a joint replacement surgery for which their care provider can obtain a bundled payment.

In 2024, CMS announced a bundled payment model that would allow Medicare beneficiaries to be attributed to an acute care bundled payment model while enrolled in a Medicare ACO. The new model is called Transforming Episode Accountability Model or TEAM and focuses on five surgical episodes. A key focus of TEAM is to reduce care fragmentation and encourage improvement in care transitions after surgery [13].

29.5 Types and Examples of ACOs

The diversity of ACOs reflects their adaptability to various healthcare settings:

- **Medicare Shared Savings Program (MSSP) ACOs**: Traditional Medicare ACO introduced in 2012 and written into healthcare law
- **Commercial ACOs**: Introduced by commercial insurers for Medicare Advantage, employer-sponsored and/or individual insurance plans
- **Specialty ACOs**: Designed for specific populations or conditions, such as oncology-focused ACOs
- **CMS ACO REACH:** Medicare ACO introduced by the CMS Innovation Center in 2021 with aim to help address the healthcare needs of medically underserved populations

An example of a successful ACO is Advocate Health Care's initiative, which significantly reduced costs while improving patient outcomes through robust care coordination and data-driven strategies [14].

29.6 Metrics in ACO Participation

Metrics used to evaluate ACO performance often align with frameworks like ASPIRE (Anesthesiology-focused Safety and Performance Improvement and Reporting Exchange), MPOG (Multicenter Perioperative Outcomes Group), and AQI (Anesthesia Quality Institute). Examples of key performance indicators include:

- Hospital-wide, 30-day, all-cause, unplanned readmission rate
- CAHPS patient experience survey
- Hemoglobin A1c Control
- Risk-standardized hospital admission rates for patients with multiple chronic conditions
- Preventive care and screening (e.g., screenings, vaccinations)
- Timely follow-up and transitional care management
- Total cost of care

29.6.1 Challenges in Meeting Metrics

Providers often face challenges in influencing metrics beyond their direct control, such as population-wide vaccination rates or long-term chronic disease outcomes. Collaborative efforts and patient engagement strategies are crucial to address these gaps [15].

29.7 Defining Upside and Downside Risk

Risk-sharing is central to ACO participation:

- **Upside Risk**: Providers share in savings if expenditures fall below established benchmarks while meeting quality metrics.
- **Downside Risk**: Providers assume financial responsibility for exceeding cost benchmarks, creating incentives to manage resources effectively. Two-sided risk models are increasingly favored to align provider incentives with patient outcomes [16] (Fig. 29.2).

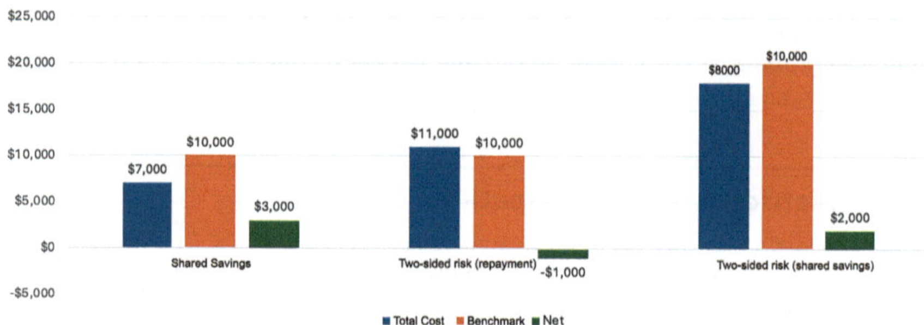

Fig. 29.2 An illustration of shared savings and two-sided (upside and downside) risk. The bar chart on the left illustrates shared savings under an upside-only model, where the provider receives a predetermined percentage of net savings if total costs fall below the benchmark, but faces no penalty if costs exceed the benchmark. The bar chart in the center demonstrates a two-sided risk model where the provider must issue a repayment since total cost exceeded the benchmark. The bar chart on the right demonstrates a two-sided risk model where the provider is issued a shared savings payment since total cost where less than the benchmark

29.8 IT and Data Management for ACOs

Robust information technology infrastructure is essential for ACO success. Effective participation requires:

- **Data Integration**: Seamless sharing of electronic health records (EHRs) across providers.
- **Analytics Platforms**: Tools to monitor quality metrics, identify care gaps, and forecast cost trends.
- **Third-Party Partners**: Data conveners and analytics firms play critical roles in managing complex datasets and ensuring compliance with regulatory standards [17]. A data convener refers to an entity (often a third-party health IT vendor) that aggregates, standardizes, and shares clinical and administrative data from multiple sources to support population health management, quality reporting, and value-based care contracts.

As technology progresses, future states for ACOs could involve remote patient monitoring equipment and other such innovations to create metrics that extend the exposure and spectrum of perioperative care.

29.8.1 Innovations in Data Management

Emerging technologies, such as artificial intelligence, predictive analytics, and remote patient monitoring technology, are revolutionizing how ACOs utilize data. These tools enable more precise risk stratification and personalized care planning, enhancing overall performance [18].

29.9 Payment Models under ACOs

ACOs employ diverse payment models to incentivize value-based care:

- **Shared Savings**: Providers receive a portion of savings generated by reducing costs below benchmarks.
- **Bundled Payments**: Fixed payments for episodes of care, promoting efficiency within specific care pathways.
- **Capitation Models**: Providers receive a per-member, per-month payment, shifting the focus to preventive and holistic care [19].

29.10 Cost Accounting and ACOs

Accurate cost accounting enables providers to identify inefficiencies and align resources with quality improvement initiatives. Understanding cost drivers and their relationship to outcomes is essential for financial sustainability in an ACO [20]. One approach to cost accounting that can be used in ACOs is time-driven activity-based costing (TDABC). Using TDABC allows perioperative teams to delineate activities involved in caring for patients and more closely reflect associated staff and fixed costs. As anesthesiologists become more involved in value-based care models such as ACOs, they should understand how to account for activities that enhance patient outcomes and may not be accurately valued in traditional time-based billing [21].

29.11 The Anesthesiologist's Role in ACO Membership

Anesthesiologists are pivotal in achieving ACO goals, contributing through:

- **Perioperative Efficiency**: Streamlining surgical workflows and minimizing delays
- **Reducing Complications**: Employing evidence-based practices to lower infection rates and other adverse events
- **Enhancing Patient Satisfaction**: Effective pain management and clear communication improve patient experiences
- **Perioperative Optimization:** Having patients in optimal medical condition in the perioperative period to reduce same day cancellations and other wasteful metrics that add to overall cost savings and better outcomes

29.11.1 Expanding the Scope of Influence

Anesthesiologists can also impact broader ACO objectives by engaging in population health initiatives, such as preoperative optimization programs, smoking cessation efforts, and addressing social determinants of health [22].

29.12 Factors in Negotiating ACO Participation

Negotiating ACO contracts requires careful consideration of:

- **Payment Distribution**: Ensuring equitable allocation of shared savings among providers.
- **Patient Attribution**: Ensuring that patients are appropriately assigned to the proper ACO providers.
- **Performance Expectations**: Aligning metrics with provider capabilities and organizational goals.

- **Risk Tolerance**: Assessing the financial implications of two-sided risk models [23].
- **Data Sharing:** Seamless and encrypted sharing of data is essential for ACO participation; analyzing risks and costs incurred for this are essential prior to participation.

29.13 Driving ACO Participation Through Perioperative Optimization

Anesthesiologists can drive ACO success by addressing non-traditional metrics. Some examples include:

- **Regional Anesthesia**: Reduces blood loss and shortens recovery times.
- **Smoking Cessation**: Improves surgical outcomes and reduces postoperative complications.
- **Multimodal Pain Management**: Decreases opioid dependence and shortens length of stay (LOS) [24].

29.13.1 Collaborating with Other Specialties

Collaboration with surgeons, primary care providers, and care managers enhances the impact of anesthesiologists' efforts on ACO performance metrics and can drive other metrics germane to overall hospital performance, further establishing the value of the anesthesiologist.

29.13.2 Challenges in ACO Participation

Despite its potential, ACO participation presents challenges:

- **Alignment with Fee-for-Service Models**: Transitioning from volume to value requires cultural and operational shifts.
- **Metric Relevance**: Many ACO quality measures, such as vaccinations or retinal exams, fall outside anesthesiologists' direct influence.
- **Financial Incentives**: Modest savings distributions may not justify the additional administrative burdens for some providers [25].
- **Alignment with Physician Compensation Models:** Many physician compensation models are still fee-for-service based and do not take into account newer quality-based paradigms.
- **Data Fidelity and Analytics:** Ensuring data is both available and in the proper format, outlining real-time progress toward ACO objectives and performance forecasts.

29.14 The Future of ACOs

The future of ACOs is promising as value-based care models gain traction. Anticipated developments include:

- **Technological Innovations**: Enhanced analytics and interoperability will improve performance tracking.
- **Policy Reforms**: Continued adjustments to participation rules will expand access and refine incentives.
- **Increased Prevalence**: As payors and providers recognize the benefits of ACOs, their adoption is expected to grow.
- **Increased Sharing of Downside Risk**: As healthcare expenditures continue to increase, payors will likely be increasingly looking to share downside risk as a means of cost containment.

Due to their ubiquitous role in acute and increasingly ambulatory perioperative care settings, anesthesiologists are well positioned to lead the evolution of perioperative culture toward alignment with ACO goals in their respective health care organizations. As ACO models shift to align with specialty care models (i.e., CMS TEAM), anesthesiologists will further demonstrate their value in ACO success by driving perioperative efficiencies, leading perioperative medicine efforts, and contributing to better patient outcomes and experience [26].

References

1. Centers for Medicare & Medicaid Services. Medicare shared savings program fact facts [Internet]. Baltimore: CMS; 2025. [cited 2025 Jan 30]. Available from: https://www.cms.gov.
2. MedPAC. Report to the Congress: Medicare and the Health Care Delivery System. Chapter 6: Accountable Care Organizations [Internet]. Washington, DC: MedPAC; 2025. [cited 2025 Jan 30]. Available from: https://www.medpac.gov/wp-content/uploads/import_data/scrape_files/docs/default-source/reports/jun19_ch6_medpac_reporttocongress_sec.pdf.
3. Fisher ES, McClellan MB, Bertko J, Lieberman SM, Lee JJ, Lewis JL, et al. Fostering accountable health care: moving forward in Medicare. Health Aff (Millwood). 2009;28:w219–31. https://doi.org/10.1377/hlthaff.28.2.w219.
4. Burke T. Accountable care organizations. Public Health Rep. 2011;126(6):875–8. https://doi.org/10.1177/003335491112600614.
5. CMS. Pioneer ACO Model [Internet]. Baltimore: Centers for Medicare & Medicaid Services; 2025. [cited 2025 Jan 30]. Available from: https://www.cms.gov/priorities/innovation/innovation-models/pioneer-aco-model.
6. CMS. Advance Payment ACO Model [Internet]. Baltimore: Centers for Medicare & Medicaid Services; 2025. [cited 2025 Jan 30]. Available from: https://www.cms.gov/priorities/innovation/innovation-models/advance-payment-aco-model.
7. CMS. Next Generation ACO Model [Internet]. Baltimore: Centers for Medicare & Medicaid Services; 2025. [cited 2025 Jan 30]. Available from: https://www.cms.gov/priorities/innovation/innovation-models/next-generation-aco-model.

8. CMS. AIM Model Final Report [Internet]. Baltimore: Centers for Medicare & Medicaid Services; 2025. [cited 2025 Jan 30]. Available from: https://www.cms.gov/priorities/innovation/data-and-reports/2020/aim-final-annrpt.
9. Fisher ES, McClellan MB, Safran DG. Building the path to accountable care. N Engl J Med. 2011;363:2445–7.
10. CMS. Innovation Center Strategy Direction White Paper [Internet]. Baltimore: Centers for Medicare & Medicaid Services; 2025. [cited 2025 Jan 30]. Available from: https://www.cms.gov/priorities/innovation/strategic-direction-whitepaper.
11. Health Catalyst. The past, present, and future of ACOs and CINs [Internet]. Health Catalyst; 2025. [cited 2025 Jan 30]. Available from: https://www.healthcatalyst.com/learn/insights/acos-cins-past-present-future.
12. Shortell SM, Casalino LP. Clinically integrated networks: a new approach to health care. Health Aff. 2013;32(1):68–74.
13. CMS. Transforming Episode Accountability Model (TEAM) [Internet]. Baltimore: CMS Innovation Center; 2025. [cited 2025 Oct 8]. Available from: https://www.cms.gov/priorities/innovation/innovation-models/team-model.
14. Advocate Health. Advocate's ACO success story [Internet]. Advocate Health; 2025. [cited 2025 Jan 30]. Available from: https://advocatehealth.com.
15. Anesthesia Quality Institute. Quality measures in ACOs [Internet]. Anesthesia Quality Institute; 2025. [cited 2025 Jan 30]. Available from: https://www.aqihq.org.
16. CMS Innovation Center. Next generation ACO model fact sheet [Internet]. Baltimore: CMS Innovation Center; 2025. [cited 2025 Jan 30]. Available from: https://innovation.cms.gov.
17. Koury J, Lieu TA. Data integration for value-based care. Health Care Financ Rev. 2020;37(4):59–72.
18. Obermeyer Z, Emanuel EJ. Predicting the future of healthcare with AI. JAMA. 2016;315(7):691–2.
19. Berwick DM, Hackbarth AD. Eliminating waste in US healthcare. JAMA. 2012; 307(14):1513–6.
20. Newton D, Bader AM. Value-based health care in perioperative medicine: process maps and costing to determine best practices. Anesthesiol Clin. 2024;42(1):75–86. https://doi.org/10.1016/j.anclin.2023.08.005. Epub 2023 Sept 15. PMID: 38278594.
21. Kaplan RS, Porter ME. How to solve the cost crisis in health care. Harv Bus Rev. 2011;89(9):46–52.
22. Lee TH. Anesthesiologists' role in population health. Anesth Analg. 2018;126(3):1073–6.
23. Bleser WK, Muhlestein DB, Saunders RS. Key factors in ACO success. Health Aff. 2017;36(11):1027–33.
24. St Sauver JL, Warner DO, Yawn BP. Anesthesiology's contribution to ACO goals. Mayo Clin Proc. 2019;94(2):345–50.
25. Jha AK, Joynt KE, Orav EJ. Financial incentives and quality metrics in ACOs. Health Aff. 2012;31(7):1565–72.
26. Glickman SW, Peterson ED. Innovations in ACO design and implementation. JAMA. 2017;318(8):745–6.

30 Advancing Research in Anesthesiology: A Comprehensive Review

Jiang-Hong Ye, Wanhong Zuo, and Zhiyi Zuo

30.1 Introduction

Anesthesiology is a rapidly evolving field with advances in technology, pharmacology, pathophysiology, and perioperative management. Research is pivotal in driving these advances, improving patient safety, and optimizing outcomes during and after surgery. Research in anesthesiology spans from basic science investigations to clinical and translational research, translating laboratory findings into clinical applications. This chapter will explore the importance of advancing research in anesthesiology, the differences between basic and clinical research, the logistics involved in conducting both types of research, the integration of research training into clinical education programs, and the essential components of a successful research program.

30.2 Importance of Advancing Research in Anesthesiology

Research in anesthesiology has a broad and significant impact on medical practice. Anesthesiologists' roles extend beyond the operating room, as they are involved in intensive care, pain management, and resuscitation, among countless other essential functions in the hospital. These diverse roles require anesthesiologists to be well-versed in the latest research to implement evidence-based practices that improve patient safety and care quality. Moreover, research efforts in anesthesiology

J.-H. Ye (✉) · W. Zuo
Department of Anesthesiology, Rutgers University, New Jersey Medical School, Newark, NJ, USA
e-mail: ye@njms.rutgers.edu

Z. Zuo
Department of Anesthesiology, University of Virginia, Charlottesville, VA, USA

G. Tewfik (ed.), *The Anesthesiologist as Perioperative Leader*,
https://doi.org/10.1007/978-3-032-18058-2_30

contribute to a better understanding of human physiology, pharmacology, and pain mechanisms, thereby improving treatment protocols for various conditions.

30.2.1 Enhancing Patient Safety

One of the main objectives of research in anesthesiology is to enhance patient safety. Rigorous research has led to many advances in anesthetic drugs, monitoring technologies, and perioperative protocols. These advances reduce the incidence of complications such as awareness during anesthesia, postoperative cognitive dysfunction, and intraoperative morbidity and mortality. Research also focuses on optimizing anesthesia for high-risk populations, such as the elderly and those with chronic diseases, where standard protocols may be inadequate.

30.2.1.1 Role of Basic Science Research

Basic research focuses on uncovering foundational knowledge about anesthesia mechanisms and safety. It often involves experimental studies investigating the physiological and molecular impacts from anesthetics. For instance:

Testing Anesthetics in Animal Models: Studies in animals allow researchers to understand the pharmacokinetics and pharmacodynamics of new anesthetic drugs, ensuring that they are safe before human trials. For example, testing the safety profile of propofol in rodents helped establish its dosage limits and potential side effects.

Understanding Neurological Mechanisms: Research using cellular and molecular models sheds light on how anesthetics like sevoflurane or isoflurane interact with receptors in the brain, helping understand how anesthesia status occurs and facilitate the development of better anesthetics.

30.2.1.2 Role of Clinical Research

Clinical research bridges the gap by testing interventions in human populations. This often involves large-scale studies and innovative technologies like electronic health records (EHRs). Examples include:

Using EHRs for Safety Analysis: Researchers can analyze EHR datasets to identify trends in perioperative complications and refine clinical protocols accordingly. For example, they can study intraoperative hypotension data across hospitals to establish safer blood pressure thresholds during surgery.

Optimizing Protocols for High-Risk Populations: Clinical trials focusing on elderly patients or those with cardiovascular conditions help develop tailored anesthetic approaches. For instance, a study comparing spinal versus general anesthesia in elderly patients with hip fracture revealed better postoperative outcomes with spinal anesthesia.

Basic science and clinical research complement each other—basic science studies provide the foundation for innovation, while clinical studies validate and translate these discoveries into practice, ensuring safer patient outcomes.

30.2.2 Innovation in Pain Management

Chronic pain management is a significant focus within the field of anesthesiology, with research contributing to the development of novel pain management techniques and therapies. Advances in understanding pain pathways at the molecular and neurophysiological levels, combined with clinical trials of new drugs and techniques, have led to the creation of safer and more effective treatment protocols for patients suffering from chronic pain.

Innovation in pain management in anesthesiology is evolving at an unprecedented pace. Researchers and clinicians are merging fundamental insights into pain pathways with cutting-edge technology to develop novel pain management therapies. These innovations not only aim to reduce patients suffering from chronic pain but also enhance the safety and efficacy of interventions in clinical settings.

30.2.3 Advanced Pain Management Techniques

Recent breakthroughs have deepened our understanding of pain at molecular and neurophysiological levels. As a result, translational research has paved the way for therapies that target specific pain circuits, ushering in treatments that are both safer and more effective. For instance, advances in neuroimaging and biomarker discovery provide new opportunities to personalize patient care. Clinical trials combining pharmacological innovations with precision monitoring validate these strategies, ensuring that interventions directly translate scientific insights into real-world benefits.

30.2.4 The Need for Anesthesia Depth Monitoring

Accurate monitoring of anesthesia depth is crucial for avoiding complications such as intraoperative awareness or overdose. Traditional metrics like the bispectral index (BIS) or entropy monitoring offer valuable insights into the brain's response during anesthesia. However, deeper integration of these monitoring techniques is needed to tailor anesthetic delivery based on each patient's unique neurophysiological response. By capturing subtle changes in brain activity, clinicians can better adjust anesthetic dosages in real time, minimizing potential side effects and optimizing recovery times.

30.2.5 Beyond Pulse Oximetry: Detecting Tissue Ischemia and Hypoxia

Conventional pulse oximetry, while indispensable, provides a limited view—primarily reporting on global arterial oxygen saturation. It does not reveal the local nuances of tissue perfusion or oxygenation. Modern advancements are targeting this gap with techniques that can detect and quantify local tissue ischemia and hypoxia:

- **Near-Infrared Spectroscopy (NIRS)**: This non-invasive technique monitors regional tissue oxygenation by measuring the absorption of near-infrared light. It has been increasingly used in neurosurgery and cardiac procedures, and its application in anesthesia monitoring could significantly enhance the detection of localized hypoxic events.
- **Laser Doppler Flowmetry**: By assessing microvascular blood flow, this technology helps gauge perfusion at the capillary level. It offers insights into tissue viability that far exceed the capabilities of a standard pulse oximeter.
- **Advanced Imaging Modalities**: Emerging systems such as hyperspectral imaging and laser speckle contrast imaging provide detailed maps of tissue oxygenation and perfusion in real time. These techniques could assist anesthesiologists in identifying regions of tissue distress before irreversible damage occurs.

30.2.6 Integrating Multimodal Monitoring

Integrating anesthesia depth monitoring with advanced tissue perfusion technologies provides a multidimensional perspective on patient status. For example, during surgeries where both brain function and tissue viability are critical, the combined use of BIS, NIRS, and laser-based perfusion imaging can offer a coherent picture of both central and peripheral conditions. This integration is particularly vital in patients with underlying conditions—such as peripheral vascular disease or diabetes—where tissue ischemia is a common complication.

In summary, the future of pain management and anesthesiology lies in harnessing a suite of advanced technologies. These tools not only address the challenges of effective pain modulation but also ensure that anesthetic care continually adapts to the dynamic needs of the patient. By embracing these innovations, the field is well on its way to transforming patient outcomes through more personalized and responsive care.

30.3 Differences Between Basic Science and Clinical Research

Anesthesiology research can be categorized into basic, clinical, and translational research. Each type plays a crucial role in advancing knowledge and improving clinical practice, but they differ significantly in their approach, scope, and outcomes.

30.3.1 Basic Research

Basic science research in anesthesiology focuses on understanding fundamental biological processes. This type of research is often conducted in laboratories using cell cultures, animal models, and biochemical techniques to investigate the mechanisms of anesthesia, pain, and consciousness. Basic research aims to answer questions about how anesthetics affect the nervous system, how different drugs interact with receptors in the body, and how pain signals are transmitted and processed in the brain.

- **Example:** Investigating how specific anesthetic agents affect ion channels in neurons to understand the molecular basis of anesthesia-induced unconsciousness.

Basic research is essential because it provides the foundation for clinical applications. However, it often takes years, if not decades, for findings from basic research to influence clinical practice.

30.3.2 Who Conducts Basic Science Research?

Basic science research in anesthesiology is often carried out by diverse teams composed of:

- **Dedicated Research Departments**: Many academic institutions and hospitals have specialized departments focusing exclusively on basic science research. These departments consist of scientists, postdoctoral fellows, and graduate students trained in specific methodologies.
- **Interdisciplinary Collaborations**: Basic science research often involves partnerships between disciplinaries, such as anesthesiology and physiology, pharmacology, or biochemistry. For example, studies investigating how anesthetics impact cardiovascular function may include collaboration between anesthesiology and physiology experts.
- **Role of Clinicians**: While scientists often conduct basic science research without direct patient involvement, clinicians play a key role by providing insights from clinical practice. Their observations of patient responses to anesthetics can inspire basic science research questions or hypotheses, and some clinicians actively engage in research themselves through dual roles as physician-scientists.

30.3.3 Economic Impacts of Basic Science Research

Basic science research drives economic benefits for institutions and society in several ways:

- **Grant Funding**: Research activities often attract substantial funding from governmental bodies like NIH or private organizations. These grants support the studies and enable the hiring of additional personnel, such as research assistants and technicians, boosting employment.
- **Commercialization**: Discoveries from basic science research can lead to the development of new drugs, medical devices, or technologies. For instance, understanding anesthetic mechanisms has led to innovations like target-controlled infusion systems for anesthetic delivery. The commercialization of such products generates revenue for institutions and stimulates broader economic growth.
- **Institutional Prestige and Investment**: Successful basic science research can enhance the reputation of the supporting institution, attracting further investments and collaborations from industry and academia.

While basic science research often requires long-term investment and patience, its impact on clinical advancements, institutional development, and economic growth is profound.

30.3.4 Interdisciplinary Collaborations

1. **Pharmacology and Anesthesiology**:
   - Research into the mechanisms of intravenous anesthetics, such as propofol, often involves collaboration between pharmacologists and anesthesiologists. Pharmacologists help determine how drugs interact with cellular targets, while anesthesiologists contribute clinical observations regarding efficacy and side effects. For example, studies exploring the modulation of GABA receptors have led to safer strategies to anesthetize patients with the combination of medications of different targets.
2. **Neurobiology and Anesthesiology**:
   - Teams specializing in neurobiology often collaborate with anesthesiology departments to study postoperative cognitive dysfunction (POCD). For instance, research investigating the impact of anesthetics on the development of POCD involves both neurobiologists focusing on cellular signaling and anesthesiologists refining protocols to minimize cognitive impacts, especially in elderly patients.
3. **Engineering and Anesthesiology**:
   - Developing advanced monitoring tools like depth-of-anesthesia monitors or brain activity sensors requires collaboration between bioengineers and anesthesiologists. For example, engineers designing EEG-based devices work closely with anesthesiology experts to ensure these tools effectively measure anesthesia depth.

30.3.5 Commercialized Innovations

1. **Depth-of-Anesthesia Monitors**:
   - The creation of devices like the Bispectral Index Monitor (BIS) monitor represents the successful translation of basic science research into commercial products. This tool analyzes EEG patterns and provides real-time feedback on anesthesia depth, reducing the risk of awareness under anesthesia. Commercializing such devices has generated significant revenue for institutions and improved perioperative patient safety.
2. **Target-Controlled Infusion (TCI) Systems**:
   - TCI systems automate the delivery of intravenous anesthetics, such as propofol, based on patient-specific pharmacokinetics. These systems stem from research into drug metabolism and personalized medicine and have been widely adopted, transforming the anesthetic delivery landscape while boosting economic returns for manufacturers.
3. **Novel Anesthetic Agents**:
   - The introduction of drugs like dexmedetomidine, an alpha-2 adrenergic agonist, highlights the commercialization of molecular mechanism research. Initially studied for its sedative and analgesic properties in basic science research, dexmedetomidine is now widely used in clinical anesthesia practices, generating substantial market growth.

These examples highlight the constructive collaboration between interdisciplinary research and commercial applications, emphasizing how fundamental discoveries drive advancements in patient care and economic growth.

30.3.6 Clinical Research

Clinical research, on the other hand, focuses on applying knowledge gained from basic science research to improve patient care. It involves human subjects and assesses the safety, efficacy, and outcomes of anesthetic techniques, drugs, and devices. Clinical trials are critical to clinical practice, as they provide evidence that guides clinical decision-making.

- **Example:** A clinical trial comparing the effectiveness of a new opioid-sparing analgesic technique to traditional opioid-based pain management in postoperative patients.

Clinical research bridges the gap between the laboratory and the bedside, ensuring that discoveries are tested and validated in real-world clinical settings before being implemented in standard practice.

30.3.7 Personnel Involved in Clinical Research

Clinical research requires a collaborative, multidisciplinary team to ensure rigorous study design, execution, and analysis:

1. **Principal Investigators (PIs)**: These are often experienced clinicians or physician-scientists responsible for leading the research project, overseeing ethical adherence, and interpreting results.
2. **Clinical Research Coordinators (CRCs)**: CRCs manage day-to-day operations, such as recruiting participants, obtaining informed consent, and ensuring protocol compliance.
3. **Statisticians/Data Scientists**: These experts are essential for analyzing data to ensure that study findings are statistically robust and meaningful.
4. **Specialists in Related Fields**: Clinical researchers may collaborate with professionals from other specialties depending on the study. For example, an anesthesiology trial might involve cardiologists for studies on perioperative cardiovascular risks.
5. **Institutional Review Boards (IRBs)**: IRB members evaluate and approve studies to ensure that ethical and safety standards are met for all participants.

30.3.8 Financial Impacts of Clinical Research

Clinical research has far-reaching financial implications that benefit institutions and society:

1. **Increased Grants and Funding**:
   - Clinical research often attracts substantial grants from governmental organizations like the NIH or private entities such as pharmaceutical companies. These funds not only cover study costs but also provide resources for personnel and infrastructure.
   - Large-scale trials involving innovative technologies may receive even higher funding due to their significance for public health.
2. **Commercialization Opportunities**:
   - Findings from clinical research often led to the development of new medical devices, drugs, or software systems. For example, studies validating the efficacy of a new anesthetic agent can pave the way for its FDA approval and subsequent commercialization.
   - Commercialization generates revenue for researchers and supporting institutions, fostering long-term economic growth. For instance, products like opioid-sparing analgesics shown by clinical trials have since gained significant market traction.

3. **Institutional Growth and Prestige**:
    - Successful clinical research enhances the reputation of the hosting institution, attracting further investments, collaborations, and patients who seek innovative care.

Despite its complexity, clinical research is an invaluable process that bridges science and patient care while driving medical progress and economic development.

30.3.9 Translational Research

Translational research serves as a bridge between basic science and clinical research. It focuses on translating laboratory findings into clinical applications. In anesthesiology, translational research might involve developing new monitoring technologies or creating novel drug delivery systems that improve the efficacy and safety of anesthesia care. It also includes studies identifying biomarkers predicting patient outcomes, allowing for more personalized anesthetic care.

- **Example:** Developing a real-time monitoring system based on basic science research findings about brain activity during anesthesia to prevent intraoperative awareness.

30.3.10 Who Is Involved in Translational Research?

1. **Multidisciplinary Teams**:
    - **Basic Scientists**: Researchers specializing in neuroscience, pharmacology, or bioengineering often make fundamental discoveries. For example, findings about brain wave patterns during anesthesia come from neuroscientists studying synaptic activity.
    - **Clinical Researchers**: Anesthesiologists and clinicians are critical in applying these discoveries to patient care. Their insights ensure that monitoring systems meet practical needs in the operating room.
    - **Engineers and Technologists**: Developing real-time systems like EEG-based anesthesia monitors requires collaboration with engineers who design algorithms and hardware.
    - **Data Scientists and Statisticians**: These professionals analyze collected data to refine monitoring systems and validate effectiveness.
    - **Institutional Leadership**: Hospital administrators or department chairs often coordinate funding, ethics approval, and partnerships to support translational efforts.

2. **Cross-Departmental Collaborations**:
   - This research frequently involves partnerships between anesthesiology, neurology, biomedical engineering, and computer science departments, fostering interdisciplinary innovation.

30.3.11 Bridging the Gap Between Science and Clinical Practice

Translational research is the engine that powers innovation in medical care. In anesthesiology, it means taking insights from studies of brain activity, pharmacology, and physiology and converting them into tangible improvements such as real-time monitoring systems designed to prevent intraoperative awareness. This not only enhances patient safety but also sets the stage for more personalized anesthetic protocols that tune treatment to individual patient needs.

30.3.12 The Power of Multidisciplinary Collaboration

The success of translational research hinges on a diverse team:

- **Basic Scientists** dive deep into the molecular underpinnings of anesthesia, elucidating processes like synaptic activity and neuronal connectivity. Their discoveries lay the groundwork for new biomarkers and potential therapeutic targets.
- **Clinical Researchers** then take these insights to the bedside, ensuring that innovations align with real-world patient needs. Their direct involvement in the operating room helps refine and validate emerging technologies.
- **Engineers and Technologists** are crucial for designing the hardware and developing the algorithms required for sophisticated monitoring systems—like EEG-based tools—that capture and interpret subtle neurophysiological signals.
- **Data Scientists and Statisticians** transform massive streams of data into actionable insights by optimizing algorithms and validating clinical outcomes.
- **Institutional Leadership** plays a strategic role by coordinating resources, navigating ethical and regulatory landscapes, and fostering partnerships across departments.

These groups often collaborate across disciplines—bringing together anesthesiology, neurology, biomedical engineering, and computer science—to drive innovation and ensure the research remains both practical and groundbreaking.

30.3.13 Opportunities for Deepening Translational Research

- **Navigating the "Valley of Death":** Many promising laboratory findings encounter a perilous gap—where regulatory hurdles, funding limitations, or logistical challenges impede progress from bench to bedside. Delving into strategies for

overcoming these hurdles, such as streamlined approval processes and targeted funding initiatives, can provide valuable insights.
- **Bridging Differing Timelines:** Laboratory research can progress at a pace that often does not match the urgent timelines in clinical settings. Outlining strategies to align these timelines, for example, through iterative prototyping and real-time clinical feedback—would provide a pragmatic roadmap for researchers.
- **Data Integration and Standardization:** As translational research increasingly leverages big data and machine learning, addressing challenges related to data quality, interoperability, and integration becomes essential. Highlighting case studies or innovative practices in data management could enrich the discourse.
- **Patient-Centered Approaches:** Incorporating patient feedback early and throughout the research process can help refine outcomes and ensure that innovations truly address clinical needs. Discussing frameworks for integrating patient-reported outcomes into research design could further enhance the translational model.

30.3.14 Looking Ahead

Translational research in anesthesiology is not merely a bridge between basic science and clinical practice—it is a dynamic interplay where each discipline fuels and informs the other. By embracing interdisciplinary collaboration and addressing the practical challenges in implementation, this research paradigm holds immense potential to revolutionize patient care.

30.3.15 Potential Financial Benefits to a Department

1. **Revenue from Innovation**:
   - Successful translation of research into commercial products, like an intraoperative brain activity monitor, can lead to licensing agreements and royalties. These revenues support further departmental growth and research activities.
   - For example, the commercialization of Bispectral Index (BIS) technology significantly boosted the standing of institutions involved in its development.
2. **Attracting Grants**:
   - Departments engaging in impactful translational research often secure substantial funding from NIH, private foundations, or industry partners. These grants support research, cover additional personnel salaries, purchase advanced equipment, and enhance departmental infrastructure.

3. **Enhanced Reputation and Recruitment**:
    - Successful translational research elevates a department's prestige, attracting top-tier faculty, collaborators, and students. It also establishes the department as a leader in innovation, drawing patients and funding for other projects.

30.3.16 Funding for Translational Research

Translational research is typically funded through a combination of:

1. **Government Grants**:
    - Agencies like the NIH often support projects that promise tangible patient care advancements, offering robust funding opportunities.
2. **Industry Partnerships**:
    - Pharmaceutical or medical device companies invest in translational research, seeing potential commercial applications for products like monitoring systems.
3. **Institutional and Philanthropic Support**:
    - Hospitals, universities, or foundations may allocate internal funds or donations for projects with high clinical or financial promise.
4. **Venture Capital**:
    - Innovative, high-impact projects sometimes attract venture capitalists interested in funding groundbreaking technologies for commercialization.

Translational research fosters significant advancements, such as developing intraoperative monitoring systems, while bringing financial and reputational gains to the departments involved.

30.4 Logistics of Pursuing Basic Science Versus Clinical Research

Whether the research is basic science, clinical, or translational, it involves complex logistics, including funding, collaboration, compliance with ethical standards, and data management. The logistical challenges of pursuing basic science and clinical research differ significantly, and understanding these challenges is crucial for trainees and early-career researchers. It is also essential for associated clinicians and administrators who may participate directly or indirectly in research endeavors.

30.4.1 Basic Science Research Logistics

Basic science research typically takes place in a laboratory setting, which requires specialized equipment, access to animal models or cell cultures, and a team of researchers with expertise in molecular biology, pharmacology, or physiology.

Funding for basic science research often comes from government grants, private foundations, or institutional support. Applying for funding is highly competitive, and securing long-term funding can be challenging.

Navigating the funding world can be daunting, but securing support for impactful research is possible with the right approach and resources. We break it down step-by-step:

30.4.2 How to Find Funding

1. **Institutional Resources**:
   - Start by exploring internal funding opportunities at your institution, such as seed grants offered by your department or university. These are often less competitive and provide initial support for early-stage projects.
2. **Government Agencies**:
   - In the USA, agencies like the National Institutes of Health (NIH), National Science Foundation (NSF), and the Department of Defense (DoD) are major sources of research funding for medicine-related projects.
   - Look into specific funding programs aligned with your research, such as the NIH's R01 grants for independent investigators or small R03 grants for pilot projects.
3. **Foundations and Nonprofits**:
   - Organizations such as the American Heart Association (AHA), the Anesthesia Patient Safety Foundation (APSF), Foundation for Anesthesia Education and Research (FAER), and the Welcome Trust provide grants for research with clear clinical or public health implications.
4. **Industry Partnerships**:
   - Pharmaceutical companies or medical device manufacturers often fund research that aligns with their product pipelines. Collaborating with industry can also open doors for commercialization.
5. **Online Databases**:
   - Tools like Grants.gov, Pivot, and Research Professional offer searchable databases of funding opportunities tailored to specific fields.

30.4.3 Tips for Writing a Grant Proposal

1. **Start with a Strong Idea**:
   - Begin with a focused and innovative research question. The proposal should address a specific problem and demonstrate how your research will contribute to solving it.
2. **Understand the Audience**:
   - Tailor your proposal to the funding agency's priorities. Review past grant recipients to understand their value and follow the guidelines closely.

3. **Build a Clear Structure**:
    - Typical components include:
        - **Abstract**: Summarize concisely the research objectives.
        - **Specific Aims**: Outline your goals and the significance of your project.
        - **Background**: Provide context and highlight gaps in existing knowledge.
        - **Methods**: Describe your approach, including study design, data collection, and analysis.
        - **Budget**: Break down the costs and justify each expense.
        - **Timeline**: Show realistic milestones for your project.
4. **Collaboration and Review**:
    - Involve mentors or colleagues to provide feedback on your proposal. They may spot gaps or areas for improvement.
5. **Be Realistic**:
    - Ensure your goals, methods, and budget align with the scope and duration of the funding.

30.4.4 Potential Funding Sources

Here is a mix of well-known and specialized sources:

- **Government**: NIH, NSF, Centers for Disease Control and Prevention (CDC)
- **Foundations**: APSF, AHA, Gates Foundation, Howard Hughes Medical Institute
- **Professional Societies**: American Society of Anesthesiologists (ASA), International Anesthesia Research Society (IARS)
- **Industry**: Pharmaceutical companies like Pfizer, or device makers like Medtronic

30.4.5 How to Structure a Grant Budget

1. **Direct Costs**:
    - This includes salaries, supplies, equipment, travel, and participant recruitment. Each expense should directly support the research.
2. **Fringe Benefits**:
    - These cover additional costs for personnel, such as health insurance, retirement, and payroll taxes. Fringe rates vary by institution and are usually provided by the finance office.
3. **Indirect Costs**:
    - Also known as "overhead." These cover institutional support for research (e.g., utilities, administration). The institution and the funding agency typically negotiate the indirect cost rate.

4. **Justification**:
   - Provide a detailed explanation for each budget line item to demonstrate necessity and alignment with the project goals.

Securing funding is no small feat, but breaking the process into manageable steps can make it less overwhelming.

Researchers must also navigate regulatory hurdles, such as obtaining approval from Institutional Animal Care and Use Committees (IACUC) for studies involving animals. Additionally, data generated from basic science research must be rigorously analyzed and documented, as it forms the foundation for future clinical trials.

30.4.6 Regulatory Hurdles

1. **Ethical Approvals**:
   - **Animal Studies**: Any use of animal models in basic science research must comply with regulations set by institutional animal care committees and laws such as the Animal Welfare Act. Approval from the Institutional Animal Care and Use Committee (IACUC) is required in the USA.
   - **Human Tissue or Samples**: Research using human-derived materials requires Institutional Review Board (IRB) approval to ensure ethical handling and informed consent.
2. **Compliance with Safety Standards**:
   - Laboratories must follow Occupational Safety and Health Administration (OSHA) regulations for handling hazardous chemicals, biological materials, or anesthetic agents.
   - Biosafety levels (BSL) may apply depending on the materials studied.
3. **Data Integrity and Reporting**:
   - Many funding agencies, such as the NIH, require strict data management protocols, including FAIR principles (Findable, Accessible, Interoperable, Reusable).
   - Mismanagement of data or deviation from approved research protocols can lead to severe penalties or loss of funding.
4. **Grant Reporting and Renewals**:
   - Researchers must document and report milestones to funding agencies. Delays or lack of compliance with grant conditions may hinder long-term funding.

30.4.7 Internal Regulations

1. **Fringe Rates**:
   - **What It Is**: Fringe rates are the additional costs associated with employing personnel, such as health benefits, retirement contributions, and payroll taxes. Each institution has specific fringe rates, which must be included in grant budgets to cover personnel costs fully.
   - **How to Handle It**: Your institution's finance or grant management office typically provides current fringe rates, which must be accurately calculated and documented in budget proposals.
2. **Indirect Costs (Overhead)**:
   - Institutions often apply an indirect cost rate to research budgets, covering administrative support, facilities, and utilities. This rate is negotiated between the institution and funding agencies and must be factored into proposals.

30.4.8 Establishing a Basic Science Research Laboratory

Setting up a laboratory involves careful planning, funding acquisition, and collaboration. Here is how:

1. **Define Research Focus**:
   - Identify specific areas of interest that align with departmental priorities, such as the mechanisms of anesthetic action or neurological impacts of anesthesia.
2. **Secure Funding**:
   - Initial funding may come from departmental seed grants, larger institutional grants, or external sources like the NIH, private foundations, or industry sponsors. Start-up packages for new faculty often include initial laboratory support.
3. **Infrastructure and Equipment**:
   - Basic research laboratories require specialized equipment such as spectrophotometers, imaging systems, or electrophysiological tools. Collaboration with other departments (e.g., physiology or pharmacology) can help share resources.
4. **Personnel Recruitment**:
   - Key team members include lab technicians, graduate students, postdoctoral fellows, and occasionally clinical staff for translational projects.
5. **Regulatory Compliance**:
   - Ensure that the laboratory meets biosafety standards, adheres to chemical handling protocols, and maintains all required licenses or certifications.
6. **Foster Collaboration**:
   - Collaboration with other departments or institutions helps share expertise, attract funding, and drive impactful research.

Setting up and running a basic science research laboratory is challenging but immensely rewarding. It creates opportunities for groundbreaking discoveries and innovation.

30.4.9 Clinical Research Logistics

Clinical research involves human subjects and requires Institutional Review Board (IRB) approval to meet ethical standards. Researchers must obtain informed consent from participants, ensure patient safety, and manage the logistics of patient recruitment, randomization, and follow-up. Clinical trials, especially large-scale randomized controlled trials, require significant financial resources, often necessitating collaboration with industry partners or government agencies.

30.4.10 How Do these Partnerships Work?

1. **Funding and Resource Allocation**:
    - **Industry Partners**: Pharmaceutical companies or medical device manufacturers often fund clinical trials to test their products, such as new anesthetic agents or surgical tools. They contribute capital, provide study materials (like drugs or devices), and sometimes offer personnel support.
    - **Government Agencies**: Organizations like the NIH or FDA provide grants and regulatory oversight. They often prioritize funding for trials with significant public health implications, such as optimizing anesthesia for elderly patients or reducing postoperative morbidity.
    - **Academic Institutions**: Universities and hospitals often act as trial sites, providing infrastructure, expertise, and patient recruitment.
2. **Shared Responsibilities**:
    - Industry partners focus on product-specific aspects (e.g., manufacturing or marketing), while academic institutions and clinicians handle study design, implementation, and analysis.
    - Regulatory bodies ensure ethical compliance, safety, and validity through protocol reviews and site inspections.
3. **Collaborative Agreements**:
    - Partnerships are typically governed by legal agreements outlining responsibilities, intellectual property (IP) rights, and revenue-sharing plans in the case of commercialization.

30.4.11 Economic Value for Participants

1. **Access to Innovation**:
   - Hospitals and academic institutions conducting trials gain early access to innovative drugs, devices, or procedures, enhancing their reputation for offering advanced care.
   - Clinicians and researchers involved in trials can generate publications, patents, or professional recognition, boosting career growth.
2. **Grant Revenue**:
   - Participation in government-funded trials provides institutions with substantial financial support, enabling them to invest in infrastructure, personnel, and future research.
3. **Patient Recruitment**:
   - Clinical trials often attract patients seeking experimental or specialized treatment, which can increase hospital utilization rates and revenue.

30.4.12 Economic Value for Investors

1. **Reduced Development Costs**:
   - Industry partners benefit from access to academic expertise, clinical settings, and real-world patient data, which can streamline product development and reduce costs.
2. **Faster Regulatory Approvals**:
   - Well-designed randomized clinical trials (RCTs) validate product safety and efficacy, expediting regulatory approval for commercialization. For example, new anesthetic agents developed through trials can be fast-tracked for FDA clearance.
3. **Revenue and Market Expansion**:
   - Once a product is approved, it generates substantial returns for industry partners. For instance, drugs like dexmedetomidine gained massive market success after clinical trials proving their safety and efficacy.
4. **Intellectual Property (IP) Rights**:
   - Collaboration agreements often include shared intellectual property (IP) rights, ensuring revenue generation for all parties involved.

30.4.13 Broader Economic Impacts

These partnerships stimulate local economies by creating jobs, attracting investment, and generating technological advancements. For example, institutions conducting groundbreaking trials may lead to spin-off companies commercializing innovations, further driving economic growth.

Data management in clinical research is complex, as it involves tracking patient outcomes, adverse events, and long-term follow-up. Researchers must adhere to Good Clinical Practice (GCP) guidelines and ensure data is accurately reported to regulatory agencies such as the Food and Drug Administration (FDA) and Clinicaltrials.gov.

Table 30.1 summarizes the key differences between basic science and clinical research logistics.

30.4.14 Key Features of Translational Research Logistics

1. **Interdisciplinary Coordination**:
   - Translational research often involves collaborations across basic sciences, clinical disciplinaries, engineering, and biostatistics.
   - Logistically, this requires coordinated meetings, aligned timelines, and shared facilities to facilitate communication and resource sharing between teams with varied expertise.
2. **Access to Both Preclinical and Clinical Data**:
   - Translational studies need access to data generated from animal models (basic science research) and early-phase human trials (clinical research). Ensuring secure and ethical data sharing between these domains is a logistical priority.
3. **Prototype Development and Testing**:
   - For innovations like devices or monitoring tools, translational research often involves prototype development. This step requires access to specialized resources such as bioengineering laboratories, medical equipment, and fabrication facilities.
   - Testing prototypes in controlled but clinically relevant environments add another layer of logistical complexity.
4. **Regulatory Compliance Across Domains**:
   - Translational research must navigate dual regulatory frameworks:
     - Preclinical requirements (e.g., Institutional Animal Care and Use Committee approvals for animal studies).

Table 30.1 Key differences in basic science vs. clinical research logistics

Aspect	Basic research	Clinical research
Setting	Laboratory, often using animal models or cell cultures	Clinical environment involving human subjects
Regulatory oversight	IACUC (for animal studies)	IRB, FDA approval
Funding sources	Government agencies, foundations	Industry partnerships, government agencies
Data collection	Laboratory data, molecular or physiological measures	Patient outcomes, adverse events, and clinical measures

- Early-phase human studies (e.g., IRB approvals for ethical human testing).
- Bridging these frameworks smoothly demands robust regulatory expertise.

5. **Industry and Academic Partnerships**:
   - Effective translational research often involves partnering with industry to commercialize findings or develop technologies. Establishing clear agreements regarding intellectual property and funding distribution is a logistical task.

30.4.15 Logistical Challenges and Solutions

1. **Funding and Resource Allocation**:
   - Translational research may require combined funding from grants, private foundations, and industry sponsorships. Managing these multiple streams and ensuring accountability are critical.
   - Unlike basic science research, translational studies often involve budgeting for laboratory work and clinical pilot studies, doubling the need for meticulous financial planning.
2. **Infrastructure and Technology**:
   - Researchers may need access to preclinical tools (e.g., molecular assays and imaging) and clinical resources (e.g., electronic health records or patient recruitment systems).
   - Sharing or expanding facilities to support dual domains can strain budgets and timelines.
3. **Team Management**:
   - Translational teams are often more extensive and diverse than those focused solely on basic science or clinical research. This requires careful delegation of responsibilities and effective communication channels.
4. **Scaling Up from Bench to Bedside**:
   - Translating laboratory findings to patient care often involves multiple iterations of refinement, requiring time and the ability to scale up operations (e.g., producing larger quantities of drugs, devices, or materials for clinical testing).

30.4.16 Comparison with Basic Science and Clinical Research

Aspect	Basic research	Clinical research	Translational research
Goal	Generate fundamental knowledge	Test interventions in human populations	Apply basic science findings to create real-world solutions
Team composition	Scientists, technicians	Clinicians, statisticians	Interdisciplinary teams across science and medicine

Aspect	Basic research	Clinical research	Translational research
Infrastructure	Laboratory-based equipment	Clinical settings (e.g., hospitals, EHR systems)	Combination of laboratory and clinical environments
Regulations	Laboratory safety, IACUC approvals	IRB, FDA guidelines	Dual compliance with laboratory and clinical standards
Funding complexity	Research grants	Government/industry funding	Combined grants, private, and industry funding

Translational research, while complex, is an exciting and crucial part of medical advancement.

30.5 Integrating Research into Training Programs

Training future anesthesiologists to be proficient in research is critical for advancing the field. Incorporating research into fellowship, postdoctoral, and residency programs gives trainees the skills to contribute to medical knowledge and improve patient care. It also allows clinicians to review and integrate innovative research into patient care. Residents and trainees may be better able to critically evaluate the results presented in peer-reviewed research when they receive dedicated training in the related discipline from active investigators.

30.5.1 Residency Programs

Residency programs in anesthesiology are increasingly incorporating research opportunities for residents. Some programs offer dedicated research tracks or electives, allowing residents to pursue research projects during training. This firsthand experience is invaluable for residents interested in academic careers or clinical research. Residency programs can also foster mentorship relationships between residents and experienced researchers, providing guidance and support for young investigators.

30.5.1.1 Examples

Duke University's Academic Career Enrichment Scholars (ACES) Program

The ACES program is an exemplary model of integrating clinical training with academic development. By combining residency with research block, this initiative aims to cultivate anesthesiologists who are skilled clinicians and innovative researchers. The program provides mentorship, research opportunities, and leadership training, preparing participants for careers in academic anesthesiology and advancing patient care through research.

Foundation for Anesthesia Education and Research (FAER)
FAER is a nationally recognized organization dedicated to advancing education and research in anesthesiology. Some highlights of FAER's programs include:

- **Research Grant Opportunities**: FAER offers grants for physician-scientists, supporting projects that improve perioperative care, patient safety, and pain management.
- **Mentoring and Development Programs**: FAER actively engages anesthesiology residents and early-career professionals, fostering their transition into academic and research-focused roles.
- **Annual Research Grants**: Designed to fund innovative studies in anesthesiology and related fields. The foundation significantly contributes to fostering groundbreaking advancements.

30.5.2 Other Nationally Recognized Organizations

1. **International Anesthesia Research Society (IARS)**:
   - IARS is committed to advancing anesthesia research and education globally. They provide grants, organize conferences, and publish the prestigious journal *Anesthesia & Analgesia* to disseminate innovative findings. Their programs are ideal for anesthesiologists pursuing academic and research careers.
2. **Association of University Anesthesiologists (AUA)**:
   - AUA promotes academic anesthesiology through education, research, and collaboration. Its members include anesthesiology research and education leaders, fostering a community of innovation and discovery.

These initiatives provide valuable opportunities for anesthesiologists to engage in research, access funding, and gain mentorship, enhancing academic anesthesiology's impact on patient care.

30.5.3 Fellowship and Postdoctoral Programs

Fellowship and postdoctoral programs provide an opportunity for more in-depth research training. Programs like the NIH T32 Postdoctoral Fellowship offer rigorous training in research fundamentals and techniques, preparing fellows for careers in academic anesthesiology or clinical research [1]. These programs often include protected research time, allowing fellows to focus on their research projects without the demands of clinical work.

- **Example:** The NIH T32 program offers postdoctoral fellows access to cutting-edge research tools and mentorship from senior investigators [1].

30.5.4 Medical Students

Exposing medical students to research early in their training is crucial for fostering a research mindset. Many medical schools offer research electives or summer research programs that allow students to work in a laboratory or clinical research setting. These experiences provide valuable research skills and help students develop critical thinking and problem-solving abilities that are essential for their future medical careers.

- **Example:** Programs that allow medical students to conduct basic or clinical research, fostering an early interest in academic anesthesiology [2].

30.6 Skills Acquired by Trainees Through Research

Participating in research offers trainees a range of skills beneficial for those pursuing academic careers and clinical practice. These skills, as shown in Fig. 30.1, include:

1. **Critical Thinking:** Research requires analyzing data, identifying trends, and drawing conclusions. These critical thinking skills are transferable to clinical practice, where anesthesiologists must make quick decisions based on patient data.
2. **Problem-Solving:** Research often involves troubleshooting experiments, analyzing unexpected results, and developing new hypotheses. These critical thinking skills are essential for handling complex clinical cases.
3. **Data Management:** Trainees learn to manage large datasets, maintain accurate records, and use statistical tools to analyze results. In clinical practice, these skills help anesthesiologists track patient outcomes and improve the quality of care.

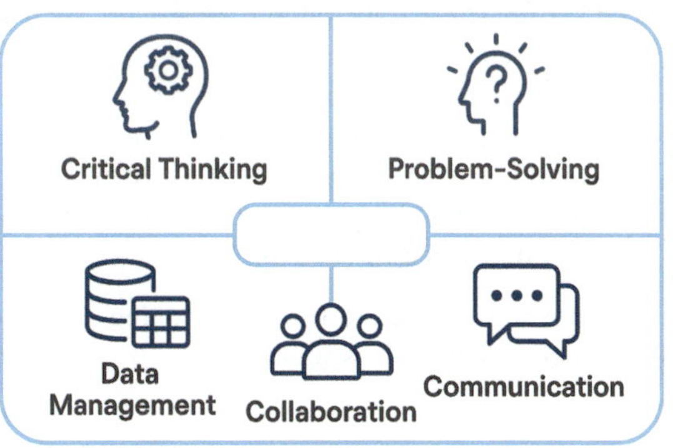

Fig. 30.1 Core competencies developed through research training include critical thinking, problem-solving, data management, collaboration, and communication—skills essential for success in academic and professionalenvironments.

4. **Collaboration:** Research often involves working with a team of investigators, technicians, and clinicians. Learning to collaborate effectively is crucial in both research and clinical settings, where multidisciplinary teams are common.
5. **Communication:** Writing research papers, presenting findings at conferences, and explaining complex ideas to colleagues are all essential communication skills that trainees develop through research. These skills are critical for communicating effectively with patients, colleagues, and the broader medical community.

30.7 Essential Components of a Successful Research Program

Building a successful research program in anesthesiology requires several key components, including:

1. **Strong Leadership:** A successful research program needs visionary leaders who can inspire and guide trainees and junior investigators. Research mentors are critical in fostering a culture of inquiry and supporting early-career researchers.
2. **Collaboration:** Interdisciplinary collaboration is essential for successful research in anesthesiology. Anesthesiologists must work closely with surgeons, intensivists, pharmacists, and basic scientists to design studies that address clinically relevant questions.
3. **Infrastructure:** A strong research program requires adequate infrastructure, including laboratory space, equipment, and access to clinical data. Institutions should invest in state-of-the-art facilities that support both basic science and clinical research.
4. **Funding:** Securing funding is one of the most significant challenges for research programs. Successful programs often have dedicated staff who can assist investigators in applying for grants from government agencies, private foundations, and industry partners.
5. **Mentorship and Training:** Developing the next generation of anesthesiologists requires mentorship programs that give trainees the guidance and support to succeed. Formal research training programs, such as fellowships and residency research tracks, are essential for cultivating research talent.
6. **Dissemination of Research:** Publishing research findings in peer-reviewed journals and presenting them at conferences is crucial for advancing knowledge and improving clinical practice. Successful programs prioritize the dissemination of research and support investigators in publishing their work.

   As summarized in Table 30.2.

Here are some effective research training strategies that can help enhance the skills and knowledge of researchers:

Table 30.2 Components of a successful research program

Component	Description
Leadership	Strong, visionary leaders who inspire and guide junior investigators
Collaboration	Interdisciplinary teams work together to address complex clinical questions.
Infrastructure	Access to laboratory space, equipment, and clinical data
Funding	Supporting staff to assist with grant applications
Mentorship	Formal mentorship programs that provide guidance and support
Dissemination	Prioritizing publication and presentation of research findings

1. **Identify Training Needs**: Assess your research team's specific skills and knowledge gaps through surveys, performance reviews, or direct feedback.
2. **Develop a Comprehensive Training Plan**: Create a structured plan that outlines the training objectives, methods, and timelines. This plan should be tailored to meet your team's needs and goals.
3. **Utilize Diverse Training Methods**: Incorporate a mix of training methods, such as workshops, seminars, online courses, and firsthand practice. This variety can cater to different learning styles and keep the training engaging.
4. **Promote Open Science and Reproducibility**: Encourage practices that support open science, such as sharing data and methodologies. Training in these areas can improve the transparency and reproducibility of research.
5. **Incorporate Cognitive Strategies**: Use evidence-based cognitive strategies, such as spaced practice, interleaving, and retrieval practice, to enhance learning and retention.
6. **Monitor and Evaluate Training Effectiveness**: Regularly assess the impact of the training through feedback, performance metrics, and follow-up sessions. This helps in making necessary adjustments to improve the training program.
7. **Foster a Collaborative Learning Environment**: Encourage research collaboration and knowledge sharing. This can be facilitated through group projects, peer reviews, and discussion forums.
8. **Leverage Technology**: Utilize digital tools and platforms to provide flexible and accessible training options. Online resources, virtual laboratories, and e-learning modules can be particularly effective.

The financial aspects of research are central to its sustainability and success. They touch every stage, from securing initial funding to leveraging research outputs for economic growth.

1. **Obtaining and Ensuring funding**

   Securing funding is a fundamental step for research, and it requires a strategic approach:

   - **Identifying Funding Sources.**
     - **Government Grants**: Agencies like NIH, NSF, and others provide robust funding for innovative projects. Specific grants, such as R01 (research project grant) or T32 (training grant), cater to projects and researcher development.

  - **Private Foundations**: Organizations like the Gates Foundation or APSF often support research that is aligned with their mission, providing alternative funding opportunities.
  - **Industry Partnerships**: Collaborating with pharmaceutical companies or medical device manufacturers can provide funding and access to specialized resources.
  - **Institutional Support**: Universities and hospitals often offer seed grants or matching funds to support early-stage projects.
- **Grant Proposal Writing**:
  - Crafting a compelling proposal is crucial. Key tips include clearly defining the research question, aligning it with funder priorities, providing realistic budgets, and emphasizing potential impact.
  - Securing letters of support and demonstrating feasibility through preliminary data are also highly effective strategies.
- **Sustaining Funding**:
  - Researchers can establish long-term funding by demonstrating consistent success in delivering impactful results, publishing papers, and maintaining relationships with funding bodies.

2. **Added Financial Benefits of Research**

   Research activities bring numerous economic benefits, both directly and indirectly:

   - **Grant Revenue**:
     - Large grants can provide significant revenue streams to departments, covering research costs, salaries, equipment, and institutional overhead.
   - **Economic Impact on Institutions**:
     - Successful research enhances an institution's reputation, attracting more funding, collaboration opportunities, and higher student enrollment or residency applications.
   - **Job Creation**:
     - Research projects often involve hiring assistants, technicians, postdoctoral fellows, and administrative staff, contributing to local job markets.
   - **Professional Growth**:
     - For individual researchers, successful projects lead to promotions, recognition, and an increased ability to attract future funding.

3. **Opportunities for Financialization of Research.**

   Research findings can be leveraged to generate additional financial value:

   - **Commercialization of Innovations**:
     - Discoveries from research can be patented and developed into marketable products like medical devices, drugs, or software. Licensing agreements or spin-off companies can create significant revenue streams for institutions and researchers.
     - Example: Real-time monitoring systems for anesthesia were developed based on research and later became highly profitable commercial products.

- **Public-Private Partnerships**:
  - Collaborating with industry on commercial ventures ensures that research has real-world applications while providing financial incentives to institutions.
- **Consulting and Advisory Roles**:
  - Researchers who are subject-matter experts can consult for industry or policy-making organizations, creating supplemental income while guiding practical applications of their work.

4. **Financial Management and Oversight.**
   Effective financial management ensures sustainability:
   - **Budgeting and Fringe Rates**:
     - Careful planning ensures that all project costs, including salaries and benefits (calculated via fringe rates), are adequately covered.
   - **Indirect Costs**:
     - Institutions often charge indirect costs (overhead) for using their facilities. Proper structuring of grants helps secure enough funding to support both direct and indirect costs.
   - **Continuous Assessment**:
     - Regularly reviewing budgets, expenditures, and return on investment helps maintain financial health and identify growth opportunities.

Research is not only a scientific endeavor but also an economic engine. The ability to attract and manage funding, while translating discoveries into real-world applications, creates long-term value for researchers, institutions, and society.

Implementing these strategies can significantly enhance the effectiveness of research training. Here are some recent case studies that highlight the efficacy of basic science, clinical, and translational research, demonstrating how the principles discussed above contributed to their success:

1. **Basic Science Research: Gene Therapy for Spinal Muscular Atrophy (SMA)**
   - **Overview**: Years of basic science research into the molecular mechanisms of SMA, a genetic condition causing muscle weakness, led to the development of RNA-based therapies like nusinersen.
   - **Key Principles in Action**:
     - **Critical Thinking**: Researchers identified the genetic mutation responsible for SMA and explored how it disrupted protein production.
     - **Collaboration**: Molecular biologists, geneticists, and pharmacologists worked together to design RNA-based interventions.
     - **Economic Impact**: The commercialization of nusinersen has provided life-changing treatment for thousands of patients while generating significant revenue for its developers.
2. **Clinical Research: Maternal Morbidity Study at Duke University and** University of North Carolina **(UNC).**

- **Overview**: A collaborative study between Duke University and the University of North Carolina examined risk factors for severe maternal morbidity (SMM) and racial disparities in outcomes.
- **Key Principles in Action**:
  - **Data Management**: Researchers analyzed large datasets from hospital records to identify trends in SMM rates.
  - **Problem-Solving**: The team developed targeted interventions to address disparities in maternal health outcomes.
  - **Collaboration**: Clinicians and public health experts collaborated to translate findings into actionable recommendations.

3. **Translational Research: HemeChip for Sickle Cell Disease.**
   - **Overview**: The HemeChip, a low-cost point-of-care diagnostic device for sickle cell disease, exemplifies successful translational research.
   - **Key Principles in Action**:
     - **Prototype Development**: Basic science research on hemoglobin variants informed the design of the HemeChip.
     - **Interdisciplinary Collaboration**: Engineers, clinicians, and public health experts collaborated to refine the device and validate its efficacy.
     - **Economic Impact**: The device has improved access to diagnostics in low-resource settings while creating opportunities for commercialization [3].

These examples highlight how integrating critical thinking, collaboration, and effective data management can drive impactful research across all stages.

30.7.1 Barriers to Successful Research Programs

1. **Lack of Protected Time**:
   - Clinicians and researchers often struggle to balance patient care with research activities, leaving insufficient time to focus on meaningful projects.
   - Without dedicated time, research progress can be delayed, and the quality of the work may suffer.
2. **Absence of Basic Science Departments**:
   - Non-academic or community facilities frequently lack dedicated basic science infrastructure, limiting opportunities for fundamental research.
   - The absence of specialized resources like laboratories, equipment, and expert faculty can impede exploratory or innovative studies.
3. **Data Silos**:
   - Fragmented systems prevent effective sharing and integration of research data across institutions or departments.
   - These silos can slow down progress, hinder collaboration, and reduce the ability to draw actionable insights from large datasets.

30.7.2 Solutions to Address Roadblocks

1. **Develop Research Tracks**:
   - **Structured Programs**: Create research tracks within residency or fellowship programs to protect time for research while integrating it into career development.
   - Example: Programs like Duke's ACES offer clear paths for combining clinical duties with academic pursuits, providing mentorship and structured time allocation.
2. **Integrate System-Wide Innovation Programs**:
   - **Centralized Support**: Institutions can implement system-wide innovation hubs that provide shared resources, mentorship, and funding opportunities for researchers across departments.
   - Example: University-wide initiatives often foster interdisciplinary collaboration, making accessing expertise from basic sciences or engineering easier.
3. **Leverage Academic–Private Partnerships**:
   - **Collaboration**: Partnerships with private organizations, such as pharmaceutical companies or biotechnology firms, can provide financial backing, shared resources, and commercialization opportunities.
   - These collaborations can offset infrastructure deficits in community facilities and create mutually beneficial relationships.
4. **Improve Data Integration**:
   - **Standardization**: Implementing standardized data management systems, such as electronic health record (EHR) interoperability, facilitates better sharing of research findings across institutions.
   - **Open Science Practices**: Encourage practices that promote data transparency and accessibility, helping to reduce the barriers created by silos.

Addressing these barriers requires institutional commitment, innovative solutions, and collaboration across sectors.

30.8 Conclusion

Advancing research in anesthesiology is essential for improving patient care, developing innovative treatments, and ensuring patient safety during anesthesia and perioperative period. By integrating basic science and clinical research into training programs, anesthesiology departments can equip the next generation of anesthesiologists with the skills they need to make meaningful contributions to the field. A successful research program relies on strong leadership, collaboration, adequate infrastructure, funding, and a commitment to mentoring trainees. Through these efforts, anesthesiologists can continue to lead the way in research that transforms perioperative care and pain management.

References

1. Logistics of learning: L&D's pursuit of managing training. https://trainingorchestra.com.
2. Research Blog. Clinical vs. basic science research for medical students.
3. Qua K, Swiatkowski SM, Gurkan UA, Pelfrey CM. A retrospective case study of successful translational research: Gazelle Hb variant point-of-care diagnostic device for sickle cell disease. J Clin Transl Sci. 2021;5(1):e207. https://doi.org/10.1017/cts.2021.871.

31 Consulting in Perioperative and Anesthesiology Services: Optimizing Operations, Strategy, and Value

Jason Klopotowski, Kristen Conway, Leslie Meyer Basham, Supriya Patel, and Joshua S. Miller

31.1 Background and History: The Evolution of Consulting in Healthcare

The field of healthcare consulting has undergone significant transformation over the past several decades. Since the early 2000s, consulting services have expanded to address the increasingly complex obstacles that hospitals and health systems face, including operational inefficiencies, rising costs, and evolving regulatory requirements [1]. In particular, the perioperative and anesthesiology spaces have emerged as critical areas where specialized consulting can drive substantial improvements.

In its early stages, healthcare consulting primarily focused on general operational assessments and high-level strategy. Over time, the field evolved to offer more targeted solutions tailored to specific service lines, including surgical services. By leveraging national and international expertise, consulting firms have become trusted partners in helping healthcare organizations navigate their most pressing challenges. These issues often include improving operating room (OR) throughput, managing anesthesiology costs, maximizing revenue, planning strategic integration/alignment, and addressing staffing shortages; all of which have direct implications for patient safety, financial performance, and provider satisfaction [2, 3].

J. Klopotowski (✉) · L. M. Basham · S. Patel · J. S. Miller
Surgical Directions, Chicago, IL, USA
e-mail: jklopotowski@surgicaldirections.com

K. Conway
Surgical Directions, Chicago, IL, USA

Queens University, Knight School of Communication, Charlotte, NC, USA

G. Tewfik (ed.), *The Anesthesiologist as Perioperative Leader*,
https://doi.org/10.1007/978-3-032-18058-2_31

31.2 Key Players in Healthcare Consulting

Several major consulting firms have played a pivotal role in shaping the landscape of perioperative and anesthesiology consulting. Prominent names such as Kaufman Hall, Deloitte, McKesson, and Huron have been instrumental in offering a range of traditional services to hospitals and ambulatory surgery centers (ASCs) [4, 5]. Historically, these firms have provided support in areas such as:

- **Operational efficiency**: Streamlining workflows and processes to optimize resource utilization [6].
- **Cost containment**: Identifying cost-saving opportunities in areas such as staffing models, supply chain, and contract negotiations [7].
- **Governance and strategy**: Assisting organizations in creating governance structures that support long-term sustainability and collaboration among stakeholders [8].

While these traditional offerings have been valuable, the field has also seen the emergence of specialized consulting firms that focus exclusively on perioperative and anesthesiology services. These firms bring unique insights and peer-to-peer collaboration models, which empower them to more effectively address the nuanced problems within these critical areas. By engaging clinicians, including physicians and nurses as part of their consulting teams, these specialized firms provide actionable recommendations grounded in real-world experience [9].

31.3 The Rise of Specialized Perioperative and Anesthesiology Consulting

Specialized consulting in perioperative operations and anesthesiology has expanded in response to the growing complications of healthcare delivery in these areas. As hospitals and ASCs strive to improve OR efficiency, reduce costs, and enhance patient outcomes, their success requires expertise beyond traditional operational consulting. This need has driven the growth of firms that focus specifically on:

- **Anesthesiology costs and staffing models**: Addressing the rising costs associated with anesthesiology and developing innovative staffing solutions [10, 11].
- **OR throughput**: Improving scheduling, block utilization, and turnaround times to maximize OR capacity [12, 13].
- **Governance structures**: Establishing frameworks for effective collaboration between administrators, surgeons, and anesthesia providers [14, 15].

This specialized focus allows consulting firms to offer tailored strategies that align with the unique needs of perioperative and anesthesiology departments. By drawing on best practices and benchmarking data, these firms help organizations achieve sustainable improvements that benefit both patients and providers [16].

31.4 Logistics of a Consulting Partnership

As the healthcare consulting industry has evolved, so too have the models of engagement used to address the specific needs of hospitals and health systems. Modern consulting partnerships often follow a phased approach, designed to adapt to the unique challenges and goals of each organization. Firms such as Deloitte, Huron, Kaufman Hall, and Surgical Directions have refined their methodologies to offer a range of engagement models, each with distinct characteristics and benefits.

1. **Assessment and diagnostics**: Most consulting engagements begin with a comprehensive assessment phase. Consultants collaborate with hospital administrators and clinical leaders to identify inefficiencies, analyze operational data, and pinpoint areas for improvement. For example, Kaufman Hall employs detailed benchmarking and performance metrics to establish a baseline, while Surgical Directions emphasizes on-site observations to gather insights directly from perioperative and anesthesiology teams [9, 16].
2. **Customized solutions**: Unlike early consulting models that relied on standardized templates, modern approaches prioritize tailored recommendations. Deloitte, for instance, leverages advanced analytics and predictive modeling to create customized strategies for improving OR throughput and cost management [4]. Similarly, Surgical Directions' peer-to-peer model ensures that solutions are not only clinically relevant but also practical for implementation within the unique cultural context of the organization [16].
3. **Implementation and collaboration**: Effective consulting partnerships extend beyond recommendations to include hands-on implementation support. Huron's consulting model emphasizes collaboration with multidisciplinary teams to ensure that changes are sustainable and integrated into daily workflows [5]. Surgical Directions distinguishes itself by embedding clinical consultants—such as anesthesiologists and OR nurses—into client organizations, fostering a collaborative environment where stakeholders work together to achieve defined goals [16].
4. **Governance and sustainability**: Modern consulting engagements often include a focus on governance structures to ensure long-term success. Kaufman Hall and Surgical Directions both advocate establishing clear governance frameworks that empower clinical leaders and administrators to sustain improvements over time [9, 16]. This approach drives accountability while also fostering a culture of continuous improvement.

31.5 Cost Structures of Consulting Engagements

The cost structure of consulting engagements in perioperative operations and anesthesiology varies widely depending on the type of firm, the scope of the project, and the engagement model. Typically, consulting firms employ one or more of the following cost structures:

1. **Hourly or daily rates**: This traditional model is often used for short-term projects or advisory services. Firms may charge by the hour or day for specific deliverables, such as data analysis or strategy development [4, 5]. While straightforward, this model can become expensive if projects extend beyond initial timelines.
2. **Flat fees for defined projects**: Many consulting firms, including Kaufman Hall, offer flat-rate pricing for specific projects, such as comprehensive perioperative assessments or contract negotiations with anesthesia providers [9]. This model provides clarity and predictability, making it a popular choice for hospitals with constrained budgets.
3. **Contingency-based fees**: Some firms, particularly those focused on financial performance, structure their fees based on the results achieved. For example, consulting fees may be tied to measurable improvements in OR utilization, cost reductions, or revenue enhancements. This approach aligns incentives between the consulting firm and the hospital, but it requires clear definitions of success metrics [6].
4. **Retainer agreements**: Retainer models are often used for long-term partnerships where ongoing support is needed. Surgical Directions, for example, might engage with a hospital on a retainer basis to provide continuous guidance on perioperative governance and operational improvements [16].
5. **Hybrid models**: Many consulting engagements employ a combination of the above approaches. For instance, a project may begin with a flat fee for the assessment phase, transition to hourly rates for implementation, and include contingency-based bonuses for achieving predefined outcomes.

Hospitals and health systems must carefully evaluate the cost structures of potential consulting engagements to ensure alignment with their financial goals and operational priorities. Transparency in pricing, as well as a clear understanding of the value delivered, is essential for building successful partnerships.

31.6 Goals and Challenges in Modern Healthcare Consulting

The overarching goal of engaging a consulting firm for perioperative and anesthesiology services is to improve patient care through more efficient and cost-effective operations. This involves enhancing OR throughput, ensuring fair access to surgical services, and maintaining high safety and quality standards. By optimizing resource utilization and governance structures, consulting firms help hospitals deliver care that is both sustainable and aligned with their financial priorities [4, 9].

However, modern healthcare faces numerous challenges that complicate these goals:

1. **Staffing shortages**: A critical issue in the perioperative and anesthesiology sectors is the shortage of qualified staff, including anesthesiologists, anesthetists, OR nurses, and support personnel. Consulting firms often assist in developing innovative staffing models to mitigate these shortages while maintaining quality of care [16].
2. **Rising costs**: The increasing costs of anesthesia services and surgical supplies put pressure on hospital budgets. Consultants help identify cost-saving opportunities without compromising patient outcomes [10].
3. **Surgeon access and block scheduling**: Ensuring equitable and efficient use of OR time is a persistent challenge. Consulting firms bring expertise in redesigning block scheduling systems to improve access for surgeons while maximizing throughput [9, 16].
4. **Governance and culture**: Sustainable improvements require a shift in organizational culture and governance. Consultants play a key role in fostering collaboration among stakeholders, establishing clear roles and responsibilities, and creating accountability frameworks [4, 16].

By addressing these challenges, consulting firms can improve operational efficiency within facilities and enhance patient safety, surgeon satisfaction, and overall quality of care. Their expertise provides hospitals with the tools and strategies needed to navigate the complexities of modern healthcare while remaining financially and operationally viable.

31.7 Perioperative Consulting

31.7.1 Introduction, Facts, and Data

Perioperative consulting is an essential component of modern healthcare management, focused on optimizing surgical services to improve patient outcomes, enhance operational efficiency, and achieve financial sustainability. Surgical services represent a significant portion of hospital expenditures, with the OR often accounting for up to 60% of hospital revenue and nearly 40% of total costs [1]. Hospitals across the United States are increasingly seeking the expertise of perioperative consultants to address challenges such as surgeon access, staffing shortages, anesthesia cost containment, and overall process efficiency.

A recent report from Kaufman Hall discussed how optimizing perioperative efficiency can lead to a 20%–30% improvement in OR utilization and a significant reduction in overtime expenses [2]. The growing demand for perioperative consulting is fueled by the need to improve key performance indicators (KPIs) such as first case on-time starts, turnover times, and block utilization rates, which can directly impact patient satisfaction and hospital profitability.

31.7.2 Definitions

Perioperative consulting encompasses a broad spectrum of services aimed at optimizing surgical workflows from preoperative to postoperative care. The perioperative period consists of three main phases:

- **Preoperative phase**: Involves patient preparation, scheduling, and resource allocation to ensure smooth workflow leading up to surgery.
- **Intraoperative phase**: Focuses on OR efficiency, including surgeon scheduling, anesthesia management, and equipment availability.
- **Postoperative phase**: Addresses recovery, discharge planning, and ensuring continuity of care to reduce readmissions and complications.

Consultants provide tailored solutions to hospitals and ASCs, assessing the current state of operations and implementing strategies to enhance throughput, minimize costs, and improve patient safety. The use of data analytics tools such as Merlin™ by Surgical Directions allows hospitals to track and analyze surgeon productivity, case volume, and turnover times to inform decision-making [3].

31.7.3 Offerings in the Market and Logistics of Partnerships

The perioperative consulting market includes a variety of firms offering specialized services, ranging from large, multinational consultancies such as Deloitte and Kaufman Hall to boutique firms with a focused perioperative niche such as Surgical Directions.

Key Offerings in the Market
1. **Operational assessments**: Comprehensive evaluations of OR processes, including first case start times, turnover times, and block utilization rates.
2. **Governance structure development**: Establishing collaborative physician-led governance committees to improve decision-making and accountability.
3. **Cost optimization**: Strategies to manage anesthesia provider contracts, surgical supply chains, and staffing models.
4. **Digital innovation**: Implementing data analytics and decision-support tools to enhance scheduling and resource allocation.
5. **Workforce planning**: Addressing staffing shortages through inventive models, such as flex scheduling and better resource utilization.

Logistics of Partnerships A typical perioperative consulting engagement begins with an in-depth assessment phase, lasting 1–2 weeks, during which consultants collaborate with hospital leadership to analyze current performance metrics and identify areas for improvement. Engagements often follow a phased approach:

1. **Initial assessment**: Data collection and stakeholder interviews to establish baseline performance.
2. **Implementation phase**: Rollout of customized solutions, including governance enhancements and process changes.
3. **Continuous monitoring**: Regular review and reporting to track progress and adjust strategies as needed.

Hospitals that partner with consulting firms benefit from structured governance and accountability frameworks, ensuring sustained improvements in perioperative efficiency [4].

31.7.4 Results (Internal and External Data)

Hospitals that have implemented perioperative consulting solutions report significant improvements across key operational metrics. Internal data from Surgical Directions' engagements show the following:

- **Twenty percent increase in OR primetime utilization within 6–12 months** [5].
- **Reduction in first case delays by up to 35%, improving overall surgical volume throughput** [6].
- **Decrease in turnover times by an average of 25%, resulting in additional cases accommodated per day** [7].

Case Studies

1. **450+ Bed Acute Care Hospital in the Southeast**: A hospital achieved a 10% increase in primetime OR utilization and identified a $19 million return on investment (ROI) over 5 years through perioperative optimization initiatives [8].
2. **Large Southeast Rural Health System**: Facing significant patient safety concerns, a health system in this geographic region improved primetime utilization by up to 12% and first case on-time starts by up to 65% after implementing comprehensive perioperative strategies [9].

A study published by the American Hospital Association corroborates these findings, noting that effective perioperative management can lead to an annual cost savings of up to $5 million for mid-sized hospitals by reducing inefficiencies and improving scheduling accuracy [10].

Additionally, cultural transformations facilitated by consulting engagements contribute to improved staff morale and retention rates. Creating a collaborative, non-retaliatory environment where all surgical team members are aligned with operational goals has been found to be a critical success factor [12].

Hospitals that implement robust perioperative governance structures have also observed:

- More predictable OR schedules, reducing staff burnout, and improving satisfaction, retention, and recruitment.
- Enhanced surgeon engagement and alignment with hospital goals.
- Improved compliance with sterilization and infection control protocols.

31.7.5 Perioperative Consulting Conclusion

Perioperative consulting is an invaluable resource for hospitals seeking to enhance surgical efficiency, reduce costs, and improve patient outcomes. Through data-driven strategies, structured governance, and continuous improvement initiatives, consulting firms empower hospitals to optimize their perioperative services and maintain long-term success. As hospitals continue to face workforce shortages, rising costs, and increasing patient demand, the role of perioperative consulting will remain vital in ensuring sustainable healthcare delivery.

31.8 Anesthesiology Consulting

31.8.1 Introduction, Facts, and Data

Anesthesiology consulting has become an increasingly critical service in healthcare, addressing the financial, operational, and workforce challenges that hospitals and healthcare systems face in maintaining anesthesiology services. Historically, anesthesiology departments operated as revenue-generating centers, often managed by private practice groups that were financially self-sustaining [17]. However, over the past 10–15 years, significant shifts in reimbursement models, workforce shortages, and rising provider compensation have placed substantial pressure on hospitals and anesthesia groups alike [1, 18].

The COVID-19 pandemic accelerated these challenges [3]. Hospitals faced a supply-and-demand mismatch for anesthesia providers, with increasing burnout among anesthesiologists and certified registered nurse anesthetists (CRNAs). A growing number of healthcare organizations sought consulting expertise to reevaluate staffing models, implement care team approaches, and analyze anesthesia stipends to mitigate financial strain [2]. According to Kaufman Hall, anesthesiology-related expenses have risen by over 25% since 2020, contributing to a growing need for cost containment and operational efficiency in surgical services [3].

31.8.2 Definitions

Anesthesiology consulting encompasses a wide range of services designed to optimize the delivery of anesthetic care in hospitals and ASCs. The primary focus areas include the following:

Financial Optimization	Analyzing anesthesiology stipends, reimbursement models, and revenue cycle efficiency
Staffing Models	Assessing the feasibility of care team models, optimizing CRNA and anesthesiologist ratios, and implementing flexible workforce strategies
Operational Efficiency	Improving first case on-time starts, reducing turnover times, and ensuring appropriate anesthesia coverage for procedural care
Regulatory Compliance	Ensuring adherence to guidelines set forth by the American Society of Anesthesiologists (ASA) and Centers for Medicare & Medicaid Services (CMS)

31.8.3 Offerings in the Market and Logistics of Partnerships

The anesthesiology consulting market includes a range of firms specializing in financial, operational, and workforce solutions. Major players such as Deloitte, Kaufman Hall, and Surgical Directions provide data-driven insights and customized solutions to help hospitals navigate the complexities of anesthesia service management.

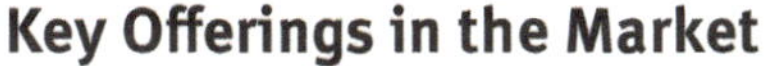

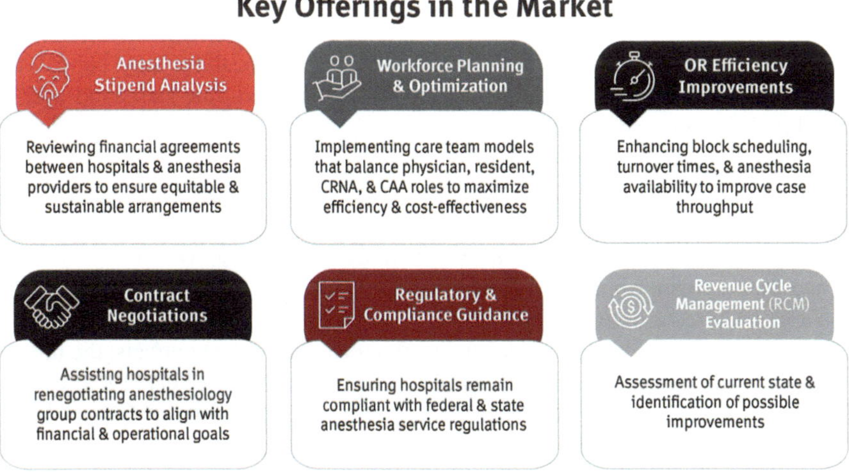

Logistics of Consulting Partnerships

A typical anesthesia consulting engagement follows a structured approach:

1. **Assessment phase**: Data collection, stakeholder interviews, and financial analysis to evaluate current anesthesia service performance.
2. **Strategic planning**: Development of tailored recommendations, including staffing model adjustments, cost-saving initiatives, and operational enhancements.

3. **Implementation and execution**: Collaboration with hospital leadership, anesthesiology groups, and OR teams to implement recommended changes.
4. **Monitoring and continuous improvement**: Ongoing assessment of performance metrics and refinement of strategies as needed [5].

Hospitals that engage in anesthesiology consulting benefit from structured governance models that support sustainable financial and operational improvements.

31.8.4 Results (Internal and External Data)

Hospitals that have implemented anesthesiology consulting strategies have observed measurable improvements in financial sustainability and operational efficiency. Key results include the following:

- **Reduction in anesthesia stipends**: Hospitals have achieved stipend reductions of 15%–30% by restructuring financial agreements with anesthesia providers [6, 19, 20].
- **Workforce efficiency gains**: Implementation of care team models has increased anesthesia provider coverage by 20%–25% without additional staffing costs [7].
- **Enhanced OR throughput**: Hospitals leveraging anesthesiology consulting have reported a 10%–15% improvement in first case on-time starts and a 12% reduction in turnover times [8].

Case Studies

1. **Large Southeastern Academic Medical Center**: Faced with a $12 million anesthesia stipend burden, a hospital in this geographic region partnered with Surgical Directions to analyze staffing models and financial agreements. By implementing a care team model and restructuring provider contracts, the hospital reduced stipend costs by 22% while maintaining quality of care [9, 21].
2. **Midwestern Regional Health System**: Struggling with anesthesia provider shortages, a health system worked with consultants to optimize CRNA and anesthesiologist utilization. By adjusting scheduling models and introducing tele-anesthesia solutions, the system improved provider efficiency by 30%, reducing reliance on locum tenens staffing [10, 22].
3. **West Coast Community Hospital**: Experiencing high turnover rates among anesthesiologists, a hospital engaged consultants to address provider burnout and workload balance. Through scheduling improvements and work-life balance initiatives, the hospital increased retention rates by 18% within a year [12, 23].

31.8.5 Anesthesiology Consulting Conclusion

In summary, anesthesiology consulting serves as a cornerstone in advancing surgical care quality. By integrating expert knowledge, cutting-edge technology, and tailored strategies, these services not only enhance patient outcomes but also drive operational excellence within healthcare facilities.

31.9 Consulting Careers in Healthcare—Opportunities in Healthcare Consulting

Healthcare consulting has emerged as a vital field for professionals seeking to improve hospital operations, enhance financial sustainability, and optimize patient care. With the increasing complexity of the healthcare landscape, the demand for experts in perioperative and anesthesia consulting has surged. Consultants work with hospitals, ASCs, and healthcare systems to address workforce shortages, reimbursement challenges, and operational inefficiencies [1].

The U.S. Bureau of Labor Statistics projects a 14% growth in healthcare management roles by 2032, reflecting the rising demand for consultants who can guide hospitals in strategic decision-making and regulatory compliance [2]. Key areas of opportunity within healthcare consulting include the following:

- **Operational consulting**: Focused on improving hospital efficiency, OR throughput, and clinical workflow optimization.
- **Financial consulting**: Assisting hospitals in negotiating contracts, optimizing anesthesiology stipends, and improving revenue cycle management.
- **Workforce planning**: Addressing shortages by designing staffing models, incorporating care teams, and optimizing anesthesia provider coverage.
- **Digital health and innovation**: Implementing analytics tools such as Surgical Directions' Merlin™ to track performance metrics and inform data-driven decisions [3].

31.9.1 Work/Life Balance in Healthcare Consulting

A career in healthcare consulting offers a dynamic work environment, blending clinical expertise with business strategy. Unlike traditional hospital roles, consultants typically operate on a project-based schedule, often traveling to multiple client sites. While travel demands can be significant, many firms now offer hybrid consulting models, allowing professionals to work remotely for portions of their engagements [4].

Work-life balance in consulting varies depending on firm size and project scope. Large firms like Deloitte and Kaufman Hall may require frequent travel and high-intensity client engagement, while boutique firms such as Surgical Directions provide more flexibility and direct peer-to-peer collaboration with hospital leadership [5].

Despite potential travel demands, consulting careers provide the following:

- **Diverse work environments**: Exposure to a variety of healthcare settings and leadership structures.
- **Professional growth**: Opportunities to engage with hospital executives and influence systemic changes.
- **High earning potential**: Compensation varies by experience, with senior consultants earning $150,000–$300,000 annually, depending on specialization and firm affiliation [6].

31.9.2 Requirements, Education, and Experience

Healthcare consulting careers typically require a combination of clinical experience, business acumen, and analytical skills. Common backgrounds include the following:

- **Medical and clinical professionals**: Physicians, anesthesiologists, CRNAs, and OR nurses who transition into consulting roles to leverage their firsthand healthcare experience.
- **Healthcare administrators**: Individuals with experience in hospital leadership, operations, or finance.
- **Business and analytics experts**: Professionals with expertise in healthcare economics, data analytics, and strategic planning.

Educational Pathways

- Bachelor's degree in healthcare administration, business, finance, or related fields.
- Master's degree in healthcare administration (MHA), business administration (MBA), or public health (MPH) preferred.
- Certifications such as Fellow of the American College of Healthcare Executives (FACHE) or Certified Healthcare Financial Professional (CHFP) can enhance credentials [7, 24].

Experience Requirements

- Entry-level consultants often have 3–5 years of experience in healthcare operations, nursing, or hospital administration.
- Senior consultants typically have 10+ years of experience and may have previously served in hospital executive roles.
- Strong data analysis and project management skills are essential, especially for consultants working in financial or digital health sectors.

31.9.3 Consulting Careers Conclusion

Healthcare consulting presents a rewarding career path for professionals eager to drive meaningful change in surgical services, anesthesiology management, and hospital operations. With growing demand for expertise in operational efficiency, financial strategy, and workforce planning, consulting firms provide diverse opportunities for clinicians and administrators alike. As hospitals continue to face economic and staffing challenges, the role of healthcare consultants will remain critical in shaping the future of the industry.

31.10 Overall Conclusion

As hospitals and healthcare systems navigate an increasingly complex landscape, the role of consulting in perioperative and anesthesiology services has become essential. By leveraging expertise in operational efficiency, financial sustainability, and workforce optimization, consulting firms help healthcare organizations address critical challenges such as OR throughput, anesthesia staffing shortages, and cost containment. Data-driven solutions, structured governance models, and strategic workforce planning have proven to enhance hospital performance, increase patient access to care, and improve provider satisfaction. Additionally, consulting careers offer healthcare professionals a dynamic and impactful pathway to influence systemic improvements, blending clinical insight with business acumen. As the healthcare industry continues to evolve, consulting will remain a vital driver of innovation and efficiency, empowering hospitals to achieve long-term success in delivering high-quality, cost-effective care.

References

1. IBISWorld. Healthcare consultants in the US. Available from: https://www.ibisworld.com/united-states/industry/healthcare-consultants/5496/.
2. Consulting.us. Top consulting firms in the US by industry expertise: healthcare. Available from: https://www.consulting.us/rankings/top-consulting-firms-in-the-us-by-industry-expertise/healthcare.
3. Kaufman Hall. Perioperative consulting services overview. Available from: https://www.kaufmanhall.com.
4. Deloitte. Strategies for improving hospital operations. Available from: https://www.deloitte.com.
5. Inven AI. Top 19 healthcare consulting companies in the US. Available from: https://www.inven.ai/company-lists/top-19-healthcare-consulting-companies-in-the-us.
6. Anesthesiology Consulting. Practice management. Available from: https://anesthesiologyconsulting.com.
7. Sullivan Healthcare Consulting. Anesthesia consulting services. Available from: https://sullivanhealthcareconsulting.com/anesthesia-consulting-services/.
8. Kaufman Hall. 2023 Healthcare workforce report. Available from: https://www.kaufmanhall.com.

9. U.S. Bureau of Labor Statistics. Healthcare management job growth. Available from: https://www.bls.gov.
10. Surgical Directions. The impact of data-driven consulting. Available from: https://www.surgicaldirections.com.
11. Deloitte. Strategies for anesthesia cost containment. Available from: https://www.deloitte.com.
12. Deloitte. Trends in healthcare consulting careers. Available from: https://www2.deloitte.com.
13. Mayo Clinic. Improving OR throughput with anesthesia strategies. Available from: https://www.mayoclinic.org.
14. American College of Healthcare Executives. Guide to healthcare consulting. Available from: https://www.ache.org.
15. Kaufman Hall. 2023 Healthcare performance improvement report. Available from: https://www.kaufmanhall.com.
16. Becker's Hospital Review. Compensation trends in healthcare consulting. Available from: https://www.beckershospitalreview.com.
17. American Society of Anesthesiologists. Workforce and financial trends in anesthesia. Available from: https://www.asahq.org.
18. Centers for Medicare & Medicaid Services (CMS). Anesthesia services regulations. Available from: https://www.cms.gov.
19. Surgical Directions. Anesthesia consulting case studies. Available from: https://www.surgicaldirections.com.
20. Surgical Directions. Stipend reduction strategies. Available from: https://www.surgicaldirections.com.
21. Surgical Directions. Large academic medical center case study. Available from: https://www.surgicaldirections.com.
22. Kaufman Hall. Regional health system anesthesia optimization report. Available from: https://www.kaufmanhall.com.
23. American Hospital Association. Retention strategies for anesthesia providers. Available from: https://www.aha.org.
24. Healthcare Financial Management Association. Certified Healthcare Financial Professional (CHFP) overview. Available from: https://www.hfma.org.

Advocacy in Action: The Anesthesiologist's Role in Shaping Healthcare Policy and Patient Safety

32

Stacey Watt, Joseph R. Current, John R. Kraus, and Charles J. Assini Jr.

32.1 Advocacy

32.1.1 What Is Meant by "Advocacy"?

Advocacy can be defined as achieving public support for, or recommendation of, a particular cause or policy. The main purpose of advocacy is to engage decision-makers in dialogue to effect a change or to preserve safe anesthesia standards and practices.

Why is it important for physicians to become engaged?

Special interest groups (e.g., hospital associations) that promote their own causes have been very powerful voices in advocating for policies that effectively serve to create a two-tier anesthesia delivery system, eliminating the guarantee of a standard of care. As an example of this dichotomy, hospitals with larger populations of patients insured by Medicaid may opt not to have a physician anesthesiologist caring for patients within their operating rooms, while another hospital only a few miles away will offer different levels of care with physician anesthesiologist-led care teams. This could be accomplished by enacting legislation aimed at eliminating the statewide requirement that physician anesthesiologists continue to directly administer and/or supervise anesthesia care (in other words, permit nurse anesthetists to practice independently).

Supplementary Information The online version contains supplementary material available at https://doi.org/10.1007/978-3-032-18058-2_32.

S. Watt (✉) · J. R. Current · J. R. Kraus
University at Buffalo, Jacobs School of Medicine and Biomedical Sciences, Buffalo, NY, USA
e-mail: swatt@buffalo.edu

C. J. Assini Jr.
New York State Society of Anesthesiologists, New York, NY, USA

G. Tewfik (ed.), *The Anesthesiologist as Perioperative Leader*,
https://doi.org/10.1007/978-3-032-18058-2_32

Some special interest groups advocate for non-physician healthcare providers to be entitled to introduce themselves as "doctor," resulting in patient confusion and a degradation of trust in the healthcare system. Patients who misunderstand the roles of their providers may make medical decisions at the recommendation of non-physician providers without knowing their place in the team. When this causes disagreement among the care team, miscommunications about treatment modalities, or complications in patient care, patients receive suboptimal care that may affect their relationship with all medical providers going forward.

Other special interest groups may advocate for maintaining legal precedents on non-competition clauses in contracts. Non-competition clauses restrict physicians from joining another practice within "close proximity" upon separation from employment, even if the separation was not of the physician's choosing. Despite lacking a legitimate reason to impose such a restriction, barring a physician from finding employment in "close proximity" to their existing practice may force physicians to relocate from their homes and communities to practice elsewhere. This tactic results in increased stress on physicians who may have decided to change their practice due to changing family needs or newly acquired skills/credentials. Beyond this, physicians may need to find new payor networks at lower reimbursement rates while the communities they leave behind sustain reduced availability of physicians.

The above examples demonstrate how advocacy may impact the safe delivery of anesthesia services.

For centuries, physicians have proudly stood among the most influential advocates in society. Positioned uniquely due to their medical expertise and the inherent respect attributed to the profession, physicians have embraced this role across many settings. Advocacy is an integral part of the ethical foundation of medicine. Historical and ongoing efforts led by physicians to safeguard and advance public health have delivered significant and lasting benefits to society. Current and historical physician-led efforts to secure public health advancements have provided innumerable benefits to society and the safety of the public at large.

Advocacy comprises individual and societal components, with the most successful physicians advocating to ensure their patient receives necessary care while simultaneously working to guarantee that systems of healthcare delivery can empower them in that mission. Recently, there has been an ever-increasing awareness that comprehensive advocacy also demands addressing the broader social determinants of health that create barriers to well-being. The dual role as clinicians and agents of societal change places physicians at a unique intersection of clinical care and public policy.

For anesthesiologists, advocacy is of paramount importance. Practicing at the critical juncture of multiple surgical departments and inpatient vs. outpatient settings, they are uniquely positioned to understand individual elements of care and systemic shortcomings. The American Society of Anesthesiologists (ASA) underscores the importance of advocacy in safeguarding patient safety and advancing public health. In conjunction with state anesthesia societies, the ASA works to preserve the highest standards of anesthesia care and ensure policies align with evidence-based best practices [1].

Effective advocacy in anesthesiology requires a structured approach to translate issues into action. It begins with identifying a problem that can be addressed through systemic change, such as ensuring equitable reimbursement or preserving high standards in patient safety. Defining the problem with clarity and supporting it with evidence establishes credibility and focus, ensuring its relevance to stakeholders and decision-makers. Advocacy efforts are strengthened by engaging strategic partners, such as professional organizations, to align resources and messaging.

The landmark passage of the Affordable Care Act in 2010 was in large part due to the combined efforts of physician professional organizations working together with policymakers and the public. A well-developed action plan with clear objectives and timelines guides efforts, while an effective communication strategy tailored to diverse audiences ensures the message resonates and garners support [2]. Through this deliberate process, advocacy becomes a practical tool for driving meaningful change in anesthesiology and healthcare at large.

32.1.2 What Are Some Advocacy Roles for the Physician Anesthesiologist?

Physician anesthesiologists can advocate for best practices in anesthesia care through various means: seeking leadership roles in medical associations; serving on government planning or political action committees created by medical associations that create and execute political agendas; engaging in grassroots lobbying activities; attending and testifying at government hearings; supporting elected officials; serving on state boards of medicine or physician disciplinary boards; and serving on hospital committees (e.g., credentialing committee and bylaws committee).

These important positions demonstrate the valuable role physicians play in the health and well-being of the communities they serve. This presence during vital discussions, offering their expertise, and sharing their time and insight on important healthcare issues, allows physicians to use their knowledge and skills to change medicine and public health for the better. In some cases, this is done by playing defense against private interest groups that attempt to dismantle the current standards of care. In raising awareness, sharing concern, and providing their insight into policies, physicians are uniquely qualified to guide decisions concerning healthcare.

32.1.3 What Entities Are Reliable in Establishing "Best Practices"?

The American Society of Anesthesiologists (ASA) has adopted numerous best practice statements and guidelines that are evidence-based in peer-reviewed content and provide recommendations for best practices in the delivery of anesthesia care. For example, the ASA has adopted a statement on the Anesthesia Care Team (ACT) [3]. The essence of this statement is that anesthesia is the practice of medicine, and the physician anesthesiologist is the physician with the specialized education, training, and extensive clinical experience necessary to serve as the patient's primary anesthesia provider and advocate throughout all phases of the anesthesia care process. The anesthesia care process includes the preoperative patient evaluation, the intraoperative phase (when immediate medical intervention may be necessary), postoperative care in the PACU, and chronic pain management.

The physician anesthesiologist is the best qualified to direct the ACT and is responsible for leading anesthesia care administered by qualified members of the ACT team (e.g., physician residents, physician fellows, nurse anesthetists, anesthesiologist assistants, and students engaged in anesthesia training) [4]. To meet the medical direction standard embodied in the ASA ACT statement, the physician anesthesiologist must perform (i) the pre-anesthesia evaluation, (ii) make a medical determination of the patient whether to proceed or not to proceed with the procedure, (iii) prescribe the anesthetic plan for periprocedural care, and (iv) manage post-anesthesia care. Furthermore, compared to other forms of medical consultation, anesthesiology consultation is the practice of medicine that may not be delegated to non-physicians. Physician anesthesiologists also ensure the assignment and delegation of tasks for clinicians for each patient and procedure. When complications arise, physician anesthesiologists must be available to take over direct patient care as needed to resolve the problem.

32.2 Critical Issues of Importance to Physician Anesthesiologists

32.2.1 Truth in Advertising

Advocating for legislation that requires healthcare professionals to clearly represent their licensure by wearing identification badges and proper introductions to patients and families is essential for transparency and to the benefit of public health for the following reasons:

1. There are several categories of healthcare professions, including those with doctoral degrees (including nurse anesthetists) who increasingly introduce themselves to patients as "Doctors" in hospital settings.
2. Patients can be confused, and often feel misled, about the differences in qualifications of various types of healthcare providers. Misuse of titles can cause patients to mistakenly believe they are meeting with a physician when they are, in fact, meeting with a member of the healthcare team who does not hold the same credentials. This may influence patient decision-making and bear the risk of increased frequency in medical error for various reasons, including disagreement among the care team, miscommunications about treatment modalities, or direct complications in patient care.
3. Requiring healthcare providers to communicate and display their proper titles, credentials, and capabilities allows patients to make informed choices about

healthcare. Patients deserve to have increased clarity and transparency in the education and training of all healthcare professionals involved in their care as a part of informed consent of care.

Healthcare teams are made up of several different members, each playing a specific role. To fit into each essential part of the medical team, healthcare training must be divergent among different careers in medicine to develop professionals into these specialized roles. For example, physician anesthesiologists are trained to think critically, problem-solve, and lead patient care teams after completing a bachelor's degree (3–4 years of college), 4 years of medical school (which is not available in an online format), 4 years of residency training, and often 1–3 additional years of fellowship training. Along this journey, physicians accumulate 12,000–16,000 h of patient care experience and training for this specialized role. The stark differences in training length and rigor between different careers in medicine are shown in Table 32.1.

Many programs grant doctoral degrees to graduates after completion, awarding honorifics such as the title "Doctor" for use in personal and professional settings. Originally, this title comes from the Latin word for "to teach" and has become a

Table 32.1 Comparison of training length/rigor between different careers in healthcare [4]

Position (*title*)	Years of school	Online option?	Years of post-graduate training	Hours of patient care experience
Physician Anesthesiologist (*MD, DO, or equivalent*)	3–4 College 4 Medical school	No	4 years residency 1–3 years fellowship (optional) Anesthesiology board-certified	12,000–16,000
Nurse Practitioner (NP) and Certified Registered Nurse Anesthetist (CRNA) (*BSN, MSN, DNP*)	4 College 1.5–3 Graduate school (optional)	Yes	1 year critical care nursing (CRNAs only) No anesthesiology board certification	500–2500
Certified Anesthesiologist Assistant (CAA) (*MSA, MMScA*)	3–4 College 1.5–2.5 Graduate school	No	No requirement No board certification	1200–2000
Physician Assistant (PA) (*MPAS, DMSc*)	3–4 College 2–4 Graduate school	Yes	No requirement	1000–4000
Pharmacist (*PharmD*)	2–4 College 4 Pharmacy school	Yes	No requirement	1740
Optometrist (*OD*)	3–4 College 4 Optometry school	No	No requirement	2500
Psychologist (*PsyD, PhD*)	3–4 College 4–6 Graduate school	Yes	1-year internship	1500–2000

name of respect for those who are experts within their field of study. In the clinical setting, the term "Doctor" is used synonymously with "physician" among practitioners and patients, referring to a professional with the degree MD, DO, or equivalent earned by completing a prescribed course of study from a credentialed school of allopathic or osteopathic medicine. Using this term to refer to other professionals holding doctoral degrees in the clinical setting, such as those non-physicians listed above, can be very confusing and misleading to patients due to this connotation. This deception—be it intentional or not—disrupts the inherent trust between patients and providers, influences patients' treatment decisions, and violates legislation such as the Lanham Act, which prohibits false advertising that "misrepresents the nature, characteristics, qualities, or geographic origin" of goods and services (15 U.S.C § 1225(a)) [5]. This view is shared by virtually every specialty society of physicians—including ASA, American College of Emergency Physicians (ACEP), and more—and is even acknowledged by the Academy of Doctoral Physician Assistants (PAs), which states that while PAs "can technically use the title 'Dr.'," they recommend reserving this title for "academic or administrative settings to avoid confusion in patient care" or using a full title such as "Dr. [Name], PA-C" to distinguish themselves from physicians [6]. However, some mid-level practitioners seek to be identified using "doctor" and referred to as physicians or equal counterparts by patients to take advantage of the historical trust placed in physicians by patients, despite the disparity in training length/rigor and patient outcomes. Some groups, including CRNAs, have taken title misappropriation a step further, seeking to be called "anesthesiologist" [7]. They justify equal rank to physicians in title and scope of practice with studies showing that clinical care delivered by NPs is "as effective, and in some cases, even more effective, for patients as physicians" [8]. However, just as in the scope of practice argument, these groups use biased studies (i.e., studies that have not been peer-reviewed and/or have been underwritten by nurse anesthetists' associations) to make their arguments seem legitimate [9].

> Ensuring clarity in medical professional titles is essential to maintaining safety, trust, and transparency in the patient care process, ultimately empowering patients to understand who is responsible for their anesthesia care. [10]

The consequences of title misappropriation are difficult to measure since they extend well beyond patient care outcomes. These deceptive practices impact the quality of patient care, affect advanced practice provider (APP) scope of practice, influence patient decision-making, and dismantle the trusting relationship between physicians and patients. Education transparency and accurate representation of healthcare provider titles are core components of informed care and consent—pillars of best practices in medicine.

32.2.2 Nurse Anesthetist (NA) and Certified Anesthesiologist Assistant (CAA) Certification and Scope of Practice

Advocating for legislation consistent with ASA best practices, as embodied in practice guidelines and the statement on the ACT, is imperative to preserve the highest standards of anesthesia care for the benefit of the patient and public health. At the state level, these policies are endorsed by state medical associations, such as the New York State Society of Anesthesiologists, Inc. (NYSSA).

The government, consisting of elected officials, not an administrative body such as the Board of Nursing, has a constitutional obligation and duty to promote the welfare of its citizens. This includes the responsibility to define the scope of practice of healthcare professionals, including nurse anesthetists and anesthesiologist assistants. For example, the administration of potentially lethal drugs qualifies as a matter of public concern that affects the welfare of citizens. Why is this an important example? Proponents of unsupervised anesthesia care (including nurse anesthetists' independent practice) have repeatedly attempted to circumvent the role of the legislature in defining their scope of practice by collaborating with nursing boards—who are not subject to public scrutiny or debate—which can result in regulatory boards inappropriately expanding a nurse anesthetists' scope of practice and dismantling the physician anesthesiologist-led care team. This has included initiatives to create, without legislative approval, a Nurse Practitioner (NP) category for nurse anesthetists, which incorporated a "collaboration" standard of care. The "collaboration" standard meant the physician anesthesiologist did not need to be physically present nor directly involved in the patient's anesthesia care. This fundamentally counters the ASA statement on the ACT, which includes the standard of physician anesthesiologists in a supervisory role, ensuring they must be physically present and immediately available to perform medical tasks and make medical interventions as needs arise. After all, "anesthesia remains a process of controlled poisoning, because all of the drugs are lethal if given improperly" [11]. Physician supervision and participation are most important in cases of emergency, when seconds count in medical decision-making.

There are many lessons to be learned that ought to guide future advocacy. It important to ensure that the Board of Nursing agendas are being monitored to assess whether there is an attempt to circumvent the legislature. All must be prepared to lobby the body that oversees the Board of Nursing in any attempts to circumvent the legislature by seeking meetings with these officials and preparing advocacy counter-position papers.

One of the first steps in advocacy in the legislative process is to identify and recruit legislators who appreciate the important role of physician-led anesthesia care. These legislators must be willing to sponsor legislation to create defining certifications with scopes of practice for nurse anesthetists and certified anesthesiologist assistants, both consistent with the ASA ACT statement. It is equally important to identify the sponsors of legislation that would dismantle physician-led anesthesia care, as stated above.

The next step in advocacy is monitoring the legislation and participating in meetings with legislators. Legislators are not trained in medicine but are experts in government policy and affect change in different industries using this tool. Creating a partnership with legislators allows physician anesthesiologists a firm hand in guiding change in our own industry. It is our responsibility to educate legislators on the nuance involved in problems faced in medicine so that they may understand the importance of each issue and help us to advocate for changes consistent with our goals.

By attending and participating in meetings with legislators, there is an opportunity to advocate for the preservation of safe anesthesia standards by identifying the differences in training goals, rigor, and length, as well as clinical hours, such as those in Table 32.1, as well as emphasizing the physician anesthesiologist's ability to immediately make medical interventions when a patient undergoing anesthesia is most at risk. Nurse anesthetists play a critical role in the ACT, but their role is different from the role a physician anesthesiologist assumes. Physicians are their own best advocates by explaining their roles and the importance of maintaining physician-led anesthesia care. This care team model saves patients' lives.

It is not possible to define the scope of practice of a nurse anesthetist without defining the role of the physician anesthesiologist. The physician anesthesiologist is the physician specialist involved in all phases of the delivery of anesthesia care. Direct medical involvement of the physician anesthesiologist in the patient's care and leading the ACT prevents patient complications and is considered the safest, most effective care model [12]. The key difference responsible for the disparity in complications between physician-led and nursing-led ACTs is how training is conducted. While nurses may have experience with diagnosis through pattern recognition in their line of work, physicians receive robust training in medical and social sciences, research, quality improvement, and therapeutic skills that equip them much more appropriately for diagnosis and treatment, especially in critical and time-sensitive situations that are often faced in the field of anesthesiology. This message is highlighted by the ASA in their "When Seconds Count… Physician Anesthesiologists Save Lives" advertisement, which provides a real example of when the training of an experienced physician anesthesiologist made the difference in life or death for a patient in a complex and dangerous situation in the OR [13]. This example represents cases that occur every day across the country. Physician anesthesiologists evaluate patients' overall health and identify, prepare for, and respond to underlying medical conditions (and their exacerbations). The superiority of the physician-led ACT in quality and safety of care delivery is included in supporting memoranda and serves as a talking point when meeting with legislators, staff, and government regulators.

It is important to understand that proponents of unsupervised anesthesia care by a nurse anesthetist are asserting that: (i) the physician supervision and direction standard creates barriers to the nurse anesthetist's practice and is unnecessary, and (ii) the unsupervised practice of nurse anesthetists will alleviate the shortage of anesthesia providers in rural areas. The proponents of unsupervised anesthesia care by nurse anesthetists use biased studies (i.e., studies that have not been peer-reviewed and/or have been underwritten by nurse anesthetists' associations) that allege there is no difference in surgical outcome whether the physician anesthesiologist directs or personally performs the care or a nurse anesthetist performs the care [8, 9]. However, what these arguments do not explain is that the expansion of nurse anesthetists' scope of care, especially in rural areas, creates differences in the quality of care based on geography and other social determinants of health in exchange for accessibility concerns. Preserving existing standards guarantees that patients—regardless of geography, payor status, or other social determinants of health—will have the benefit of a physician leading their anesthesia care.

Strong advocacy requires preparation of robust counterarguments to proponents of unsupervised anesthesia care. For example, some healthcare associations representing hospitals promote unsupervised nurse anesthetists' practice because their members state they cannot recruit physician anesthesiologists when, in fact, the real reason is their members desire the flexibility to disregard best practices and eliminate the role of physician anesthesiologists to achieve savings at the patient's expense. However, there are a myriad of ways to address these multifactorial accessibility concerns that do not surrender quality of care, including to incentivize physicians to practice in geographical areas with physician shortages, increase the number of residency training positions allotted by the federal government, or break down non-compete contracts preventing physicians from working in specific geographic areas that need providers. Incentives that recruit physicians should not come at the cost of patients' quality of care. When the proponents of nurse anesthetists' independent practice claim there are currently "barriers" to their practice, it must be understood that these so-called barriers actually protect patients from having nurse anesthetists practice beyond their training and clinical capabilities. They protect patients from allowing nurse anesthetists unrestricted prescription authority and prohibit the adoption of an entirely new, untested anesthesia delivery model of care.

Note *For a recent illustration of when practice barriers are disregarded, see the attached memorandum on the CMS investigation of two California hospitals that allowed unsupervised nurse anesthetist anesthesia care.*

These same arguments can be made regarding the scope of practice for Certified Anesthesiology Assistants (CAAs). We must support legislation that defines the roles of all members of the ACT, including policy to create an anesthesiologist assistant certification and to define the CAA's scope of practice consistent with the ASA ACT statement. CAAs, like nurse anesthetists, play an important role in the delivery of anesthesia care but must work under the supervision of practicing anesthesiologists to maintain quality of care and safety for patients.

Proponents of CRNA-independent practice argue it will expand anesthesia services in rural areas, but empirical studies largely refute this claim. A recent analysis of US hospitals found no significant increase in anesthesia access in states that opted out of physician supervision, with researchers reporting that such "opt-out" policies do not improve access in rural counties and further noted no increase in surgical services nor a reduction in travel distance for patients in states granting

CRNAs autonomy compared to states maintaining physician oversight [14]. Notably, this pattern extends to other non-physician providers; evidence suggests that expanding nurse practitioners' scope of practice has not automatically drawn more providers to underserved communities, as NPs with full practice authority still tend to work in the same areas as physicians rather than dispersing to rural shortage areas [15]. These findings suggest that simply removing supervision requirements has not, on its own, solved provider shortages or improved anesthesia access, or other medical care, in rural America.

While eliminating physician supervision for CRNAs does not contribute to solving the challenges in rural regions, addressing other systemic factors, like restrictive physician contracts, may help.

Restrictive covenants—more often referred to as "non-competes"—are agreements barring doctors from practicing in a geographic area for a period after leaving an employer. These clauses significantly constrain physician mobility and subsequent patient access to care. Surveys estimate that upward of 45% of physicians have non-competes, a practice that especially hampers early-career doctors by limiting their job opportunities and even preventing them from continuing to care for patients in their community if they change employers [16]. Such restrictions may disrupt continuity of care and exacerbate provider shortages; the AMA Code of Medical Ethics cautions that non-competes "restrict competition, can disrupt continuity of care, and may limit access to care." These concerns become particularly acute during public health emergencies, where workforce flexibility is essential for effective patient care. For instance, during the COVID-19 pandemic, physicians who spoke out about patient safety concerns sometimes faced termination [16]. In such instances, restrictive non-compete clauses further compounded the problem by preventing physicians from relocating or immediately resuming practice, thereby leaving local communities without timely access to care. Recognizing these harms, professional organizations have called for curbing physician non-competes. This push to limit non-compete agreements reflects a growing consensus that physician workforce mobility is vital for maintaining adequate access and continuity of care for patients.

32.2.3 Insurance Reimbursement

Hospital systems across the country have been fighting to increase insurance reimbursement rates, or at minimum not have them reduced, often to the detriment of the physicians who are also billing services on the healthcare encounters of patients within their healthcare system. This battle for the proverbial piece of the pie has resulted in a fight between hospital systems and physicians to gain a foothold in fair insurance reimbursement rates. Historically, hospital systems' lobbying efforts have been more effective than individual physicians in securing higher reimbursement rates. This disparity is evident in healthcare expenditure trends; between 1997 and 2012, hospital services reimbursement rose by 149%, compared to a 55% increase for physician services over the same period [17].

Hospitals are paid facility fees based on the procedure performed, including costs for equipment, supplies, and resources such as staff, space, and time. Similarly to the anesthesiologists, the hospitals are paid depending upon the time spent in the procedure, the complexity of the procedure, and the billing code(s).

Recent proposed changes to this system of payment may change the landscape of financial payments, opting for a system that is more in alignment with our surgical colleagues. The proposed system would have an estimated time for each procedure and, therefore, provide a set payment for the procedure listed with a reduction in modifiers available for increased payment. In this new system, hospitals and physicians would receive set amounts, and any additional time spent within the operating room would not be factored into payments.

Reimbursement for anesthesia care is based upon time and a conversion factor, which is predetermined by the insurance payor. The payment for anesthesia services is traditionally based on Anesthesia Time Units (ATUs). Services provided by an anesthesiologist are billed based on the amount of time the physician spends with the patient and includes the time from the start of anesthesia care to the end of the procedure, including the time the patient spends in the recovery room post-procedure. The reimbursement rate is typically based on a fee schedule that assigns a monetary value to each ATU. The fee schedule is updated annually to reflect changes in the cost associated with providing service. In addition to the ATU, a physical status modifier is often applied. This modifier takes into account the higher level of services an anesthesiologist must provide to patients with advanced medical conditions who require additional levels of care and resources to be cared for safely within the operating room.

Additional challenges to physician reimbursement have come from an increase in "out of network" reimbursement assignments to many anesthesiologists. As patients receive surgical care, they may be notified that their anesthesiologist is out of network. The out-of-network designation from the insurance company results in patients being forced to pay for a larger portion of the cost of care. This is what is often referred to as a "surprise bill" due to the unexpected high costs incurred by patients who had previously thought their care was covered under their current insurance coverage plans.

32.3 Importance of Creating a Multifaceted Advocacy Strategy

Physicians are critical collaborators in all facets of government advocacy. The components of advocacy include strong and effective physician leadership. Physician leadership needs to embrace the importance of promoting legislation that is consistent with best practices and defeating legislation that dismantles the ACT, such as defining the roles of nurse anesthetists and CAAs, clarifying what truth in advertising means in the healthcare sector, addressing non-compete clauses that amplify the physician shortage, and emphasizing the importance of fair insurance reimbursement.

These efforts should be conducted at all levels, starting with a physician's practice and expanding to the hospital; hospital system; local community; and regional, state, and national levels. The impact is magnified as the scope of advocacy is broadened, as local communities are often governed by regional legislation, which is consistent with state policy, and so on. Physician leadership must make this an advocacy priority and commit resources to support the following:

1. Ensure the engagement of a qualified lobbyist with no conflicts of interest. Effective "boots on the ground" lobbying requires constant intelligence of developments in the halls of the Capitol.
2. Ensure engagement of a qualified legislative counsel responsible for preparing strong and effective advocacy memorandums. Factual arguments continue to be a very effective advocacy component. This information can be shared during interactive meetings, on podcasts, in books, on pamphlets, and across the web in advertisements, social media, and organization websites. Sharing this mission with many people, especially those who can affect change, is critical to successful advocacy.
3. Grassroots involvement: physician members of a society/association must be actively involved and meet with the lawmakers where physicians provide patient care. In particular, emphasis must be made on how physician anesthesiologists practice safe and effective anesthesia in hospitals located in the member's district. The use of personal anecdotes and local data can be very helpful to connect with legislators in ways beyond logical arguments and facts.
4. Collaborating with the ASA. Learn what other states are doing to advance their agendas so that you may mimic or build upon these efforts in your own area. There are many tools offered by the ASA to address problems faced by anesthesiologists across the country.
5. Attend meetings and work with state medical societies and other medical specialty societies. Legislators may be more inclined to be persuaded by healthcare experts' perspectives that rely on physician anesthesiologists every day in the operating room. Power comes in numbers, especially when different specialties in medicine agree on similar causes. Recruitment of physicians within your medical society is another way to show support in masses for the aforementioned causes. It is much more difficult to disagree with groups than to disregard an individual.
6. Involve residents and even medical students, who can serve as other important ways to supplement the stream of recruitment of future physicians and can offer different perspectives on ways to address the issues we advocate for.
7. Conduct effective social media campaigns. Promote and introduce to the public some prominent physician anesthesiologists who make a difference. Public opinion can be a powerful tool in influencing government, as it is designed to represent the people. *See the attached campaign.*
8. Create a strong Political Action Committee (PAC). Financial reserves can make a world of difference in today's political state, and a committee with funds

dedicated to advocacy is a way to ensure that the interests of physicians are at the table rather than on the menu.

32.3.1 Working with Your Local Officials

Advocacy within your practice, group, hospital, hospital system, and local community has the greatest impact on your direct colleagues, staff, and patients. Physicians advocating within their locale often do so by organizing quality improvement and service projects to create evidence for change or by climbing the administrative ladder to raise concerns about current practices and bring evidence-based solutions directly to the attention of decision-makers. Securing a seat on decision-making boards and committees can have a real impact on policy in the local area.

Residents and medical students play many important roles in healthcare advocacy. Both groups offer a fresh perspective by offering creative solutions to existing problems faced by physicians and identifying new inefficiencies that physicians may have grown habituated to. They are the backbone of the academic healthcare system, spending nearly a decade working and training with diverse patients across a variety of specialties and environments. This exposure gives residents and medical students insight into novel strategies for advocacy that physicians working in the same group or hospital system may not be exposed to. Additionally, residents and medical students may have an edge in appealing to diverse audiences of decision-makers due to their inherent diversity in age, locale, and cultural background. Lastly, residents and medical students bring enthusiasm for learning to the table, making it easy to involve them in advocacy. One of the best ways to amplify the voice we share now, and ensure advocacy work continues to expand, is to train residents and medical students to work alongside physicians in advocacy by exposing them to current efforts and teaching them how to contribute. Developing strong relationships with medical school leaders and residency program directors provides an opportunity to pipeline new physicians into the advocacy campaign and avoid deterioration in advocacy efforts with decreasing recruitment.

32.3.2 Working Within Your Jurisdiction

Organized medicine divides responsibility over a group of physicians who work toward the same cause. The strength of organized medicine lends itself to the cliché "power in numbers" in advocacy just as much as it does in negotiating reimbursement contracts with insurance companies. In the larger theatres of policy at the regional, state, and national levels, the voice of one physician sounds much quieter than it can in a local community or hospital. Uniting all of the physicians in a geographical region to advocate for the same cause can provide strength in advocating for policies that uphold standards of care. Just as evidence supports these arguments, maintaining a united front eliminates secondary options that compromise the values of patient or provider experience and population health for reduced costs.

Grassroots movements, organized medicine policies, and legislative lobbying are all examples of the united front that is foundational to successful advocacy work. Messaging is a critical component to effective advocacy in all of these forms. Physicians must be actively involved and meet with the lawmakers where physicians provide patient care, learn from what other states and regions are doing to advance their agendas, and replicate these efforts by discussing them with other physicians in organized medical societies. The ASA Advocacy Toolkit is a great place to start for resources [18].

Strong Political Action Committees (PACs) provide crucial financial reserves that make advocacy possible, especially at higher levels. Advocacy involves travel for face-to-face meetings between physicians, lobbyists, and legislators to discuss topics of importance. It also requires the gathering of evidence to support these efforts, either through first-hand accounts or through second-hand acquisition from peer-reviewed research. Enthusiasm, time, and resources are needed for advocacy to occur, and PACs are key in providing these resources. Physicians who may not have the time to advocate personally can still contribute to advocacy by supporting these PACs, enabling those with the time to conduct the work.

32.3.3 Patient-Based Advocacy

While leveraging colleague physicians, residents, medical students, lawyers, lobbyists, and legislators is core to any advocacy campaign, one group of people that may be overlooked is a cohort of patients. Our work directly or indirectly impacts our patients' experiences with each encounter with the healthcare system, whether it is through a guaranteed standard of care, truth in advertising, or paying the bill (with or without insurance). Nothing stands in the way of patients advocating for themselves. One must ask—what role do physicians play in this? In one word, the answer is "empowerment." Our responsibility to our patients goes beyond advocating on their behalf and is a foundational part of providing healthcare. As physicians, we can educate patients about medicine, the healthcare system, and the care we provide. We may inform them of the policies that play a role in care delivery and how we are advocating for them. These conversations—which may take place anywhere from 1-on-1 s in the office to organized healthcare rallies and social media campaigns—may invite patients to become involved and encourage them to advocate with us. When we keep patient care at the forefront of our advocacy efforts, we will always have similar interests to our patients. Public opinion can be a powerful tool in influencing government, as it is designed to represent the people. Decision-makers and physicians alike, at one point or another, may serve as patients themselves. The concerns we raise become more personal by reminding decision-makers of this fact, which may supplement our logical approach with emotional icing, often just enough to spark a fire and create an impetus to act, especially in those decision-makers who may be more reserved in the face of plain facts and evidence.

32.4 Conclusion

As anesthesiologists, residents, and medical students, our responsibility extends beyond direct patient care. Advocacy is a powerful tool that must be leveraged to shape the future of patient care, public health, and the integrity of our profession by preserving high standards of quality care and "best practices" in medicine. Whether championing patient safety, influencing healthcare policy, or mentoring the next generation, these voices matter. It is our duty to engage hospital administrators, medical societies, and lawmakers to create policies that align with patient interests by educating them on issues we currently face, such as truth in advertising, APP scope of practice, non-compete contracts, and insurance reimbursement, among many other topics. Whether through grassroots movements, policy lobbying, or patient-centered initiatives, our efforts strengthen the role of physicians as leaders in healthcare, ensuring that every patient receives compassionate, equitable, and high-quality care. This must be a call to action: step forward, speak up, and make a difference. We must commit to being informed, involved, and united because our advocacy today shapes the care of tomorrow.

References

1. American Society of Anesthesiologists Public Relations. Made for this moment advocacy toolkit. 2025. https://www.asahq.org/member-center/state-component-resources/mftm-advocacy-toolkit. Accessed 16 Mar 2025.
2. Earnest MA, Wong SL, Federico SG. Perspective: Physician advocacy: what is it and how do we do it? Acad Med. 2010;85(1):63–7.
3. American Society of Anesthesiologists Governance Committee on Anesthesia Care Team. Statement on the Anesthesia Care Team. 2023. https://www.asahq.org/standards-and-practice-parameters/statement-on-the-anesthesia-care-team. Accessed 16 Mar 2025.
4. O'Reilly KB. Physicians and nonphysicicans: what are the differences? 2024. https://www.ama-assn.org/practice-management/scope-practice/physicians-and-nonphysicians-what-are-differences#:~:text=Meanwhile%2C%20nurse%20practitioners%20have%20no,patient%2Dcare%20hours%20in%20training. Accessed 16 Mar 2025.
5. Justia Consumer Protection Law Center. False advertising under Consumer Protection Laws. 2024. https://www.justia.com/consumer/deceptive-practices-and-fraud/false-advertising/ Accessed 16 Mar 2025.
6. The Academy of Doctoral PAs. Can a doctorate PA use the title "Dr" at work? 2024. https://www.padoc.org/faq. Accessed 16 Mar 2025.
7. Conte AH. Title misappropriation in anesthesia. 2023. https://www.anesthesiologynews.com/Multimedia/Article/01-23/Title-Misappropriation-in-Anesthesia/69201. Accessed 16 Mar 2025.
8. Bruise C. Some doctoral-prepared nurses use the title, "Doctor" and it's causing a heated debate. 2020. https://nurse.org/articles/doctoral-prepared-DNP-nurses-use-title-doctor/#:~:text=In%20sheer%20technical%20terms%2C%20anyone,come%20together%2C%E2%80%9D%20she%20added. Accessed 16 Mar 2025.
9. American Association of Nurse Practitioners. Quality of nurse practitioner practice. 2023. https://www.aanp.org/advocacy/advocacy-resource/position-statements/quality-of-nurse-practitioner-practice. Accessed 16 Mar 2025.

10. American Society of Anesthesiologists Governance Committee on Anesthesia Care Team. Statement on title misappropriation. 2024. https://www.asahq.org/standards-and-practice-parameters/statement-on-title-misappropriation. Accessed 16 Mar 2025.
11. Stoelting RK, Miller RD, Larson MD. Chapter 1: History of anesthesia. In: Basics of anesthesia. 5th ed. Philadelphia: Churchill Livingstone; 2007. p. 1–10.
12. Burns ML, Saager L, Cassidy RB, et al. Association of anesthesiologist staffing ratio with surgical patient morbidity and mortality. JAMA Surg. 2022;157(9):807–15.
13. American Society of Anesthesiologists, Arnold S. When seconds count… Physician Anesthesiologists save lives. 2014. https://www.asahq.org/~/media/sites/asahq/files/public/newsroom/news/asa-wsc-media-planet-ad.pdf?la=en. Accessed 16 Mar 2025.
14. Feyereisen S, McConnell W, Puro N. Revisiting the effects of state anesthesia policy interventions: a comprehensive look at certified registered nurse Anesthetist service provision in U.S. hospitals from 2010 to 2021. J Rural Health. 2024;41(1):1–11.
15. Hesgrove B, Zapata D, Bertane C, et al. The graduate nurse education demonstration project: final evaluation report; 2019. p. 80–3. https://www.cms.gov/priorities/innovation/files/reports/gne-final-eval-rpt.pdf. Accessed 16 Mar 2025.
16. Robeznieks A. AMA backs effort to ban many physician noncompete provisions. 2023. https://www.ama-assn.org/medical-residents/transition-resident-attending/ama-backs-effort-ban-many-physician-noncompete#:~:text=Unfair%20noncompete%20clauses%20are%20extensive,economically%20or%20socially%20marginalized%20communities. Accessed 16 Mar 2025.
17. Rosenthal E. Chapter 2: The age of hospitals. In: An American sickness: how healthcare became big business and how you can take it back. New York: Penguin Books; 2017. p. 23.
18. American Society of Anesthesiologists, Deanna. Advocacy tools. 2022. https://www.asahq.org/advocacy-and-asapac/advocacy-tools. Accessed 16 Mar 2025.

Practice Guidelines and Best Practices in Perioperative Care

33

Karen B. Domino

Practice guidelines and best practice statements help assure up-to-date, high-quality perioperative care of patients. National guidelines and advisories produced by the American Society of Anesthesiologists (ASA) and anesthesia subspecialty societies synthesize a large body of research via systematic reviews and meta-analyses to form the scientific basis of recommendations for patient care. Expert opinion and consensus-based best practice recommendations also may provide clinical advice when scientific evidence is lacking. Teams of anesthesia subspecialists and surgeons also produce best practice statements for perioperative care that may be applied at local practice settings. These statements are instructional and are vital to ensure quality of care by anesthesia providers who infrequently care for subspecialty patients, such as neurosurgery, transplant, laser-surgery, and obstetric patients. These documents summarize local "best practices" and are available on departmental website for ready access during clinical care.

This chapter will focus upon the methodology and examples of practice parameters produced by the ASA, and its membership of physician anesthesiologists. ASA practice guidelines and advisory provide guidance for perioperative care of patients within the United States. While the ASA methodology is very rigorous and time-consuming, principles discussed can also be adapted and implemented on a local institutional level for internal guidelines of care when other guidelines, advisories, or best practice statements are not available, and when new research is available.

K. B. Domino (✉)
University of Washington, Seattle, WA, USA
e-mail: kdomino@uw.edu

G. Tewfik (ed.), *The Anesthesiologist as Perioperative Leader*,
https://doi.org/10.1007/978-3-032-18058-2_33

33.1 ASA Practice Parameters

The ASA develops and distributes three types of practice parameters: practice standards, practice guidelines, and practice advisories. Practice standards are accepted principles of anesthetic management that provide minimal *requirements* for perioperative anesthesia care. Standards may be modified only under unusual circumstances or emergencies. The ASA has three standards of care, each aimed at the three phases of anesthesia care: preoperative care [1], monitoring requirements during intraoperative care [2], and postoperative care [3]. The "Basic Standards for Preanesthesia Care" describe requirements for medical record review, history and focused physical exam, anesthesia consent, and documentation in the medical record. The "Standards for Basic Anesthetic Monitoring" sets requirements for the presence of anesthesia personnel during the conduct of anesthesia and requirements for continual monitoring of the patient's oxygenation, ventilation, circulation, and temperature. The "Standards for Postanesthesia Care" describe requirements for transport from the procedural area to the post-anesthesia care unit by a member of the anesthesia team, handoff of care to the nurse, and physician discharge of a patient.

In contrast, practice guidelines and advisories provide *recommendations* for perioperative care that are not requirements. Anesthesiologists may choose to adhere to the recommendations in caring for patients based upon their clinical judgment. However, practice guidelines and advisories summarize new evidence and provide very helpful recommendations for clinical care.

33.2 Development of Practice Guidelines and Advisories

Practice guidelines and advisories are evidence-based documents based upon standards to form clinical practice guidelines. The practice guideline standards include transparency, resolving conflicts of interest, development group composition, systematic review conduct, ratings for strength of recommendations, articulation of recommendations, external reviews, and updates [4]. ASA practice guidelines and advisories adhere to the standards for trustworthy guidelines. They provide transparency, strict disclosure, and management of potential conflicts of interest, which had been an issue in the past with some professional societies.

Although practice guidelines and advisories utilize similar approaches and methodologies, the evidence base supporting practice guidelines is stronger in quantity, quality, and consistency compared to practice advisories. The ASA prioritizes use of randomized clinical trials for making recommendations in its practice parameters. Non-randomized studies are used to assess adverse outcomes or when sufficient randomized clinical trials are not available.

The Practice Guideline on the Monitoring and Antagonism of Neuromuscular Blockade is an example of a guideline [5]. This document was produced as a guideline due to the high quality of evidence in the area with multiple randomized clinical trials yielding consistent results. While practice advisories also summarize scientific evidence and provide suggestions for perioperative care, the breadth of the scientific evidence may be poorer. There may be fewer randomized clinical trials or only nonrandomized clinical studies. However, practice advisories aid anesthesiologists in decision-making. Examples of practice advisories include the Practice Advisory for Perioperative Visual Loss Associated with Spine Surgery 2019 [6], Practice Advisory for Perioperative Management of Patients with Cardiac Implantable Electronic Devices [7], and Practice Advisory for Perioperative Care of Older Adults Scheduled for Inpatient Surgery [8].

The ASA practice guidelines and advisories use a comprehensive systematic review, careful formulation of clinical questions, formal study inclusion and exclusion criteria, risk of bias assessments, outcome assessment, and determination of strength of evidence by methodologists. Recommendations based upon the scientific findings are made by the task force consisting of experts, generalists, methodologists, and a patient representative. Figure 33.1 illustrates the systematic review process and development of recommendations.

Formulation of Clinical Questions The first step in the process is to develop formal clinical questions for the review. These questions are formatted using PICOTS (population, interventions, comparators, systematic review, and evidence synthesis) which guide the systematic review. Patient outcomes are ranked according to importance for decision-making and must include patient preferences and values. A formal study protocol is developed showing details of the population, interventions at various anesthetic phases, comparators, and outcomes of importance. Although outcomes important to patients are most important, these are unfortunately frequently absent from many anesthesia studies. An example of an analytic framework to guide systematic review and data analysis is shown in Fig. 33.2.

Systematic Review A systematic review is performed by a medical librarian to identify studies for review by methodologists. Duplicates are removed. Screening of titles and subsequently screening of abstracts are performed to determine the full-text studies to be assessed for eligibility. After applying inclusion and exclusion criteria, studies are selected for synthesis of evidence. Study data, including

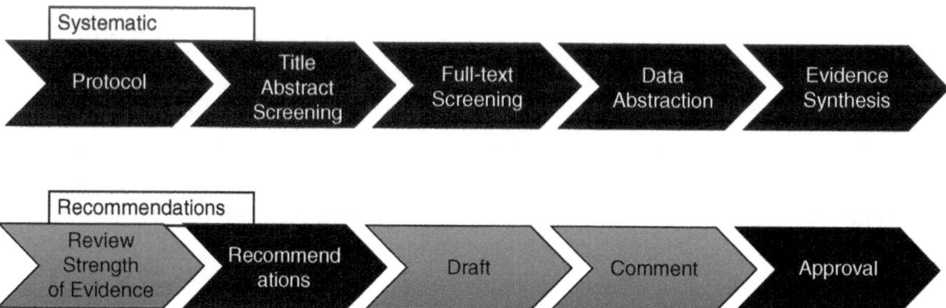

Fig. 33.1 Summary of the processes involved in a systematic review and formulation of recommendations

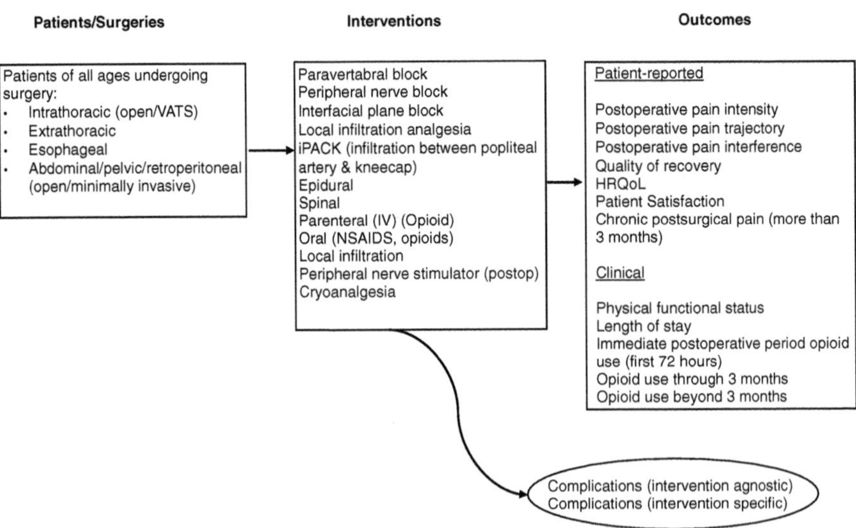

Fig. 33.2 Analytic framework for a systematic review of regional analgesia for truncal surgeries

subjects, age, ASA status, surgery, and outcomes, is abstracted and synthesized by using quantitative and qualitative approaches.

The systematic review process is documented using a PRISMA flow diagram (Preferred Reporting Items for Systematic Reviews and Meta-Analyses) [9]. This diagram shows the number of studies identified, screened, included, and excluded (with associated reasons for these decisions) at various stages of the systematic review. Data is summarized in tables and analyzed by meta-analyses as appropriate.

The methodologists analyze the strength of evidence by tools to assess if results are believable and internally valid. The methodologists grade the quality of evidence based on the evidence hierarchy and certainty of evidence. The evidence hierarchy rates systematic reviews and meta-analysis of randomized clinical trials as the highest level of convincing evidence. Certainty of evidence is judged by the quality, quantity, and consistency of the scientific evidence.

Evaluation of Strength of Evidence and Recommendations The ASA utilizes the GRADE (Grades of Recommendation, Assessment, Development, and Evaluation) system to evaluate strength of evidence and guide subsequent wording of recommendations [10]. While some evaluation systems rely solely on the hierarchy of evidence based upon the study design, GRADE also evaluates quality of evidence based upon the overall body of evidence, not just individual studies. Rating the strength of evidence takes into consideration risk of bias, consistency of results, directness, precision, and publication bias. Consistency of evidence refers to the degree of similarity in the direction of effects and magnitude of effects. Direct evidence directly compares interventions of interest in populations of interest and measures patient-oriented outcomes. Evidence is indirect if the tested intervention, study population, and/or outcomes differ from those of primary interest or if treatment comparisons have not been evaluated in head-to-head comparisons. Precision is the degree of certainty surrounding an estimate of effect with respect to an outcome. Precision is assessed by examining the 95% confidence interval around the summary effect size.

The GRADE system rates certainty of evidence as high, moderate, low, or very low (Table 33.1). Randomized clinical trials are rated at a higher quality of evidence and then downgraded for lack of certainty of evidence. Studies using non-randomized designs start at a lower quality of evidence and are downgraded in the GRADE rating for lack of certainty of evidence. Unfortunately, even most randomized clinical trials in anesthesiology suffer from a low quality of evidence. Improving the number, diversity, and quality of randomized clinical trials is needed to improve the quality of evidence in perioperative care overall [11].

GRADE links the strength of recommendation to the level of evidence. Rating of recommendations uses specific wording related directly to the level of evidence (Table 33.2). For instance, a strong recommendation can be made if the level of evidence is high or moderate. For low to very low levels of evidence, GRADE uses the word "conditional" in the recommendation. However, in rare circumstances, a strong recommendation may be made in a life-threatening situation if low quality of evidence suggests benefit, while high-quality evidence suggests harm. A conditional recommendation reflects the lack of robust evidence. However, a conditional recommendation should not be interpreted as dismissing the potential benefit of a recommendation. GRADE also permits the use of good or best practice statements for important recommendations without formal ratings of quality of evidence. GRADE also permits the inclusion of no recommendations when evidence is insufficient.

Public Comment Drafts of ASA practice guidelines and advisories are posted on the ASA website, reviewed by the ASA Committee on Practice Parameters, the ASA Board of Directors, and other interested parties. Suggested revisions are incorporated into the document. Practice guidelines and advisories are submitted to ANESTHESIOLOGY where they undergo peer review and revision prior to acceptance by the society's premier scholarly journal. Final approval by the ASA House of Delegates is required prior to publication.

Table 33.1 GRADE strength of evidence definitions

GRADE	Interpretation
High	We are very confident that the true effect lies close to that of the estimate of the effect
Moderate	We are moderately confident in the effect estimate: The true effect is likely to be close to the estimate of the effect, but there is a possibility that it is substantially different
Low	Our confidence in the effect estimate is limited: The true effect may be substantially different from the estimate of the effect
Very low	We have very little confidence in the effect estimate: The true effect is likely to be substantially different from the estimate of effect

Table 33.2 Strength of recommendations definitions

Strength of recommendation	Level of evidence	Interpretation
Strong	High to moderate	Task force believes that all or almost all clinicians would choose (or not) the specific action or approach
Conditional	Low to very low	Task force believes that most, but not all, would choose (or not choose) the action or approach
Best practice statements	Ungraded	Best practice statements are statements for which there is sparse direct evidence or limitations in the available evidence that does not make them amenable to the GRADE process. However, they may be valuable for anesthesiologists to consider in the management of patient care

33.3 Local Adaptation of Systematic Reviews and GRADE Technology

ASA, subspecialty, and relevant other specialty guidelines and advisories only make specific recommendations in select areas of perioperative care. However, individual local anesthesia departments can utilize a few aspects of the GRADE system to produce recommendations for local care if published guidance is lacking. A local medical librarian can perform a literature search with examples of key references as a guide to reduce the number of citations to review. Focusing on published meta-analyses if available is particularly helpful. Local recommendations can be made using GRADE to assess the strength of evidence. If the literature is insufficient to utilize GRADE, multidisciplinary local expert consensus groups can review the literature and formulate local best practice statements to provide up-to-date quality care.

33.4 Conclusion

Clinical practice guidelines, advisories, and best practice statements provide useful recommendations to improve the quality and consistency of patient care in the perioperative setting. The American Society of Anesthesiologists, as the premier organization of physician anesthesiologists, plays an invaluable role in the development and dissemination of these standards of care for the practice of perioperative medicine. While national/international guidelines are most highly trusted, they may not cover all aspects of perioperative care. Locally produced best practice statements can improve quality of care when subspecialists are not available or when evidence is lacking, to supplement societal guidance. Physician anesthesiologists play a crucial role in the implementation of practice guidelines and best practices in local practice to produce patient care of the highest caliber.

References

1. Basic standards for preanesthesia care. https://www.asahq.org/standards-and-practice-parameters/basic-standards-for-preanesthesia-care. Accessed 25 Sept 2025.
2. Standards for basic anesthetic monitoring. https://www.asahq.org/standards-and-practice-parameters/standards-for-basic-anesthetic-monitoring. Accessed 25 Sept 2025.
3. Standards for postanesthesia care. https://www.asahq.org/standards-and-practice-parameters/standards-for-postanesthesia-care. Accessed 25 Sept 2025.
4. Graham R. Clinical practice guidelines we can trust. Washington, DC: National Academies Press; 2011.
5. Thilen SR, Weigel WA, Todd MM, et al. 2023 American Society of Anesthesiologists practice guidelines for monitoring and antagonism of neuromuscular blockade: a report by the American Society of Anesthesiologists Task Force on neuromuscular blockade. Anesthesiology. 2023;138(1):13–41.
6. Apfelbaum JL, Roth S, Rubin D, et al. Practice advisory for perioperative visual loss associated with spine surgery 2019: an updated report by the American Society of Anesthesiologists Task Force on perioperative visual loss, the north American neuro-ophthalmology society, and the Society for Neuroscience in Anesthesiology and critical care. Anesthesiology. 2019;130(1):12–30.
7. Apfelbaum JL, Schulman PM, Mahajan A, et al. Practice advisory for the perioperative management of patients with cardiac implantable electronic devices: pacemakers and implantable cardioverter-defibrillators. Anesthesiology. 2020;132:225–52.
8. Seiber F, McIsaac DI, Deiner S, et al. 2025 American Society of Anesthesiologists practice advisory for perioperative care of older adults scheduled for inpatient surgery. Anesthesiology. 2025;142(1):22–51.
9. PRISMA. https://www.prisma-statement.org. Accessed 25 Sept 2025.
10. Andrews J, Guyatt G, Oxman AD, et al. GRADE guidelines: 14. Going from evidence to recommendations: the significance and presentation of recommendations. J Clin Epidemiol. 2013;66:719–25.
11. Neuman MD, Apfelbaum JL. Clinical practice guidelines in anesthesiology: adjusting our expectations. Anesthesiology. 2021;135(1):9–11.

34 Professional Citizenship: How Anesthesiologists Advance Medicine Through Society Engagement

Lois A. Connolly, Kraig S. de Lanzac,
and Matthew Popovich

34.1 Introduction

The American Society of Anesthesiologists (ASA) is the primary medical association representing anesthesiologists in the United States. The ASA Mission is "Advancing the Practice and Securing the Future." Its vision is "A world leader improving health through innovation in quality and safety." ASA's values are "Patient Safety, Physician-led Care and Scientific Discovery." A common and prominent feature of ASA's logo and ethos is the Lighthouse. The Lighthouse was originally placed on the Society's seal in 1932 and represents "ASA's commitment to physician anesthesiologists around the world to organize and form a union of sharp minds, kind hearts and steady hands to protect patients during their most vulnerable moments."

L. A. Connolly (✉)
Department of Anesthesiology, Medical College of Wisconsin, Milwaukee, WI, USA
e-mail: l.connolly@asahq.org

K. S. de Lanzac
Department of Anesthesiology, Tulane University School of Medicine,
New Orleans, LA, USA

Tulane Lakeside Hospital,, Metairie, LA, USA

American Society of Anesthesiologists, Washington, DC, USA
e-mail: k.delanzac@asahq.org

M. Popovich
American Society of Anesthesiologists, Washington, DC, USA
e-mail: m.popovich@asahq.org

G. Tewfik (ed.), *The Anesthesiologist as Perioperative Leader*,
https://doi.org/10.1007/978-3-032-18058-2_34

ASA is one of hundreds of medical specialty associations in the United States and is a distinct association from other anesthesiology associations. ASA includes state component societies and supports several foundations and related organizations: Foundation for Anesthesia Education and Research (FAER), Wood Library Museum (WLM), Charitable Foundation (CF), Anesthesia Foundation (AF), Anesthesia Patient Safety Foundation (APSF), and Anesthesia Quality Institute (AQI). FAER supports and funds research initiatives. FAER has been dedicated to developing the next generation of physician-investigators through mentoring physician-investigators and providing grants to support medical students, residents, and early career investigators. WLM's mission is to advance Anesthesiology by preserving and sharing its heritage and knowledge. AQI houses three registries: Anesthesia Incident Reporting System, Closed Claims, and National Anesthesia Clinical Outcomes Registry (NACOR). Founded by the ASA in 1985, Anesthesia Patient Safety Foundation (APSF) mission is to improve the safety of patients during anesthesia care. The ASA collaborates and supports the work of APSF in patient safety activities. ASA holds that no patient should be harmed by anesthesia. A list of all ASA Foundations and related organizations is found on the ASA website.

Although ASA often has strong relationships with subspecialty societies of anesthesiology, ASA is managed and administered separate and distinct from the organizations listed below (list may not be inclusive). Many ASA members belong to these associations and participate in their educational, networking, and professional events:

Anesthesiology Subspecialty Organizations
American Society of Regional Anesthesia and Pain Medicine (ASRA)
Association of Anesthesia Clinical Directors (AACD)
Association of University Anesthesiologists (AUA)
International Anesthesia Research Society (IARS)
Society for Airway Management (SAM)
Society of Ambulatory Anesthesia (SAMBA)
Society of Cardiovascular Anesthesiologists (SCA)
Society for Education in Anesthesia (SEA)
Society for Neuroscience in Anesthesiology & Critical Care (SNACC)
Society for the Advancement of Transplant Anesthesia (SATA)
Society of Academic Associations of Anesthesiology and Perioperative medicine (SAAAPM)
Society of Critical Care Anesthesiologists (SOCCA)
Society for Obstetric Anesthesia and Perinatology (SOAP)
Society for Pediatric Anesthesia (SPA)
Trauma Anesthesiology Society (TAS)

As physicians and leaders of the Anesthesia Care Team, anesthesiologists ensure safety and strive to deliver the best outcomes for all patients. Anesthesiologists apply their expertise to identify and mitigate patient risks before surgery, prevent complications and respond to emergencies in the operating room, and enhance their patients' postoperative recovery. Anesthesiologists benefit from, and contribute to, the continued improvement in anesthesia care by participating in their medical association.

34.2 Benefits to Members and the Responsibility of the Members to the Professional Association

34.2.1 Personal Growth

Medical association membership is an expression of professional citizenship. For many, it is essential to their identity as a physician. Although most physicians belong to private practices or are employed by institutions, those organizations may not provide the rich and diverse benefits of a medical society membership. Professional societies, such as ASA, offer the opportunity for lifelong learning, development, and personal growth. This includes not just formal continuing medical education but career-long learning through the incorporation of evolving practice. Publications, online modules, and meetings provide members with the type of ongoing education they want to pursue. Members receive education but also may become creators of the education themselves. These opportunities lead to collaboration and a widening of the physician's professional and, often, social network.

According to Sheepers, happy and healthy physicians improve patient care and satisfaction [1]. A sense of belonging goes a long way to physician satisfaction. Professional society membership allows for that community [2, 3]. Through in-person meetings, virtual collaborations, and the online community, physicians can interact with others from around the world or right down the street. Utilizing these interactions, association members realize the shared challenges faced by their profession, inspiring some to address these challenges for the organization and the benefit of the specialty. By engaging the society, members develop relationships, which broaden their professional and social network, bringing further benefit to the member [4].

34.2.2 Professional Recognition

Professional societies bring recognition to work and other efforts that may otherwise go unnoticed. These organizations often facilitate the publication of research and clinical findings. Founded in 1940, *Anesthesiology* is the official journal of the American Society of Anesthesiologists, operating with complete editorial autonomy. The journal mission is to promote scientific discovery and knowledge in perioperative, critical care, and pain medicine to advance patient care. *Anesthesiology* leads the world in publishing and disseminating the highest quality work to inform daily clinical practice and transform the practice of medicine in the specialty with a Journal Impact Factor: 9.3*—the highest among all anesthesiology journals.

ASA members may also contribute through the official news publication of the ASA, the *ASA Monitor.* Published monthly, the *ASA Monitor* presents the latest specialty and industry news, and practice-changing clinical information to the perioperative healthcare community. Often, a theme of the month prompts evidence-based articles curated by experts from ASA committees.

Both academic and private practice physicians benefit from the professional recognition that medical societies can provide. Academic institutions recognize faculty leadership and engagement in regional and national activities [5, 6]. Professional societies develop and publish programs and courses to enhance the leadership skills among their members, whether in academic or private practice.

Professional societies reward achievements in research, teaching, and professional expression. Fellowship in an organization can highlight the contributions of a member to their specialty. The ASA offers the designation of Fellow of the American Society of Anesthesiologists (FASA) to recognize member achievements in the areas of professionalism, leadership, advocacy, and education (Fig. 34.1). These professional recognitions are not the purpose of the activities, but rather an acknowledgment of achievement and commitment.

34.2.3 Career Advancement

The goals and purposes of membership evolve over a career and throughout one's lifetime [7]. Professional societies serve as a gateway for medical students, residents, fellows, and early career members to contribute to the future of their chosen specialty, while deriving benefits themselves [7]. ASA membership as a student or resident provides a glimpse of the issues facing anesthesiologists, clinical advances, and a wide array of practice opportunities within the field. For them, membership allows the individual to assimilate, becoming a part of their specialty, charged with the future of the specialty.

Early career members are often concerned with achieving board certification and starting practice. ASA engages with early career members through its Early Career Membership Program, a 3-year initial membership, which allows members the opportunity to experience many of the more popular features of ASA membership at a lower membership fee (Fig. 34.2). Engaging with the community that professional societies offer, members can develop formal or informal mentor-mentee relationships. The national reach of professional societies allows for matching of professional interests, resulting in a suitable mentor-mentee fit [8]. ASA offers a very successful mentorship program matching individuals with similar interests.

As members mature in their practice, their focus may change to career advancement, transition, leadership development, or a focus on a wider set of clinical and professional issues. With the confidence of a few years practice experience, members may choose to express their voices, and professional societies can provide resources and experience. In the later phases of one's career, professional society

FASA

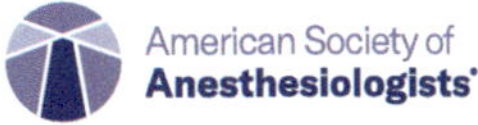

Fellow of the American Society of Anesthesiologists

FASA Eligibility Criteria

- Active ASA and state component membership for the past five years, or if a retired member, in the five years leading into retirement
- Unrestricted medical license
- Board certified by the ABA, the AOBA, or a recognized international body
- Two letters of endorsement from ASA Active Members
- CV and optional bibliography
- Dedication in the three areas outlined at right within the past five years demonstrated by meeting six total requirements, with at least one from each category

PROFESSIONALISM AND LEADERSHIP

- Leadership or participation in ASA, ASA committees or components or other ASA entity
- Participated in local/community leadership position/activities related to the field of medicine
- Held a hospital/practice leadership position
- Held a leadership position with a subspecialty or any medical society
- Involvement in the ASA Foundations
- Held a military/government leadership position

ADVOCACY

- Attend ASA Legislative Conference
- Active participation in state-level advocacy efforts
- Active participation in ASA advocacy efforts

EDUCATION AND SCHOLARLY ACTIVITIES

- Active involvement in teaching or mentoring activities
- Conducted research in anesthesiology
- Published in journals, web content or teaching materials
- Served as a board examiner, exam program development
- Involved in education program development
- Held a faculty position for ASA or other educational programs or meetings
- Served as an editor for publications
- Subspecialty or other medical board certification
- Participation in the Maintenance of Certification in Anesthesiology (MOCA)
- Participation or attendance at three ASA or ASA component society live educational events within the past five years

Fig. 34.1 ASA Fellow of the American Society of Anesthesiologists (FASA) designation criteria and qualifications. (FASA® is a registered trademark of the American Society of Anesthesiologists (ASA). (2025). Used with permission from ASA)

membership is also meaningful. Not only do late-career members continue to benefit from advances in the field, but professional societies can assist with resources for career transitions. Furthermore, professional societies offer an opportunity for members to leave a legacy through their actions and contributions to the specialty. Shaping the specialty's future and protecting the field's integrity are important for those that follow.

34.2.4 How Members Influence Societies

Physicians must decide if membership provides value, but their actions and expectations for involvement within the society determine its true value. The benefit side of the value equation is increased when members take advantage of their membership through active engagement. Organizations improve with member engagement, transforming the relationship from a transactional one where members pay dues and have the privilege to call themselves a member, to one where members pay dues and

American Society of Anesthesiologists
ASA Early-Career Membership Program
A three-year membership, PLUS:
Free Online Education
• Anesthesiology Continuing Education (ACE)
• Summaries of Emerging Evidence (SEE)
• Fundamentals of Patient Safety
In-person Meetings
• One free registration to ANESTHESIOLOGY® annual meeting
• One free registration to ASA® ADVANCE: The Anesthesiology Business Event
Curated Early-Career Member Resources
• Career and specialty
• Wellness
• Mentoring
• Financial
• Clinical practice and patient safety
ASA Membership Benefits
Continuing Medical Education
Practice and Patient Safety Resources
Advocacy
Career Advancement
Community
Guidelines, Standards, and Statements
Leadership Devlopment
Professional Engagement Opportunities
Wellness Resources

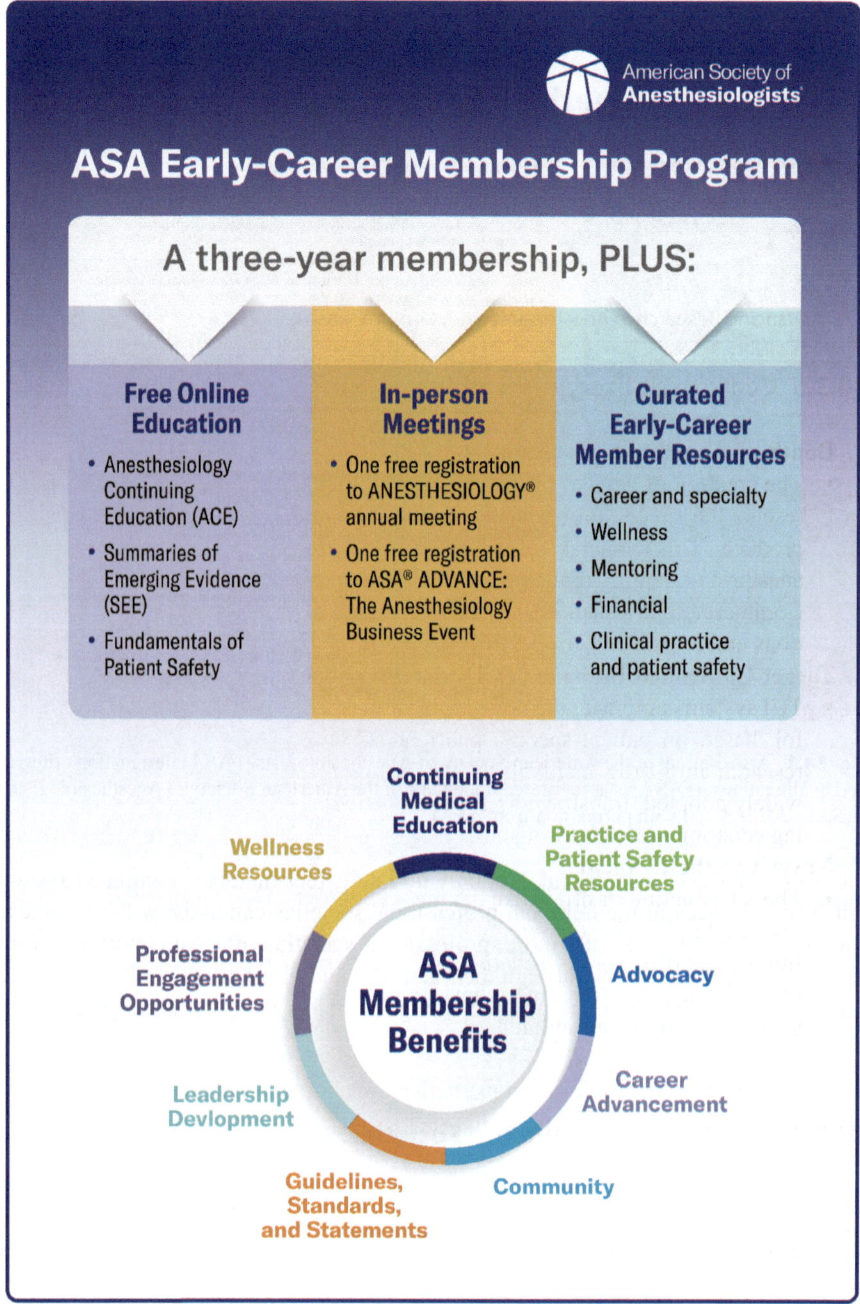

Fig. 34.2 ASA Early Career Membership Program (ECMP). This membership is available to any US-based anesthesiologist in the first 3 years of practice after the completion of training. (American Society of Anesthesiologists (ASA). (2025). Early-Career Membership Program (ECMP). Used with permission from ASA)

see membership as a resource engine to derive the value they want from their professional society.

Engagement with a professional medical association starts with membership (Fig. 34.3). Active engagement begins with reading communications from ASA and responding to calls to action for volunteers, survey responses, or engaging in regulatory and legislative issues. Members develop areas of interest that can be further explored by involvement in local components. Through committee activity, governance, or through direct communication with state and national leaders, members can address their concerns and develop solutions. The ASA has component societies in every state, the District of Columbia, Puerto Rico, and one each for military members, medical students, and residents. Components offer numerous volunteer opportunities ranging from governance, communication, membership, meeting planning, and scientific and political activity. Component societies enable members to act locally and gain necessary leadership experience and policy understanding. Engagement allows members to grow their network across the country and in some cases internationally.

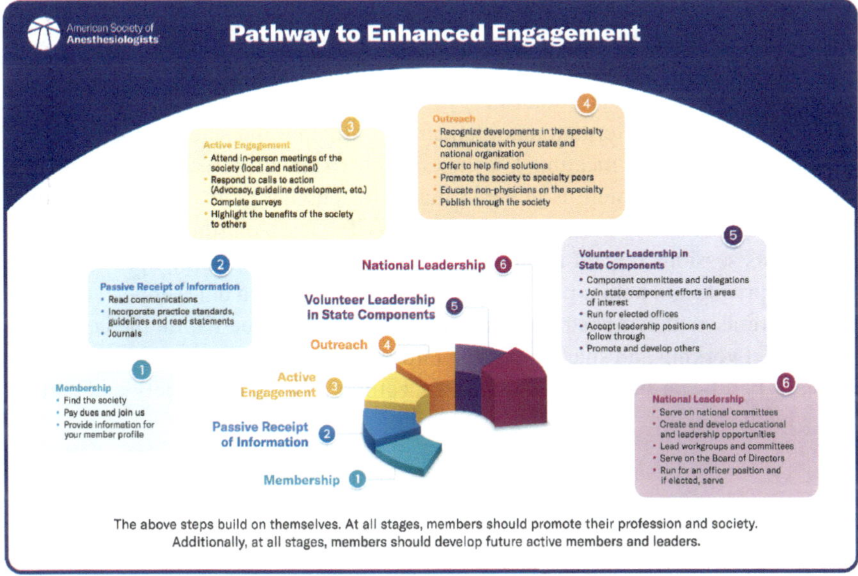

Fig. 34.3 Pathway to Enhanced Engagement in a professional medical society. This illustrates one potential pathway for professional medical society involvement. (American Society of Anesthesiologists (ASA). (2025). Pathway to Enhanced Engagement. Reproduced with permission from ASA)

34.3 Key Functions and Benefits for Joining a Professional Society

Professional societies serve several functions that benefit the members of the society, though some members may be unaware of the vast resources available to them.

34.3.1 Networking Opportunities

ASA facilitates communication and networking opportunities between anesthesiologists, often through in-person or virtual events. Most anesthesiologists share clinical knowledge or best practices through online forums, in-person meetings, educational events, and publications. Within the ASA, members have the opportunity to participate in an extensive committee structure (Fig. 34.4) that allows members to serve on a committee that aligns with their expertise. Committees often work to promulgate best practices and ASA policy through the development and updating of statements, committee resources, and guidelines that drive standard of care in the profession.

Conferences hosted nationally and locally provide physicians with the opportunity to share their work and perspectives and engage with their peers. The ASA hosts conferences and events such as ANESTHESIOLOGY, the ASA's annual meeting, and ADVANCE: The Anesthesiology Business Event. The ANESTHESIOLOGY meeting draws large international attendance, enriching the scientific and clinical content presented at the meeting. For those unable to attend all sessions, educational and clinical session content is made available for purchase OnDemand, the online content portal. Among other topics, ADVANCE: The Anesthesiology Business Event hosts sessions related to anesthesia quality and patient safety, practice management, private and public payors, contracting, optimization of revenue, workforce considerations, and demonstrating an anesthesiologist's value within the healthcare system. Networking and sharing clinical information and innovative ideas and solutions are significant benefits of in-person meetings to both the society and participating members.

34.3.2 Professional Development

ASA provides a vast array of professional development resources for anesthesiologists to maintain and advance their clinical knowledge and skill sets. Anesthesiologists will find numerous Continuing Medical Education (CME) and certificates of expertise opportunities through the ASA, including proprietary programs like ACE (Anesthesiology Continuing Education), Anesthesia SimSTAT Simulated Anesthesia Education, SEE (Summaries of Emerging Evidence), Anesthesiology Journal CME, Diagnostic POCUS Certificate Program, PeRLS (Perioperative Resuscitation and Life Support), and Live Simulation Training. Other, more targeted modules and courses allow anesthesiologists to earn credit at times

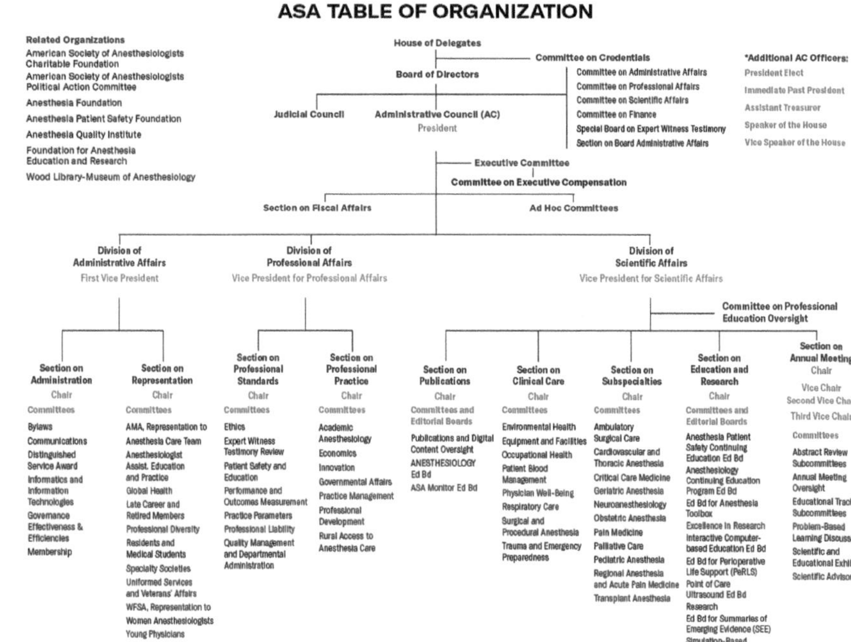

Fig. 34.4 ASA Table of Organization 2025 ASA. Center for Workforce Studies (CAWS), Center for Perioperative Medicine (CPMed), and Center for Anesthesia Perioperative Economics (CAPE) are not represented in this figure. (American Society of Anesthesiologists (ASA). (2025) Used with permission from ASA)

convenient for their schedule. American Board of Anesthesiology (ABA) Maintenance of Certification in Anesthesiology (MOCA) is supported by the educational programs developed and maintained by the ASA. ASA has become the home for many anesthesiologists to track and claim their CME credits, Patient Safety credits, and ABA Quality Improvement points.

ASA provides further opportunities for members to learn more about their specialty and important topics through podcasts and webinars [9]. The *Central Line* podcast features leaders in anesthesiology discussing a wide variety of challenges and opportunities vital to our practice and our profession. *Residents in the Room* features anesthesiologists-in-training from across the country, discussing anesthesiology topics important to younger physicians, including their hopes, fears, and expectations for residency and beyond. The ASA journal, *Anesthesiology*, hosts a podcast providing a monthly overview of new content that highlights research through author and editor interviews.

ASA and other medical associations understand that many physicians desire leadership positions within their facilities and healthcare systems. According to a recent study, physician leadership has been independently associated with higher average quality ratings [10]. Physician-led healthcare organizations tend to have improved clinical outcomes, patient satisfaction, and greater operational efficiency than those managed by nonphysicians [11, 12]. ASA encourages members to pursue leadership positions within their organizations and offers resource education and tools to support these career paths. Among other courses, ASA hosts a Leadership Academy and Center for Physician Leadership Excellence courses. ASA partners with other societies such as the American College of Healthcare Executives (ACHE). Partnership also exists with the American Association for Physician Leaders (AAPL) to provide courses that lead to the Certified Physician Executive (CPE) designation or a Master of Business Administration (MBA).

34.3.3 Advocacy and Representation

Professional medical societies represent members' and their patients' interests in the legislative and regulatory arena. These efforts are complicated requiring subject matter experts, advocates, and supportive elected and appointed officials to achieve desired results. Individual anesthesiologists and practice groups would be very challenged to stay informed and influential without the expertise and influence of ASA. ASA lobbies for policies beneficial to anesthesiology and in alignment with the ASA mission [13]. ASA has dedicated resources for policymakers, patients, and other stakeholders to facilitate their understanding of complex anesthesiology issues. This includes brochures, checklists, tip sheets, and other materials to provide non-anesthesiologists with information on anesthesia, pain management, and anesthesiologists, the medical experts committed to delivering patient safety and high-quality care before, during, and after surgery, procedures, and other treatments.

ASA advocates and influences health system transformation to integrate care and collaborates with various stakeholders to optimize patient care and outcomes [14]. As a society of 59,000 members, ASA's voice in federal as well as state-level decisions carries significant weight. Although many often think of scope of practice challenges when advocacy is mentioned, ASA is involved in many different legislative and regulatory efforts that affect anesthesiologists and their patients. For example, regarding quality and patient safety, ASA ensures that the actions of anesthesiologists are well documented and understood by regulators, facility executives, and patients. Within the current Center for Medicare and Medicaid (CMS) Quality Payment Program (QPP), ASA advocates for the use of anesthesia-specific quality measures and appropriate attribution of other measures that determine an anesthesiologist's or their group's performance. For patient safety purposes, the ASA advocates for appropriate regulations that protect both patients and anesthesiologists. Engaging with accrediting organizations and state regulators, ASA leaders and staff will act upon trends found during onsite accreditation surveys to offer training and education programs to members.

At the same time, anesthesiologists and ASA staff understand that several regulations are either outdated, no longer reflect clinical care, or are burdensome without contributing to patient safety or quality. In those cases, ASA physicians and staff align policy statements with policy initiatives to improve physician workflow without compromising patient safety. For example, as information sharing and artificial intelligence become more prominent, ASA must be nimble enough to understand proposed regulation and to shape regulation and legislation to the benefit of both anesthesiologists and patients. ASA also advocates for patient-friendly policy positions, including those that affect out-of-network payments through the No Surprises Act (NSA) and prior authorization obstacles faced by surgical patients as well as pain medicine physicians.

ASA advocates for its members to ensure appropriate payments and opportunities to participate in delivery and alternative payment models that capture and express the value of an anesthesiologist's work. Too often, payments for anesthesia services are constrained by legislative short-sightedness and apathy. Laws and regulations established several decades ago directly influence the economic viability of anesthesia practice and the specialty. Specifically, budget-neutrality constraints on Medicare physician payment rates for anesthesia services have resulted in anesthesia payments far below 33% of commercial insurance payment rates. The combination of previously passed laws and regulations with the lack of an inflation adjustor for Medicare physician payments unfortunately locks the specialty into Medicare Conversion Factor (CF) cuts every year. ASA advocacy operations have been working across medical specialties to support bills that would address these annual payment cuts by adding inflation adjustments and revising budget neutrality requirements.

Legislative actions, unfortunately, sometimes result in unintended consequences or flawed implementation. ASA tracks and attempts to remedy these challenges for anesthesiologists and their patients, improving group and practice viability. For example, legislators and other societies originally saw the CMS QPP as one solution to address payment shortcomings with enhanced focus on quality and measurement. The QPP was originally meant to offset payments by rewarding exceptional performance in quality domains, but the program never yielded much financial gain for anesthesiologists or other medical professionals [15, 16]. Additionally, the No Surprises Act has been a win in protecting patients from surprise billing, but the backend process for adjudicating claims between insurers and physicians has required lawsuits, extensive rulemaking, and unnecessary financial expenditure (https://www.cms.gov/nosurprises/policies-and-resources/reports). As the professional society for anesthesiologists, ASA has been intensively engaged in examining the results of these legislative actions and has worked with stakeholders to advocate for the best possible implementation and operability of these processes for anesthesiologists.

34.3.4 Standards, Guidelines, and Statements

Members and the general healthcare system benefit from having clear standards and practice guidelines. ASA develops and maintains professional standards and promulgates best practices through its guidelines and statements. ASA guidelines are developed and facilitated by the Committee on Practice Parameters. Guidelines are developed through rigorous scientific processes, including the use of librarians, statisticians, methodologists, and others who use best practices for developing guidelines, including the use of the GRADE rating system. Once approved by the ASA House of Delegates and published in *Anesthesiology*, guidelines are often used by accrediting organizations and regulatory agencies as well as local anesthesia departments and hospitals to set policy.

34.3.5 Practice Quality Benchmarking

ASA members also have access to the Anesthesia Quality Institute (AQI) and its three clinical registries to track their performance locally. The AQI is a recognized Agency for Healthcare Research and Quality (AHRQ) Patient Safety Organization (PSO) that collects and analyzes data voluntarily reported by healthcare providers to help improve patient safety and healthcare quality [17]. AQI Anesthesia Incident Reporting System (AIRS) allows anesthesiologists and other healthcare professionals to confidentially submit cases that may have experienced a near miss or adverse event. The Anesthesia Closed Claims Program's goal is to identify anesthesia-related major safety concerns, patterns of injury, and prevention strategies in areas where anesthesiologists provide care. The National Anesthesia Clinical Outcomes Registry (AQI NACOR) is a clinical data warehouse designed to elevate anesthesia care through focus on patient outcomes and quality improvement. NACOR is a CMS-designated Qualified Clinical Data Registry (QCDR) for members to participate in CMS QPP by Merit-Based Incentive Program (MIPS) reporting.

34.4 Public Awareness of the Profession and Society

Outside of a professional society, there are few opportunities to promote and support your profession, especially in anesthesiology. All anesthesiologists should strive to engage with their patients and demonstrate their critical role in healthcare. Still, membership in ASA provides a collective voice for public relations and patient education support. Professional societies allow members to amplify their voices on important issues.

Communications and public relations efforts highlight patient safety concerns presented by anesthesiologists. Professional societies allow members to amplify their voices on important issues, supplying various media outlets with accurate healthcare information well beyond the scope of individual physicians [18]. ASA produces public relation and educational resources for all anesthesiology practices independent of size or affiliations and delivers that message on a grander scale.

Patients may not always understand the risks and safety of modern anesthesia and often are not knowledgeable about the importance of an anesthesiologist leading their care. At the point of patient care, this message can be difficult to deliver, despite best efforts [19]. Large-scale public relations campaigns can inform patients, legislators, healthcare leaders and our colleagues in a way that individuals cannot.

With the assistance of members, ASA develops concise, consistent, understandable messages for appropriate audiences regarding issues that affect anesthesiologists and their patients. ASA public relations and communication efforts support the work of individual anesthesiologists at the bedside.

34.5 Conclusion

Every member of the ASA has the opportunity to contribute to the future direction of anesthesiology and improvements to patient safety and quality. Career-long membership unlocks opportunities that would otherwise not be available. Professional societies offer the opportunity for lifelong learning, development, and personal growth. Leadership and career advancement opportunities exist within professional societies. Leadership often starts at a local or regional level with the state components' boards, committees, and officer positions. Further engagement leads to national involvement in committees or representation within the ASA House of Delegates or the Board of Directors. Dedication, passion, and diligence can lead to further leadership opportunities that range from national committee leadership positions, through ASA section and division leadership, all the way to elected office on the ASA Administrative Council and possibly, the ASA presidency. At every stage of engagement, actively participating anesthesiologists derive benefits not just for themselves, but for the patients and facilities they serve. Specialty society membership and involvement allow physicians a broader, more forward-facing view of the specialty and insight into where the future challenges and advancements lie. The expertise and wisdom present within a national specialty society can be harvested and applied to every physician's practice. Expertly vetted guidelines, practice parameters, and solutions to clinical and financial challenges are available within a specialty society membership, and if accessed and appropriately applied, are extremely beneficial to practices, hospital systems, and the patients under our care.

Whether you aspire to be a medical society leader or simply want to participate, membership in a professional medical society such as ASA provides innumerable benefits and opportunities. Membership is what you make of it. Coupled with the benefits of clinical practice, membership in ASA and other professional medical societies enriches the careers and lives of physicians.

References

1. Scheepers RA, et al. A systematic review of the impact of physicians' occupational well-being on the quality of patient care. Int J Behav Med. 2015;22(6):683–98. https://doi.org/10.1007/s12529-015-9473-3.
2. Beck DE. Role of professional societies in career development. Clin Colon Rectal Surg. 2011;24(2):106–8. https://doi.org/10.1055/s-0031-1278406.
3. Persaud A, Bilal M. Involvement in National Gastroenterological Societies for professional development and career advancement: tips for trainees. Dig Dis Sci. 2023;68(11):4073–80. https://doi.org/10.1007/s10620-023-08103-z.

4. Theodosiou NA, et al. Professional societies can play a vital role in career development. Dev Biol. 2020;459(1):5–8. https://doi.org/10.1016/j.ydbio.2019.10.038.
5. Ansmann L, et al. Career development for early career academics: benefits of networking and the role of professional societies. Patient Educ Couns. 2014;97(1):132–4. https://doi.org/10.1016/j.pec.2014.06.013.
6. Liang PS, Andres SF, Perumpail RB, Shah R, Strauss AT, Pointer S. The importance of professional societies as academic homes. Clin Gastroenterol Hepatol. 2023;21(10):2450–6. https://doi.org/10.1016/j.cgh.2023.05.005.
7. Mata H, et al. Benefits of professional organization membership and participation in National Conferences: considerations for students and new professionals. Health Promot Pract. 2010;11(4):450–3. https://doi.org/10.1177/1524839910370427.
8. Vail EA, et al. The role of professional organizations in fostering the early career development of academic intensivists. Ann Am Thorac Soc. 2020;17(4):412–8. https://doi.org/10.1513/AnnalsATS.201908-573PS.
9. Madara J, Miyamoto S, Farley JE, Gong M, Gorham M. Clinicans and professional societies COVID-19 impact assessment: lessons learned and compelling needs. Discussion paper. National Academy of Medicine; 2021. p. 1–28. https://doi.org/10.31478/202105b
10. Tasi MC, Keswani A, Bozic KJ. Does physician leadership affect hospital quality, operational efficiency, and financial performance? Health Care Manag Rev. 2019;44(3):256–62. https://doi.org/10.1097/HMR.0000000000000173.
11. See H, Shreve L, Hartzell S, Daniel S, Slonim AD. Comparison of quality measures from US hospitals with physician vs nonphysician chief executive officers. JAMA NetwOpen. 2022;5(10):e2236621. https://doi.org/10.1001/jamanetworkopen.2022.36621.
12. Gupta AK. Physician versus non-physician CEOs: the effect of a leader's professional background on the quality of hospital management and health care. J Hosp Admin. 2019;8(5):47–55. https://doi.org/10.5430/jha.v8n5p47.
13. Welchman J, Griener GG. Patient advocacy and professional associations: individual and collective responsibilities. Nurs Ethics. 2005;12(3):296–304. https://doi.org/10.1191/0969733005ne791oa.
14. Indar A, et al. Exploring how professional associations influence health system transformation. Int J Integr Care. 2023;23(2):1–11. https://doi.org/10.5334/ijic.7017.
15. Hayden R-L, Zirui S, Zhu JM. Value-based payment and vanishing small independent practices. JAMA. 2024;332(11):871–2. https://doi.org/10.1001/jama.2024.12900.
16. Glance LG, Thirukumaran CP, Feng C, Lustik SJ, Dick AW. Association between the physician quality score in the merit-based incentive payment system and hospital performance in hospital compare in the first year of the program. JAMA Netw Open. 2021;4(8):e2118449. https://doi.org/10.1001/jamanetworkopen.2021.18449.
17. Cunningham FC, et al. Health professional networks as a vector for improving healthcare quality and safety: a systematic review. BMJ Qual Saf. 2012;21:239–49. https://doi.org/10.1136/bmjqs-2011-000187.
18. Park H, Reber BH. Using public relations to promote health: a framing analysis of public relations strategies among health associations. J Health Commun. 2010;15(1):39–54. https://doi.org/10.1080/10810730903460534.
19. Kopp VJ, Shafer A. Anesthesiologists and perioperative communication. Anesthesiology. 2000;93(2):548–55. https://doi.org/10.1097/00000542-200008000-00035.

Part VII

Transforming the Business and Future of Perioperative Care: Innovation, Partnerships, and the Strategic Evolution of Anesthesiology

The Hidden Economy of Anesthesiology: Unpaid Work That Sustains Healthcare

35

Thanh-Giang Vu

35.1 Introduction

Anesthesiologists serve as consultants in the medical field, bringing expertise in physiology, pharmacology, and team-based care. The perioperative environment is a significant source of revenue for medical systems, with physician anesthesiologists at the core. In 2014, surgical care represented an estimated 51% of Medicare spending or $124.9 billion [1]. Nearly 100 million procedures are performed annually in both the inpatient and ambulatory settings [2, 3]. Anesthesia care is an indispensable component of perioperative care. The scope of work for anesthesiologists, however, is not always fully understood nor appropriately appreciated or compensated.

35.2 The Anesthesiologist Role

The cultural role of physicians of all specialties has long been represented as someone knowledgeable, respected, and virtuous [4]. This perspective has led to expectations of exceptional work, including a physical on-site presence beyond the typical workday and being on-call virtually at all hours to respond directly to patient messages and requests [5]. Although this increased access is a benefit for improved healthcare delivery, allowing patients to be more active in their own well-being and to receive information in a timelier fashion, it has led to increased responsibilities, expectations, and availability that may not be compensated accordingly. One study identified that primary care physicians spent an additional 1.4 h in the electronic medical record after clinic hours, with inbox management (responding to messages) accounting for nearly a quarter of that time [6]. Another study analyzed time spent

T.-G. Vu (✉)
Washington Permanente Medical Group, Kaiser Permanente, Seattle, WA, USA
e-mail: tgvu@uw.edu

G. Tewfik (ed.), *The Anesthesiologist as Perioperative Leader*,
https://doi.org/10.1007/978-3-032-18058-2_35

in the electronic medical record for total joint arthroplasty patients demonstrating an average of 76.8 min of preoperative time was spent by the surgical care team per case [7].

Anesthesiologists often care for patients at the most vulnerable times in their lives. They are responsible for maintaining the safety and comfort of their patients while they undergo medical procedures and surgeries [8]. The needs vary greatly between patients, procedures and surgeries, and clinical environments, and the anesthesiologist is expected to uphold a set of standards as set forth by the American Board of Anesthesiology. Vigilance is presumed throughout care provision. Anesthesiologists know their patients' medical history in detail via knowledge obtained during preoperative review that precedes intraoperative care [9]. Time spent reviewing these records, looking at imaging and cardiac studies, or consulting with other providers (among countless other activities) is not captured in compensation models for anesthesiologists.

Traditional compensation models favor physical time spent in an operating room. Nonetheless, these invaluable actions are necessary for adequate care provision for patients. A visit to a preoperative clinic staffed by an anesthesiologist, for example, has been shown to reduce in-hospital postoperative mortality [10]. Therefore, many practices are increasingly moving toward a model where a preoperative assessment is performed in advance of the day of surgery to encourage optimization and thereby reduce perioperative events and case cancellations. Nevertheless, this does not reduce the time needed for each anesthesiologist to review their own cases in preparation for patient care on or around the day of the procedure, activities which remain uncompensated [11].

As the demand for surgery and anesthesia increases while the supply of providers fails to meet those needs, physicians are expected to see more patients in less time. Operating room turnover is a closely followed metric by hospital administrators, and it is a target for optimization and enhanced scrutiny. However, it is during this uncompensated time that may be the first and only time a patient remembers meeting and speaking with their anesthesiologist [12]. Each minute of operating room is valued at $36–$37/min, with emphasis on minimizing turnover time in the name of efficiency and to maximize revenue [12–14]. One high-volume center reported turnover times of 6–18 min [15]. This increasingly brief amount of time requires the anesthesiologist to perform a medical evaluation, hold a thorough consent discussion, and to provide reassurance to the patient.

Anesthesiologists often do not have the added benefit of the continuity of a preoperative visit in clinic similar to that of their surgical colleagues. These office visits provide an additional opportunity to gain insightful patient history, perform an exam, and develop a relationship with a patient, but are often a luxury not available to anesthesiologists. This amplifies the importance of the preoperative consultation, performed during the turnover time. Yet time spent with the patient in excess of an institution's goal case-turnover metric may penalize providers, despite the fact that patients often have nearly the same amount of fear for anesthesia as they do for surgical procedures [16, 17]. Anesthesiologists are generally compensated only for intraoperative time; therefore, these critical, patient-oriented, and time-consuming preoperative consultations and discussions become one of the myriads of uncompensated activities performed by an anesthesiologist [18, 19].

Anesthesiologists also often serve as the primary airway expert in a facility [20–22]. This requires not only additional stress, but often means an ongoing presence in the facility, including covering nocturnal shifts that may not have weighted pay. A lack of compensation for off-hours coverage neglects to recognize the known challenges of working overnight: circadian rhythm misalignment with reduced sleep duration and impaired alertness, impaired cognitive function, increased risk of metabolic syndrome and other cardiometabolic diseases, relationship deterioration, and increased burnout, anxiety, and depression [23]. Overnight work often also requires performing additional roles that are understaffed during a nocturnal shift: Anesthesiologists may be working without the support of additional assistants or anesthesia technicians, increasing patient risk, and requiring these highly trained providers to also clean the operating room after a case and to re-stock equipment [24]. When an anesthesiologist is serving as the airway manager in a facility, they may be expected to cover both operating-room care and provide airway services in the emergency room, intensive care unit, or elsewhere in the hospital—essentially serving multiple roles while being compensated for one.

Some institutions utilize an anesthesia care team model with a combination of anesthesiologists, certified registered nurse anesthetists (CRNA), and certified anesthesiologist assistants (CAAs) ([25]). There is an uncomfortable reality, however, in which these clinicians may operate with separate billing practices. In cases of CRNA absence, anesthesiologists are often expected to cover the anesthesia care needs without additional compensation. CRNAs have been shown to have higher rates of unscheduled absences when compared with physician anesthesia providers (including anesthesiologists, residents, and fellows) [26]. As such, physician practices may bear undue costs. There is an additional cost to patients in some of these mixed models: As staffing ratios adjust to match an increasing need for anesthesiologists, patients have an increased risk of morbidity and mortality [27].

The provision of anesthesia staffing demands maintenance of appropriate training, licensure, and credentialing. Although requirements vary from institution to institution, board certification by the American Board of Anesthesiology requires a series of at least three separate exams totaling more than $4000 [28–30]. Maintenance of this board certification requires an annual completion of 50–60 continuing medical education credits, 120 maintenance of certification (MOCA) questions, and quality improvement activities meeting predefined goals [31]. Fees for these activities vary but require the anesthesiologist to re-certify every 5 years at a cost of at least $350 annually [31]. The time taken to complete additional unaffiliated certifications, including Advanced Cardiac Life Support, may not only be uncompensated but may also require the anesthesiologist to pay out-of-pocket. These activities have term limits and must be renewed and repeated, some annually. Maintenance of certification and remaining up-to-date on current anesthesia practices also may require attendance at professional meetings. Although these events allow anesthesiologists to meet and collaborate with others, the costs may be high and uncompensated;

attendance at the meeting, potential travel, lodging, food, and time may all exceed thousands of dollars individually.

35.3 Outside the Operating Room

In private practices, anesthesiologists not only practice clinical work but may be directly responsible for the success of their business in an ownership model [32]. Financial acumen is necessary to maintain profitability despite the increasingly complex world of healthcare. These anesthesiologists must spend time negotiating stipend contracts with hospitals while also meeting the clinical requirements of such agreements [32]. Providers who serve as partners may also be involved in hospital administrative meetings and may need to spend time maintaining relationships with contract stakeholders to ensure sustained longevity and success of the practice [32].

Academic anesthesiologists comprise approximately 20% of practicing anesthesiologists [33]. In academic practice, anesthesiologists are expected to serve the pillars of education, research, and clinical practice. As the healthcare model shifts (and clinical burdens increase), academic anesthesiologists may be expected to work clinically on par with their private practice colleagues. These conflicting responsibilities may erode the time and funding available for academicians to make progress on education or research and may make a non-academic practice more appealing [34]. Academic anesthesiologists are expected to perform their educator, researcher, and clinical roles with excellence to achieve successful promotion, nonetheless challenging their ability to advance professionally when clinical performance pressure is also present [35]. In addition, as research grants wane, time spent on developing lecture materials and coursework and writing and submitting manuscripts for publication may be uncompensated and may even require the anesthesiologist to self-fund, further challenging issues of diversity in the workforce [36].

As perioperative leaders, anesthesiologists possess a skillset that extends naturally into institution-level responsibilities [37]. Hospital committee work often involves managing and improving on safety, patient experience, care delivery, and census throughput; these metrics benefit greatly from anesthesiologist expertise based on their clinical role. Hospital performance has been linked to physician leader status suggesting opportunity for anesthesiologists [38, 39]. Given the unique perspective anesthesiologists provide in the perioperative world, it is a natural fit for many anesthesiologists to go on to serve in hospital administration. Anesthesiologists work in team-based environments, transferring their collaboration, problem-solving, and negotiation skills out of the OR to offer high value and impact to the healthcare system [40]. Hospital administration positions are generally salaried, though, and the expectations of the role, including availability and degree of responsibility, may not be reflected in this compensation. In addition, physician leaders may still be burdened with a high (if not same) degree of clinical productivity, creating further discrepancy.

Similarly anesthesiologists engaging in advocacy may be working passionately to support their profession, which some consider a core competency [41].

Anesthesiology advocates recognize the special role occupied by the profession, promoting the work and educating others in order to shape its future [42]. Healthcare advocacy has a wider reach that may extend into general healthcare access and patient safety as a whole. Although it offers professional satisfaction and growth, advocacy is usually performed without financial support [42].

Anesthesiologists enter their specialty with a desire to provide the best care for patients. This compassion and altruism may lead many to become involved in humanitarian outreach. An estimated 5 billion people worldwide do not have access to safe surgical and anesthesia care, which contributes to approximately 1.5 million deaths a year in low- and middle-income countries [43]. Funding to reduce these global health disparities is grossly inadequate to fully support the efforts [44]. The global surgical disease burden is estimated at 30%, yet anesthesia and surgical care development assistance comprises less than 1% [43]. Much global health work involves long-term investment in infrastructure building and helping to increase and train a local workforce. For some, volunteerism or involvement in mission trips allows temporary and acute provision of anesthesia care in under-resourced settings [43]. These anesthesiologists ultimately donate their time to not only delivering clinical care on the ground at these sites but often serve critical roles in procuring supplies and funds, and transport of these goods, to ensure success of the trip. Volunteerism acts, by their very nature, are wholly uncompensated.

35.4 The Cost of Uncompensated Activity

The costs associated with not recognizing work performed are high. Physician burnout has gained increasing attention in recent years, often cited as a reason for provider attrition amidst an increased need for patient care [45]. Burnout can be characterized by emotional exhaustion and depersonalization, and when a low sense of personal accomplishment is added, burnout syndrome exists [45]. The ability to continue to provide excellent care suffers when providers are burned out, decreasing productivity, and placing a system dependent on anesthesiologists and their altruism in peril. At an individual level, burnout is associated with depression, anxiety, and suicidality [46]. Other studies have similarly identified that anesthesiologists are at a high risk for suicide with one identifying anesthesiologists were twice as likely to die by suicide when compared with other physicians [47, 48].

Anesthesiologists operate under stressful conditions in a fast-paced environment. This often means supporting patient care in many different models, with varying demands, which unfortunately means their work may go unrecognized and puts them at risk of being undervalued. Corrective models to improve physician well-being recognize the need for humanism and boundary development [49]. This shift may have profound effects for anesthesiologists and other physicians as these efforts should improve compassion, connection, and community [49]. Healthcare systems will need to prepare for these changes and adapt in order to protect the valuable space filled by anesthesiologists.

References

1. Kaye DR, Luckenbaugh AN, Oerline M, et al. Understanding the costs associated with surgical care delivery in the Medicare population. Ann Surg. 2020;271(1):23–8. https://doi.org/10.1097/SLA.0000000000003165.
2. CDC National Center for Health Statistics. Inpatient surgery. CDC. https://www.cdc.gov/nchs/fastats/inpatient-surgery.htm. Last reviewed 5 Apr 2013. Last accessed 28 Sept 2025.
3. Hall MJ, Schwartzman A, Zhang J, Liu X. Ambulatory surgery data from hospitals and ambulatory surgery centers: United States, 2010. Natl Health Stat Rep. 2017;102:1–17.
4. Dopelt K, Bachner YG, Urkin J, et al. Perceptions of practicing physicians and members of the public on the attributes of a "good doctor". Healthcare (Basel). 2021;10(1):73. https://doi.org/10.3390/healthcare10010073.
5. Ofri D. Opinion: the business of healthcare depends on exploiting doctors and nurses. New York Times. 2019. p. 8. https://www.nytimes.com/2019/06/08/opinion/sunday/hospitals-doctors-nurses-burnout.html. Last accessed 26 Sept 2025.
6. Arndt BG, et al. Tethered to the EHR: primary care physician workload assessment using EHR event log data and time-motion observations. Ann Fam Med. 2017;15(5):419–26.
7. Mohler SA, et al. Electronic medical record audit time logs as a measure of preoperative work before total joint arthroplasty. J Arthroplast. 2021;36(7):2250–3. https://doi.org/10.1016/j.arth.2021.01.050. Epub 2021 Jan 23.
8. American Society of Anesthesiologists. Made for this moment: role of anesthesiologist. American Society of Anesthesiologists. https://madeforthismoment.asahq.org/. Last accessed 10 Oct 2025.
9. Wijeysundera DN, Finlayson E. Chapter 28: Preoperative evaluation. In: Gropper MA, Eriksson LI, Fleisher LA, Cohen NH, Leslie K, Johnson-Akeju O, editors. Miller's anesthesia. 10th ed. Elsevier; 2024. p. 808–72.
10. Blitz JD, Kendale SM, Jain SK, et al. Preoperative evaluation clinic visit is associated with decreased risk of in-hospital postoperative mortality. Anesthesiology. 2016;125(2):280–94. https://doi.org/10.1097/ALN.0000000000001193.
11. Edwards AF, Slawski B. Preoperative clinics. Anesthesiol Clin. 2016;34(1):1–15. https://doi.org/10.1016/j.anclin.2015.10.002.
12. MacMillan L, Madura GM, Elliot M, et al. What affects operating room turnover time? A systematic review and mapping of the evidence. Surgery. 2025;181:109263. https://doi.org/10.1016/j.surg.2025.109263. Epub 2025 Mar 6.
13. Childers CP, Maggard-Gibbons M. Understanding costs of care in the operating room. JAMA Surg. 2018;153(4):e176233. https://doi.org/10.1001/jamasurg.2017.6233. Epub 2018 Apr 18.
14. Goldhaber NH, Schaefer RL, Martinez R, et al. Surgical pit crew: initiative to optimise measurement and accountability for operating room turnover time. BMJ Health Care Inform. 2023;30(1):e100741. https://doi.org/10.1136/bmjhci-2023-100741.
15. Parrott J. Speed up room turnovers. Outpatient Surgery Magazine: A Division of AORN. https://www.aorn.org/outpatient-surgery/article/2022-September-room-turnovers. Published 15 Sept 2022. Last accessed 28 Sept 2025.
16. Eberhart L, Aust H, Schuster M, et al. Preoperative anxiety in adults—a cross-sectional study on specific fears and risk factors. BMC Psychiatry. 2020;20(1):140. https://doi.org/10.1186/s12888-020-02552-w.
17. Ruhaiyem ME, Alshehri AA, Saade M, et al. Fear of going under general anesthesia: a cross-sectional study. Saudi J Anaesth. 2016;10(3):317–21. https://doi.org/10.4103/1658-354X.179094.
18. ASA Committee on Economics. Distinguishing between a pre-anesthesia evaluation and a separately reportable evaluation and management service. American Society of Anesthesiologists. https://www.asahq.org/quality-and-practice-management/managing-your-practice/timely-topics-in-payment-and-practice-management/

distinguishing-between-a-pre-anesthesia-evaluation-and-a-separately-reportable-evaluation-and-management-service. Published Nov 2020, revised Mar 2023. Last accessed 10 Oct 2025.
19. Nelson H. Anesthesiology billing primer. MSN Healthcare Solutions. https://msnllc.com/anesthesia-billing-primer/. Published 6 Mar 2022. Last accessed 28 Sept 2025.
20. Grissom TE, Samet RE. The anesthesiologist's role in teaching airway management to non-anesthesiologists. Adv Anesth. 2020;38:131–56. https://doi.org/10.1016/j.aan.2020.08.002.
21. Root CW, DuCanto J. Review articles: strategies for airway management in patients encountered in atypical situations: the floor airway. Anesthesiol News. https://www.anesthesiologynews.com/Review-Articles/Article/07-23/Strategies-for-Airway-Management-in-Patients-Encountered-in-Atypical-Situations-The-Floor-Airway/70738. Published 2 Aug 2023. Last accessed 28 Sept 2025.
22. Sollid SJM, Mellin-Olsen J, Wisborg T. Emergency airway management—by whom and how? Acta Anaesthesiol Scand. 2016;60(9):1185–7. https://doi.org/10.1111/aas.12759.
23. Boivin DB, Boudreau P, Kosmadopoulos A. Disturbance of the circadian system in shift work and its health impact. J Biol Rhythm. 2022;37(1):3–28. https://doi.org/10.1177/07487304211064218.
24. de Cordova PB, Phibbs CS, Schmitt SK, Stone PW. Night and day in the VA: associations between night shift staffing, nurse workforce characteristics, and length of stay. Res Nurs Health. 2014;37(2):90–7. https://doi.org/10.1002/nur.21582. Epub 2014 Jan 9.
25. ASA Committee on Anesthesia Care Team. Statement on the Anesthesia Care Team. American Society of Anesthesiologists. https://www.asahq.org/standards-and-practice-parameters/statement-on-the-anesthesia-care-team. Published 26 Oct 1982, Revised 18 Oct 2023. Last accessed 27 Oct 2025.
26. Dexter F, Epstein RH, Marian AA. Comparisons of unscheduled absences among categories of anesthesia practitioners, including anesthesiologists, nurse anesthetists, and anesthesia residents. Perioper Care Oper Room Manag. 2020;21:100139. https://doi.org/10.1016/j.pcorm.2020.100139. Epub 2020 Oct 17.
27. Burns ML, Saager L, Cassidy RB, et al. Association of anesthesiologist staffing ratio with surgical patient morbidity and mortality. JAMA Surg. 2022;157(9):807–15. https://doi.org/10.1001/jamasurg.2022.2804.
28. The American Board of Anesthesiology. The basic exam. American Board of Anesthesiology. https://www.theaba.org/certification-exam-type/basic-exam/. Accessed 28 Sept 2025.
29. The American Board of Anesthesiology. The advanced exam. American Board of Anesthesiology. https://www.theaba.org/certification-exam-type/advanced-exam/. Accessed 28 Sept 2025.
30. The American Board of Anesthesiology. The APPLIED exam. American Board of Anesthesiology. https://www.theaba.org/certification-exam-type/advanced-exam/. Accessed 28 Sept 2025.
31. The American Board of Anesthesiology. Information for newly certified physicians. American Board of Anesthesiology. https://www.theaba.org/wp-content/uploads/2023/04/Digital_diplomate_welcome_kit.pdf. Accessed 28 Sept 2025.
32. Dutton RP, Koehler R. Foundations for success in the transition to private practice. Adv Anesth. 2020;38:41–61. https://doi.org/10.1016/j.aan.2020.07.003. Epub 2020 Sept 12
33. Toledo P, Lewis CR, Lange EMS. Women and underrepresented minorities in academic anesthesiology. Anesthesiol Clin. 2020;38(2):449–57. https://doi.org/10.1016/j.anclin.2020.01.004.
34. Tran BW, May KA, Pal N. Academic anesthesiology: what does it mean for most of us? Anesth Analg. 2024;138(4):e15–6. https://doi.org/10.1213/ANE.0000000000006898.
35. Eichhorn JH. Chapter 2: Scope of practice. In: Barash PG, Cullen BF, Stoelting RK, et al., editors. Clinical anesthesia. 8th ed. Wolters Kluwer PE; 2017. p. 26–64.
36. Kwan JM, Gross CP. Improving support for physician scientists-mind the (funding) gap. JAMA Netw Open. 2023;6(9):e2332982. https://doi.org/10.1001/jamanetworkopen.2023.32982.
37. Conroy JM, Lubarsky D, Newman MF. Anesthesiologists as health system leaders: why it works. Anesth Analg. 2022;134(2):235–40. https://doi.org/10.1213/ANE.0000000000005845.

38. Goodall AH. Physician-leaders and hospital performance: is there an association? Soc Sci Med. 2011;73(4):535–9.
39. Gupta AK. Physician versus non-physician CEOs: the effect of a leader's professional background on the quality of hospital management and health care. J Hosp Admin. 2019;8(5):47–51.
40. Mathis MR, Schonberger RB, Whitlock EL. Opportunities beyond the anesthesiology department: broader impact through broader thinking. Anesth Analg. 2022;134(2):242–52. https://doi.org/10.1213/ANE.0000000000005428.
41. Kothari R, Ke JXC, Bainbridge D, McKeen DM. Professional advocacy and citizenship: a continuing journey that begins during residency. Can J Anaesth. 2020;67(11):1493–6. https://doi.org/10.1007/s12630-020-01795-1. Epub 2020 Aug 14.
42. Dutton RP, Zaafran S, Azam M. Advocacy for anesthesiologists. Adv Anesth. 2022;40(1):223–39. https://doi.org/10.1016/j.aan.2022.07.006.
43. Asnake B, Law T, Lilaonitkul M, et al. Chapter 2: Anesthesia and global health equity. In: Gropper MA, Eriksson LI, Fleisher LA, Cohen NH, Leslie K, Johnson-Akeju O, editors. Miller's anesthesia. 10th ed. Elsevier; 2024. p. 10–47.
44. Bishen S. Why we need innovation and new funding models in the face of falling global health spend. World Econ Forum. https://www.weforum.org/stories/2025/05/falling-global-health-spend-innovation-new-funding-models/. Published 19 May 2025. Last accessed 29 Sept 2025.
45. Afonso AM, Cadwell JB, Staffa SJ, Sinskey JL, Vinson AE. U.S. attending anesthesiologist burnout in the postpandemic era. Anesthesiology. 2024;140(1):38–51. https://doi.org/10.1097/ALN.0000000000004784.
46. Ryan E, Hore K, Power J, Jackson T. The relationship between physician burnout and depression, anxiety, suicidality and substance abuse: a mixed methods systematic review. Front Public Health. 2023;11:1133484. https://doi.org/10.3389/fpubh.2023.1133484. eCollection 2023.
47. Dutheil F, Aubert C, Pereira B, et al. Suicide among physicians and health-care workers: a systematic review and meta-analysis. PLoS One. 2019;14(12):e0226361. https://doi.org/10.1371/journal.pone.0226361. eCollection 2019.
48. Huang J, Brenner A. Our own safety. Anesth Patient Saf Found. 2019;33(3):82–3.
49. Shanafelt T. Physician well-being 2.0: where are we and where are we going? Mayo Clin Proc. 2021;96(10):2682–93. https://doi.org/10.1016/j.mayocp.2021.06.005.

Redesigning Perioperative Care Through Telemedicine and Data Integration

36

Saul Abreu and Dennis Grech

36.1 Introduction

Telemedicine is defined by the Health Resources and Services Administration (HRSA) as the use of electronic information and telecommunication technologies to support long-distance clinical health care, patient and professional health-related education, public health, and health administration [1]. The technologies that underpin telemedicine include Internet platforms, video conferencing, store-and-forward imaging, streaming media, and landline or wireless communications—tools that enable both synchronous (real-time) and asynchronous (delayed) interaction between providers and patients.

The Institute of Medicine (IOM) further clarifies that telemedicine is not a new form of medical care, but rather a delivery mechanism for applying traditional medical expertise across geographic distances [2]. Its central value lies in facilitating greater access, continuity, and efficiency of care, especially for underserved or remote populations. The IOM emphasized that when applied appropriately, telemedicine can reduce disparities, improve clinical decision-making, and serve as a complement to in-person care—not a replacement.

In anesthesiology, the scope of telemedicine has expanded significantly beyond its early associations with critical care consults and postoperative follow-up [3, 4]. It now includes a range of preoperative functions, such as triage assessments, medication reconciliation, informed consent discussions, and increasingly, airway evaluations. Through the use of still images or live video, anesthesia providers can assess key anatomic features relevant to airway difficulty, including Mallampati classification, thyromental distance, and cervical spine mobility [5, 6]. These virtual assessments have been shown to be feasible, safe, and accurate alternatives to traditional

S. Abreu (✉) · D. Grech
Rutgers New Jersey Medical School, Newark, NJ, USA
e-mail: sa1545@njms.rutgers.edu

G. Tewfik (ed.), *The Anesthesiologist as Perioperative Leader*,
https://doi.org/10.1007/978-3-032-18058-2_36

face-to-face examinations, especially when standard protocols and image quality are maintained [5, 7].

By offering a platform for remote airway screening, telemedicine helps anesthesiologists better prepare for operative interventions while also reducing the burden on patients to attend in-person pre-admission testing. This model not only improves clinical safety and efficiency but also contributes to measurable cost savings by streamlining workflow and reducing resource utilization. In this way, telemedicine underscores the broader role of anesthesiologists as perioperative physicians whose responsibilities begin long before intubation and extend into preventive, consultative, and systems-based care.

36.2 History of Telemedicine

The historical arc of telemedicine began in the 1960s with satellite-based consults developed by NASA in partnership with the Indian Health Service and the US Public Health Service. These early initiatives were designed to provide care to geographically isolated populations, such as Native American communities and astronauts, marking some of the first formal uses of remote medical consultation [2]. Around the same time, the Department of Veterans Affairs (VA) began piloting telemedicine programs to extend care into rural areas, leveraging videoconferencing to connect patients with specialists without requiring travel to centralized hospitals.

By the 1980s and 1990s, the US government began funding broader rural outreach programs that employed the "hub-and-spoke" model of telemedicine, where a central academic or specialty center served as the hub providing services to smaller, rural, or correctional facilities acting as spokes. These programs helped establish the feasibility of using telecommunication technologies for clinical care, especially for populations with limited access to health professionals [2].

In anesthesiology, a key milestone occurred in 2004 with a prospective, randomized controlled pilot study comparing telemedicine-based and in-person preadmission anesthesia consultations [5]. The study enrolled 50 patients scheduled for ambulatory surgery, who were randomly assigned to receive either a traditional in-person consultation or a real-time two-way video consultation. The investigators assessed multiple outcomes, including completeness of consultation, technical feasibility, patient satisfaction, and provider acceptance. The results showed that remote evaluations were comparable in thoroughness to in-person visits, with no adverse events related to missed findings. Patients reported high levels of satisfaction with the virtual experience, citing convenience and confidence in the quality of care. Providers also expressed strong support, emphasizing the clinical viability of telemedicine within preoperative workflows. This study was among the first to demonstrate that remote pre-anesthetic evaluations could achieve the same clinical efficacy and satisfaction outcomes as traditional consultations, even in a tertiary academic setting. It helped establish a foundational framework for expanding the role of tele-anesthesia in perioperative care.

The COVID-19 pandemic catalyzed a dramatic expansion of telemedicine use by clinicians. In response to urgent safety concerns and the need to limit in-person interactions, institutions rapidly scaled telehealth platforms to conduct preoperative assessments—including airway evaluations—via smartphone images and live video consults. A narrative review synthesized available evidence and issued structured recommendations for implementing telemedicine in preoperative anesthetic care during the pandemic. The authors emphasized telemedicine's safety, feasibility, and ability to be rapidly implemented. They proposed its integration as a long-term strategy beyond crisis response to improve access and efficiency in routine care [8].

These developments reflect an evolution from experimental and logistical innovation to structured, scalable platforms with broad clinical utility. Telemedicine in anesthesiology has matured into a viable tool for preoperative planning, airway risk stratification, and perioperative consultation, reshaping the traditional geographic and temporal boundaries of patient care.

36.3 Technology

Telemedicine applications for preoperative airway evaluation primarily rely on two modes of data transmission: asynchronous (store-and-forward) and synchronous (real-time video). Both have distinct advantages and limitations in clinical practice, particularly for assessing anatomical predictors of difficult intubation or mask ventilation.

In the store-and-forward model, patients or clinicians capture and transmit still images of key anatomical features—such as Mallampati view, thyromental distance, dentition, and neck extension—to be reviewed later by the anesthesiologist. This method allows for greater flexibility in scheduling, supports documentation for the medical record, and facilitates review by multiple providers. A 2017 study demonstrated the feasibility and clinical utility of integrating standardized airway photographs into the electronic health record. The researchers implemented a protocol for capturing still images of the upper airway during pre-anesthetic evaluations and embedding them directly into the patient's chart. This allowed providers to reference anatomical findings at later time points—including intraoperatively—and enabled consistent assessment across team members. The approach was shown to enhance safety, improve reproducibility of documentation, and support better-informed airway management decisions [9]. However, this approach requires high-quality image capture with proper lighting, positioning, and resolution. Inconsistent image quality may compromise diagnostic accuracy, particularly when patients lack assistance or guidance during image acquisition.

Conversely, synchronous video-based consultations offer a more interactive and comprehensive approach. Anesthesiologists can directly observe dynamic maneuvers such as jaw protrusion, cervical spine mobility, and patient cooperation. A 2014 study evaluated the use of preoperative video and photographic images to assess airway characteristics—including Mallampati class, inter-incisor distance, and jaw mobility—in a virtual setting. These remote assessments were compared to traditional in-person evaluations and showed high concordance. The findings demonstrated that real-time video could effectively capture subtle dynamic movements critical to airway evaluation, supporting the reliability of virtual airway screening [6].

Similarly, a 2019 study evaluated a synchronous telemedicine workflow for presurgical assessment, emphasizing operational efficiency and patient satisfaction. The implementation of real-time virtual consultations led to reduced wait times and improved provider workflow, while maintaining clinical effectiveness and a positive patient experience. The results demonstrated that live video-based preoperative evaluations could match the quality of traditional in-person visits while offering logistical and operational advantages [10].

The technical requirements for both still-image and video-based telemedicine assessments differ, but both benefit from high-resolution cameras, proper lighting, stable Internet connections, and clear patient instructions. To ensure clinical reliability, structured protocols, consistent image quality, and provider and patient training are essential. These measures help minimize variability, enhance safety, and support scalable implementation—even under time-sensitive conditions such as during a public health crisis [8, 11]. Importantly, survey data also show that anesthesiologists themselves report high satisfaction and feasibility when integrating telemedicine into perioperative workflows [12]. This professional acceptance underscores that telemedicine is not only technically feasible but also clinically embraced by those best positioned to implement and oversee it.

Together, these modalities provide complementary approaches to airway evaluation, allowing flexibility in how and when assessments are performed. When integrated into the broader pre-admission testing workflow, both synchronous and asynchronous tools contribute to safer, more accessible anesthetic planning—particularly in remote, underserved, or high-risk populations.

36.4 Use of Telemedicine Pre-COVID

Prior to 2020, the use of telemedicine in anesthesiology and perioperative care was limited in scale but steadily expanding, supported by growing evidence across both clinical practice and academic exploration. As early as 1996, the IOM recognized the potential of telemedicine but also identified key barriers that hindered its adoption, including unclear reimbursement policies, interstate licensing restrictions, data security concerns, and limited mechanisms for tracking outcomes [2]. These challenges contributed to telemedicine's confinement to niche applications and pilot initiatives throughout the late twentieth and early twenty-first centuries.

Foundational studies, including early trials on video-based preoperative evaluations, confirmed that telemedicine could be used to conduct essential components of the anesthesia consult—such as airway assessment and surgical risk stratification—with reliability and high patient satisfaction [5]. In 2000, a study evaluated the use of telemedicine within a chronic pain clinic by implementing real-time video conferencing to facilitate follow-up consultations between patients and multidisciplinary care teams. The approach enabled physicians, psychologists, and physical therapists to remotely evaluate patient progress, adjust treatment plans, and provide coordinated care—without requiring patients to return for in-person visits. This was particularly beneficial for individuals living in rural or underserved areas, where access to specialty care was limited. The study emphasized telemedicine's value in enhancing continuity of care, reducing travel-related delays, and maintaining adherence to treatment regimens. By demonstrating that remote consultations could effectively support complex, multidisciplinary management, this work helped establish the viability of telemedicine in specialty and longitudinal care settings [13].

Zetterman et al. (2011) further validated the concept of a "virtual preoperative clinic" by demonstrating that remote consultations were equivalent to in-person evaluations in terms of safety, completeness, and patient satisfaction. Their pilot study showed that essential elements of the preoperative assessment—such as airway visualization, comorbidity review, and medication reconciliation—could be reliably conducted via secure digital platforms, even in tertiary care settings [14]. This work helped establish the clinical credibility of virtual anesthetic evaluations before the pandemic, when its use expanded dramatically across all disciplines.

Further, Jacobs et al. (2012) investigated the ergonomics of early telehealth platforms, highlighting the importance of interface usability, audio-visual quality, and screen design—factors critical to anesthesiologists who depend on nuanced visual and auditory cues [15]. Additionally, work by Chatrath et al. and Bridges et al. emphasized that pre-pandemic telemedicine applications had already extended into several functional areas: preoperative assessments (including history-taking, Mallampati scoring, and airway evaluation), informed consent discussions, postoperative follow-up, intraoperative tele-mentoring for complex cases, and remote education of junior clinicians or international teams [3, 4].

Despite the clinical promise of these efforts, systemic adoption remained fragmented due to persistent logistical and regulatory hurdles. Bandwidth limitations, lack of reimbursement frameworks, concerns about patient privacy, and inconsistent electronic medical record (EMR) integration hampered widespread implementation. As a result, most pre-COVID use of telemedicine in anesthesia remained siloed within academic studies, rural outreach initiatives, or specialty-driven pilot projects.

Nonetheless, these early developments collectively demonstrated that telemedicine could safely and effectively extend anesthetic services beyond traditional clinical boundaries. They laid the conceptual and operational groundwork for the rapid, large-scale adoption that would occur during the COVID-19 pandemic.

36.5 Telemedicine and COVID-19

The onset of the COVID-19 pandemic in early 2020 forced health systems worldwide to minimize in-person contact and strive to preserve hospital resources. This urgency catalyzed an unprecedented expansion of telemedicine across medical disciplines—including anesthesiology- where preoperative evaluations and airway assessments had traditionally required face-to-face interaction. Virtual airway screening quickly evolved from a novel adjunct to a clinical necessity, offering a means to maintain perioperative safety, conserve personal protective equipment, and reduce viral transmission risk.

In 2020, Mihalj et al. issued structured recommendations for conducting remote airway evaluations, outlining best practices for patient positioning, lighting, and communication to ensure accuracy and reliability in the virtual setting [8]. These guidelines reflected lessons drawn from earlier feasibility trials, such as Applegate et al.'s (2013) randomized pilot study, which demonstrated that telemedicine-based pre-anesthesia evaluations were comparable to in-person consultations in terms of clinical utility, patient satisfaction, and efficiency [16]. They also aligned work showing that smartphone-captured images—particularly for Mallampati views and neck anatomy—could be reliably used as a tool in airway risk assessment when patients were appropriately guided [6]. This research in aggregate helped to validate telemedicine's readiness for broader clinical adoption and to standardize practices during a time of urgent need.

At the institutional level, Kamdar et al. (2020) detailed the development, implementation, and evaluation of a system-wide telemedicine preoperative evaluation program at a major academic medical center. In response to the COVID-19 pandemic, their team rapidly transitioned hundreds of patients from in-person to virtual consultations within weeks. The rollout involved integration into the electronic health record, creation of standardized workflows for airway exams, and structured training for providers and support staff. Patients were evaluated through synchronous video platforms, with providers assessing speech, dentition, Mallampati class, and neck mobility. Over a six-month period, the program achieved a 95% completion rate for scheduled evaluations, high patient satisfaction scores, and no increase in day-of-surgery cancellations. Importantly, they reported sustained success beyond the peak of the pandemic, citing telemedicine's operational efficiency, safety, and positive reception as justification for its integration as a permanent fixture in perioperative care [11].

The pandemic transformed telemedicine from a convenience into a clinical imperative. It forced the anesthesia community to adopt and optimize remote assessment strategies, which have since demonstrated long-term value for patient safety, provider efficiency, and access to care.

36.6 Post-COVID Use

Following the initial waves of the COVID-19 pandemic, many institutions chose to retain and refine their telemedicine platforms, taking advantage of the technology. The crisis had not only demonstrated the feasibility of virtual preoperative evaluations, but had also provided a recalibration of traditional workflows, accelerating the normalization of tele-anesthesia in clinical practice [11].

Bridges et al. (2020) explored this transformation in their forward-looking review, "To Infinity and Beyond," which examined the technological and cultural shift within anesthesiology toward remote care. They described how pandemic-driven tele-anesthesia programs helped clarify the role of anesthesiologists beyond intraoperative care, emphasizing preoperative optimization, triage, and risk stratification. The authors argued that, with continued innovation in image quality, EMR integration, and patient accessibility, telemedicine would likely remain a cornerstone of perioperative care moving forward [4].

Prior to 2020, studies had demonstrated that telemedicine workflows improved operational efficiency, patient throughput, and provider satisfaction. Pre-surgical teleconsults reduced appointment wait times and travel burdens while maintaining clinical efficacy. As systems restructured post-pandemic, these benefits provided strong justification for making telemedicine a permanent offering, especially in large health networks with geographically dispersed patient populations [10].

Today, as telemedicine transitions from pandemic necessity to institutional standard, anesthesiology departments are leveraging its capabilities to expand patient reach, support perioperative coordination, and reduce system strain. The post-COVID landscape has proven that virtual care is not a temporary workaround but rather a scalable, patient-centered solution with enduring clinical and economic value.

36.7 Use for Pre-admission Airway Evaluation

The pre-admission airway evaluation is a critical component of perioperative planning, enabling anesthesiologists to anticipate intubation difficulties, select appropriate equipment, and prepare adjunctive airway strategies. Traditionally, these evaluations required in-person assessments, but advancements in telemedicine have made remote airway screening a reliable and practical alternative, especially for preoperative clinics managing high volumes or distant patients.

A validation pilot study by Reddy et al. (2021) confirmed that still images obtained via telemedicine can reliably capture essential features such as Mallampati classification, jawline profile, and neck mobility, with strong inter-rater agreement between virtual and in-person evaluators. These photographs—captured using smartphone cameras—provided sufficient resolution to allow clinicians to assess airway risk and document findings in the medical record [7].

While still-image review is beneficial for static anatomical evaluation, real-time video consultations add clinical value by allowing for dynamic assessments such as mouth opening, dental inspection, speech clarity, and patient cooperation. These synchronous interactions help clinicians identify subtle predictors of difficult airway management that may not be evident in photos alone, such as limited temporomandibular joint excursion or abnormal phonation. The potential of tele-anesthesia in this context was recognized well before the COVID-19 era. Chatrath et al. (2010) reported early success with telemedicine-enabled anesthesia consultations, noting that key airway features could be assessed reliably and that remote evaluations improved efficiency, accessibility, and continuity of care. Their findings helped lay the foundation for broader adoption of telemedicine in pre-admission workflows, especially for surgical patients in rural or resource-limited settings [3].

The emerging body of evidence demonstrates that telemedicine—whether via still images, live video, or hybrid models—can support safe, effective airway evaluation. When integrated into pre-admission testing, it reduces logistical burdens for patients while maintaining the clinical rigor needed for anesthetic planning.

36.8 Telemedicine for Preadmission Testing Airway Exam

Telemedicine airway evaluations can be effectively performed using both still and video images, each offering unique advantages. These approaches allow anesthesiologists to assess patient anatomy remotely, ensuring timely risk stratification for airway management before surgery.

36.8.1 Still Images

Still images, when captured with standardized protocols, can offer consistent and reproducible assessments across providers. These images are typically used to evaluate static predictors of difficult airway such as Mallampati score, dental anatomy, jaw profile, and neck circumference. The ability to store and forward these images (asynchronous communication) makes them especially useful in settings with limited Internet connectivity or where provider schedules do not allow for synchronous interaction. One study demonstrated that integrating standardized airway photographs into the electronic medical record (EMR) was both feasible and effective, providing reliable visual documentation of patient anatomy. These images proved especially valuable when reviewed by multiple team members, enhancing consistency in preoperative assessment and promoting continuity of care [9].

36.8.2 Video Images

Real-time video consultations (synchronous telemedicine) provide a more dynamic and interactive evaluation. They allow providers to observe speech, tongue protrusion, inter-incisor distance, and cervical range of motion, enabling a more comprehensive airway assessment. Live interaction also permits clarification of unclear findings and adjustment of patient positioning or lighting to optimize visibility.

Dilisio et al. (2014) pioneered the use of video-based preoperative airway screening and found high agreement between virtual and in-person assessments for several airway predictors, including Mallampati score and mouth opening [6]. In a larger implementation, Kamdar et al. (2020) integrated video airway exams into a major academic center's telehealth platform and reported not only high reliability but also improved patient satisfaction and workflow efficiency [11].

Both still and video modalities benefit from high-quality cameras, proper lighting, and patient education or coaching to ensure optimal image acquisition. As telemedicine expands, the use of hybrid approaches—leveraging asynchronous image submission with optional synchronous follow-up—may further optimize remote airway evaluation.

36.9 How Telemedicine Improves Healthcare Delivery in Preadmission Testing

Telemedicine has significantly expanded access to preoperative airway evaluation by reducing geographic, socioeconomic, and logistical barriers. In the context of anesthesia care, this modality has demonstrated particular value in supporting vulnerable populations who often experience limited access to in-person preadmission testing. By integrating both asynchronous and synchronous platforms, preoperative telehealth can provide equitable and efficient care tailored to a patient's environment and limitations.

36.9.1 Underserved Communities

The HRSA and the IOM have consistently emphasized the role of telehealth in mitigating healthcare access disparities. One of telemedicine's principal benefits lies in its ability to offset specialist shortages in urban health deserts and lower-resource populations by providing remote consultative services. Findings from a systematic review by Ekeland et al. (2010) reinforced that telemedicine implementations tend to improve healthcare equity by reducing disparities in access and outcomes. Their analysis highlighted that patients in rural or underserved regions benefited from increased access to specialty care, improved care coordination, and greater satisfaction with services—effects consistently supported across multiple independent reviews [17]. These findings are consistent with HRSA's stance that telehealth strengthens healthcare delivery by supporting long-distance care coordination and clinical access [1].

36.9.2 Rural Communities

Patients in rural areas often face travel distances of several hours for surgical clearance or anesthesia evaluations. Telemedicine addresses this challenge by enabling real-time or store-and-forward preadmission assessments directly from primary care sites or patient homes. Early pilot studies demonstrated the feasibility of using telemedicine for remote anesthesia consultations, showing that virtual evaluations could match in-person visits in terms of clinical completeness and provider confidence [5]. Similarly, Roberts et al. (2015) found that patients in rural Australia responded positively to preoperative teleconsultations, citing increased convenience and satisfaction [18].

36.9.3 Elderly Patients

Older adults are among the top beneficiaries of tele-anesthesia. The integration of caregiver support and easy-to-navigate platforms has improved usability among elderly patients, particularly those with reduced mobility or sensory limitations. Studies have shown that virtual preoperative consults reduced the stress of travel, increased family participation, and supported timely clinical decision-making from home [10, 11].

36.9.4 Incarcerated Patients

The incarcerated population represents one of the earliest and most successful use cases of telemedicine. As cited in the IOM's foundational reports on telehealth, correctional facilities successfully adopted remote specialty evaluations—particularly anesthetic and surgical clearance—to avoid the high costs and security risks of inmate transportation. This model laid the groundwork for broader applications of telemedicine in constrained environments and remains an example of cost-effective, high-quality care delivery via virtual means [1].

36.10 Economic Impact of Telemedicine in Preoperative Care

Beyond clinical benefits, telemedicine has demonstrated substantial economic value. One early study reported cost savings of $180–$270 per consult in remote preoperative anesthesia evaluations by eliminating patient travel and improving workflow efficiency [5]. Another pilot trial found that integrating telemedicine into pre-anesthesia assessments reduced per-patient evaluation costs by nearly 50%, due to improved scheduling and decreased reliance on physical clinic space [16]. Additional institutional reports noted an average savings of $137 per visit and a projected cost reduction exceeding $64,000 within 6 months of implementation [10, 11]. These savings compound at scale, making telemedicine a cost-effective strategy in both urban and rural healthcare systems.

36.11 Conclusion

As telemedicine continues to evolve from a contingency solution into a standardized component of perioperative care, its impact on anesthesiology becomes increasingly clear. Remote airway evaluations, once experimental, now offer clinically validated tools to enhance safety, efficiency, and accessibility—especially for vulnerable populations. With continued investment in high-fidelity imaging, EMR integration, and provider training, tele-anesthesia holds the potential to redefine perioperative workflows while addressing long-standing disparities in healthcare access.

Physician anesthesiologists are essential to this transformation. Their expertise in perioperative medicine ensures that virtual airway evaluations and preoperative assessments are implemented with clinical rigor, integrated seamlessly into hospital systems, and leveraged to optimize patient outcomes [3, 12]. Multiple studies and institutional programs demonstrate that tele-anesthesia maintains safety and satisfaction while improving access and operational efficiency, providing anesthesiologists a proven platform to lead value-based perioperative innovation [5, 7, 10, 11, 16, 18]. Rather than replacing the traditional bedside exam, telemedicine modernizes its principles into a technology-driven format—one that anesthesiologists are uniquely positioned to implement, underscoring their ability to innovate and lead perioperative care while reducing inefficiencies such as unnecessary in-person visits and day-of-surgery cancellations, thereby adding measurable economic value.

References

1. Health Resources and Services Administration (HRSA) [Internet]. What is telehealth? | HRSA. 2022 [cited 2025 June 16]. Available from: https://www.hrsa.gov/telehealth/what-is-telehealth.
2. Telemedicine: a guide to assessing telecommunications for health care [Internet]. Washington, DC: National Academies Press; 1996 [cited 2025 June 16]. Available from: http://www.nap.edu/catalog/5296.
3. Chatrath V, Attri J, Chatrath R. Telemedicine and anaesthesia. Indian J Anaesth. 2010;54(3):199.
4. Bridges KH, McSwain JR, Wilson PR. To infinity and beyond: the past, present, and future of tele-anesthesia. Anesth Analg. 2020;130(2):276–84.
5. Wong DT, Kamming D, Salenieks ME, Go K, Kohm C, Chung F. Preadmission anesthesia consultation using telemedicine technology: a pilot study. Anesthesiology. 2004;100(6):1605–7.
6. Dilisio RP, Dilisio AJ, Weiner MM. Preoperative virtual screening examination of the airway. J Clin Anesth. 2014;26(4):315–7.
7. Reddy K, Awuku K, Shah YM, Tewfik G, Xiong M, Spivack E, et al. A validation pilot study comparing telemedicine images to a face-to-face airway exam for conducting the anesthesia preoperative airway evaluation. Open J Anesthesiol. 2021;11(07):207–18.
8. Mihalj M, Carrel T, Gregoric ID, Andereggen L, Zinn PO, Doll D, et al. Telemedicine for preoperative assessment during a COVID-19 pandemic: recommendations for clinical care. Best Pract Res Clin Anaesthesiol. 2020;34(2):345–51.
9. Incorporating airway examination photography into the electronic record. Rom J Anaesth Intensive Care [Internet]. 2017 [cited 2025 June 16];24(1). Available from: http://www.jurnalul-anestezie.ro/archive/y2017/n1/a2.
10. Mullen-Fortino M, Rising KL, Duckworth J, Gwynn V, Sites FD, Hollander JE. Presurgical assessment using telemedicine technology: impact on efficiency, effectiveness, and patient experience of care. Telemed E-Health. 2019;25(2):137–42.
11. Kamdar NV, Huverserian A, Jalilian L, Thi W, Duval V, Beck L, et al. Development, implementation, and evaluation of a telemedicine preoperative evaluation initiative at a major academic medical center. Anesth Analg. 2020;131(6):1647–56.
12. Umeh UO, Roediger F, Cuff G, Romanenko Y, Vaz A, Hertling A. Satisfaction with telemedicine among anesthesiologists during the COVID-19 pandemic. Trends Anaesth Crit Care. 2022;45:32–6.
13. Burton R, Boedeker B. Application of telemedicine in a pain clinic: the changing face of medical practice. Pain Med. 2000;1(4):351–7.

14. Zetterman CV, Sweitzer BJ, Webb B, Barak-Bernhagen MA, Boedeker BH. Validation of a virtual preoperative evaluation clinic: a pilot study. Stud Health Technol Inform. 2011;163:737–9.
15. Jacobs K, Blanchard B, Baker N. Telehealth and ergonomics: a pilot study. Technol Health Care. 2012;20(5):445–58.
16. Applegate RL, Gildea B, Patchin R, Rook JL, Wolford B, Nyirady J, et al. Telemedicine pre-anesthesia evaluation: a randomized pilot trial. Telemed E-Health. 2013;19(3):211–6.
17. Ekeland AG, Bowes A, Flottorp S. Effectiveness of telemedicine: a systematic review of reviews. Int J Med Inform. 2010;79(11):736–71.
18. Roberts S, Spain B, Hicks C, London J, Tay S. Telemedicine in the Northern Territory: an assessment of patient perceptions in the preoperative anaesthetic clinic: telemedicine in the Northern Territory. Aust J Rural Health. 2015;23(3):136–41.

After the RFP: Building Sustainable Partnerships Between Anesthesia Practices and Hospitals

37

Shena J. Scott, Jason Greenberg, Joseph W. Szokol, and Jay Mesrobian

37.1 Introduction

It is imperative that every anesthesia practice, either big or small, continually demonstrates its value proposition to its partner healthcare organization, highlighting service, efficiency, patient care, quality, and patient experience. Even the best anesthesia practices may see the facility with which they partner solicits a request for proposal (RFP) for anesthesia services. Whether you are the incumbent group or a new practice seeking an opportunity, it is critical to view the process unemotionally and seek to both understand the motivations behind the RFP and how best to respond to the RFP. It is vital that the responding practice consider what resources are available to best manage the next steps. This may be as simple as utilizing internal resources or may require the help of external resources familiar with these proposals. Understanding the competition and best positioning a response is critical to a favorable outcome. Finally, it is important that the respondent has a strong relationship with facility's administration and providers,

S. J. Scott
Scott Healthcare Consulting, Inc., Melbourne, FL, USA

J. Greenberg
Department of Anesthesia and Perioperative Care, University of California San Francisco, San Francisco, CA, USA

J. W. Szokol (✉)
David Geffen School of Medicine at UCLA, Department of Anesthesiology and Perioperative Medicine, UCLA Health, Los Angeles, CA, USA

American Society of Anesthesiologists, Schaumberg, IL, USA

Department of Anesthesiology, Critical Care, and Pain Medicine, NorthShore University HealthSystem, Evanston, IL, USA

J. Mesrobian
Advocate Aurora Health, Milwaukee, WI, USA

G. Tewfik (ed.), *The Anesthesiologist as Perioperative Leader*,
https://doi.org/10.1007/978-3-032-18058-2_37

has a well-defined value proposition, and positions themselves for success. Whichever practice is ultimately selected must realize that the work has just begun. The transition is just as important as the pitch, and continuing to strengthen and communicate your value proposition is key.

37.2 Discussion

Consider this (not uncommon) scenario: Clueless Anesthesia Group (CAG) has been providing exclusive services at Hospital XYZ for over 15 years, and suddenly they learn that the hospital has put out a request for proposal (RFP) for anesthesia services. CAG feels caught off guard, hurt, and angry—what should they do?

Find the trigger The first step is to assess what are the motivations behind the hospital publishing an RFP. Finding out the contents of the RFP is essential. The group needs to know why the facility is considering changing partners and what specific concerns triggered this decision. Possibilities include:

1. The hospital may have requested services (more operating room coverage, additional non-operating room locations, a perioperative surgical home [PSH], a more robust quality program, or other service enhancements) that the group has been slow, or unwilling, to provide.
2. The hospital may not realize the full extent of current services provided. For instance, the group may be providing PSH or enhanced quality services but failed to communicate to the hospital its "value adds." The CAG has failed to demonstrate its value proposition. It is critical to demonstrate how your group is better than the competition and support the assertion with data that align with facility's values.
3. The hospital may be frustrated with group communication. Perhaps group leaders do not engage well or are not visible to hospital leadership. The group may not schedule regular meetings with hospital leadership, including the Chief Executive, Operations, Medical, Nursing, Information Officers, etc. The reality is that an RFP will often not be surprising to the incumbent group if it is regularly communicating with the C-Suite. If the C-Suite is unhappy about something, the group should be hearing about it before an RFP is issued.
4. The group may not manage itself well, allowing disruptive behavior or failing to act upon recurring complaints about physicians. When a physician group fails to manage its own liabilities, often the onus falls on the facility partner to manage this risk, which may quickly sour the relationship.
5. "Wild Cards" that may be buried in as RFP: requirements to be in-network with all hospital payers; requirements to accept hospital-negotiated rates; selection of leadership; performance metrics. If a group does not contract with all insurers, it will throw some patients out of network and lead to potential complaints to the facility.

6. The group may have recently requested additional support and/or terminated the contract "to put the negotiation on a timeline." Often significantly increased subsidy needs will in itself trigger the facility to "consider its options."
7. The hospital may have new leadership that is trying to level-set service requirements or define the market rate. Understanding the trigger will help the group determine what to emphasize if deciding to respond to the RFP, which is really its first decision point to address. Other, relevant questions will often follow. Does the group want to provide a response? If the group has been unwilling or unable to meet the hospital's needs, is it willing and/or capable of making the necessary changes to win the bid now? Are the parties aligned in their mission and/or goals for the anesthesia service? And if the hospital has unreasonable cost expectations for the service level it is requesting, how far will the group go to maintain the contract?

Respond professionally Successfully responding to an RFP means putting forth your best offer and showcasing your strengths, but it also provides the incumbent group an opportunity to assess their own weaknesses. It is important not to get emotional about the hospital's business decision to explore its options. And it is essential to concentrate in a positive way on your value proposition as it compares to potential competitors. Ultimately, the group must understand that a hospital contract is a business agreement, and periodic due diligence is a reasonable practice for both stakeholders.

Evaluate your organization's capabilities in the context of competitor performance An incumbent group facing a RFP must understand not only its own strengths and weaknesses, but those of potential competitors. This framing must be assessed from the perspective of the hospital or facility administration. Strengths may include positive relationships with surgeons and administrators, ability to recruit regionally, collaborative staffing, and reliable revenue cycle management with strong payer contracts. On the other hand, weaknesses may include strained relationships with surgeons, inability to recruit, inflexible staffing, and outdated revenue cycle management. To form a solid value proposition and competitive bid, the incumbent group must assess its weaknesses honestly and address how it will address them clearly.

Given workforce and recruitment challenges in anesthesiology, the incumbent group should understand the market for services when forming its bid. A group needs to consider the competitive landscape. Perhaps you are a large multispecialty group in a high-cost, extremely tight anesthesia market. Anesthesiology in 2025 is facing significant shortages in the United States and it may be difficult, or near impossible, to replace an incumbent group. Additionally, a large multispecialty group may be hard to replace based on its coverage of many hospital services, such as pain, ICU, regional blocks, and other specialty services. What is the reasonable likelihood another group could truly replace your group? If that is the case, weigh your leverage in your response. Alternatively, if your market is flush with resources, your group is small, and your facility is considered desirable, you will have less leverage.

Engage consultants While many smaller groups are reluctant to spend the money, it may be "penny wise and pound foolish" not to engage professional help in this situation. There are consultants who have experience with this type of work. An unbiased and experienced outsider can ask the tough questions and help the group assess what items and services it needs to emphasize in its response. An experienced professional can assist in determining an optimal staffing model and appropriate cost structure, as well as how to best market yourself and create a presentation that showcases your strengths and ability to partner with the facility.

Understand what may be called for in an RFP Essential elements that are common to almost any RFP: staffing levels and model; quality program; pro forma development; type of financial support (cost plus, revenue guarantee, fixed subsidy).

Create an exceptional proposal Once the group understands which strengths to emphasize/weaknesses to acknowledge (and, more importantly, solutions to offer), responding to the RFP becomes straightforward. Read carefully through the questions and gather your documentation for answers. Be sure to note any restrictions to the process, such as timelines and prohibitions against speaking with members of hospital administration and/or the medical staff about the RFP. This element regarding communication is critical for all group members to understand, as one person having a prohibited conversation could jeopardize the group's bid. Often, the document will ask for background about the group and its members. This is an opportunity for an incumbent group to highlight past efforts to advance hospital causes. Do not assume that the RFP evaluators know any history, and do not feel defensive about needing to explain your past contributions. Take time to update requested CVs into a uniform, professional format. Be sure to highlight specialty training like fellowships and certifications, and emphasize your clinicians' depth/strength to handle key services such as regional anesthesia or high-risk obstetrics.

Highlight your leadership The value of strong and effective leadership cannot be overstated. The hospital must trust in the group's leadership. This leadership must be demonstrated in the operating rooms, non-operating room anesthesia (NORA), in patient safety, and in its relations with hospital administration. The RFP will likely ask about leadership. If you know that the hospital has issues with an incumbent leader, your group may need to assess its current leadership and consider changes for group survival. Make certain you include viable alternatives and/or a transition plan to include someone that you know will be more acceptable.

Many groups find that a hospital has put out an RFP because they are unhappy with several members of the group which it finds disruptive. If you have a physician who you know is considered "problematic," explain your action plan to address that.

Better yet, demonstrate actionable changes to your governing documents to facilitate proactive management of future disruptive group members.

Highlight your quality Often, an RFP will ask about quality initiatives and group willingness to tie some reimbursement to performance. If you have not had a strong quality performance program in the past, provide a detailed description of the program you will create. Know that you cannot make empty promises—the RFP response is often binding, but even if not, a group should honor commitments. You will likely have an opportunity to talk about efficiency initiatives—from the past or for the future. If the hospital has asked for a small group of "anesthesiologists in charge," but your group has not developed a plan for this, do so now. The same applies to other service indicators—explain what you have done and how you will expand these efforts in the future. Many small groups provide elements of a PSH (assisting with preoperative testing protocols and clearance, enhanced recovery after surgery [ERAS] protocols, and/or developing a strong regional anesthesia program to improve ambulation and reduce length of stay) even if they have not marketed it as such. Now is the time to explain what you have done and how you will expand your efforts. If you have data to support how you have reduced cancellations and/or length of stay to improve the hospital's bottom line, be sure to share that in your response and presentation.

Consider all options The RFP will likely include a detailed description of services to be covered. It is critically important to look at different ways to staff the service and compare costs. For example, if you are an all-physician group, you need to consider pricing a care team model as well because you know that competitors will. Even if your group does not want to staff it as a care team should it win the bid, you need to put forward the most competitive price if you want the opportunity to provide the service, with the understanding that hiring of CRNAs or Certified Anesthesiologists Assistants (CAAs) may be difficult in this market and setting reasonable expectations for a timeline to execute.

If the request is for less service than the group currently provides, mention this fact and highlight the value adds that are not being considered in the current request. If you think the data supplied is unworkable based upon experience, provide your answer based upon the information supplied to facilitate "apples to apples" comparison with competitors (who lack experience to identify the discrepancy and will answer based upon data provided). But also consider providing a second response explaining the discrepancy and how that will influence your bid. Valuation of services can be particularly difficult for small- or medium-sized groups. Most physicians have little experience assessing full time equivalent (FTE) needs, understanding benchmarks, and weighing that against hospital expectations. If you have never enlisted professional help, now may be the time to do so. Finally, be sure to include transition costs if you will be expecting facility assistance. Particularly as the incumbent, you may have an advantage if you already have the staff, but locums are expensive and hiring can take time, so be realistic in considering those costs if you have lost staff because of delayed negotiations or due to the RFP process itself.

The bottom line Be sure that both your written response and presentation are concise, well-written (avoid grammatical or spelling mistakes), and presented in an appealing, professional format. A consultant will be very helpful in providing exemplars of previous RFP responses. This is your chance to market yourself, so put your best foot forward. Do not anticipate an opportunity to negotiate after the fact, as you may not win the bid. Offer the most competitive price that you can, include all the services you can reasonably provide, and then allow the process to commence. If someone else is willing to do it for less than your best offer, they will likely sacrifice quality, take a loss, or fail. You have not lost if you have put forth your best assessment and could not match the winning bid. At that point, it might be better to move on or go to work for that person and let them pay your salary rather than using your salary to supplement payment to others because of "winning" a below-market award.

After the award If your group is selected, know that this is just the beginning, not the end. Bear in mind what triggered this process and begin working on strengthening and communicating your value proposition to avert a future RFP. It is critically important to understand that the hospital wants a partner in the perioperative environment and the group that meets that expectation will succeed.

37.3 Subtopic: Our Group Was Awarded the Contract. Now What?

In 2022, Dr. Szokol, Dr. Greenberg, and Ms. Scott wrote an article titled "Your Hospital Put Out an RFP—What Do You Do Now?" The articleended with a simple statement: "If your group is selected, know that this is the beginning, not the end. Bear in mind what triggered this process and begin working on strengthening and communicating your value proposition to avert a future RFP."

In most RFP processes, the client will identify the key needs and expectations that underlie the need for the RFP. They will identify what services are desirable in a new partner. Yet even in a thorough RFP process, the level of detail provided by the client can vary greatly. There are always issues that are not revealed during the RFP process and likely to surface after start of a new contract. The new group also will not have had the chance to meet many of the key stakeholders, clinical and nonclinical, with whom it will be working.

After a decision is made to transition to a new anesthesiology group or employment model, it is critical that the client and anesthesiology group put in place a foundation—processes and communication—that allows both to share information, build relationships, and support a successful partnership. Below is one description of how to build a foundation, based upon one key underlying principle: consistent and structured communication between the client and practice.

37.4 Work Toward a Smooth Transition

The primary goal is to ensure that on day one, your team is ready to provide services with no or minimal disruption. Key steps include:

- Establish an onboarding team that will work with the client using agreed upon milestones and timelines up to and after the contract start date. This team will identify and work with key contacts at the facility related (but not limited) to:
  - Clinician privileging
  - Payer contracting
  - EHR training
  - On-site orientation
  - Quality reporting
  - Mandatory training, if applicable, around human resources and compliance
- Ensure clinical and operational leaders meet the incumbent anesthesiologists and anesthetists. This meeting should take place as soon as feasible, ideally soon after the transition is announced. Depending upon the RFP process, the incumbent clinicians may have had little or no knowledge of the change until it became public. This meeting may be the new leadership's first opportunity to start building trust with the clinicians and is critical for a successful transition. Key elements include:
  - Hold the meeting in person and, unless prohibited, involve client leadership to demonstrate a unified partnership around shared goals.
  - Describe your group's history, experiences, and culture around anesthesiology practice management.
  - Listen and gain understanding of how the clinicians view their challenges. Acknowledge that you do not know everything about the practice but are committed to partnering with them to address the needs identified by the client.
  - Describe your approach to group leadership and management. Will you keep existing leadership in place? Will you honor already scheduled call and vacation? How do you support clinicians?
  - Be prepared to review compensation and benefits. If you have had the chance to review existing compensation, commit to sending the clinicians detailed proposals after the meeting. If you have not had the chance to review existing compensation, commit to doing so within a specified time period.
  - Set up recurring scheduled meetings with both practice leaders and clinicians.
  - Meet with key surgeon and proceduralist stakeholders to gain additional perspective and understanding.
  - Be prepared to discuss how you will provide site leadership and sufficient staffing should some of the incumbent clinicians opt not to join your practice.
- Set realistic and honest expectations with the client around key aspects of the transition, including retention of existing group, potential (and likely) use of part-time and/or locums tenens clinicians during transition, and financial impact. Establishing (if necessary) strong and reliable transitional leadership onsite is essential for success.

37.5 Establish and Review Quarterly Goals with Client Senior Leadership

The primary purpose is to mutually identify quarterly goals with client senior leadership. Participants should include senior practice leaders (e.g., Practice President/ Senior Vice-President, Chief Operating Officer, Chief Financial Officer) and the client's C-suite (e.g., CEO, CMO, CNO, COO, CFO) as applicable.

- The focus of this meeting is highly strategic and is designed around client needs and goals.
- Identify the client's goals with respect to recruitment, financial performance, operational performance, program development, and clinical quality.
- At each quarterly meeting, share progress toward the goals. Collaboratively discuss progress, resources, and tools necessary to advance the work.
- Benefits of this strategic meeting include:
  - Clearly identifying the resources that the practice and/or client may need to deploy
  - Establishing practice leadership as the clinical and operational "experts and problem solvers" at the facility
  - Creating joint accountability between the practice and client
  - Updating the client on high level issues around litigation, payer strategies, or legislative/regulatory changes
- After each meeting, the practice should send a summary email to the C-suite stakeholders, including key discussion points, decisions made, and relevant data.

37.6 Establish Monthly Communication with Client Clinical and Operational Leadership

The purpose of this meeting is to provide standardized tactical communication to the client around key clinical and operational issues. Participants may include practice leaders (e.g. Department Chief, Chief Anesthetist, Vice-President Operations) and client leaders and/or key managers (e.g. Director Perioperative Services; Chair-Department of Surgery; Director-Quality and/or CMO/CNO).

- The practice should prepare a standard client-facing report including updates on the following performance indicators:
  - Recruitment and retention
  - Staffing
  - Quality metrics (e.g. Merit-based Incentive Payment System [MIPS], contract performance metrics)
  - Operational metrics (OR utilization, workforce optimization)
  - Financial performance (revenue, clinician expense, premium labor)

- The practice can also use this meeting to update the client on specific value-added initiatives related to clinical quality, clinical operations, patient experience, or education.
- The practice can provide insight into opportunities around wellness, recognition, clinician support.
- Benefits of this monthly meeting include:
  - Joint review of performance metrics and identification of opportunities to improve performance.
  - Opportunity to show a solutions-based mindset: introduce new ideas around recruitment, staffing, perioperative operations, quality, or performance improvement.
  - Confirm the practice is responding to the client's needs and issues.
  - Provide peer recognition for both clinicians and staff.
- Again, after each meeting, the practice should send a summary email to the C-suite stakeholders, including key discussion points, decisions made, and relevant data.

37.7 Summary

Once a practice is awarded a new contract, its work is just beginning. While this work will differ depending upon practice size, complexity, and culture, it always will be necessary for a new practice to create alignment between both client and clinicians. Consistent and transparent communication, a solutions-oriented approach, and willingness to address problems promptly are foundational pieces of a reliable partnership between client and practice.

References

1. Greenberg J, Scott S, Szokol J. Your hospital put out an RFP-what do you do now? ASA Monit. 2022;86(8):1–7. https://doi.org/10.1097/01.ASM.0000855608.56982.30.
2. Creating and Communicating Your Value Proposition. RFP Response Essentials. American Society of Anesthesiologists. Committee on Practice Management. 2022. https://www.asahq.org/quality-and-practice-management/managing-your-practice/value-proposition. If not, an ASA member material excerpted from The Compendium: Creating and Communicating Your Value Proposition RFP Response Essentials/2023. Developed by: The American Society of Anesthesiologists Committee on Practice Management. Contact info@asahq.org for access to the materials.
3. Requesting Hospital Assistance for Undercompensated Services. American Society of Anesthesiologists. 2024. https://www.asahq.org/about-asa/governance-and-committees/asa-committees/committee-on-practice-management/requesting-hospital-assistance-for-undercompensated-services. If not, an ASA member material excerpted from The Compendium: Creating and Communicating Your Value Proposition RFP Response Essentials/2023. Developed by: The American Society of Anesthesiologists Committee on Practice Management. Contact info@asahq.org for access to the materials.

Anesthesiologists in Hospital Leadership: Bridging the Gap with Regulatory and Accrediting Organizations

38

Michael Simon and Matthew Popovich

38.1 Introduction

Hospitals operate and compete in an environment defined by clinical excellence, operational efficiency, and adherence to a vast array of regulatory and accreditation standards. Administrators are constantly striving to meet regulatory burdens, avoid payment penalties, and remain in the top tier of rated institutions within their geographic location. It is impossible for facilities to do this without the contributions of physicians, nurses, and other health care professionals. Compliance with ever-changing regulatory requirements takes buy-in and cooperation from every division and department within an institution.

Among the diverse team of health care professionals, anesthesiologists stand out as pivotal figures, uniquely positioned to guide hospital leadership in navigating regulatory requirements set forth by federal authorities like the Centers for Medicare & Medicaid Services (CMS), state agencies, and accrediting organizations like The Joint Commission (TJC), Det Norske Veritas (DNV), and others.[1] This chapter explores how anesthesiologists, with their multifaceted expertise, contribute indispensable value to hospital leadership in maintaining compliance and achieving excellence in patient care, care coordination, operating room management, infection control, and other features of regulatory compliance. You will find that their reach extends far beyond the individual operating theater and touches the majority of the institution.

The health care industry is subjected to an ever-growing number of regulations designed to ensure patient safety, quality care, and operational accountability. These

[1] Insert names of accrediting organizations.

M. Simon (✉)
HCA Florida Memorial Hospital, Jacksonville, FL, USA

M. Popovich
American Society of Anesthesiologists, Washington, DC, USA

G. Tewfik (ed.), *The Anesthesiologist as Perioperative Leader*,
https://doi.org/10.1007/978-3-032-18058-2_38

regulations originate from federal, state, and standard setting organizations, creating a complex web that healthcare facilities must navigate to receive reimbursement and maintain licensure and accreditation status. Adherence to these requirements is complex and requires partnership between clinical and non-clinical staff as well as continuous attention to detail.

38.2 Federal and State Legislative Oversight in Accreditation

Facility accreditation is not governed solely by private accrediting organizations, but rather it is also influenced by federal and state oversight to shape the standards and enforcement mechanisms. Federal and state entities ensure that accrediting organizations, healthcare facilities, and health care professionals meet minimum standards for adherence to laws, the safeguarding of public health, and the support of patient safety.

38.2.1 Federal Oversight

CMS, housed within the US Department of Health and Human Services (HHS), is the federal authority overseeing accreditation through its Conditions of Participation (CoPs). CMS often applies standards and regulations from other HHS departments within the CoPs. Other HHS agencies establish overarching healthcare policies, including regulations for patient privacy (Health Insurance Portability and Accountability Act [HIPAA]), compliance with the Affordable Care Act (ACA), and initiatives aimed at reducing healthcare disparities. The Occupational Safety and Health Administration (OSHA) sets standards for workplace safety, including those affecting healthcare workers and patient environments. The Food and Drug Administration (FDA) regulates medical devices and pharmaceuticals that are integral to hospital operations and accreditation compliance. Each of these federal agencies influences the criteria used by Medicare and accrediting organizations to evaluate healthcare facilities, ensuring alignment with federal laws and national healthcare priorities.

38.2.2 State Oversight

State governments play a complementary role in healthcare regulation by setting licensing requirements, conducting inspections, and enforcing compliance with state-specific health codes. State health departments issue licenses to hospitals, ambulatory surgery centers, and other facilities. These licenses are often prerequisites for accreditation and participation in Medicare and Medicaid programs. States implement health programs targeting issues such as infection control, vaccination, and emergency preparedness. States may also mandate reporting of adverse events, infection rates, and other critical metrics, which are often reviewed during accreditation surveys. Anesthesiologists should work with their facility compliance staff to understand state-specific regulations prior to any accreditation survey.

38.2.2.1 CMS and the Conditions of Participation

CMS regulations set the baseline standards that healthcare organizations must meet to participate in Medicare and Medicaid programs. Established in 1965 and expanded to incorporate changes in health care delivery over the past 60 years, the CoPs focus on patient safety, quality of care, and operational excellence. There are more than two dozen CoPs and related Conditions of Coverage administered by CMS. Anesthesiologists typically encounter CoPs related to Hospitals, Ambulatory Surgery Services, and Critical Access Hospitals although other CoPs touch upon Psychiatric Hospitals, Rural Health Clinics, and other locations where anesthesia services may be delivered. Although CMS and state agencies have the power to survey health care facilities, they are unable to survey thousands of facilities for compliance with federal regulations. Due to the sheer volume of institutions, accrediting organizations have been granted "deeming" authority to survey and ensure compliance with the federal CoPs.

The CoPs range in size and focus. Regulations related to hospital accreditation are more than 450 pages in length, while ambulatory surgery center accreditation regulations are just over 150 pages in length. An accrediting organization will survey the facility, its policies and procedures, and medical staff on many issues. In general, there are six key areas for which anesthesiologists should be aware:

1. **Patient Rights:** Ensuring respect for patient autonomy, privacy, and access to care
2. **Quality Assurance and Performance Improvement (QAPI):** Mandating continuous monitoring and improvement of care processes
3. **Infection Control:** Establishing protocols to prevent healthcare-associated infections (HAIs)
4. **Emergency Preparedness:** Requiring readiness for natural disasters, pandemics, and other emergencies
5. **Medical Staff:** Defining credentialing, privileging, and oversight of healthcare providers
6. **Physical Environment:** Ensuring that facilities are safe and meet regulatory standards

CMS, however, must also conduct its due diligence on the work of accrediting organizations. CMS collaborates with accrediting organizations that have deeming authority, and the agency also conducts its own "validation surveys" to verify the effectiveness of accrediting organizations' evaluations. During these surveys, CMS surveyors will focus on facility documentation, observing clinical processes and workflows and interviewing staff to assess their understanding of regulations and protocols.

38.2.2.2 Deeming Authority

A critical concept in healthcare regulation is "deeming authority." This refers to the power granted by CMS to accrediting organizations to assess and determine whether healthcare facilities comply with the CoPs. Organizations with CMS deeming authority serve as intermediaries, ensuring that hospitals adhere to federal standards while also fostering quality and safety.

Deeming authority streamlines the regulatory process. Rather than undergoing multiple inspections, hospitals can focus on meeting the standards of a single accrediting body, which in turn reports compliance to CMS. This framework underscores the importance of collaboration between hospital leadership and accrediting organizations with anesthesiologists playing a vital role in ensuring that operational and clinical practices align with these requirements.

38.2.2.3 The Joint Commission (TJC)

Established through a collaboration of the American College of Surgeons (ACS), the American Medical Association (AMA), the American Hospital Association (AHA), and the Canadian Medical Association (CMA), The Joint Commission on Accreditation of Hospitals (JCAH) was founded in 1951 with a mission aimed to create a comprehensive framework for assessing hospital quality. Over the decades, JCAH's role expanded to include other healthcare settings, leading to its rebranding as The Joint Commission (TJC) in 1987.

Today, TJC is an independent, nonprofit organization that accredits nearly 22,000 healthcare organizations in the United States. It is governed by a Board of Commissioners comprised of individuals selected by the founding members as well as public members whose skillsets and abilities fulfill needs of the Board. Its accreditation process includes rigorous, unannounced, and announced surveys conducted by teams of experts in healthcare quality, management, and safety.

Hospitals under The Joint Commission's purview must meet additional requirements that exceed those outlined by the CoPs. Those requirements include adherence to National Patient Safety Goals (NPSGs) and other evidence-based practices that improve clinical outcomes. TJC uses its Elements of Performance (EPs) by which it assesses institutions. These standards have made The Joint Commission a global influencer in patient safety and quality improvement. The organization's history underscores its commitment to evolving with the healthcare landscape, continually updating its standards to address emerging challenges such as electronic health records, telemedicine, and population health management.

38.2.2.4 DNV Healthcare (Det Norske Veritas)

DNV Healtcare's origin dates back to 1864 in Oslo, Norway. Although DNV began in the shipping industry, assessing and inspecting merchant marine vessels, their expertise grew into other industries, including healthcare. DNV became experts in assessing and mitigating risk, an expertise that has many applications. DNV integrates the ISO 9001 Quality Management System standards into its accreditation process. This methodology emphasizes continuous improvement, risk management, and organizational resilience. DNV's focus on fostering a culture of quality aligns closely with the goals of many progressive healthcare institutions. Through their unique process, DNV is able to assess clinical excellence with operational efficiency, supporting hospitals in achieving long-term sustainability.

38.2.2.5 Accreditation Commission for Health Care (ACHC)

Hospital accreditation from the Accreditation Commission for Health Care (ACHC) has evolved in recent years as the organization acquired other accrediting organizations and a number of facilities they accredit. ACHC focuses on a commitment to quality improvement, ensuring their accredited facilities deliver "consistent, safe, high-quality care to their patients."

38.2.2.6 Accreditation Association for Ambulatory Health Care (AAAHC)

AAAHC is a leading accreditor of ambulatory care facilities, including surgery centers and outpatient clinics. It focuses on promoting high-quality, patient-centered care in non-hospital settings.

38.2.2.7 Center for Improvement in Healthcare Quality (CIHQ)

CIHQ has enjoyed deeming authority since 1999. They advertise themselves as a more cost-effective alternative providing accreditation services to hospitals and other healthcare facilities. CIHQ places a strong emphasis on ensuring compliance with CMS standards.

38.2.2.8 Institute for Medical Quality (IMQ)

IMQ, another newer player in the accreditation space, focuses on accrediting outpatient facilities, particularly in California. Its standards emphasize infection prevention, clinical competency, and patient-centered care, making it a trusted partner for many ambulatory surgery centers.

38.2.2.9 QUAD A

Originally named the American Association for Accreditation of Ambulatory Surgery Facilities or "AAAASF," the QUAD A focuses on office-based and ambulatory surgery centers.

38.3 Role of State Departments of Health

State departments of health are critical regulators in the healthcare ecosystem. They oversee licensing and certification, conduct inspections, and ensure compliance with both state and federal laws. These departments often collaborate with accrediting organizations to streamline the regulatory process. For example, a hospital may undergo a state inspection in conjunction with an accreditation survey to ensure comprehensive compliance. When national accreditors find issues during a survey, they may involve the individual state department of health, triggering additional surveys and scrutiny. Additionally, state health departments play a vital role in public health initiatives, emergency preparedness, and infection control, areas where anesthesiologists often contribute their expertise. The rules and regulations promulgated by each state's department of health can vary greatly. While anesthesiologists often focus on national accreditation requirements, anesthesiologists must always remain mindful of local statutes first.

38.4 Anesthesiologists, Anesthesia Departments, and the Accreditation Survey

Accreditation surveys may occur as part of a three-year review cycle, as a follow-up for cited deficiencies or for other issues that may come to the attention of federal and state regulators as well as accrediting organizations. Anesthesiologists and their groups should be knowledgeable of facility-level compliance requirements as well as perioperative and operating room policies and procedures. For a successful survey, anesthesiologists and their departments should be aware of the CoPs as well as how the hospital implements those policies.

Facility-wide policies and procedures span a range of topics, including the staff organization and by-laws, physician leadership structure, infection control, patient intake and discharge, and documentation requirements. Surveyors may also ask health care personnel to describe where certain physician equipment is available, such as the location of fire extinguishers, call buttons, or emergency exits. Surveyors may also ask about facility-wide policies on infection prevention, patient safety, or patient engagement features. Facility-wide policies and procedures are often developed by multidisciplinary groups composed of physicians and non-clinical staff. When appropriate and relevant, anesthesia departments should identify a specific representative to sit on and participate in those committees and meetings.

Surveyors are required to review policies and procedures across individual departments throughout the hospital, and those reviews often intersect with anesthesiologist actions. A review of pharmaceutical services by a surveyor may indicate facility-wide training is required on aseptic technique within the hospitals policies and procedures. A review of surgical services will look at surgical consent forms. However, anesthesiologists may be required to provide their anesthesia consent forms as well if included in hospital policies and procedures. Reviews of credentialing or privileging criteria may also require anesthesiologist to ensure compliance with hospital policies. Infection control and prevention are also sources for enhanced scrutiny during accreditation surveys. Anesthesia departments should identify those cross-department policies and procedures and identify committees or compliance professionals for further understanding how anesthesiologists can contribute to a successful survey of the hospital and other departments.

Most anesthesiologists and their departments will encounter surveys within the perioperative environment and in the administration of anesthesia services. Anesthesia services are located within federal statute at §482.52. CMS and its deeming organizations will review adherence to those rules and regulations as well as any hospital and department implementation policies and procedures on file.

Anesthesia departments, including anesthesiologists and members of the anesthesia care team, should be aware of these regulations and local policies and procedures.

Anesthesia services require a physician, typically an anesthesiologist, to be in charge of "all anesthesia administered in the hospital." The CoPs clearly define different types of anesthesia, paraphrasing American Society of Anesthesiologists (ASA) guidance, and who may administer anesthesia to patients. The CoPs also define medical direction and supervision requirements, offering facilities and anesthesia departments-specific direction on establishing and implementing an anesthesia service. Those rules and regulations also govern preoperative and postoperative evaluation requirements as well as intraoperative anesthesia records.

In developing anesthesia-specific policies and procedures, anesthesia departments and facilities often build off those base requirements found in the CoPs with supplemental standards, guidelines, and standards from the ASA and other anesthesia specialty societies. Anesthesia departments may also work across the ASA and among peers to understand best practices and processes when official policy of the ASA or other subject matter organization does not exist. Supplementing policies and procedures with recent literature or best practices ensures that anesthesiologists are adhering to practices well beyond the CoPs.

Surveyors may negatively cite the facility based upon their review of anesthesia services. When a citation occurs, anesthesiologists and their departments should work with their compliance officers and others to understand how to address the citation and implement a corrective action plan. For anesthesiologists, citations may occur on any number of actions within the hospital, but citations are likely to occur when the practice does not follow local policies and procedures. Citations sometimes include, but are not limited to, documentation requirements, adherence to pre- and post-anesthesia evaluation processes, surgical attire, open supplies, hand hygiene, cleaning of the anesthesia cart between cases, and other infection control scenarios.

Other citations may be related to either new or novel workflows or equipment that is used outside of the manufacturer's or hospital's guidance. In recent years, anesthesiologists have debated the costs and benefits of reusable and disposable laryngoscopes. In those cases, facilities and anesthesia departments need to find a common solution to follow and ensure the policy is implemented. Technology also plays a role, especially regarding patient access to records. Facilities and anesthesiologists need to clearly define when an anesthesia record should be made available to the patient or their caregiver, especially if the technology allows for near real-time access to records during the intraoperative period. Regardless of the cause for a citation, after the survey is completed, anesthesia departments should work with their facility compliance officers on addressing these citations and creating a corrective action plan or other materials to meet CoPs, local policy, and procedure requirements.

38.4.1 The Anesthesiologist as a Systems Thinker

Anesthesiologists are trained to think holistically. While one of their primary responsibilities lies in managing patient care in the operating room, procedural area, and throughout the perioperative period, their expertise extends to areas such as patient safety, infection control, critical care, and pain management just to name a few. These competencies make them uniquely equipped to address the cross-disciplinary challenges posed by regulatory and accrediting organizations.

1. Patient Safety Advocates

Patient safety is a cornerstone of accreditation standards. Anesthesiologists are inherently patient safety advocates, as their role demands vigilance in monitoring physiological parameters, preventing adverse events, and managing crises. Their commitment to safety aligns seamlessly with the goals of accreditation bodies, making them effective partners in:

- **Developing and Implementing Protocols:** Anesthesiologists often lead the creation of evidence-based protocols for managing surgical site infections, venous thromboembolism, airway emergencies, trauma, and mass casualty events. These protocols are critical for meeting the patient safety goals outlined by accrediting organizations.
- **Root Cause Analysis:** When adverse events occur, anesthesiologists' clinical expertise and analytical skills are vital for conducting root cause analyses and developing actionable solutions.

2. Leaders in Quality Improvement

Quality improvement (QI) is a shared priority for accrediting bodies and hospital leadership. Anesthesiologists, with their data-driven approach to patient care, are natural leaders in QI initiatives. They play a key role in:

- **Measuring Outcomes:** By analyzing metrics such as surgical morbidity and mortality, post-operative complications, and anesthesia-related adverse events, anesthesiologists provide actionable insights that drive QI efforts.
- **Championing Evidence-Based Practices:** Their familiarity with the latest research enables the anesthesiologist to advocate for, and implement, practices that improve patient outcomes and align with accreditation standards.
- **Fostering Interdisciplinary Collaboration:** The anesthesiologists' ability to work across departments makes them effective facilitators of hospital-wide QI initiatives. This is an advantage other disciplines and providers often lack, giving anesthesiologists a very unique perspective.

3. Compliance with National Patient Safety Goals (NPSGs)
For Institutions that utilize The Joint Commission for their accreditation, an adherence to NPSGs is required. This is an example of going beyond the COPs. The NPSGs address critical areas such as infection prevention, medication safety, and communication. Anesthesiologists contribute to compliance by:

- Ensuring proper handoff communication during perioperative care
- Implementing measures to prevent wrong-site surgeries and retained surgical items
- Advocating for best practices in antimicrobial stewardship

38.4.1.1 Anesthesiologists and Operational Excellence

Beyond their clinical contributions, anesthesiologists are instrumental in achieving operational excellence. Their role encompasses:

1. Optimization of Perioperative Services
The perioperative environment is one of the most resource-intensive areas of a hospital. Anesthesiologists are critical to its optimization, ensuring both efficiency and compliance with regulatory standards. Their contributions include:

- **Surgical Scheduling:** By balancing case complexity, patient acuity, and staff availability, anesthesiologists help maximize operating room utilization while minimizing delays.
- **Enhanced Recovery Pathways:** Anesthesiologists lead initiatives such as Enhanced Recovery After Surgery (ERAS), which improve patient outcomes and reduce length of stay—aligning with a focus on value-based care.

2. Emergency Preparedness and Risk Management
Both The Joint Commission and DNV emphasize the importance of emergency preparedness. Anesthesiologists, with their expertise in crisis management, play a crucial role in:

- **Developing Response Plans:** Their experience in managing critical events, such as trauma, malignant hyperthermia, or massive transfusions, informs hospital-wide emergency protocols.
- **Simulation Training:** Anesthesiologists often spearhead simulation-based training for high-risk scenarios, enhancing the readiness of interdisciplinary teams.

38.4.1.2 The Bridge Between Clinical Care and Leadership

Hospital leadership often grapples with translating clinical realities into strategic decisions that satisfy accrediting bodies. Anesthesiologists serve as a vital bridge in this process, offering a unique perspective.

1. Clinical Expertise in Strategic Decision-Making
Anesthesiologists' deep understanding of clinical workflows and patient care dynamics allows them to:

- Advocate for investments in technologies and practices that enhance compliance with accreditation standards
- Provide insights into the implications of policy changes on clinical care

2. Education and Training
Compliance with regulatory standards requires continuous education. Anesthesiologists contribute by:

- Leading training sessions that are often multidisciplinary on topics such as infection control, safe medication practices, and patient handoffs.
- Mentoring other clinicians in adopting practices that align with accreditation goals.
- Anesthesiologists oversee all hospital sedation. They are responsible for establishing guidelines for sedation training. In addition there must be regular queries of outcomes and complications associated with sedation.

3. Data-Driven Leadership
The reliance on data in modern healthcare cannot be overstated. Anesthesiologists leverage their familiarity with data collection and interpretation to:

- Develop dashboards that track key performance indicators relevant to accreditation.
- Identify trends and opportunities for improvement. These may be varied and wide-reaching, allowing anesthesiologists to effect positive change throughout the institution.

38.4.1.3 The Role of the American Society of Anesthesiologists (ASA)

The American Society of Anesthesiologists (ASA) is a professional organization dedicated to advancing the practice and science of anesthesiology. One of its crucial roles is supporting its members in navigating the complexities of regulatory compliance and accreditation. The ASA provides an array of resources and tools tailored to help anesthesiologists prepare for accreditation surveys and improve outcomes in their institutions.

Anesthesiologists and their local departments benefit from ASA Standards, Guidelines, and Statements. Updated each year in November and December, these publicly available resources are used by anesthesia departments, hospitals, and other stakeholders to update their policies and procedures. According to its 2021 Statement on Practice Parameters, "Practice standards provide rules or minimum requirements for clinical practice. They are regarded as generally accepted principles of patient management. Standards may be modified only under unusual circumstances, e.g., extreme emergencies or unavailability of equipment." ASA labels practice guidelines as providing "Recommendations for patient care that describe a basic management strategy or a range of basic management strategies."

Practice guidelines include recommendations that are developed based on a systematic review that assesses the quality, quantity, and consistency of evidence.[2] "Evidence-based practice guidelines are not offered or intended as standards or minimum requirements." Practice advisories "provide guidance to assist decision-making in areas of patient care where there is insufficient published research." ASA practice advisories "are based on a systematic review but supported by evidence of limited quality, quantity, or consistency. Practice advisories are not offered or intended as standards, minimum requirements, or guidelines."[3] According to the ASA Administrative Procedures, ASA Statements are guidance documents that do not meet the practice parameter development requirements and are often developed based on a collective opinion or consensus of a convened expert panel. Statements must be approved by the ASA House of Delegates, are updated every 5 years, and are publicly available.[4]

ASA offers several education programs that will assist anesthesiologists and their departments in maintaining compliance with local credentialing and privileging requirements. ASA hosts webinars, workshops, and continuing medical education (CME) courses that focus on regulatory updates, accreditation standards, and quality improvement strategies. These programs equip anesthesiologists with the knowledge needed to lead compliance initiatives effectively. ASA also offers course credit for non-anesthesiologist professionals, including other members of the Anesthesia Care Team, proceduralists, and sedation nurses.

The Anesthesia Quality Institute offers two registries that are beneficial for anesthesiologists and their departments. The AQI National Anesthesia Clinical Outcomes Registry (NACOR) allows groups to benchmark their data against national averages. For those in TJC programs, NACOR can be used support Ongoing Professional Practice Evaluation (OPPE) and Focused Professional Practice Evaluation (FPPE) activities. AQI NACOR can also be used by anesthesiologists to track their performance as it contributes to hospital-based measures required by federal authorities and accrediting organizations. The Anesthesia Incident Reporting System (AIRS) allows any health care professional, including anesthesiologists, to report patient safety, adverse events, or near misses. As a Patient Safety Organization, AQI follows national standards for confidentiality and quality improvement.

ASA provides advocacy and policy support for members through its engagement with accrediting organizations. ASA and its physician experts actively engage with

---

[2] Eden J: *Finding what works in health care: standards for systematic reviews*, National Academies Press, 2011.

[3] American Society of Anesthesiologists. Statement on Practice Parameters. https://www.asahq.org/standards-and-practice-parameters/statement-on-practice-parameters. October 13, 2021. Accessed March 24, 2025.

[4] American Society of Anesthesiologists. Administrative Procedures. November 5, 2024. P. 197.

accrediting organizations and regulatory bodies to ensure that anesthesiology perspectives, workflows, and recent guidelines are considered in accreditation policy development. By advocating for reasonable and effective standards, the ASA helps its members navigate the regulatory landscape more efficiently.

ASA members also have access to collaboration opportunities and sharing of information and best practices. Anesthesiologists and their departments may not realize that the concerns at one facility may also be of concern at other facilities and locations where anesthesiologists work. The ASA fosters collaboration among its members through forums and committees that focus on quality improvement and accreditation readiness. The ASA communities dashboard also allows members to communicate with one another on professional, educational, and clinical issues. Each of these networks allow anesthesiologists to share insights and strategies for meeting regulatory standards.

By leveraging the resources and support offered by the ASA, anesthesiologists are better equipped to lead accreditation efforts and enhance their institutions' compliance with regulatory requirements.

38.4.1.4 The Anesthesiologist's Role in CMS Compliance

Anesthesiologists play a critical role in meeting CMS standards by:

1. **Supporting Quality Assurance Programs:**
   - Leading Quality Assurance and Performance Improvement (QAPI) initiatives focused on perioperative safety and efficiency
   - Monitoring outcomes, such as rates of surgical site infections and anesthesia-related complications, to identify areas for improvement
2. **Enhancing Infection Control Practices:**
   - Implementing evidence-based protocols for sterilization, hand hygiene, and antimicrobial stewardship
   - Educating perioperative staff on infection prevention strategies
3. **Ensuring Documentation Compliance:**
   - Ensuring that anesthesia records, informed consent forms, and other critical documents meet CMS requirements
   - Supporting accurate and complete reporting for quality measures and reimbursement purposes
4. **Participating in Emergency Preparedness:**
   - Contributing expertise to the development of emergency protocols for events such as mass casualties or natural disasters
   - Leading simulation training exercises to enhance readiness

5. **Engaging During Surveys:**
    - Assisting surveyors by providing insights into clinical workflows and quality improvement efforts
    - Demonstrating compliance through examples of successful initiatives, such as Enhanced Recovery After Surgery (ERAS) protocols

By aligning their clinical expertise with CMS requirements, anesthesiologists not only enhance patient safety and outcomes but also ensure their institutions maintain eligibility for Medicare and Medicaid funding.

38.4.1.5 Anesthesiologists' Role in Legislative Compliance

Anesthesiologists play a key role in ensuring that their institutions comply with federal and state regulations. Their contributions include:

1. **Advocating for Compliance:**
    - Monitoring changes in legislation and advising hospital leadership on necessary adaptations to meet new requirements
    - Leading efforts to align clinical protocols with legal and regulatory standards
2. **Participating in Legislative Advocacy:**
    - Engaging with professional organizations, such as the American Society of Anesthesiologists (ASA), to influence policy decisions that affect accreditation and patient care
    - Providing expert testimony or consultation on matters related to perioperative care and patient safety

38.4.1.6 Where Can Anesthesiologists Make a Difference?

Anesthesiologists and their departments play an essential role in **enhancing survey readiness**. Anesthesiologists and their groups must ensure that policies and procedures are not only compliant with accrediting body standards but also with state and federal laws. Anesthesiologists should also act as a liaison between hospital leadership and regulatory agencies during surveys and inspections, especially in perioperative locations. By bridging the gap between legislative requirements and clinical practice, anesthesiologists help their institutions navigate the intricate regulatory landscape, ensuring both compliance and the highest standards of patient care.

The following are examples of the impact of anesthesiologists on hospital compliance and leadership.

38.4.1.7 Enhancing Preoperative Assessment Efficiency

Preoperative delays due to incomplete patient evaluations may lead to increased costs and patient dissatisfaction. Anesthesiologist-led initiatives can streamline the preoperative process by introducing standardized electronic assessment tools and checklists. The results can lead to reductions in surgical delays and improved patient satisfaction scores.

A. Reducing Opioid Dependence in Postoperative Care
Anesthesia departments may seek to address high rates of postoperative opioid use. By championing the implementation of multimodal pain management strategies, including regional anesthesia and non-opioid analgesics, these efforts may lead to reductions in opioid prescriptions, aligning with both accreditation standards and public health goals.

B. Mitigating Risks in Blood Product Utilization
Concerns over inappropriate blood product usage are common. By developing evidence-based, anesthesia-led transfusion protocols and conducting staff training sessions, it is possible to reduce unnecessary transfusions by 25%, enhancing patient safety and meeting accreditation standards.

C. Preventing Surgical Site Infections
Surgical site infections (SSIs) present continued challenges to institutions. In multiple instances, anesthesiologists have spearheaded opportunities to enhance sterile techniques, optimize intraoperative ventilation, and implement evidence-based wound care protocols.

38.4.2 The Survey

This is the moment for the anesthesiologist to shine!

38.5 Conclusion

Anesthesiologists play an indispensable role in hospital leadership, especially to navigate the complex landscape of regulatory and accreditation standards. Their expertise in patient safety, quality improvement, and operational efficiency positions them as vital contributors towards successful compliance with organizations like TJC, DNV, ACHC, AAAHC, CIHQ, IMQ, and state departments of health. By bridging the gap between clinical care and strategic leadership, anesthesiologists not only ensure regulatory compliance, but also drive continuous improvement in healthcare delivery.

Bibliography

1. American Association for Accreditation of Ambulatory Surgery Facilities (AAAASF). About us. https://www.aaaasf.org. Accessed Jan 2025.
2. Accreditation Association for Ambulatory Health Care (AAAHC). Advancing quality in ambulatory health care. https://www.aaahc.org. Accessed Jan 2025.
3. Centers for Medicare & Medicaid Services (CMS). Conditions of Participation (CoPs) and deeming authority. https://www.cms.gov. Accessed Jan 2025.

4. Centers for Medicare & Medicaid Services (CMS). Deeming authority and accreditation of health care providers and suppliers. Federal Register.
5. Center for Improvement in Healthcare Quality (CIHQ). About us. https://www.cihq.org. Accessed Jan 2025.
6. Det Norske Veritas (DNV). Healthcare accreditation and certification. https://www.dnv.com. Accessed Jan 2025.
7. Healthcare Facilities Accreditation Program (HFAP). Standards and accreditation services. https://www.hfap.org. Accessed Jan 2025.
8. Institute for Medical Quality (IMQ). Accreditation services. https://www.imq.org. Accessed Jan 2025.
9. The Joint Commission. About the joint commission. https://www.jointcommission.org. Accessed Jan 2025.
10. The Joint Commission. National patient safety goals. https://www.jointcommission.org/standards/national-patient-safety-goals. Accessed Jan 2025.
11. Enhanced Recovery After Surgery (ERAS) Society. ERAS protocols and guidelines. https://www.erassociety.org. Accessed Jan 2025.

Anesthesiology and Artificial Intelligence: Leading the Next Transformation in Perioperative Medicine

39

Chris Eixenberger and Vikas O'Reilly-Shah

39.1 Introduction

Artificial intelligence (AI) is rapidly reshaping the landscape of many industries, including healthcare. It is no longer a futuristic concept, but a broad set of tools that are already gaining traction in clinical settings and influencing the delivery of healthcare whether directly or indirectly [1–3]. As health systems race to integrate these AI tools, the question is no longer whether these tools will be implemented, but *how*, *where*, and by *whom*.

The success of AI in healthcare hinges on thoughtful implementation, clinical relevance, and continuous oversight. It is crucial to bridge clinical expertise in medicine and health systems with continuously evolving data science. Among all medical specialties, anesthesiologists are uniquely qualified to guide this connection. Anesthesiologists bring a distinct combination of technical fluency, a systems-wide view, collaborative practice, and strong clinical judgement.

This chapter explores the growing role anesthesiologists can, and should, play in shaping the future of AI in medicine, not simply as users of algorithms, but as designers, validators, and stewards of responsible innovation. Their value extends beyond the operating room and into the boardroom, which is evidenced by a growing body of research demonstrating anesthesiology teams' active involvement in developing and validating AI tools. Many of the applications discussed in this chapter emerged directly from these initiatives. Finally, this chapter addresses the risks and challenges inherent in AI, underscoring why anesthesiologists' leadership is critical for responsible integration.

C. Eixenberger (✉) · V. O'Reilly-Shah
Department of Anesthesiology and Pain Medicine, University of Washington, Seattle, WA, USA
e-mail: chriseix@uw.edu

G. Tewfik (ed.), *The Anesthesiologist as Perioperative Leader*,
https://doi.org/10.1007/978-3-032-18058-2_39

39.1.1 AI's Relevance in Perioperative Medicine

Artificial intelligence in healthcare encompasses a wide array of technologies, including machine learning (ML), natural language processing (NLP), and computer vision. The most powerful of these tools fall broadly into the category of, and are driven by, artificial neural networks (ANNs). Perioperative medicine, with its abundant data generation and real-time decision making, is ripe for AI innovations. AI tools are already entering perioperative medicine as anesthesiologists, surgeons, and nursing staff are beginning to encounter them in daily practice [4]. Historically, some of the most effective innovations in both AI and medical devices have come directly from these users. Yet, the clinician's perspective is often underrepresented in the development and implementation of these systems, even though their workflows are frequently among the first impacted by AI deployment.

39.1.2 A Growing Market Opportunity

The integration of AI into healthcare presents an immense economic opportunity. Within healthcare, AI is expected to reduce annual US healthcare costs by $150 billion by 2026 [3]. Meanwhile another study estimates annual savings in the USA to be up to $450 billion [5]. The anticipated growth is mirrored by increased venture capital and industry investment, with healthcare AI startups consistently among the most funded in digital health [6]. As healthcare becomes more digitalized, the volume of data will dramatically expand. However, this data is nothing more than noise if it cannot be analyzed efficiently, which leaves a market gap to be addressed by AI.

This surge in demand reflects a common recognition of AI's potential to transform healthcare, especially in the perioperative space where hospitals generate much of their revenue. Accordingly, academic and industry researchers alike have begun identifying broad applications of AI in perioperative care [1–3]. However, without clinical leadership, technologies risk being developed in silos resulting in poor integration and misalignment with true clinical needs.

39.2 Anesthesiologists Are Naturally Positioned to Become Leaders in AI Implementation

Anesthesiologists are central to the perioperative space and are uniquely positioned to drive the iterative innovation and implementation of clinical AI. The practice of anesthesiology requires constant balancing of physiology, pharmacology, time-sensitive decision-making, and interdisciplinary collaboration. This equally broad and rare set of skills has earned them the nickname the "Swiss-Army-Knives" of medicine [7]. Such versatility allows anesthesiologists to not only understand the clinical implications of artificial intelligence, but also to shape how these technologies are adopted, interpreted, and integrated into perioperative workflows.

This culture of versatility is reinforced by a long history of anesthesiologist-driven innovation [8–10]. The Society for Technology in Anesthesia (STA), founded in 1988, has consistently grown in popularity as an outlet for anesthesiologists to study and apply new technology in the field. This tradition has led to advances in non-invasive physiology monitors, prediction algorithms, and more recently AI-driven tools [10]. This rooted interest demonstrates that anesthesiologists are active stakeholders in this marketplace and *eager* to ensure that rapidly evolving technologies like AI meet the complex demands of clinical care.

39.2.1 Technologically Savvy Specialty by Nature

Anesthesiologists are among the most technology-savvy physicians in medicine. They work daily with complex monitoring systems, ventilators, infusion pumps, and electronic health records. This familiarity with real-time data streams makes them particularly adept at understanding the fundamentals and utility of AI tools. From intraoperative physiology sensors deconstructed by ML and ANNs to regional anesthesia image guidance assisted by computer vision, anesthesiologists frequently use technology that is in the direct path of imminent AI. As the end-users of many potential AI tools, anesthesiologists are key stakeholders who can drive the iterative innovation of this emerging technology.

Anesthesiologists have already begun to push the boundaries of AI in the perioperative space. AI-related literature has rapidly increased in the last decade, leading *Anesthesia & Analgesia*, the associated journal of the STA, to publish a special edition dedicated to the topic in 2020 [10]. Additionally, anesthesiologists have created a collaborative database known as the Multicenter Perioperative Outcomes Group (MPOG), which allows hospitals from around the globe to use and share perioperative data to further research, education, and quality improvement [10, 11]. As of 2025, the program includes data for 32 million cases. While MPOG is an impressive innovation of its own, its massive repository of quality data is already feeding into AI. For example, researchers from Washington University and the University of Michigan leveraged MPOG's vast data to externally validate a ML algorithm, which estimated surgical transfusion risk significantly better than standard care practice methodology [12].

39.2.2 A Systems-Level Perspective

Unlike many specialties that interact with patients in a single phase of care, anesthesiologists are embedded throughout the entire perioperative continuum including preoperative optimization, intraoperative management, postoperative recovery, ICU care—and, by extension, management of pain, airways, and vascular access across the hospital. This system-wide view enables anesthesiologists to see the eventual outcomes, complications, and friction a patient will encounter during their progression of care. In simple terms, anesthesiologists have a vantage point to see the big-picture of a patient's care and how delays, disruptions, and gaps at one stage may ripple into the next. With this perspective, anesthesiologists are uniquely able to identify system-level gaps in care which contextualizes the application for focused AI innovations.

39.2.3 Leaders in Interdisciplinary Collaboration

The anesthesiologist's role is inherently collaborative. Whether coordinating with surgeons, nurses, pharmacists, or administrators, anesthesiologists serve as hubs of communication within the hospital. These traits translate well into leading AI implementation efforts, which require bridging the gap between various stakeholders. Anesthesiologists often participate in, or lead, multidisciplinary quality improvement, safety, and informatics committees where personal networks are further strengthened while also opening the door for AI tools to be applied. As with any clinical innovation, AI will need to be tailored to the needs of a wide spectrum of stakeholders, and anesthesiologists are in an optimal position because of their daily interaction with many of these stakeholders.

39.2.4 Strong Clinical Judgement amid Uncertainty and Complexity

AI has been hailed as a save-all tool; however, it is more realistically a tool that adds a layered perspective to a knowledgeable user [1–3, 11–13]. As these tools gain traction, users have raised consistent concerns regarding their questionable outputs ranging from lack of reproducibility to hallucinations—a phenomenon where large language model outputs are confident and plausible-sounding yet factually incorrect or even nonsensical [13, 14]. At best, AI algorithms generate probabilities, not certainties. Without viewing AI results critically and with appropriate context, these outputs can lead to harmful decisions.

Anesthesiologists are accustomed to dynamic, high-stakes environments and are well-suited to interpret evolving data pragmatically. The risk of clinicians' overreliance on algorithmic predictions, known as *automation bias*, is a concept anesthesiologists consider in their daily work flow [15, 16]. From processed electroencephalographic devices assessing depth of anesthesia to quantitative train-of-four monitors measuring depth of paralysis, anesthesiologists routinely consider data as a piece of their broader clinical judgement. As every anesthesiologist understands, these tools do not provide a single-point source of truth about the patient condition, and these tools are subject to failures of various kinds. The same mindset is essential for AI. Anesthesiologists understand the importance of human oversight and can play a critical role in ensuring that AI supports, rather than replaces, clinical judgment. In the same way that the train-of-four sticker can malfunction leading to overassessment or underdetection of electromyographic signal, AI tools are subject to errors of commission (acting upon incorrect information) or omission (acting while leaving out or ignoring key information when generating outputs). Dr. Sachin Kheterpal, an anesthesiologist at the University of Michigan and the executive director of MPOG, emphasized in a *JAMA* interview that anesthesiologists are already well-practiced in real-time risk stratification and interpretation of multimodal data. We naturally make use of a variety of data points to determine if, say, a high blood pressure is due to light anesthesia, pain, or some other factor. Their "air traffic controller" role in the OR and PACU alone positions them to design AI workflows that enhance safety without compromising human judgment [17].

39.3 Applications of AI in Perioperative Workflow

39.3.1 Risk Stratification and Predictive Analysis

AI models have shown favorable results in stratifying risk and predicting outcomes such as ASA physical status classification, PACU duration, and hospital length of stay [1–3]. For example, anesthesiologists at the University of Washington have shown natural language processing models to accurately predict unplanned ICU admission and mortality [18]. Meanwhile an anesthesiology team from the University of Alabama used machine learning tools to stratify post-operative patients by unexpected care escalation risk [19]. Such tools could complement traditional scoring systems and enhance a clinician's situational awareness. When embedded into workflows, they could support personalized care plans, optimize resource allocation, and improve team coordination.

Another specific application of AI is the prediction and prevention of surgical site infections (SSIs), which strain resources and induce poor patient outcomes. The development of SSIs increases hospital stays by roughly 10 days on average and leads to more than 90,000 readmissions annually. Collectively, SSIs are estimated to cost $10 billion annually in the United States. Importantly, it is estimated that 60% of SSIs could have been prevented with proper adherence to guidelines [20]. By deploying AI tools that assist in real-time compliance with infection control protocols, such as antibiotic timing, glucose control, and normothermia maintenance, anesthesiologists can help prevent these costly complications. Because anesthesiologists oversee many of these parameters perioperatively, they are well-positioned to contribute to AI tools and translate them into timely clinical action.

39.3.2 Real-Time Decision Support

Machine learning systems present an opportunity to analyze growing amounts of perioperative physiologic data and aid in critical decision making. One notable example is the analysis of intraoperative blood pressure to prevent hypotension. Intraoperative hypotension is linked to myocardial injury and acute kidney injury, which can progress into unexpected ICU admissions and ultimately poor clinical outcomes and institutional performance [21, 22]. Given this need, anesthesiologist researchers leveraged ML to recognize blood pressure trends and identify hypotension before it occurred, significantly reducing depth and duration of intraoperative hypotension [5]. Similar technology is now commercially available as the Acumen Hypotension Prediction Index (Edwards Lifesciences, Irvine, CA, USA)—a product which anesthesiologists helped develop [23]. Intraoperative blood pressure is just one of many parameters an anesthesiologist must simultaneously manage; by extension, it is just one application for AI to be used in real-time decision support. Depth of anesthesia, drug pharmacokinetic and pharmacodynamic profiles, and procedural image guidance are all gaining significant interest from both academia and industry [24]. As real-time data managers and decision-makers in the OR, anesthesiologists are the natural users and innovators of such tools. Their ability to interpret physiologic nuance, calibrate alerts, and guide team responses ensures these systems function as tools to assist decision-making, not replacements for clinicians.

39.3.3 Workflow Optimization

Machine learning tools are becoming increasingly practical for optimizing OR scheduling and reducing room turnover delays. AI tools have been evaluated in multiple domains such as team coordination, setup standardization, and prearrival optimization, with reported efficiency gains and cost savings [24]. ORs are among the most expensive hospital resources, costing an estimated $16.21 per minute excluding physician fees [25]. This valuable (but resource intensive) hospital commodity is hindered by inefficiencies in turnover, staffing, and PACU bottlenecks that contribute to case delays, extended work hours, and wasted resources [11, 24]. Anesthesiologists often coordinate the timing and priority of surgical cases and therefore stand as key players in the development of AI tools for OR logistics. Accordingly, anesthesiologist-researchers have found that AI-assisted OR management can yield gains in efficiency and cost savings via improved sequencing, setup, and team readiness [1, 11, 24, 26]. Translating these results from the bench to the bedside will certainly benefit from further anesthesiologist input. Their intimate understanding of intraoperative complexity, staff workflow, and perioperative variability ensures that scheduling predictions remain grounded in clinical feasibility.

39.3.4 Documentation and Administrative Support

Documentation has become a significant burden for clinicians, and it is linked to increased workloads, clinician burnout, and shortened patient encounters [12, 26–29]. NLP may facilitate streamlining for portions of clinical documentation including progress notes, operative summaries, and billing records, alleviating onerous tasks. In a focused study, researchers trained AI models to classify anesthesia-specific current procedural terminology (CPT) codes [30]. Resulting models were highly accurate, which could help reduce redundant manual data entry while streamlining reimbursement, quality improvement, and research workflows. On a larger

Table 39.1 Summary of AI applications in the perioperative workflow

Application	AI modality	Use case	Target outcome
Risk stratification and predictive analysis	Natural language processing, machine learning	Predict ASA classification, unplanned ICU admission, hospital mortality, SSI risk	Early identification of high-risk patients, reduced complications, prevention of SSIs, optimized care planning
Real-time decision support	Machine learning	Early hypotension detection, anesthesia depth monitoring, drug pharmacokinetics and pharmacodynamics modeling, image guidance	Prevent intraoperative hypotension, reduce myocardial/renal injury, improve intraoperative safety
Workflow optimization	Machine learning	OR scheduling, turnover reduction, PACU flow optimization	Increased operating room efficiency, reduced delays, cost savings
Documentation and administrative support	Natural language processing	Automated CPT coding, operative summaries, progress notes	Reduced documentation burden, improved billing accuracy, clinician time savings

scale, similar models hold high potential across all medical specialties, providing clinicians with more direct clinical time and hospitals with efficient workflows. The aforementioned applications are summarized in Table 39.1, which outlines the modalities, representative use cases, and target outcomes of AI in perioperative workflows.

39.4 Risks and Challenges

While artificial intelligence holds tremendous promise, its integration into perioperative care carries significant risks that must be carefully managed. Understanding these challenges is essential for anesthesiologists to serve as responsible stewards of AI implementation.

39.4.1 Patient Safety and Clinical Risks

The most critical concern in AI deployment is patient safety. AI prediction models often demonstrate only moderate accuracy with area under the receiver operating characteristic (AUROC) values typically ranging from 0.7 to 0.85 [15]. This imperfect performance creates risks of both over-treatment and under-treatment. For example, a false-positive hypotension prediction could lead to unnecessary fluid administration or vasopressor use, potentially causing fluid overload or acute kidney injury. Furthermore, it should be recognized that AUROC reflects the sensitivity and specificity of a test. This is important because sensitivity and specificity are measures that are **independent of incidence**. Even a test with very high sensitivity and specificity will be swamped by false positives when the test is assessing for the presence of rare events. Most of the events and outcomes that anesthesiologists are interested in are, thankfully, relatively rare. This should underscore to the reader that these tools may serve much better as screening tools rather than as oracles of truth in the domain of anesthesiology.

Automation bias may also compound these risks. Studies demonstrate that clinicians may ignore contradictory evidence when presented with confident AI assessments, potentially leading to diagnostic errors or inappropriate treatment decisions. The sophisticated presentation of AI outputs can create a false sense of certainty that undermines clinical reasoning.

39.4.2 Data Quality and Bias Concerns

The quality of clinical data feeding AI systems poses additional concerns, which can be represented by the maxim, "garbage in, garbage out" [31, 32]. For example, electronic health records often contain significant amounts of copy-pasted or outdated information while key perioperative events such as blood loss or medication administration are inconsistently documented [15]. Algorithms trained on such data may misrepresent a patient's real-time status, leading to erroneous decisions and compromised patient care. In addition, many perioperative datasets inadequately represent racial, ethnic, and socioeconomic diversity, potentially leading to skewed algorithms that perpetuate inequities in care [13, 15, 33]. For instance, hypoxemia prediction models based on pulse oximetry data may be less accurate in patients with darker skin pigmentation due to underlying sensor limitations that were not adequately considered during model development. Ultimately, poor data quality can still produce models that appear statistically robust during development but fail catastrophically in real-world implementation, potentially causing patient harm and undermining clinician trust in AI technologies.

39.4.3 Cybersecurity and Privacy Threats

As anesthesia equipment becomes increasingly networked, cybersecurity risks multiply [34]. Ransomware attacks on healthcare systems have already disrupted major medical centers, and AI-connected devices add further targets. A significant near-term risk involves clinicians unknowingly exposing sensitive patient data into public AI tools like ChatGPT, thereby violating privacy regulations. The sophisticated capabilities of these tools can create a false sense of security about their appropriate clinical use.

39.4.4 Implementation and Integration Challenges

Despite the growing research in AI and its exciting early results, most perioperative AI models remain in the development phase, with few studies demonstrating successful clinical implementation [35]. Barriers include electronic health record integration difficulties, workflow disruption, and inadequate user interface design. Algorithms also risk "model drift," which represents a long-term decay in model accuracy as clinical practices evolve, patient populations change, or data collection methods shift [36]. Many promising algorithms fail in real-world deployment due to poor consideration of end-user needs and clinical workflow realities. This is recognized within industry circles as technology founders and executives often identify the most common barrier to market entry being lack of health system knowledge [37]. This disconnect not only reduces AI accuracy but also limits adoption.

39.4.5 Regulatory and Liability Issues

The regulatory landscape for clinical AI remains complex and fragmented, which leads to a reluctance for AI adoption in healthcare. The FDA has extended Software as a Medical Device regulations to cover AI applications, but the approval process for adaptive algorithms that learn from new data remains unclear [34]. Liability is similarly unclear [38, 39]. If AI-based treatments lead to patient harm, responsibility between clinician, institution, and developer is ambiguous. The "black box" nature of many AI algorithms—that is, the lack of explainability or reproducibility of results—compounds this uncertainty [10, 13, 40].

39.4.6 Financial and Resource Challenges

AI development and implementation require substantial financial investment. Large language models can cost millions of dollars to develop and maintain, while the computational infrastructure required for clinical AI deployment represents ongoing operational expenses [35]. These costs must be balanced against uncertain clinical and financial benefits, particularly given the limited evidence for AI's impact on patient outcomes.

39.4.7 The Path Forward

These challenges are not insurmountable obstacles but rather important considerations that must inform responsible AI implementation. Success will require rigorous validation, continuous monitoring, ethical safeguards, and above all, maintaining the primacy of clinical judgment in patient care. Furthermore, what these challenges highlight is the need for clinician leadership at each stage of AI development and implementation. Healthcare needs iterative, clinically driven AI: systems that evolve in response to real-world use are embedded in clinical environments and are shaped by the people who rely on them. Historically, physicians have been at the forefront of innovation, balancing technological promise with patient-centered outcomes.

Among them, anesthesiologists are particularly well-positioned to lead this effort and ensure AI is integrated responsibly and effectively.

39.5 Conclusion

Healthcare has reached an inflection point in the development of artificial intelligence. Its implementation across industries is accelerating rapidly, yet its integration into medicine remains cautious for good reason. AI carries real risk—patient safety concerns from imperfect accuracy, automation bias, bias in underlying data, cybersecurity threats, unclear liability, and resource allocation among many others—that could derail progress if ignored.

Meanwhile, the hospitals facing economic and efficiency pressures are propelling the prospect of AI to play a growing role in perioperative care. As it evolves from novelty to necessity, its direction will inevitably be catalyzed by industry. However, it is imperative that clinicians claim their seat at the table of stakeholders, not only as users, but as co-designers, innovators, and patient advocates. This is where anesthesiologists are indispensable. Their technological fluency, systems-level perspective, collaborative role, and decisiveness under uncertainty uniquely position them to ensure that AI supports, rather than replaces, clinical judgment.

The path forward will require anesthesiologists to embrace AI as both a tool and a responsibility—guiding its design, demanding rigorous validation, embedding safeguards against bias, and maintaining human oversight at every stage. By claiming this role, anesthesiologists can help transform AI from a source of risk into a driver of safer, more efficient, and more equitable care. The question is not whether AI will enter the perioperative space, but whether it will do so responsibly—and anesthesiologists are best positioned to make sure it functions effectively and as intended.

References

1. Hashimoto DA, Phitayakorn R, Fernandez-del-Castillo C, Meireles O. Artificial intelligence in surgery: promises and perils. Ann Surg. 2018;268(1):70–6.
2. Ali O, Abdelbaki W, Shrestha A, Elbasi E, Alryalat MAA, Dwivedi YK. A systematic literature review of artificial intelligence in the healthcare sector: benefits, challenges, methodologies, and functionalities. J Innov Knowl. 2023;8(1):100333.
3. Lopes S, Rocha G, Guimarães-Pereira L. Artificial intelligence and its clinical application in Anesthesiology: a systematic review. J Clin Monit Comput. 2024;38(2):247–59. https://doi.org/10.1007/s10877-023-01088-0. Epub 2023 Oct 21. PMID: 37864754; PMCID: PMC10995017.
4. Lambert SI, Madi M, Sopka S, et al. An integrative review on the acceptance of artificial intelligence among healthcare professionals in hospitals [published correction appears in NPJ Digit Med. 2023;6(1):125. https://doi.org/10.1038/s41746-023-00874-z]. NPJ Digit Med. 2023;6(1):111. https://doi.org/10.1038/s41746-023-00852-5. Published 2023 Jun 10.

5. Wijnberge M, Geerts BF, Hol L, Lemmers N, Mulder MP, Berge P, Schenk J, Terwindt LE, Hollmann MW, Vlaar AP, Veelo DP. Effect of a machine learning-derived early warning system for intraoperative hypotension vs standard care on depth and duration of intraoperative hypotension during elective noncardiac surgery: the HYPE randomized clinical trial. JAMA. 2020;323(11):1052–60. https://doi.org/10.1001/jama.2020.0592. PMID: 32065827; PMCID: PMC7078808.
6. McNabb NK, Christensen EW, Rula EY, Coombs L, Dreyer K, Wald C, Treml C. Projected growth in FDA-approved artificial intelligence products given venture capital funding. J Am Coll Radiol. 2024;21(4):617–23. https://doi.org/10.1016/j.jacr.2023.08.030. Epub 2023 Oct 16. PMID: 37843483.
7. Jeleff A, Nh A, Keli-Barcelos G, Savoldelli G. Anesthesiologists are the Swiss army knife of the hospitals: report of experience during the COVID-19 pandemic at the Geneva University Hospitals abbreviations. CasesMed Res J. 2021;3:25–30.
8. Kwon AH, Marshall ZJ, Nabzdyk CS. Why anesthesiologists could and should become the next leaders in innovative medical entrepreneurism. Anesth Analg. 2017;124(3):998–1004. https://doi.org/10.1213/ANE.0000000000001793.
9. Chao R, Solanki P, Chelly JE, Wasan AD, Emerick T. Fostering innovation in medical education: addressing the void of entrepreneurship education in anesthesiology and pain medicine through incubator clubs. A A Pract. 2024;18(7):e01817. https://doi.org/10.1213/XAA.0000000000001817.
10. Moon JS, Cannesson M. A century of technology in anesthesia & analgesia. Anesth Analg. 2022;135(2S):S48–61. https://doi.org/10.1213/ANE.0000000000006027.
11. Colquhoun DA, Shanks AM, Kapeles SR, Shah N, Saager L, Vaughn MT, Buehler K, Burns ML, Tremper KK, Freundlich RE, Aziz M, Kheterpal S, Mathis MR. Considerations for integration of perioperative electronic health records across institutions for research and quality improvement: the approach taken by the Multicenter Perioperative Outcomes Group. Anesth Analg. 2020;130(5):1133–46. https://doi.org/10.1213/ANE.0000000000004489. PMID: 32287121; PMCID: PMC7663856.
12. Lou SS, Kumar S, Goss CW, et al. Multicenter validation of a machine learning model for surgical transfusion risk at 45 US hospitals. JAMA Netw Open. 2025;8(6):e2517760. https://doi.org/10.1001/jamanetworkopen.2025.17760. Published 2025 Jun 2.
13. Ahmed MI, Spooner B, Isherwood J, Lane M, Orrock E, Dennison A. A systematic review of the barriers to the implementation of artificial intelligence in healthcare. Cureus. 2023;15(10):e46454. https://doi.org/10.7759/cureus.46454. PMID: 37927664; PMCID: PMC10623210.
14. Xu Z, Jain S, Kankanhalli M. Hallucination is inevitable: an innate limitation of large language models. arXiv [CsCL]. 2024.
15. Elendu C, Amaechi DC, Elendu TC, Jingwa KA, Okoye OK, John Okah M, Ladele JA, Farah AH, Alimi HA. Ethical implications of AI and robotics in healthcare: a review. Medicine. 2023;102(50):e36671. https://doi.org/10.1097/MD.0000000000036671.
16. Kandaswamy S, Muthu N, Braykov N, Carter R, Blanco R, Bui T, Orenstein E, Mai M. Human performance evaluation of a pediatric artificial intelligence sepsis model. J Am Med Inform Assoc. 2025. https://doi.org/10.1093/jamia/ocaf106.
17. Abbasi J, Hswen Y. Tapping AI's strengths-from operating room safety to wearable device interpretation. JAMA. 2024;332(5):354–8. https://doi.org/10.1001/jama.2024.0802. PMID: 38967952.
18. Chung P, Fong CT, Walters AM, Aghaeepour N, Yetisgen M, O'Reilly-Shah VN. Large language model capabilities in perioperative risk prediction and prognostication. JAMA Surg. 2024;159(8):928–37. https://doi.org/10.1001/jamasurg.2024.1621. PMID: 38837145; PMCID: PMC11154375.
19. Barker AB, Melvin RL, Godwin RC, Benz D, Wagener BM. Machine learning predicts unplanned care escalations for post-anesthesia care unit patients during the perioperative period: a single-center retrospective study. J Med Syst. 2024;48(1):69. https://doi.org/10.1007/s10916-024-02085-9. PMID: 39042285; PMCID: PMC11266221.

20. Ban KA, Minei JP, Laronga C, et al. American College of Surgeons and Surgical Infection Society: surgical site infection guidelines, 2016 update. J Am Coll Surg. 2017;224(1):59–74.e1.
21. Salmasi V, Maheshwari K, Yang D, et al. Relationship between intraoperative hypotension, defined by either reduction from baseline or absolute thresholds, and acute kidney and myocardial injury after noncardiac surgery: a retrospective cohort analysis. Anesthesiology. 2017;126(1):47–65. https://doi.org/10.1097/ALN.0000000000001432.
22. Shah N, Mentz G, Kheterpal S. The incidence of intraoperative hypotension in moderate to high risk patients undergoing non-cardiac surgery: a retrospective multicenter observational analysis. J Clin Anesth. 2020;66:1–12.
23. Kouz K, Garcia MIM, Cerutti E, Lisanti I, Draisci G, Frassanito L, et al. Intraoperative hypotension when using hypotension prediction index software during major noncardiac surgery: a European multicentre prospective observational registry. (EU HYPROTECT). BJA Open. 2023;6:100140.
24. MacMillan L, Madura GM, Elliot M, Frendl DM, Jorge IA, Ven Fong Z, Hasse C, Etzioni DA. What affects operating room turnover time? A systematic review and mapping of the evidence. Surgery. 2025;181:109263. https://doi.org/10.1016/j.surg.2025.109263. PMID: 40054053.
25. Moody AE, Gurnea TP, Shul CP, Althausen PL. True cost of operating room time: implications for an orthopaedic trauma service. J Orthop Trauma. 2020;34(5):271–5. https://doi.org/10.1097/BOT.0000000000001688.
26. Bellini V, Russo M, Domenichetti T, Panizzi M, Allai S, Bignami EG. Artificial intelligence in operating room management. J Med Syst. 2024;48(1):19. https://doi.org/10.1007/s10916-024-02038-2. PMID: 38353755; PMCID: PMC10867065.
27. Kernberg A, Gold JA, Mohan V. Using ChatGPT-4 to create structured medical notes from audio recordings of physician-patient encounters: comparative study. J Med Internet Res. 2024;26:e54419. https://doi.org/10.2196/54419. PMID: 38648636; PMCID: PMC11074889.
28. Liu TL, Hetherington TC, Stephens C, McWilliams A, Dharod A, Carroll T, Cleveland JA. AI-powered clinical documentation and clinicians' electronic health record experience: a nonrandomized clinical trial. JAMA Netw Open. 2024;7(9):e2432460. https://doi.org/10.1001/jamanetworkopen.2024.32460. PMID: 39240568; PMCID: PMC11380097.
29. Bundy H, Gerhart J, Baek S, Connor CD, Isreal M, Dharod A, Stephens C, Liu TL, Hetherington T, Cleveland J. Can the administrative loads of physicians be alleviated by AI-facilitated clinical documentation? J Gen Intern Med. 2024;39(15):2995–3000. https://doi.org/10.1007/s11606-024-08870-z. Epub 2024 Jun 27. PMID: 38937369; PMCID: PMC11576703.
30. Burns ML, Mathis MR, Vandervest J, Tan X, Lu B, Colquhoun DA, Shah N, Kheterpal S, Saager L. Classification of current procedural terminology codes from electronic health record data using machine learning. Anesthesiology. 2020;132(4):738–49. https://doi.org/10.1097/ALN.0000000000003150. PMID: 32028374; PMCID: PMC7665375.
31. O'Reilly-Shah VN, Gentry KR, Walters AM, Zivot J, Anderson CT, Tighe PJ. Bias and ethical considerations in machine learning and the automation of perioperative risk assessment. Br J Anaesth. 2020;125:843–6. https://doi.org/10.1016/j.bja.2020.07.040.
32. Teno JM. Garbage in, garbage out-words of caution on big data and machine learning in medical practice. JAMA Health Forum. 2023;4:e230397.
33. Norori N, Hu Q, Aellen FM, Faraci FD, Tzovara A. Addressing bias in big data and AI for health care: a call for open science. Patterns (NY). 2021;2:100347.
34. Food and Drug Administration. Transparency for machine learning-enabled medical devices: guiding principles. Available at: https://www.fda.gov/medical-devices/software-medical-device-samd/transparency-machine-learning-enabled-medicaldevices-guiding-principles. Accessed 3 Oct 2024.
35. Harris S, Bonnici T, Keen T, Lilaonitkul W, White MJ, Swanepoel N. Clinical deployment environments: five pillars of translational machine learning for health. Front Digit Health. 2022;4:939292.

36. Feng J, Phillips RV, Malenica I, et al. Clinical artificial intelligence quality improvement: towards continual monitoring and updating of AI algorithms in healthcare. NPJ Digit Med. 2022;5:66.
37. Olaye IM, Seixas AA. The gap between AI and bedside: participatory workshop on the barriers to the integration, translation, and adoption of digital health care and AI startup technology into clinical practice. J Med Internet Res. 2023;25:e32962. https://doi.org/10.2196/32962. PMID: 37129947; PMCID: PMC10189623.
38. Price WN 2nd, Gerke S, Cohen IG. Potential liability for physicians using artificial intelligence. JAMA. 2019;322:1765–6.
39. Tewfik G, Minzter B, Chiao F, Zivot J, Wecksell M, Simpao AF, CIIT Collaborators, O'Reilly-Shah V, Berg K, Wang E, Tan JM, Ondecko K, Banoub M, Pesce M, Khatib R, Abola RE. Narrative review of electronic health record systems in anesthesia: benefits, risks, and medico-legal considerations in the United States of America. J Med Syst. 2025;49:87.
40. Lundberg SM, Nair B, Vavilala MS, et al. Explainable machine-learning predictions for the prevention of hypoxaemia during surgery. Nat Biomed Eng. 2018;2:749–60.

Index

A
Academic healthcare system, 439
Accountable Care Organizations (ACOs), 16
  and Broader Payor Landscape, 374
  and CIN, 374
  collaborating with specialties, 379
  cost accounting and, 378
  data management, innovations in, 377
  definition and prevalence of, 371
  expanding scope of influence, 378
  factors, in negotiating ACO participation, 378, 379
  future of, 380
  healthcare ecosystem, 371, 372
  history of, 372, 373
  interaction with value-based models, 374, 375
  IT and data management for, 377
  meeting metrics, challenges in, 376
  membership
    anesthesiologist's role in, 378
    benefits of, 373
  participation
    challenges in, 379
    metrics in, 375
    perioperative optimization, 379
  payment models under, 377
  types and examples of, 375
  upside and downside risk, 376
Accreditation, 498–501
Accreditation Association for Ambulatory Health Care (AAAHC), 255, 501
Accreditation Commission for Health Care (ACHC), 501
ACOG Levels of Maternal Care, 324, 325
ACS NSQIP Surgical Risk Calculator, 60, 103
Activated clotting time (ACT), 145
Active errors, 302
Active temperature management, 62
Acute kidney injury (AKI), 61
Acute normovolemic hemodilution (ANH), 143
Acute pain services, 229, 230
  complication rates, reduction in, 231, 232
  cost effectiveness, 232
  cost reduction, 230, 231
  revenue, 232
Advanced practice provider (APP), 432
Adverse event analysis, 215
  definitions and classification of, 216
  disclosure, feedback and follow-up, 224
  perioperative clinician, 216–218
  process, 218, 219, 222–224
  reporting of, 220–222
  safety culture, establishing and ensuring, 220
Advisories, 444
Advocacy, 427, 428, 433–435, 460–461, 470
  ASA, 429, 430
  physician anesthesiologists, 429
  strategy, 437, 438
Advocating for legislation, 430–433
Affordable Care Act (ACA), 107, 429, 498
Agency for Healthcare Research and Quality (AHRQ), 462
AI-driven clinical decision support, 34
AI-driven surveillance systems, 296
Airway and pulmonary management, 208
Airway evaluations, 475, 477, 478
Airway management, 208, 316
Alliance for Innovation on Maternal Health (AIM), 330
Allogeneic whole blood/blood components, 133
Alternative noninvasive physiologist monitors, 152

G. Tewfik (ed.), *The Anesthesiologist as Perioperative Leader*,
https://doi.org/10.1007/978-3-032-18058-2

Alternative payment models (APMs), 15, 293, 374
Ambulation, 177
Ambulatory surgery centers (ASCs), 39, 414
Ambulatory surgery services, 499
America's Blood Centers (ABC), 133
American Association for the Surgery of Trauma (AAST), 164
American Board of Anesthesiology (ABA), 5, 366, 469
American College of Chest Physicians (ACCP), 178
American College of Surgeons (ACS), 35, 202, 500
American Hospital Association (AHA), 500
American Medical Association (AMA), 500
American Society of Anesthesiologists (ASA), 30, 35, 294, 324, 327–329, 331–334, 364, 367, 428, 429, 443, 451, 506–508
American Society of Hematology (ASH), 178
American Society of Regional Anesthesia and Pain Medicine (ASRA), 120
Anaesthetists' Non-Technical Skills (ANTS) framework, 308
Analgesic stewardship, PACU, 208–209
Anemia, 134
Anesthesia, 29, 190
  anesthetic management, genetic profiling for, 36, 37
  care, 353, 427, 437, 467
  clinician and procedure coder communication, 357
  collaboration, communication, and flow of information, 33, 34
  developing specialized perioperative guidelines, 35
  economic contributions of, 39
  efficiency and reducing costs, 32, 33
  electronic health records, 34, 35
  equipment, 186
  ERAS, 74–75
  healthcare costs, 33, 37
  medication and formulary management, 198, 199
    cost management and service, 202, 203
    drug management, 200
    drug preparation, 201
    emergency medication management, 202
    medication safety, 199, 200
    OR, drug education in, 201
  multidisciplinary collaboration, 40
  patient safety, 31
  perioperative care, anesthesiologists in, 29, 30
  postoperative setting, preparing for, 35, 36
  preoperative evaluations, 37
  preoperative optimization programs, operational and economic impact of, 37, 38
  procedure coders, 357
  record documentation education, 348, 356, 357
  risk assessment tool, physical and clinical characteristics, 32
  services, 428
  strategic preoperative evaluation, 30
    financial waste, cost implications and avoidance of, 30, 31
    guideline-driven frameworks, 31
    patient-centered evaluation, risk mitigation through, 30
    safety outcomes, 31
  supply chain, 184, 185
  supply procurement, 187, 188
Anesthesia Incident Reporting System (AIRS), 462, 507
Anesthesia information management systems (AIMS), 7, 285–288
Anesthesia-led multidisciplinary approach, 119
Anesthesia Patient Safety Foundation (APSF), 277
Anesthesia Quality Institute (AQI), 294–295, 462, 507
Anesthesia Time Units (ATUs), 437
Anesthesiologist-administered sedation, 259
Anesthesiologist-directed OPEs, 49
Anesthesiologist-in-Charge (AIC), 242
Anesthesiologist-led preoperative evaluations, 51
Anesthesiologists, 316, 321, 363
  economic value of
    cost control, waste reduction, and efficiency, 6
    critical care, pain, and perioperative systems, 7, 8
    operating room efficiency, 6
    revenue preservation, documentation, and reimbursement, 7
    value-based care, quality, and risk mitigation, 6, 7
  institutional leaders, 20
  leadership, 57, 58, 60
  perioperative leader, 8
  systems-based role for
    leading system change, 62, 63
    multifaceted approach, 61, 62
    optimization and anesthesiologist's leadership role, 57, 58

perioperative leader and value generator, 63
prehabilitation, 59, 60
preoperative assessment, 58, 59
risk stratification, 60, 61
Anesthesiology, 453
advancing research in, 383
clinical research, 389, 390
commercialized innovations, 389
depth monitoring, 385
integrating multimodal monitoring, 386
interdisciplinary collaborations, 388
pain management, 385
patient safety, 384, 385
pulse oximetry, 386
basic science research logistics, 387, 394
funding, 395
grant budget, structure, 396, 397
internal regulations, 398
laboratory, 398
potential funding sources, 396
regulatory hurdles, 397
writing grant proposal, 395, 396
clinical research logistics, 399
broader economic impacts, 400, 401
economic value for investors, 400
economic value for participants, 400
partnerships work, 399
consulting, 414, 420
case studies, 422
definitions, 420
logistics of partnership, 421, 422
in market, 421
results, 422
evolution of
origins and pre-specialty era, 4
perioperative systems and organizational influence, 5
waters, rovenstine, and specialty movement, 5
leadership, NORA, 281
and perioperative care, 29
research program, components of, 406, 407
barriers, 410
financial benefits of research, 408
financial management and oversight, 409
obtaining and ensuring funding, 407, 408
opportunities for financialization of research, 408, 409
solutions, 411
residency program, 366
skills acquired by trainees through, 405, 406
training programs, integrating research, 403
translational research, 391
cross-departmental collaborations, 392
features of, 401, 402
funding for, 394
logistical challenges and solutions, 402
multidisciplinary collaboration, 392
multidisciplinary teams, 391
opportunities for, 392, 393
potential financial benefits, 393, 394
science and clinical practice, 392
Anesthetic care, 215
Anesthetic management, genetic profiling for, 36, 37
Antibiotic compliance, 287
Antibiotic prophylaxis, 161
Anticoagulant classes, 139
Anticoagulated patient, 138–139
Antifibrinolytic therapy, 146–147
Antithrombin III (ATIII), 145
Anxiety, 51
AQI National Anesthesia Clinical Outcomes Registry (NACOR), 507
Area under the receiver operating characteristic (AUROC) values, 519
Arterial line documentation compliance, 287
Artificial intelligence (AI), 18, 23, 36, 49, 189, 287, 296, 352, 513
clinical judgement amid uncertainty and complexity, 516, 517
documentation and administrative support, 518, 519
implementation, 514, 515
interdisciplinary collaboration, leaders in, 516
market opportunity, 514
real-time decision support, 517, 518
risk stratification and predictive analysis, 517
risks and challenges, 519
cybersecurity and privacy threats, 520
data quality and bias concerns, 520
financial and resource challenges, 521
implementation and integration challenges, 520, 521
patient safety and clinical risks, 519, 520
regulatory and liability issues, 521
in perioperative medicine, 514
systems-level perspective, 515, 516
technologically savvy specialty by nature, 515
workflow optimization, 518

Artificial intelligence investments, 359–360
ASA Committee on Anesthesia Care Team, 469
ASA Mission, 451
ASA Monitor, 454
ASA practice guidelines and advisories, 447
Aspirin, 176
Association for the Advancement of Blood and Biotherapies (AABB), 188
Association of Blood Donor Professionals (ADRP), 133
Association of University Anesthesiologists (AUA), 404
Automated dashboards, 267
Automation, 189, 359, 360, 516, 520

B
Backorders, 187
Balanced Scorecard, 109
Barcoding, 189
Bariatric and hepatobiliary surgery, 77
Behavior modification, 59
Biomedical Engineering (BioMed) department, 185
Blood loss, intraoperative minimization of, 134
Blood sampling/testing, 151, 152
Blood sampling with closed loop systems, 152
Blood transfusions, surgical site infection prophylaxis, 164, 165
Board certification, 366
Broader Payor Landscape, 374
Bundled payments, 15
Burnout syndrome, 471
Bylaws, 255

C
Call to Action, 441
Canadian Medical Association (CMA), 500
Cancellations, 87
Caprini score, 173
Carbohydrate loading, 73
Cardiac arrest, 123
Cardiac failure, 139
Cardiac surgery, 77, 173
Cardiac ultrasound, 331
Cardiologists, 316
Cardiopulmonary bypass, 143–144
Care coordination, 45
Cell salvage, 142–143
Center for Improvement in Healthcare Quality (CIHQ), 501
Centers for Disease Control and Prevention (CDC), 159
Centers for Medicare and Medicaid Services (CMS), 116, 202, 232, 254–255, 277, 460, 497–499
Certification, 241
Certified Anesthesiologist Assistant (CAA), 353, 431, 433–436, 469, 491
Certified Professional in Patient Safety (CPPS), 309
Certified registered nurse anesthetist (CRNA), 119, 279, 353, 420, 431, 435, 436, 469
Change agents, anesthesiologists, 96, 97
Childbirth-related posttraumatic stress disorder (CR-PTSD), 332
Clinical care, 505, 506
Clinical decision support (CDS), 34, 303
Clinical informatics, 287
Clinically Integrated Networks (CINs), 374
Clinical practice guidelines, 444, 448
Clinical Practice Improvement (CPI), 102
Clinical research, 384–385, 390–391, 409
Clinical Research Coordinators (CRCs), 390
Clinical research logistics, 399
    broader economic impacts, 400, 401
    economic value for investors, 400
    economic value for participants, 400
    partnerships work, 399
Closed-loop feedback system, 95
Closed loop systems, 152
Clueless Anesthesia Group (CAG), 488
CMS ACO REACH, 375
CMS compliance, anesthesiologist's role in, 508, 509
CMS Quality Payment Program (QPP), 293
Coagulation, physiology of, 140–142
Code Blue, 121
    anesthesiologist, role of, 121
    costs of rapid response system, 122–125
    protocols, 122
    rapid response teams, 125
Coding audit program, 357
Cognitive aids, 303
Cognitive biases, 302, 303
Cognitive forcing strategies, 303
Cognitive overload, 303, 304
Collaborative operational dyads, 88
Colorectal surgery, 76
Commercial ACOs, 375
Commercialization, 388
Committee on Performance and Outcomes Measurement (CPOM), 294
Committee on Trauma and Emergency Preparedness (COTEP), 247, 248

Communication failures, 308
Comparative institutional outcomes, 21
Competency, 241
Complex airway management, 242
Compliance, 353
Complication rates, reduction in, 231, 232
Computer vision, 514
Conditions of Participation (CoPs), 498
Consulting engagements, 415
Continuing medical education (CME), 367, 507
Continuous capnography, 208
Controlled Substances Act of 1970, 199
Cortisol, 71
Cost accounting, 378
Cost avoidance, 16
Cost-effective, 86
Cost effectiveness, 232
Cost management, 187, 202–203
Counseling, 72–73
COVID-19 pandemic, 420, 436
Credentialing and competency systems
  administrative and clinical components, 261–263
  implementation considerations, 265
  performance metrics tied to credentialing, 264
  purpose and guiding principles, 261
  remediation, restrictions, and suspension process, 264–265
  Sample Initial Privileging Checklist, 263–264
  Sample Proctor Observation Checklist, 264
Crew resource management, 308
Critical Access Hospitals (CAH), 116, 499
Critical care admission, 323
Critical care anesthesiologist, 315–321
Critically ill patients, 150, 315, 316, 318, 319
CRNAs, *see* Certified registered nurse anesthetist
C-Suite, 102, 103
Culture of communication, 358
Cybersecurity, 520
CYP2B6, 36
Cytochrome P450 (CYP450) enzyme, 36
Cytokine release, 71

D

Dantrolene, 115
Data analytics, 359, 418
Data collection, 266–268, 271
Data-driven decision-making leverages software, 186
Data-driven leadership, 506
Data-driven operating room, 94
Data management, 377
Data quality, 520
Day-of-surgery delays, 49
Debriefing, 308
Decision-making, 104
Decision-support tools, 18
Deeming authority, 500
Deep vein thrombosis (DVT), 61, 171, 178
Delirium precautions, 321
Delirium prevention, PACU, 209
Demand forecasting and planning, 185, 186
Difficult airway cart, 242
Difficult airway management, 240, 243
Difficult Airway Response Team (DART), 240
Difficult/failed intubation, 243
Digital health, 514
Direct oral anticoagulants (DOACs), 175, 176, 178
Distributors, 184
DNV GL Healthcare, 255
DNV healthcare, 500, 501
Documentation, 285–288, 350, 518, 519
Drug diversion, 200
Drug education, 201
Drug Enforcement Agency (DEA), 198
Drug management, 200
Drug preparation, 201
Drug shortages, 184
Duke University's Academic Career Enrichment Scholars (ACES) Program, 403
DuPont analysis, 107

E

Early tracheostomy, 316
Early warning systems (EWS), 325
Education of anesthesiologist, 365
Effective advocacy in anesthesiology, 429
Effective care, 326–331
  ERAC and quality metrics, 329
  medications and drugs, 329–330
  patient safety bundles, 330
  POCUS, 330–331
  predelivery optimization, 326–329
Efficiency and Thoroughness Tradeoff (ETTO) Spectrum, 304
Efficient care, 333, 334
Efficient information flow, 33
Electronic health records (EHRs), 34, 35, 85, 95, 186, 285–287
Electronic medical record (EMR), 263, 265, 267, 268, 285–287, 479

Elements of Performance (EPs), 500
Emergency airway management, 243
Emergency airway preparedness, 242
Emergency intubation, 241–243
Emergency medication management, 202
Emergency preparedness, 246–249
Emergent airway protection, 242
End-users of healthcare supply chains, 185
Enhanced recovery after surgery (ERAS), 20, 61–63, 351
  definition and origins of, 69
  in different surgical specialties, 75
    bariatric and hepatobiliary surgery, 77
    cardiac and thoracic surgery, 77
    challenges and outcomes, 78
    colorectal surgery, 76
    gynecologic and urologic surgery, 76
    orthopedic surgery, 76
    sinus surgery, 77
  multidisciplinary approach, 70
  perioperative care paradigms, evolution of, 69, 70
  physiologic basis of, 70
    surgical stress response, 71
    traditional approaches vs. metabolic and inflammatory implications of, 71, 72
  protocols, components of, 17, 72
    anesthesia techniques, 74, 75
    early enteral nutrition, 75
    early mobilization, 75
    education and counseling, 72, 73
    goal-directed fluid therapy, 74
    intraoperative phase, 74
    minimizing fasting times, 73
    multimodal pain management, 75
    nutritional optimization, 73
    obstructive sleep apnea, assessment of, 73, 74
    postoperative phase, 75
Enteral nutrition, 75
Equitable care, 334
Error-seeking bias, 300
Erythropoietin (EPO), 137–138
Escalation of care, 14
Ethical purchasing, 190
Ethical sourcing, supply chain, 190
European Commission, 188
Event Reporting Systems, 267
Excessive intravenous fluids, 72
Expert Recommendations for Implementing Change (ERIC) strategies, 166
Extended FAST (eFAST), 244
External transparency, 110

F

Facility accreditation, 498
Facility airway management, 240–242
Facility-wide policies, 502
Factor and fibrinogen concentrates, 145–147
Federal oversight, 498
Feedback loops, 267
Fellow of the American Society of Anesthesiologists (FASA), 454
Fellowship and Postdoctoral Programs, 404
Fibrinolysis, 142, 144
Financial accounting, 196
Financial analysis, surgical service line, 106–109
Financial waste, cost implications and avoidance of, 30, 31
First-case start accuracy, 86
Fluid management, surgical site infection prophylaxis, 164, 165
Focused Assessment with Sonography in Trauma (FAST), 244
Focused Professional Practice Evaluation (FPPE), 507
Food and Drug Administration (FDA), 183, 498
Formularies, hospital medication and formulary management, 198
Foundation for Anesthesia Education and Research (FAER), 404
Fragmentation of care, 22
Fresh frozen plasma (FFP), 145

G

Gastrointestinal (GI) endoscopy, 273
General Accepted Accounting Principles (GAAP), 106
General anesthesia, 300
Gene therapy, spinal muscular atrophy (SMA), 409
Genetic profiling transforms, 36
Global surgical disease burden, 471
GLP-1RA medication management, 35
Glycemic control, surgical site infection prophylaxis, 164
Goal-directed fluid therapy (GDFT), 62, 72, 74
Grades of Recommendation, Assessment, Development, and Evaluation (GRADE) system, 446–448
Graduated compression stockings (GCS), 174, 175
Grant funding, 388
Grassroots movements, 440, 441

Group Purchasing Organizations (GPOs), 183, 185, 186, 189
Guideline-driven frameworks, 31
Gupta Myocardial Infarction and Cardiac Arrest (MICA) index, 35
Gynecologic and urologic surgery, 76

H

Haemothorax, 244
Hand hygiene, surgical site infection prophylaxis, 162
Healthcare advocacy, 439
Healthcare associated infections (HAI), 159
Healthcare consulting
  areas of opportunity, 423
  background and history, 413
  careers in, 423, 424
  key players in, 414
  traditional offerings, 414
  work/life balance in, 423, 424
Healthcare costs, 374
Healthcare delivery, telemedicine
  elderly patients, 484
  incarcerated patients, 484
  rural communities, 483
  underserved communities, 483
Healthcare ecosystem, 371, 372
Health care industry, 497
Healthcare management, 417, 423
Healthcare organizations, 190
Healthcare quality
  effective care, 326–331
    ERAC and quality metrics, 329
    medications and drugs, 329–330
    patient safety bundles, 330
    POCUS, 330–331
    predelivery optimization, 326–329
  efficient care, 333, 334
  equitable care, 334
  patient-centered care, 331–332
  safe care, 324–327
  timely care, 332–333
Healthcare supply chains, 183–184, 355, 522
Healthcare system, 11, 461
Healthcare teams, 431
HemeChip, 410
Health economics of innovation and technology, 17
  artificial intelligence and predictive analytics, 18
  cost-benefit considerations of innovation, 19
  informatics and decision-support tools, 18
  monitoring and minimally invasive technologies, 18, 19
Health Resources and Services Administration (HRSA), 475
Health system priorities, 16
Hemodynamic stability, 208
Hemophilia A & B, 139
Hemostatic resuscitation, 245, 246
Heparin-induced thrombocytopenia (HIT), 176
Hepatobiliary surgery, 77
High-quality perioperative care, 19
High-reliability organizations (HROs), 100, 306
Hip fracture surgery (HFS), 178
Hospital Consumer Assessment of Healthcare Providers and Systems (HCAHPS), 108, 232
Hospital leadership, anesthesiologists in, 497, 498
  AAAHC, 501
  Accreditation Commission for Health Care, 501
  accreditation, federal and state legislative oversight in, 498
  American Society of Anesthesiologists, 506–508
  anesthesiologists and operational excellence, 505
  anesthesiologists, anesthesia departments, and the accreditation survey, 502, 503
  CIHQ, 501
  clinical care and leadership, 505, 506
  CMS
    compliance, anesthesiologist's role in, 508, 509
    and conditions of participation, 499
  deeming authority, 500
  DNV healthcare, 500, 501
  federal oversight, 498
  IMQ, 501
  Joint Commission, 500
  legislative compliance, anesthesiologist's role in, 509
  patient safety, 504, 505
  preoperative assessment efficiency, 509, 510
  QUAD A, 501
  quality improvement, 504
  state departments of health, 501, 502
  state oversight, 498, 499
  survey, 510
  systems thinker, 504

Hospital pharmacy, 198–203
  cost management and service, 202–203
  drug education, 201
  drug management, 200
  drug preparation, 201
  emergency medication management, 202
  medication
    and formulary management, 196–198
    safety, 199, 200
Hospital readmissions, 14
Hospital Readmissions Reduction Program (HRRP), 231
Hospital systems' lobbying efforts, 436
Hospital value-based purchasing (HVBP), 108, 293–294
Hub-and-spoke model, 476
Human factors, 348
Human factors engineering (HFE), 306
Hybrid models, 416
Hyperglycemia, 164
Hypoxia, 172

I

ICD-10 procedure, 99
Idarucizumab, 176
Immobilization, 72
IMPROVE score, 174, 175
Inferior vena cava (IVC) filters, 178
Informatics, 18
Information technology, 104, 359, 360
Informed consent, 350
Innovative care models, 318
Inpatient preoperative evaluation (IPE), 46
Inspired gas concentration, 163
Institute for Medical Quality (IMQ), 501
Institute of Medicine (IOM), 324, 475
Institutional policies, 255
Institutional reputation, 19
Institutional Review Boards (IRBs), 390
Insulin resistance, 71
Insurance reimbursement, 436, 437
Intensive care unit (ICU), 315, 316
Intensivists, 316–318
Interdisciplinary team leadership, 210
Intermittent pneumatic compression (IPC), 175, 177
International Anesthesia Research Society (IARS), 404
International Electrotechnical Commission (IEC), 187
International normalized ratio (INR), 146
Interoperability, 355, 356
Interventional radiology (IR), 244, 273
Intracranial pressure monitoring devices, 316
Intralipid®, 120
Intraoperative and postoperative anemia, 134
Intraoperative minimization of blood loss, 140, 142
Intraoperative phase
  anesthesia techniques, 74, 75
  goal-directed fluid therapy, 74
Intraoperative techniques, 142–144
Intravenous fluids, 196
Inventory management strategies, 186
Investor owned (IO), 107
Iron deficiency, 135, 136
Iron therapy, 137
Ishikawa diagrams, 104

J

Jehovah's Witness (JW) patient, 140
Joint Commission (TJC), 216, 276, 500
Joint Commission on Accreditation of Hospitals (JCAH), 500
Just Culture, 301

K

Key performance indicators (KPIs), 62, 85, 86, 106, 308–309

L

Laboratory-based transfusion, 147
Large language models (LLM), 49, 360
Laser Doppler flowmetry, 386
Latent errors, 302
Leadership, 454, 457, 459, 463
Learning organization, 102
Legislative compliance, anesthesiologist's role in, 509
Legislative process, 433
Legislature, 433
Length of stay (LOS), 14, 50
Liability, 243
Licensed Vocational Nurses (LVNs), 48
Lidocaine, 120
Lobbying, 438, 440, 441
Local anesthetic systemic toxicity (LAST), 118, 119
  clinical guidelines, 120
  CMS requirements, 119, 120
  financial considerations, 120
  protocol development, 119
Logistical management of the OR, 96

Low molecular weight heparin (LMWH), 175, 176, 178
Lung ultrasound, 331

M
Machine learning (ML), 104, 189, 287, 517
Magnetic resonance imaging (MRI), 275
Maintenance of certification in anesthesiology (MOCA 2.0) program, 296
Maintenance of certification in anesthesiology (MOCA) curriculum, 248
Malignant hyperthermia (MH), 115
  clinical guidelines, 117
  CMS requirements, 116
  financial considerations, 118
  protocol development, 116
Malignant Hyperthermia Association of the United States (MHAUS), 117
Mallampati classification, 475
Market competitiveness, 19
Massive bleeding/hemorrhage, 151
Massive transfusion protocols (MTP), 150, 151, 246
Mechanical prophylaxis, 175, 177
Mechanical ventilation, 242
Medical assistants (MAs), 48
Medical association membership, 453
Medical director of perioperative services (MDPS), 4, 88, 89
Medical school education, 364, 365
Medical students, 405
Medicare ACOs, 109
Medicare physician payment rates, 461
Medicare Shared Savings Program (MSSP), 372, 375
Medication and formulary management, 195
  anesthesia and hospital pharmacy, 198, 199
    cost management and service, 202, 203
    drug management, 200
    drug preparation, 201
    emergency medication management, 202
    OR, drug education in, 201
    safety, 199, 200
  hospital formularies, 198
  hospital pharmacy environment, 196, 197
  hospital pharmacy management and function, 197, 198
Medication errors, 304
Medicolegal considerations
  documentation, 350
  duty of care, 349
  informed consent, 350
  preoperative clearance, 351
  professional societies and guidelines, 349
  standard-of-care deviation, 349
Merit-based incentive payment system (MIPS), 293
Midwestern Regional Health System, 422
Minimal extracorporeal circulation (MECC), 144
MIPS Value Pathways (MVPs), 293
Mission control model, 94
Mitigations, 306
Mobile apps, 186
Modern consulting partnerships, 415
Modified ultrafiltration, 144
Multicenter Perioperative Outcomes Group (MPOG), 515
Multidisciplinary approach, 70
Multidisciplinary PBM teams, 134
  anticoagulated patient, 138, 139
  erythropoietin, 137, 138
  hemophilia A & B, 139
  iron therapy, 137
  Jehovah's Witness (JW) patient, 140
  preoperative anemia, 135, 136
  preoperative red cell optimization, 136
  sickle cell, 140
  thalassemias, 139, 140
Multidisciplinary perioperative teams, 21
Multidisciplinary stakeholders, 116
Multifaceted approach, 61, 62
Multimodal analgesia, 208
Multimodal monitoring, 386
Multimodal pain management, 75
Multiple scoring systems, 173
Muscle breakdown, 71
Myocardial Ischemia and Transfusion (MINT) trial, 149

N
National Anesthesia Clinical Outcomes Registry (NACOR), 280, 462
National guidelines and advisories, 443
National Partnership for Maternal Safety (NPMS), 324, 325
National Patient Safety Goals (NPSGs), 500, 505
National Shortage of Anesthesiologists, 367, 368
National Surgical Quality Improvement Program (NSQIP) Surgical Risk Calculator, 35
National systems, 188
Natural language processing (NLP), 514

Near-Infrared Spectroscopy (NIRS), 386
Near miss (NM), 216
Neuraxial labor analgesia, 332
Neuraxial procedures, 331, 332
Neurocognitive recovery, 209
Neurosurgical Intensive Care Unit (NSICU), 317
Non-anesthesiologist administered sedation, 259–260
Non-competition clauses, 428
Non-operating room anesthesia (NORA), 273, 274, 367
  comprehensive pre-procedural checklist, 276
  locations and common procedures, 274
  oversight and management
    anesthesiology leadership in, 281
    navigating regulation, 276, 277
    preoperative evaluation, 277, 278
    safety and communication concerns, 275
    scheduling and staffing, 278–280
  scheduling, challenges in, 279
Non-physician healthcare providers, 428
Nontechnical skills, 308
Nose sinuses, 77
Nurse-administered procedural sedation (NAPS), 260
Nurse Anesthetist (NA), 433–436
Nurse Practitioners (NPs), 48, 433
Nutritional optimization, 59, 73

O

Obstructive sleep apnea (OSA), 73, 74
Occupational Safety and Health Administration (OSHA), 498
Office-based sedation models, 260
Ongoing Professional Practice Evaluation (OPPE), 507
Operating room (OR) scheduling, 85, 273, 468, 470–471
  anesthesiologist's operational leadership, 91, 92
  change agents, anesthesiologists as, 96, 97
  governance and structure of, 88
    Medical Director of Perioperative Services, 89
    PSC, 88, 89
    sample perioperative dashboard layout, 90
    surgery, nursing, and administration, 89
  leveraging data and technology
    data-driven operating room, 94
    predictive analytics, 94, 95
    real-time OR management software and dashboards, 94
    workflow coordination, electronic health records in, 95
  managing emergency and after-hours cases, 96
  models and principles, 90, 91
  turnover time and throughput improvement, 93
  utilization, economics and metrics of, 85–87
Operating room (OR) fires, 125, 126
  closed claims database outcomes and areas for improvement, 126, 127, 129
  fire prevention and response protocols, 129
  Fire Triad and Fire Prevention Algorithm, 126
Operating room (OR) transfusion, 148–149
Opioid induced immunosuppression, 165
Opioid-sparing strategies, 72
Opioid stewardship, 233
Optometrist (OD), 431
Organizational shared governance, 90
Organizational structure, 196
Organization for International Standardization (ISO), 187
Organized medicine, 439, 440
Orthopedic surgery, 76
Outcome metrics, 267
Outpatient anesthesia consultation clinics (OPACs), 7
Outpatient preoperative evaluations (OPEs), 47, 51

P

PADUA score, 174
Pain management, 385
Pain, PACUU, 208, 209
Palliative care, 318–320
Paranasal sinuses, 77
Patient-Based Advocacy, 440
Patient blood management (PBM)
  anesthesiologist as perioperative physician in, 152, 153
  programs, 133–134
Patient care protocols, 317
Patient-centered care, 328, 331–332
Patient-centered evaluation, 30
Patient-centered outcomes, 24
Patient education, 45
Patient pathways, 62–63
Patient safety, 211, 218, 384, 504

active errors, 302
AI, 519, 520
clinical research, 384, 385
cognitive errors, 302–305
cognitive overload, 303, 304
history of anesthesia, 299–300
Just Culture, 301
latent errors, 302
production pressures, 304
psychological safety, 301
resilience, 305
safety culture, 301
safety-1, -2, -3 approach, 305
safety program, 305, 307
education and training, 307–308
key performance indicators, 308
leadership, 309
safety culture assessments, 309
science research, 384
Patient Safety Officer, 309
Patient Safety Organization (PSO), 462
Patient's decompensation, 319
Pay-for-performance incentives, 15–16
Percutaneous tracheostomiy, 316
Performance Improvement and Patient Safety (PIPS) committee, 245
Perioperative and anesthesiology consulting
cost structures of, 415, 416
engagement models, characteristics and benefits, 415
goals and challenges, 416, 417
growth of firms, 414
Perioperative anemia management, 21
Perioperative anesthesia and surgical screeding clinic (PASS), 101
Perioperative blood management
intraoperative minimization of blood loss and transfusion of blood products
factor and fibrinogen concentrates, 145–147
intraoperative techniques, 142–144
physiology of coagulation, 140, 142
multidisciplinary teams, 134
anticoagulated patient, 138, 139
erythropoietin, 137, 138
hemophilia A & B, 139
iron therapy, 137
Jehovah's Witness (JW) patient, 140
preoperative anemia, 135, 136
preoperative red cell optimization, 136
sickle cell, 140
thalassemias, 139, 140
tolerance of anemia and postoperative interventions
alternative noninvasive physiologist monitors, 152
blood sampling with closed loop systems, 152
critically ill patients, transfusion strategies in, 150
massive transfusion and massive transfusion protocols, 150, 151
PBM, anesthesiologist as perioperative physician in, 152, 153
transfusion algorithms and viscoelastic testing, 150
transfusion triggers, 148, 149
Perioperative care, 478, 480, 484, 485
anesthesiologists in, 29, 30
direct cost drivers in, 12
cancelations and delays, 13
medications and supply utilization, 13
operating room utilization, 12
Post-Anesthesia Care Unit (PACU) efficiency, 13
staffing models, 12
Perioperative consulting, 417
case studies, 419, 420
definitions, 418
logistics of partnerships, 418, 419
offerings in market, 418
results, 419
Perioperative economics, 11, 12
challenges and barriers, 21
economic data, limitations in, 21
fragmentation of care and misaligned incentives, 22
policy and regulatory hurdles, 22
resistance to change, 22
resource constraints, 22
comparative institutional outcomes, 21
downstream cost implications, 13, 14
length of stay, 14
postoperative complications, 14
readmissions and escalation of care, 14
surgical cancelations and throughput bottlenecks, 15
Enhanced Recovery After Surgery (ERAS) pathways, 20
health economics of innovation and technology, 17
artificial intelligence and predictive analytics, 18
cost-benefit considerations of innovation, 19
informatics and decision-support tools, 18

Perioperative economics (*cont.*)
monitoring and minimally invasive technologies, 18, 19
multidisciplinary perioperative teams, 21
patient-centered outcomes, 24
perioperative anemia management, 21
perioperative care, direct cost drivers in, 12
cancelations and delays, 13
medications and supply utilization, 13
operating room utilization, 12
Post-Anesthesia Care Unit (PACU) efficiency, 13
staffing models, 12
perioperative medicine and value-based care, 15
alignment with health system priorities, 16
bundled payments and alternative payment models, 15
cost avoidance through quality initiatives, 16
pay-for-performance incentives, 15, 16
Perioperative Surgical Homes, 23
policy and payment reform, 23
population health management, anesthesiologist's role in, 16
ERAS protocols, 17
high-risk populations, perioperative management of, 17
preoperative optimization of comorbidities, 16
preventive and longitudinal care impact, 17
predictive analytics and artificial intelligence, 23
preoperative optimization clinics, 20
strategic and institutional value, 19
anesthesiologists as institutional leaders, 20
hospital throughput and capacity management, 19
institutional reputation and market competitiveness, 19
integration with strategic priorities, 20
telemedicine and remote optimization, 23
Perioperative Enhancement Team (POET), 48, 101, 136
Perioperative leadership, 470
Perioperative management, 13
Perioperative medicine, 4, 11, 366
artificial intelligence, 514
and value-based care, 15
alignment with health system priorities, 16
bundled payments and alternative payment models, 15
cost avoidance through quality initiatives, 16
levers in, 15
pay-for-performance incentives, 15, 16
Perioperative optimization, 57
Perioperative Optimization Clinic (POC), 48
Perioperative physician, 363
Perioperative physicians, 363
Perioperative Services Committee (PSC), 88, 89
Perioperative Surgical Home (PSH), 23, 351
Peripartum cardiomyopathy, 331
Person approach, 301
Personal protective equipment (PPE), 162
Personalized care, 60–61
Pharmacist, 431
Pharmacodynamics, 315
Pharmacokinetics, 315
Pharmacologic prophylaxis, 178
Pharmacy and Therapeutics Committee (P&T committee), 202
Pharmacy leadership, 196
Phases of anesthesia care, 444
Physical/administrative barriers, 306
Physical exercise, 59
Physical Status Classification, 35
Physician anesthesiologists, 429–431
"Physician Anesthesiologists Save Lives" advertisement, 434
Physician Assistant (PA), 431
Physician authority, 3, 4
Physician burnout, 469, 471
Physician leadership academies, 4
Physicians, as hospital leaders
early hospitals and physician authority, 3, 4
medical director and departmental leadership, 4
Plasminogen activator inhibitor-1 (PAI-1), 142
Pneumatic compression devices (PCDs), 174
Pneumothorax, 244
Point-of-care ultrasound (POCUS), 330–331
Policy and payment reform, 23
Political Action Committees (PACs), 429, 438, 440
Population health, 378
Population health management, 16
ERAS protocols, 17
high-risk populations, perioperative management of, 17
preoperative optimization of comorbidities, 16

Population, interventions, comparators, systematic review, and evidence synthesis (PICOTS), 445
Post-Anesthesia Care Unit (PACU), 207
  clinical stewardship and patient management, 208
    airway and pulmonary management, 208
    hemodynamic stability, 208
    neurocognitive recovery and delirium prevention, 209
    pain, sedation, and analgesic stewardship, 208, 209
    and recovery optimization, 209
  efficiency, 13
  integration with hospital-wide initiatives, 211
  interdisciplinary team leadership and education, 210
  leadership, economic and operational value of, 211
  model for systems thinking, 212
  practice, technology and the future of, 211, 212
  quality assurance, safety culture, and governance, 209, 210
Postdural puncture headache (PDPH), 328–330, 334
Postoperative nausea and vomiting (PONV), 62, 74
Postoperative phase, 75
Practice advisories, 444, 445
Practice Guideline on the Monitoring and Antagonism of Neuromuscular Blockade, 444
Practice guidelines, 444
Practice parameters, 443, 444
Practice reporting, 359
Pre-admission testing (PAT), 29, 33
Pre-anesthesia clinic (PAC), 44, 47, 48, 59
Predictive analytics, 18, 23, 94, 95, 517
Prehabilitation, 59, 60
Preoperative anemia, 135–136
Preoperative assessment, 58, 59, 509, 510
Preoperative care, telemedicine, 484
Preoperative clearance, 351
Preoperative evaluation models
  advantages, 47
  anxiety, reduction in, 51
  day-of-surgery delays and cancelations, 49
  disadvantage, 47
  inpatient evaluations, 43–46
  length of hospital stay, reduction in, 50
  outpatient evaluations
    core functions of, 44–46
    disadvantages of, 51
    history, 43, 44
    PACs, 47, 48
  preoperative testing, reduction of, 49, 50
  technology in, 48, 49
Preoperative iron therapy, 138
Preoperative optimization, 20, 37
Preoperative red cell optimization, 136
Preoperative risk stratification, 44
Preoperative testing, 49, 50
Primary hemostasis, 140
Principal Investigators (PIs), 390
Privacy threats, 520
Process metrics, 267
Production pressure, 304
Products liability law, 352
Professional development, 458–460
Professional organizations, 99
Professional societies, 453–455, 457, 458, 461–463
Propofol, 36, 260
Prospective registries, 267
Prothrombin complex concentrates (PCCs), 145, 176
Protocol management for emergencies
  Code Blue, 121
    anesthesiologist, role of, 121
    costs of rapid response system, 122–125
    protocols, 122
    rapid response teams, 125
  local anesthetic systemic toxicity, 118, 119
    clinical guidelines, 120
    CMS requirements, 119, 120
    financial considerations, 120
    protocol development, 119
  malignant hyperthermia, 115
    clinical guidelines, 117
    CMS requirements, 116
    financial considerations, 118
    protocol development, 116
  operating room fires, 125, 126
    closed claims database outcomes and areas for improvement, 126, 127, 129
    developing fire prevention and response protocols, 129
    Fire Triad and Fire Prevention Algorithm, 126
Psychological safety, 217, 301, 303, 309
Psychological support, 59
Pulmonary critical care physicians, 317
Pulmonary embolism (PE), 61, 171

Pulmonary hypertension, 331
Pulse oximetry, 386

Q
Quality assurance (QA), 188, 209, 210, 262, 263, 265, 266, 268, 287
Quality improvement (QI), 61, 62, 504
Quality management in anesthesiology
- aligning safety and sustainability, 296
- artificial intelligence, 296
- challenges, 297
- domains, 292–293
- education, leadership, and human factor, 296–297
- historical context, 292
- informatics, 296
- measure development and data-driven improvement, 295
- national quality frameworks and programs, 293–294
- in practice, 295–296
- quality infrastructure, 294–295
- systems leader, 292

Quality of care, 443
Quality Payment Program (QPP), 460
Quality review process, 347–349

R
Radio-frequency identification (RFID), 189
Rapid Response Teams (RRT), 125
Readmissions, 14
Real-time decision support, 517, 518
Real-time documentation, 350
Real-time OR management software, 94
Real-time video consultations, 482
Red cell mass, preoperative optimization, 134
Regional anesthesia, 163, 177, 230
Registered nurses (RNs), 48
Regulatory and liability issues, 521
Regulatory compliance, 186, 506
Relative-value units-based costing, 105
Request for proposal (RFP), 487–489
- bottom line, 492
- competitor performance, organization's capabilities in, 489
- consultants, 490
- elements, 490, 493
- exceptional proposal, 490
- leadership, 490, 491
- monthly communication with client
  - clinical and operational leadership, 494, 495
- options, 491, 492
- quality, 491
- quarterly goals with client senior leadership, 494
- responding professional, 489
- smooth transition, 493
- subtopic, 492

Residency programs, 403
Resilience, 305–307
Resource constraints, 22, 246
Respiratory complications, 208
Retainer Agreements, 416
Return of spontaneous circulation (ROSC), 125
Return on equity (ROE), 106
Revenue cycle management
- automation and artificial intelligence investments, 359, 360
- coding and RCM compliance system, 356, 357
  - anesthesia clinician and procedure coder communication, 357
  - anesthesia procedure coders, coding education for, 357
  - anesthesia record documentation education, 356, 357
  - anesthesia record templates, 356
  - coding audit program, 357
- culture of communication, 358
- information technology strategic partnership, 360
- interoperability, 355, 356
- operations team hiring, 358
- practice reporting and data analytics, 359
- robust allowable monitoring, 354, 355
- system investment, 353, 354

Revised Cardiac Risk Index (RCRI), 35, 60
ReviveME campaign, 247
Risk management
- in anesthesiology, 347, 348
- supply chain, 188, 189

Risk mitigation
- patient-centered evaluation, 30
- strategies, 188

Risk-sharing agreements, 111
Risk stratification, 60, 61, 517
Robust allowable monitoring, 354, 355
Root cause analysis (RCA), 222

Rotational thromboelastometry (ROTEM), 147, 148
Rural communities, 483
Ryanodine receptor type 1 (RYR1) gene, 115

S
Safe care, 324–327
Safer transfusion practices, 133
Safety culture, 301, 304, 309
  adverse event analysis, 220
  PACU, 209, 210
Safety outcomes, 31
Safety-1 approach, 305–307
Safety-2 approach, 305
Safety-3 approach, 305
Sample transfusion ICU algorithm, 151
Scope of practice, 432–436, 441
Secondary hemostasis, 142
Sedation, 208–209
Sedation governance
  ASA and professional guidelines, 256–257
  credentialing and competency, 261–266
    administrative and clinical components, 261–263
    implementation considerations, 265
    performance metrics tied to credentialing, 264
    purpose and guiding principles, 261
    remediation, restrictions, and suspension process, 264–265
    Sample Initial Privileging Checklist, 263–264
    Sample Proctor Observation Checklist, 264
  economic and strategic value, 268–270
    alignment with value-based care, 269
    anesthesiologist's value proposition, 270
    in competitive markets, 269
    cost avoidance, 268–269
    operational efficiency, 269
  models of sedation oversight, 259–261
    anesthesiologist-administered sedation, 259
    NAPS, 260
    non-anesthesiologist-administered sedation, 259–260
    office-based sedation models, 260
    propofol administration, 260
  quality assurance and data collection, 266–268
    core principles, 266
    data collection systems, 267
    locums and multi-site environments, 268
    outcome metrics, 266, 267
    process metrics, 267
    review processes, 267–268
  regulatory and accreditation framework, 254–256
  safety concerns, 257–259
Severe maternal morbidity (SMM), 323, 324
Sickle cell disease, 140, 410
Sinus surgery, 77
Six Sigma methodologies, 93
Sleep medicine, 320, 321
Sleep order sets, 321
Sleep-wake cycle, 320
Social determinants of health (SDOH), 58
Social Security Act, 116
Society for Ambulatory Anesthesia (SAMBA), 164
Society for Obstetric Anesthesia and Perinatology (SOAP), 324–334
Society for Technology in Anesthesia (STA), 515
Society of Cardiovascular Anesthesiologists (SCA), 145
Sourcing and vendor management, 186
Southeast Rural Health System, 419
Speaking up algorithms, 308
Speaking up behaviors, 308
Specialized care units, 317
Specialized perioperative guidelines, 35
Specialty ACOs, 375
Spinal muscular atrophy (SMA), 409
Staffing models, 12, 280
Standardization, 189
Standardized handoffs, 97
Standardized scoring systems, 210
Standards for Basic Anesthetic Monitoring, 444
Standards for Postanesthesia Care, 444
Standards for Preanesthesia Care, 444
State departments of health, 501, 502
State oversight, 498, 499
Stockouts, 187
Strategic and institutional value, 19
  anesthesiologists as institutional leaders, 20
  hospital throughput and capacity management, 19
  institutional reputation and market competitiveness, 19
  integration with strategic priorities, 20
Strategic decision-making, 506

Strategic preoperative evaluation, 30
  financial waste, cost implications and avoidance of, 30, 31
  guideline-driven frameworks, 31
  patient-centered evaluation, risk mitigation, 30
  safety outcomes, 31
Structured handoffs, 210
Supply chain
  anesthesia, components of, 184, 185
  anesthesia supply procurement, challenges in, 187, 188
  demand forecasting and planning, 185, 186
  disruptions, 187
  in healthcare, 183–184
  management, technology and innovation in, 189
  procurement fundamentals, 186, 187
  quality assurance and risk management, 188
  sustainability and ethical sourcing, 190
Surgery, transfusion triggers in, 149
Surgical critical care physicians, 317
Surgical patient safety system (SURPASS) checklist, 160
Surgical readiness, preoperative evaluation, 43
Surgical service line, 99, 100, 109–111
  C-suite, 102, 103
  finance, 106–109
  operations, 104–106
  perioperative physicians' perspective, 100–102
Surgical site infections (SSIs) prophylaxis, 61, 159, 231, 517
  anesthesiologist-led initiatives, 160
  antibiotic prophylaxis, 161
  barriers and anesthesiologists, 165, 166
  checklists, 160, 161
  economic impact, 160
  fluid management and blood transfusions, 164, 165
  glycemic control, 164
  hand hygiene and personal protective equipment, 162
  inspired gas concentration, 163
  opioid induced immunosuppression, 165
  patient impact, 159, 160
  regional anesthesia, 163
  thermoregulation, 162
Surgical stress response, 71
Surgical supply chain efficiency, 105
Surgical volume, 163
Survey, 510
Sustainability, supply chain, 190
Swiss cheese model, 301, 302
Synchronous video-based consultations, 477
Systematic reviews, 443, 445, 446
System 1 thinking, 302
System 2 thinking, 302
Systems approach, 301, 302

T
Target controlled infusion (TCI) pumps, 186
TDABC Healthcare Consortium, 109
Technological innovations, 18
Telehealth, 49
Telemedicine, 475
  and COVID-19, 479–480
  healthcare delivery, in preadmission testing, 483
    elderly patients, 484
    incarcerated patients, 484
    rural communities, 483
    underserved communities, 483
  history of, 476–477
  post-COVID use, 480, 481
  pre-admission airway evaluation, 481, 482
  pre-COVID, use of, 478, 479
  preoperative care, economic impact of, 484
  and remote optimization, 23
  scope of, 475
  technology, 477, 478
Thalassemia, 139–140
The Joint Commission (TJC), 255, 294
Thermoregulation, surgical site infection prophylaxis, 162
Thoracic surgery, 77
Thromboelastography (TEG), 147, 148
Thromboprophylaxis, 174
Time-Driven Activity-Based Costing (TDABC), 104–106, 108
Timely care, 332–333
Tissue plasminogen activator (tPA), 142
Total hip arthroplasty (THA), 76, 178
Total intravenous anesthesia (TIVA), 7, 74
Total knee arthroplasty (TKA), 76, 178
Total Performance Score, 108
Tracheal intubation, 239
Traditional compensation models, 468
Transabdominal plane (TAP) blocks, 74
Transfusion
  algorithms, 147–148, 150
  of blood products, 134, 140–148
  in OR and ICU, 148, 149

in surgery, 149
viscoelastic testing, 150
Transfusion Committee (TC), 245, 246
Transfusion Requirements in Critical Care (TRICC) trial, 149
Transfusion strategies, in critically ill patients, 150
Translational research, 391, 410
cross-departmental collaborations, 392
features of, 401, 402
financial benefits, 393, 394
funding for, 394
multidisciplinary collaboration, 392
multidisciplinary teams, 391
logistical challenges and solutions, 402
opportunities for, 392, 393
science and clinical practice, 392
Trauma anesthesiologist
in drafting and implementing guidance, 245
education and clinical research in POCUS, 244
FAST, 244
hemostatic resuscitation, 245, 246
patient-centered protocols and policies, 245
trauma centers, 243–245
Trauma patient care, 202
Trauma program management, 202
Trauma Resuscitation with Low Titre O WB or Products (TROOP) trial, 246
Turnover time (TOT), 87, 93
2019 Anesthesia Closed Claims Analysis, 243

U
UK National Reporting and Learning System, 188
Uncompensated activity, 471
Undergraduate degree, 364
Underserved communities, 483
Unfractionated heparin (UFH), 175, 176
Unsupervised anesthesia care, 434
Urologic surgery, 76
U.S. Bureau of Labor Statistics projects, 423
US Department of Health and Human Services (HHS), 498
US Drug availability, 186
U.S. Pharmacopeia (USP), 201

V
Value-based care, 6–7, 15, 62–63
Value-based models, 374, 375
Value-based perioperative innovation, 485
Value-Based Purchasing Program, 107
Value chain analysis, 110, 187
Value proposition, 487–489, 492
Value stream mapping (VSM), 93
Venous thromboembolism (VTE), 137, 138, 171
cost of, 172
epidemiology and prevalence, 171, 172
pathophysiology of
pathogenesis, 172
risk factors, 172–175
prevention strategies, 175
ambulation, 177
aspirin, 176
DOACs, 176
IVC, 178
LMWH, 175, 176
mechanical prophylaxis, 177
pharmacological prophylaxis, 175
regional anesthesia, 177
summary recommendations, 178, 179
UFH, 176
vitamin K antagonists, 176
special populations
cancer patients, 179
patients with prior/existing DVTs, 179
Venout thromboembolism (VTE), 61
Virchow's triad, 172
Virtual emergency team, 96
Virtual preoperative clinic, 479
Viscoelastic testing (VET), 147–148
Vitamin K antagonists, 176

W
Wake-sleep cycle, 320
Whole blood (WB) program, 246
Workflow optimization, artificial intelligence, 518
Workforce, 366
Work-life balance, 423
World Health Organization (WHO), 183, 216, 223
World Society of Emergency Surgery (WSES), 164

GPSR Compliance

The European Union's (EU) General Product Safety Regulation (GPSR) is a set of rules that requires consumer products to be safe and our obligations to ensure this.

If you have any concerns about our products, you can contact us on ProductSafety@springernature.com

In case Publisher is established outside the EU, the EU authorized representative is:

Springer Nature Customer Service Center GmbH
Europaplatz 3
69115 Heidelberg, Germany

Batch number: 10370734

Printed by Printforce, the Netherlands